DIAGNOSTIC OBSTETRICAL ULTRASOUND

DIAGNOSTIC OBSTETRICAL ULTRASOUND

John P. McGahan, M.D.

Professor and Director
Ultrasound and Abdominal Imaging
Department of Radiology
University of California
Davis Medical Center
Sacramento, California

Manuel Porto, M.D.

Associate Professor and Director
Division of Maternal–Fetal Medicine and Center for Fetal Evaluation
Department of Obstetrics and Gynecology
University of California, Irvine
Orange, California

With 29 additional contributors

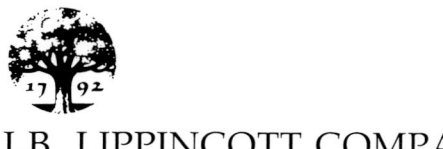

J.B. LIPPINCOTT COMPANY

Acquisitions Editor: *James Ryan*
Assistant Editor: *Wendy Greenberger-Czarnecki*
Project Editor: *Tom Gibbons*
Indexer: *Ellen Murray*
Design Coordinator: *Kathy Kelley-Luedtke*
Cover Designer: *Lou Fuiano*
Interior Designer: *Holly Reid McLaughlin*
Production Manager: *Helen Ewan*
Production Coordinator: *Kathryn Rule*
Compositor: *Bi-Comp, Inc.*
Printer/Binder: *Walsworth Publishing Company*

Text printed on acid-free paper.

6 5 4 3 2 1

Library of Congress Cataloging in Publication Data

Diagnostic obstetrical ultrasound / [edited by] John P. McGahan,
  Manuel Porto.
       p.   cm.
    Includes bibliographical references and index.
    ISBN 0-397-51320-8
    1. Fetus—Ultrasonic imaging.   2. Ultrasonics in obstetrics.
  I. McGahan, John P.   II. Porto, Manuel.
    [DNLM: 1. Ultrasonography, Prenatal.   2. Fetal Diseases—ultrasonography.
  3. Pregnancy Complications—ultrasonography.   WQ
  209 D536 1994]
  RG628.3.U58D65   1994
  618.2′2—dc20
  DNLM/DLC
  for Library of Congress   93–49755
                                                                             CIP

Contributors

Itai Bar-Hava, M.D.
Research Fellow, Department of Obstetrics and
    Gynecology of the Albert Einstein College of
    Medicine;
Research Fellow, The Jack D. Weiler Hospital of
    the Albert Einstein College of Medicine
Bronx, New York

Beryl R. Benacerraf, M.D.
Clinical Professor
Department of Obstetrics and Gynecology
Harvard Medical School;
Brigham and Women's Hospital
Boston, Massachusetts

Carol B. Benson, M.D.
Associate Professor of Radiology, Harvard
    Medical School;
Co-Director, Division of Ultrasound Department
    of Radiology
Brigham and Women's Hospital
Boston, Massachusetts

Raphael Boldes, M.D.
Shaare Zedek Medical Center
Jerusalem
Israel

Dru E. Carlson, M.D.
Director, Reproductive Genetics
Cedar-Sinai Medical Center;
Assistant Professor
University of California, Los Angeles School of
    Medicine
Los Angeles, California

Frank A. Chervenak, M.D.
Professor of Obstetrics
Cornell University Medical College;
Professor of Obstetrics
Director, Division of Maternal Fetal Medicine
The New York Hospital
New York, New York

Terry L. Coates, M.D.
Assistant Professor
Department of Radiology
University of California School of Medicine
Davis, California

Joshua A. Copel, M.D.
Professor, Obstetrics and Gynecology
Section Head, Maternal–Fetal Medicine
Yale University School of Medicine;
Chief, Obstetrics
Yale–New Haven Hospital
New Haven, Connecticut

Sidney M. Dashefsky, M.D.
Assistant Professor
University of Manitoba;
Radiologist
Health Sciences Center
Winnipeg, Manitoba
Canada

Greggory R. DeVore, M.D.
Director, Maternal–Fetal Medicine
The Genetics Institute
Pasadena, California

Michael Y. Divon, M.D.
Associate Professor of Obstetrics and Gynecology
The Albert Einstein College of Medicine;
Chief of Obstetrics and Perinatology
Jack D. Weiler Hospital of the Albert Einstein
  College of Medicine
Bronx, New York

Peter M. Doubilet, M.D., PH.D.
Associate Professor of Radiology
Harvard Medical School;
Co-Director of Ultrasound
Department of Radiology
Brigham and Women's Hospital
Boston, Massachusetts

Norman B. Duerbeck, M.D.
Director of Maternal–Fetal Medicine
White Memorial Medical Center
Los Angeles, California

Keith A. Eddleman, M.D.
Assistant Professor
Department of Obstetrics and Gynecology
Cornell University Medical Center;
Director of Prenatal Diagnosis
The New York Hospital
New York, New York

Harris J. Finberg, M.D.
Director, Diagnostic Ultrasound
Phoenix Perinatal Associates
Phoenix, Arizona

Ruth B. Goldstein, M.D.
Associate Professor of Radiology and Obstetrics
  and Gynecology
Director, Radiology Residency
University of California, San Francisco
San Francisco, California

Lawrence P. Gordon, M.D.
Associate Professor of Pathology
State University of New York Health Sciences
  Center at Syracuse;
Staff Pathologist
Crouse Irving Memorial Hospital
Syracuse, New York

Lyndon M. Hill, M.D.
Associate Professor of Obstetrics and Gynecology
Division of Maternal–Fetal Medicine
University of Pittsburgh School of Medicine;
Medical Director Ultrasound
Magee Women's Hospital
Pittsburgh, Pennsylvania

Susan C. Holt, M.D., F.R.C.P.(C.)
Staff Radiologist
Department of Radiology and Lecturer
University of Manitoba
Health Sciences Center
Winnipeg, Manitoba
Canada

Richard A. Humes, M.D.
Assistant Professor of Pediatrics
Wayne State University
Director, Echocardiography Laboratory
Children's Hospital of Michigan
Detroit, Michigan

David C. Jones, M.D.
Assistant Professor
Obstetrics and Gynecology
Division of Maternal–Fetal Medicine
Yale University School of Medicine
Yale–New Haven Hospital
New Haven, Connecticut

Keith B. Lescale, M.D.
Assistant Professor of Obstetrics and Gynecology
Cornell University Medical Center;
Attending Physician in Obstetrics and
  Gynecology
The New York Hospital
New York, New York

Clifford S. Levi, M.D.
Associate Professor
Diagnostic Radiology
University of Manitoba;
Section Head, Section of Diagnostic Ultrasound
Health Sciences Center
Winnipeg, Manitoba
Canada

Daniel J. Lindsay, M.D.
Assistant Professor
University of Manitoba
Health Sciences Center
Winnipeg, Manitoba
Canada

Edward A. Lyons, M.D., F.R.C.P.(C.), F.A.C.R.
Professor and Chairman
University of Manitoba;
Radiologist-in-Chief
Health Sciences Center
Winnipeg, Manitoba
Canada

John P. McGahan, M.D.
Professor of Radiology
University of California, Davis
School of Medicine;
Director of Abdominal Imaging and Ultrasound
University of California, Davis Medical Center
Sacramento, California

Manuel Porto, M.D.
Associate Professor and Director
Division of Maternal–Fetal Medicine
University of California, Irvine
Orange, California

Kathryn L. Reed, M.D.
Professor, Obstetrics and Gynecology
University of Arizona College of Medicine
Arizona Health Sciences Center
Tucson, Arizona

Beverly A. Spirt, M.D., F.A.C.R.
Professor of Radiology
Chief of Ultrasound
State University of New York Health Sciences
    Center at Syracuse
Syracuse, New York

Ralph M. Steiger, M.D.
Assistant Professor in Residence
Division of Maternal–Fetal Medicine
University of California, Irvine
Orange, California

Amy S. Thurmond, M.D.
Associate Professor of Radiology and Obstetrics
    and Gynecology
Director of Women's Imaging
Oregon Health Sciences University
Portland, Oregon

TABLE 1-1. Normal Endovaginal Sonographic Findings: 3.5–6.5 Weeks of Menstrual Age

Menstrual Age (approximate)	Sonographic Sign	Sonographic Features	Comments
3.5–4 weeks	Decidual thickening	Focal thickening of the echogenic decidua at the site of implantation	Sign is difficult to appreciate. Predictive value has never been published.
? After 4.5 weeks	Trophoblastic flow	High-velocity, low-impedance signal at the implantation site	Peak velocity of 8–30 cm/sec before EVS visualization of the gestational sac.
4.5–5.5 weeks	Intradecidual sign	Gestational sac within the decidua abutting the endometrial canal	Should always be seen when maternal serum β-hCG is ≥1700–2000 mIU/mL (First International Reference Preparation).
After 5.5 weeks	Double-decidual sign	Echogenic ring formed by decidua capsularis and chorion laeve surrounded by echogenic decidua vera	Vague or absent double-decidual sign is nondiagnostic.
After 4.5 weeks	Yolk sac sign	Visualization of the yolk sac within the gestational sac	The yolk sac is often seen when the MSD is 5–6 mm and should always be seen when the MSD is ≥8 mm.
5.5 weeks	Double-bleb sign	Visualization of the amnion as a 2-mm bleb adjacent to the yolk sac	A transient finding. After this stage, visualization of the amnion in the absence of a visible embryo is abnormal.
After 5–5.5 weeks	Visualization of the embryo	Visualization of the embryo adjacent to the yolk sac	The embryo should always be seen when the MSD is ≥16 mm.
After 5–5.5 weeks	Cardiac activity	Cardiac activity within embryo immediately adjacent to the yolk sac	Nonvisualization of cardiac activity may be completely normal in embryos ≤4–5 mm CRL.

earliest sonographic sign of an intrauterine pregnancy was described by Yeh and colleagues.[16] They identified a focal echogenic zone of decidual thickening at the site of implantation at 3.5 to 4 weeks of menstrual age. This sign may be difficult to appreciate, and the diagnostic value in terms of predicting the presence of an intrauterine pregnancy has never been published.

Recent data suggest that EVCFD may provide the first reliable evidence of the presence of an intrauterine gestational sac.[7,8] The EVCFD diagnosis of an intrauterine pregnancy is based on demonstrating trophoblastic flow, which is characterized by a high-velocity, low-impedance signal.[5,6] Taylor and colleagues hypothesized that the flow signature of the trophoblast is related to invasion of the decidua by chorionic villi.[6] As the chorionic villi invade the decidua, the spiral arteries shunt blood to the intervillous spaces, resulting in an arteriovenous-type waveform.

EVCFD demonstrates increased vascularity in the trophoblast immediately surrounding the gestational sac. Emerson and associates found that the peak flow velocity of peritrophoblastic flow in a normal intrauterine pregnancy ranged from 8 to 30 cm/sec before EVS visualization of the gestational sac, from 10 to 30 cm/sec with a gestational sac of 1

to 5 mm mean gestational sac diameter (MSD), and from 10 to 60 cm/sec with a gestational sac of 6 to 10 mm MSD.[8] In this series, the sensitivity of diagnosis of an intrauterine pregnancy was improved from 90% using EVS alone to 99% using EVCFD. The specificity of diagnosis of an intrauterine pregnancy with EVCFD was 99% to 100%.[8] In a separate study, EVCFD correctly identified 47 of 47 intrauterine pregnancies, compared with EVS, which identified 38 of 47 (81%).[17] The findings suggest that it is possible to demonstrate peritrophoblastic flow with EVCFD before EVS demonstration of the gestational sac.

The first reliable gray-scale sonographic evidence of an intrauterine pregnancy is visualization of the gestational sac within the thickened decidua.[16] This sign was first described by Yeh and associates and is referred to as the *intradecidual sign*[16] (Fig. 1-3). Using EVS, it is usually possible to identify the gestational sac within the decidua by about 4.5 weeks of menstrual age, when the MSD should be about 2.5 mm. To distinguish an intrauterine gestational sac from a decidual cyst, it is important to ensure that the sac abuts the endometrial canal.

The *double-decidual sign* is based on visualization of an echogenic ring formed by the decidua capsu-

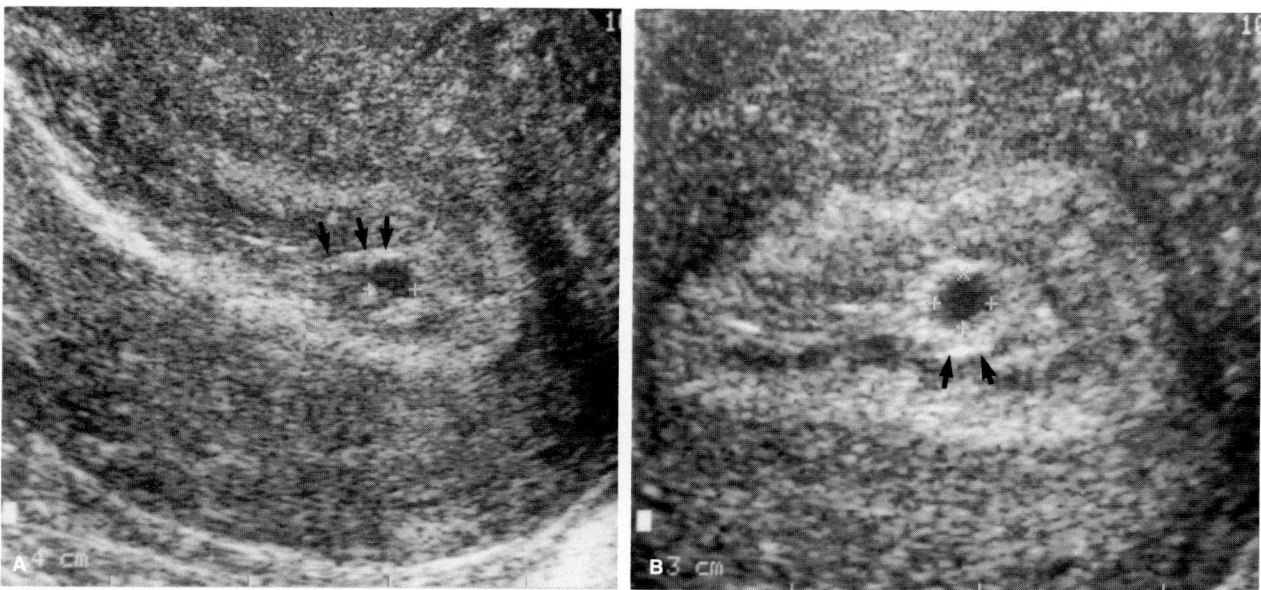

FIGURE 1-3.   Intradecidual sign. Endovaginal sonogram in the sagittal **(A)** and coronal **(B)** planes in a patient at 4.5 weeks of menstrual age. The uterus is retroverted. The 3-mm gestational sac (*electronic calipers*) is demonstrated within the decidua, abutting and slightly displacing the echogenic endometrial canal (*arrows*).

laris and chorion laeve, eccentrically located within the echogenic decidua vera[18] (Figs. 1-4 and 1-5). The decidua basalis and villous chorion complex (future placenta) may also be visualized as an area of eccentric echogenic thickening. The double-decidual sign was originally described by Nyberg and colleagues and can often be identified after 5.5 to 6 weeks of menstrual age.[18] A well-defined double-decidual sign is accurate in predicting the presence of an intrauterine pregnancy. A vague or absent double-decidual ring may be seen in some patients with ectopic pregnancies and should be considered nondiagnostic.[16]

The gestational sac can often be identified at relatively low serum β-hCG levels. The *threshold level* (lowest β-hCG level possible to identify a normal intrauterine gestational sac) has much less clinical significance than the *discriminatory level* (β-hCG level above which it is abnormal to be unable to identify a gestational sac). Two studies have identified β-hCG discriminatory levels for EVS. Bree and colleagues identified a discriminatory level of 1000 mIU/mL (First International Reference Preparation).[19] Nyberg and associates identified a discriminatory level of 1000 mIU/mL (Second International Standard), which converts to 1700 to 2000 mIU/mL First International Reference Preparation.[20] The actual discriminatory level varies depending on the resolution of the ultrasound scanner and the type of hormonal assay.

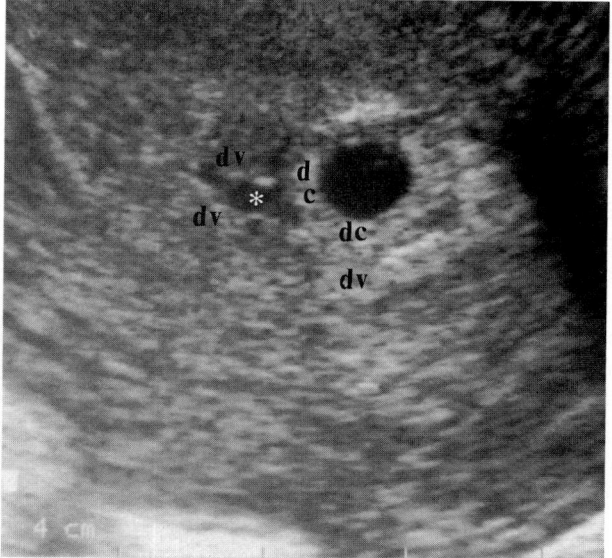

FIGURE 1-4.   Double-decidual sign (5 weeks of menstrual age). The decidua vera (dv) can be discerned from the decidua capsularis (dc) and chorion laeve surrounding the gestational sac. A small subchorionic hemorrhage (*) is present between the unapposed layers of decidua vera.

Yolk Sac

The yolk sac plays an important role in early embryonic life (Fig. 1-6). It is involved in transfer of nutrients to the embryo, hematopoiesis, and for-

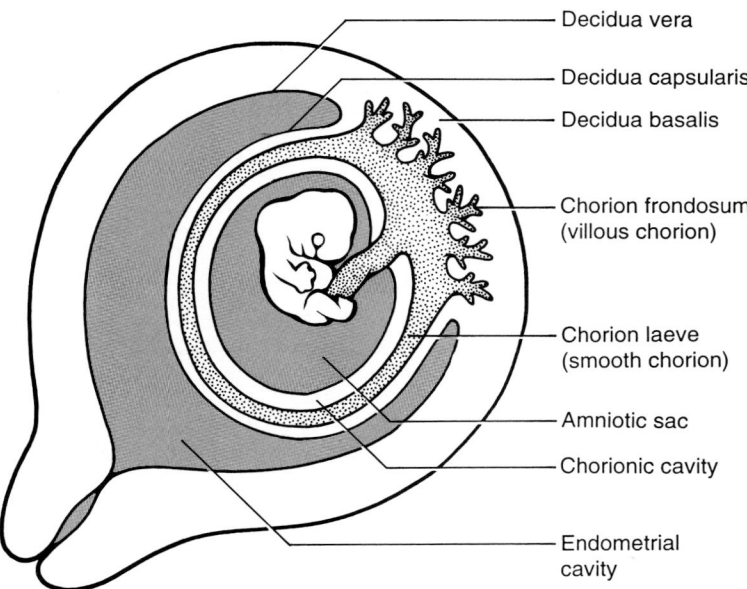

- Decidua vera
- Decidua capsularis
- Decidua basalis
- Chorion frondosum (villous chorion)
- Chorion laeve (smooth chorion)
- Amniotic sac
- Chorionic cavity
- Endometrial cavity

FIGURE 1-5. Anatomic basis for the double-decidual sign.

mation of the primitive gut.[21] The yolk sac remains connected to the mid-gut by the vitelline duct, which can often be demonstrated sonographically (Fig. 1-7).

The yolk sac is normally round or oval and has a uniformly thick, echogenic wall.[22] The yolk sac can often be demonstrated by EVS when the MSD is 5 to 6 mm, and it is often seen before the embryo or amnion (see Fig. 1-6). Although the double-decidual sign can be equivocal, the presence of a yolk sac within the gestational sac (the *yolk sac sign*) is diagnostic of an intrauterine pregnancy.[23]

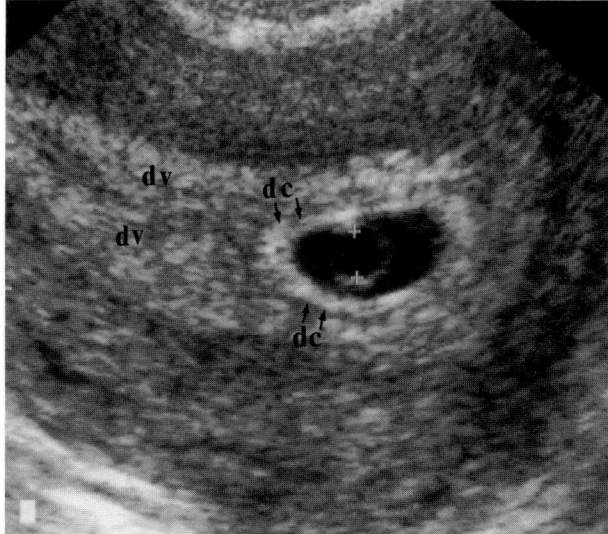

FIGURE 1-6. Gestational sac and yolk sac (5 weeks of menstrual age). A normal yolk sac (*electronic calipers*) measuring 3.1 mm in internal diameter is visualized. The embryo is not identified. The decidua vera (dv) and decidua capsularis (dc) are identified (double-decidual sign).

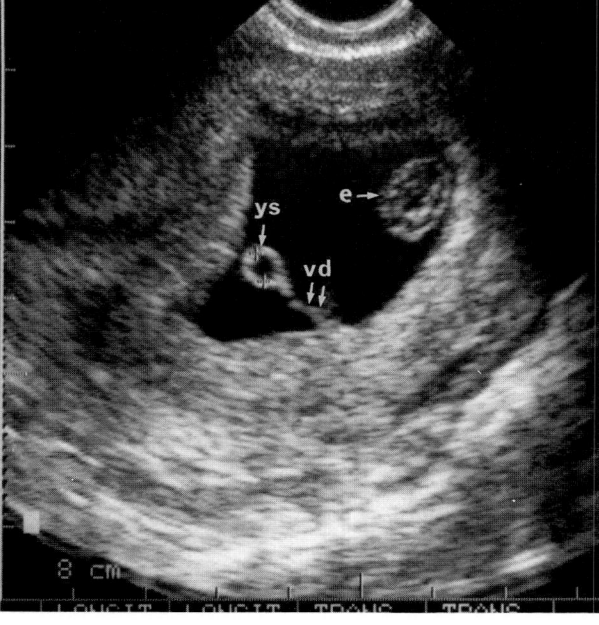

FIGURE 1-7. Normal gestation at about 9 weeks of menstrual age. The yolk sac (ys), vitelline duct (vd), and embryonic head (e) are visualized.

Using EVS, the yolk sac should always be visualized when the MSD is 8 mm.[3] The yolk sac grows at a rate of 0.1 mm per millimeter growth of the MSD before 15 mm MSD, after which it grows at a rate of 0.03 mm per millimeter growth of the MSD.[22] Bree and associates demonstrated the yolk sac in 8 of 8 patients with a serum β-hCG level of 7200 mIU/mL (First International Reference Preparation).[19]

Embryo and Amnion

At about 5.5 weeks of menstrual age, the amnion normally may be seen before the embryo as a 2-mm bleb adjacent to the yolk sac. This transient finding was originally described by Yeh and Rabinowitz and is referred to as the *double-bleb sign*.[24] Visualization of the amnion without an embryo after the double-bleb stage is abnormal.[1]

The amnion is demonstrated as a thin, filamentous, rounded membrane surrounding the embryo. The amnion is, in turn, completely surrounded by the thick, echogenic chorion.[25,26] The thinnest portion of the chorion is comprised of the decidua capsularis and chorion laeve. The yolk sac is situated between the amnion and chorion (Fig. 1-8). Chorionic fluid is often more echogenic than the essentially anechoic amniotic fluid (Fig. 1-9). Sonographic differentiation between the amnion and chorion is usually not difficult in the first tri-

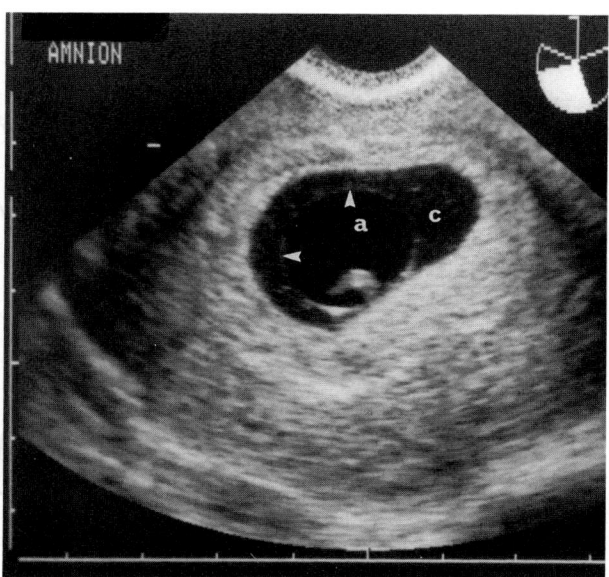

FIGURE 1-9. Relative echogenicity of amniotic and chorionic fluid. Normal gestation at about 9 weeks of menstrual age. A live embryo is present but not visualized in this scan plane. The chorionic fluid (c) is more echogenic than the amniotic fluid (a). The *arrowheads* show the amniotic membrane.

mester, allowing for reliable determination of amnionicity and chorionicity in multifetal pregnancies[25,26] (Figs. 1-10 and 1-11).

Using EVS, embryos as small as 1 to 2 mm CRL can be identified routinely.[4] Cardiac activity may be identified immediately adjacent to the yolk sac and is indicative of a live embryo.[27] The absence of cardiac activity, however, does not necessarily indicate embryonic demise. Using EVS, absent cardiac activity may be completely normal in embryos of 4 to 5 mm CRL.[4,28] Using transvesical sonography, absent cardiac activity may be normal in embryos of 9 mm CRL.[28]

In two separate studies, cardiac activity was first demonstrated at 40 days of menstrual age and was seen in all normal embryos by 46 days of menstrual age.[29,30] The reliability of using these parameters as predictors of abnormal outcome, however, has not been demonstrated. In using ultrasound landmarks as predictors of outcome, we prefer to use internal controls (eg, MSD) rather than menstrual age.

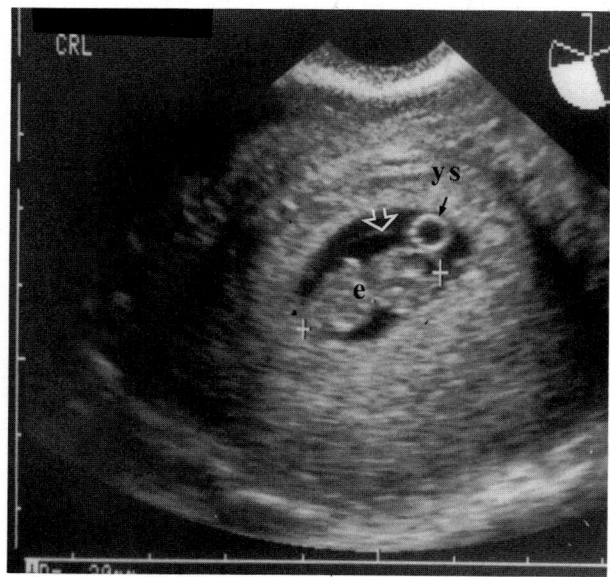

FIGURE 1-8. Amnion, yolk sac, and embryo (9 weeks of menstrual age). The yolk sac (ys) is situated within the chorionic cavity, between the amniotic membrane (*open arrow*) and chorion. The embryo (e) is within the amniotic cavity.

ECTOPIC PREGNANCY

Ectopic pregnancy accounts for 1.4% of all pregnancies and for about 15% of maternal deaths. An increase in the incidence of ectopic pregnancy has

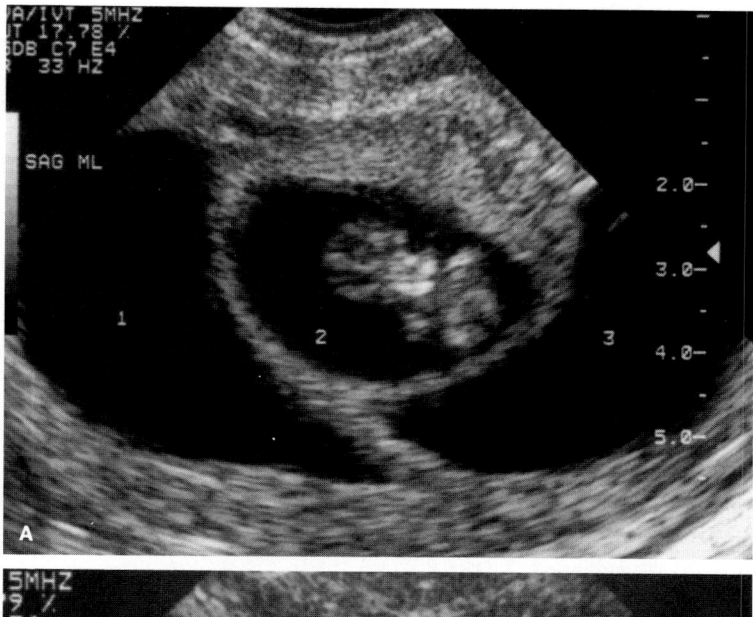

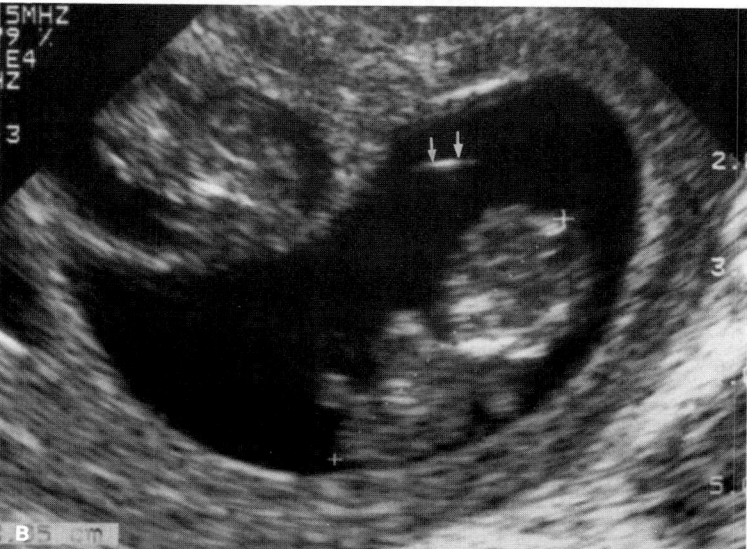

FIGURE 1-10. Trichorionic triplet pregnancy (10 weeks of menstrual age). **(A)** Endovaginal sonography showing three gestational sacs (1, 2, 3). **(B)** A magnified view of one of the gestational sacs shows an embryo (*calipers*) and an amniotic membrane (*arrows*).

occurred due to an increase in the prevalence of risk factors. The case-fatality rate, however, declined from 3.5/1000 in 1970 to less than 1/1000 in 1983, likely owing to improved diagnostic accuracy in the early stages of ectopic pregnancy and resultant earlier intervention.[31,32]

All patients in the reproductive age group are at risk for ectopic pregnancy. The prevalence of ectopic pregnancy in a clinically suspected group varies according to the patient population and the group's inherent risk factors.

Table 1-2 describes factors associated with an increased incidence of ectopic pregnancy. The common element in these risk factors is prevention or delay of transit of the zygote through the fallopian tube. Chlamydia salpingitis has been implicated as a major cause of the increasing incidence of ectopic pregnancy.[33]

A strong association exists between infertility and ectopic pregnancy. This is likely due to the shared tubal abnormalities in both conditions. The increased incidence of multiple pregnancy with ovulation induction and in vitro fertilization further increases the risk for both ectopic and heterotopic (intrauterine and ectopic) gestation. The hydrostatic forces generated during embryo transfer may also contribute to the increased risk. The frequency of heterotopic pregnancy is about 1/7000 in the general population[34] and is higher in high-risk groups.[35]

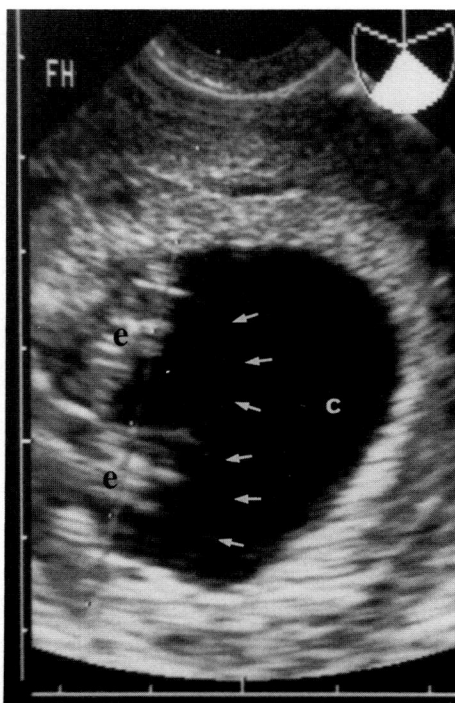

FIGURE 1-11. Monochorionic diamniotic twins (8 weeks of menstrual age). A single chorionic sac (c) is present that contains two live embryos (e). An amniotic membrane (*arrows*) is identified surrounding each embryo.

Sonographic Diagnosis

Regardless of clinical presentation, the primary goal of early first-trimester sonographic diagnosis should be to identify the location of the gestational sac. The most important contribution of EVS in the evaluation of patients presenting with suspected ectopic pregnancy is its ability to identify either a normal or abnormal intrauterine gestational sac earlier and more reliably than transabdominal ultrasound.

TABLE 1-2.   Factors Associated With an Increased Incidence of Ectopic Pregnancy

Past history of:
   salpingitis; pelvic inflammatory disease
   tubal surgery
   ectopic pregnancy
Use of intrauterine contraceptive device
Advanced maternal age
Infertility
Ovulation induction
In vitro fertilization

Because of the low incidence of heterotopic pregnancy, sonographic demonstration of an intrauterine pregnancy reduces the risk of ectopic pregnancy to an almost insignificant level. Heterotopic pregnancy, however, should be suspected in the appropriate clinical setting, especially in high-risk groups. Evaluation of the adnexa should be routine in all patients, including those with documented intrauterine pregnancies.

The demonstration of a live embryo in the adnexa is diagnostic of ectopic pregnancy. In early intrauterine pregnancy, incomplete abortion, or ectopic pregnancy, it is not always possible to identify the gestational sac. In the absence of specific sonographic findings, the probability of ectopic pregnancy can be predicted by identifying nonspecific sonographic features and by correlating those findings with the discriminatory level of serum β-hCG.[19,20] The relative risk of ectopic pregnancy and clinical status of the patient determine the need for surgical intervention or repeat sonography and conservative management.

Specific Findings (Table 1-3)
Intrauterine Pregnancy. As described in the section on normal sonographic appearances, the intradecidual sign can be used to demonstrate the presence of an intrauterine pregnancy before visualization of the yolk sac or embryo.[16] Using EVS, the double-decidual sign is usually demonstrated at about the same time that the yolk sac is visualized.[17]

In patients with ectopic pregnancies, the decidua may slough, resulting in a fluid collection within the endometrial canal, referred to as a *decidual cast* or *pseudogestational sac* (Fig. 1-12). EVS improves differentiation of the decidua, which produces the pseudogestational sac, from the choriodecidual reaction of the intradecidual and double-decidual signs.[36] A pseudogestational sac is a fluid collection within the endometrial canal surrounded by a single decidual layer, as opposed to a sac within the decidua abutting the endometrial canal (intradecidual sign) or the two concentric rings of the double-decidual sign (see Figs. 1-3 through 1-6).

Small cysts within the decidua may present as sac-like structures in patients with ectopic pregnancy.[15] These decidual cysts may be distinguished from gestational sacs in that the cysts do not abut the endometrial canal (Fig. 1-13).

Live Embryo in the Adnexa. The sonographic demonstration of a live embryo in the adnexa is specific for the diagnosis of ectopic pregnancy[37] (Fig. 1-14).

TABLE 1-3.   Diagnostic Table for Patients With Suspected Ectopic Pregnancy and Positive Pregnancy Test

Sonographic Findings (Uterine and Adnexa)	β-hCG mIU/mL*	Diagnosis
Intrauterine pregnancy; normal adnexa		Intrauterine pregnancy
Intrauterine pregnancy; adnexal mass or free fluid		Possible heterotopic pregnancy; requires clinical correlation
No intrauterine pregnancy; no adnexal abnormality	>1700	Ectopic pregnancy likely; could be incomplete abortion or abnormal intrauterine pregnancy
No intrauterine pregnancy; no adnexal abnormality	<1700	Likelihood of ectopic pregnancy depends on clinical findings
No intrauterine pregnancy; echogenic-free fluid; adnexal mass		High likelihood of ectopic pregnancy
No intrauterine pregnancy; live ectopic or trophoblastic ring		Ectopic pregnancy

* First International Reference Preparation

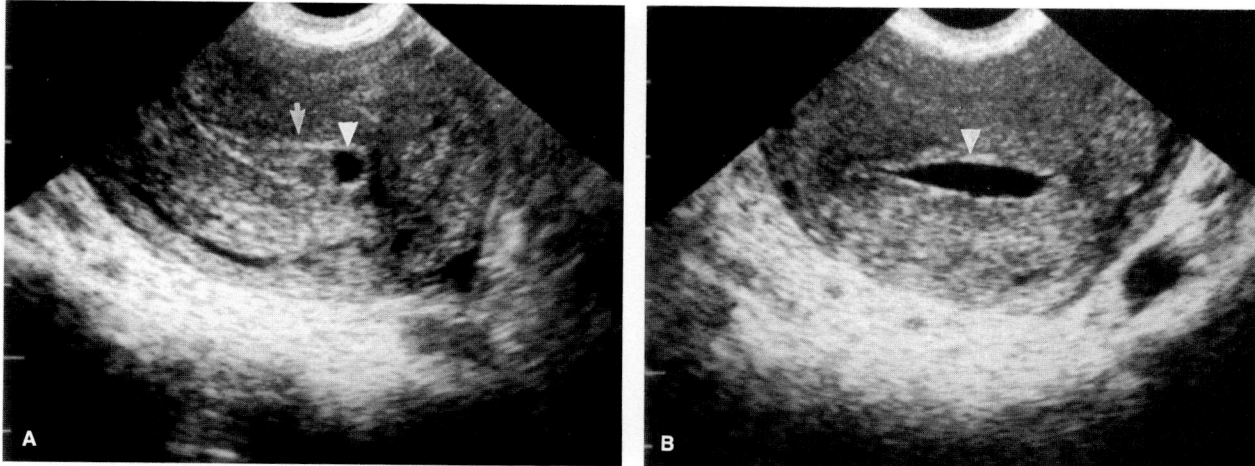

FIGURE 1-12.   Decidual cast. **(A)** Sagittal and **(B)** coronal sonograms of the uterus. The pseudogestational sac is composed of fluid (*arrowhead*) and debris (*arrow*) within the endometrium, surrounded by a single layer of decidua.

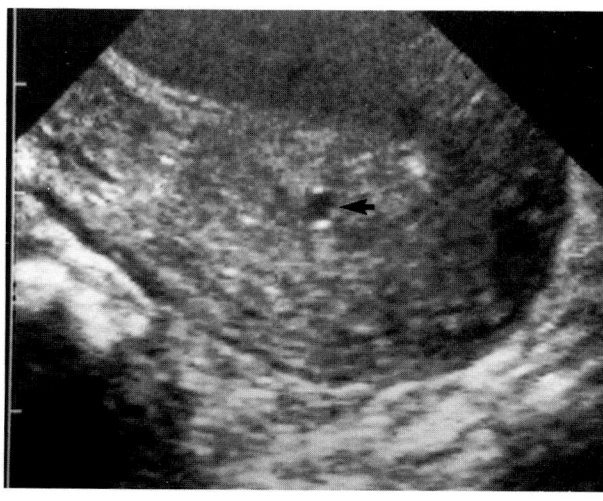

FIGURE 1-13.   Decidual cyst in a patient with ectopic pregnancy. A 3-mm cyst (*arrow*) is identified within the decidua. This cyst is not an intradecidual gestational sac because it is peripherally located within the decidua and does not abut the endometrial canal.

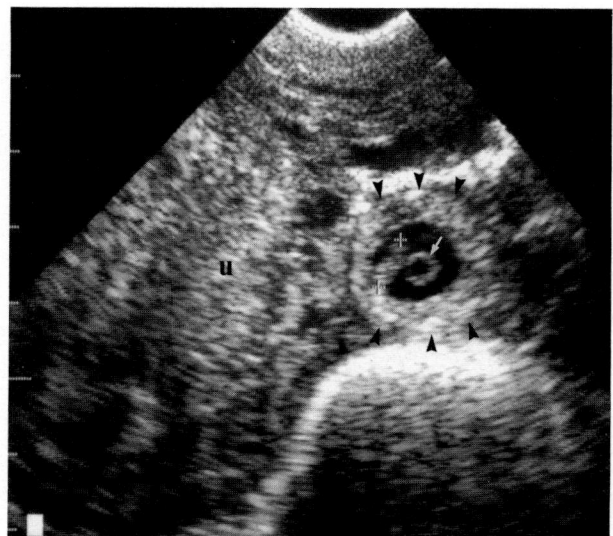

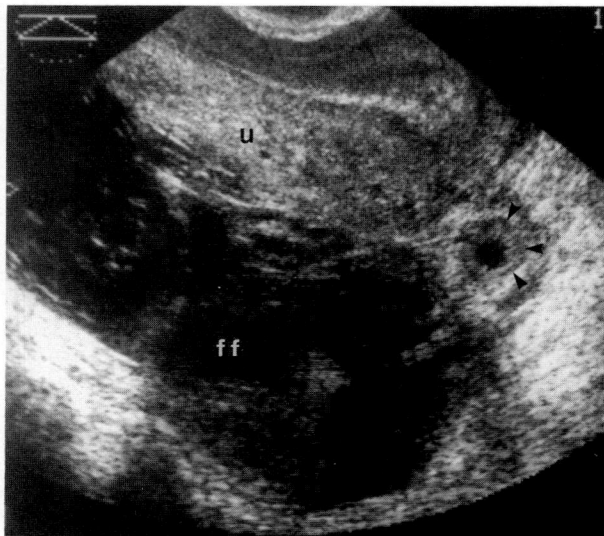

FIGURE 1-14. Live ectopic pregnancy. A 7-mm embryo (*calipers*) and yolk sac (*arrow*) are visualized within a well-defined trophoblastic ring (*arrowheads*). The sac is situated in the posterior cul de sac, adjacent to the uterus (u). Embryonic cardiac activity was identified on sonography.

FIGURE 1-15. Ectopic pregnancy: tubal ring. An extrauterine trophoblastic ring (*arrowheads*) is visualized adjacent to the uterus (u). Fluid (ff) and blood clot are present in the posterior cul de sac. The uterus is retroverted.

A live extrauterine fetus has been detected with EVS in 17% to 28% of patients with ectopic pregnancies,[2,36,38,39] compared with about a 10% detection rate using transabdominal ultrasound.[40]

Nonspecific Findings

Adnexal Mass. An adnexal mass can be found in conditions other than ectopic pregnancy and is therefore not diagnostic. The presence of an adnexal mass, however, in patients with a positive β-hCG who have no sonographic evidence of an intrauterine pregnancy has a positive predictive value of 70% to 75% for ectopic pregnancy[37] (Table 1-4).

Tubal Ring. Fleischer and colleagues reported finding a tubal ring in 49% of patients with ectopic pregnancy and in 68% of unruptured tubal pregnancies using EVS.[36] A tubal ring is an echogenic adnexal ring separate from the ovary created by the trophoblast of the ectopic pregnancy surrounding the gestational sac (Fig. 1-15). In Nyberg and

TABLE 1-4.   Ectopic Pregnancy: Extrauterine Findings

Sonographic Finding	Sensitivity (%)	Specificity (%)	Positive Predictive Value (%)	Negative Predictive Value (%)
Adnexal mass	21	93	70	58
Free fluid	63	69	63	69
Moderate to large amount of free fluid	29	96	86	62
Echogenic fluid, no mass	15	98	85	58
Adnexal mass, no fluid	22	94	75	57
Echogenic fluid plus adnexal mass	42	99	97	67

(Adapted from Nyberg DA, Hughes MP, Mack LA, Wang KY: Extrauterine findings of ectopic pregnancy at transvaginal US: Importance of echogenic fluid. Radiology 1991; 178:823–826.)

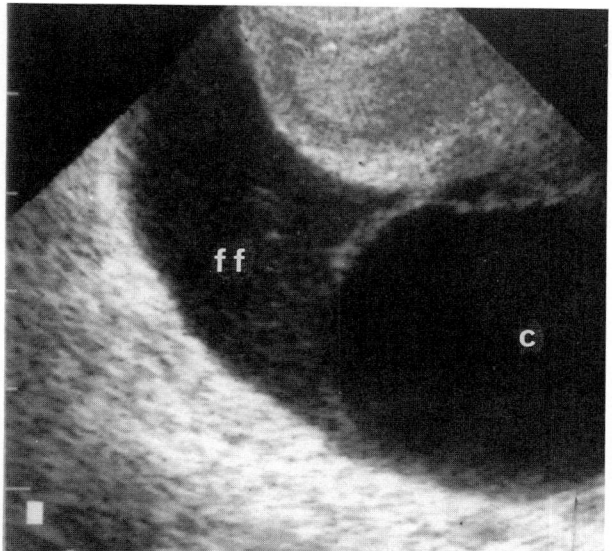

FIGURE 1-16. Ectopic pregnancy: free fluid. Echogenic free fluid (ff) is present in the adnexa adjacent to an adnexal cyst (c) in a patient with a ruptured ectopic pregnancy.

colleagues' series, the positive predictive value of a tubal ring for ectopic pregnancy was 100%.[37]

Free Fluid. The presence of free fluid is a nonspecific finding that suggests the presence of an ectopic pregnancy in the appropriate clinical setting. The presence of a large amount of free fluid or echogenic free fluid increases the positive predictive value from 63% to 86%.[37] In patients with suspected ectopic pregnancy, the combination of an adnexal mass and echogenic free fluid is associated with a 97% positive predictive value for ectopic pregnancy[37] (Figs. 1-15 and 1-16).

Normal Sonogram. Patients with ectopic pregnancy may have a completely normal pelvic ultrasound examination. In Nyberg and colleagues' series, 14.7% of patients with ectopic pregnancy had no evidence of either an adnexal mass or free fluid.[37]

Endovaginal Color Flow Doppler Diagnosis

Diagnosis with EVCFD of ectopic pregnancy is based on the identification of *adnexal peritrophoblastic flow*, defined as high-velocity, low-resistance flow separate from the ovary[7] (Figs. 1-17 and 1-18). Recent studies demonstrated that EVCFD increases the diagnostic sensitivity for ectopic pregnancy compared with EVS alone.[7,8] Furthermore, these studies suggest that EVCFD increases the percentage of initial examinations that are diagnostic of either intrauterine or ectopic pregnancy compared with EVS alone.[8]

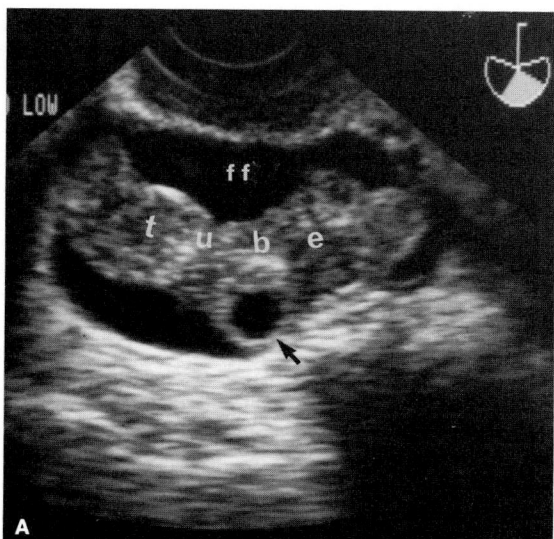
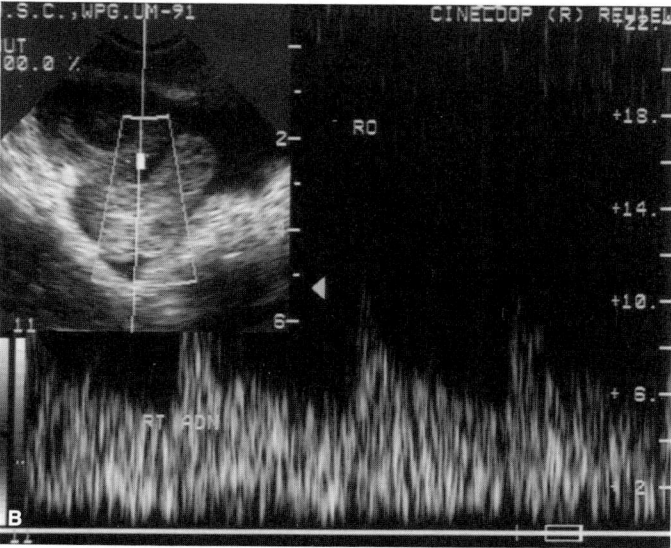

FIGURE 1-17. Ectopic pregnancy: gray-scale and Doppler findings. **(A)** Coronal sonogram through the right adnexa showing a fallopian tube (tube) filled with echogenic fluid (blood) and a trophoblastic ring (*arrow*). Echo-free fluid (ff) surrounds the tube. **(B)** Doppler interrogation of the right adnexa demonstrates high-velocity, low-resistance flow.

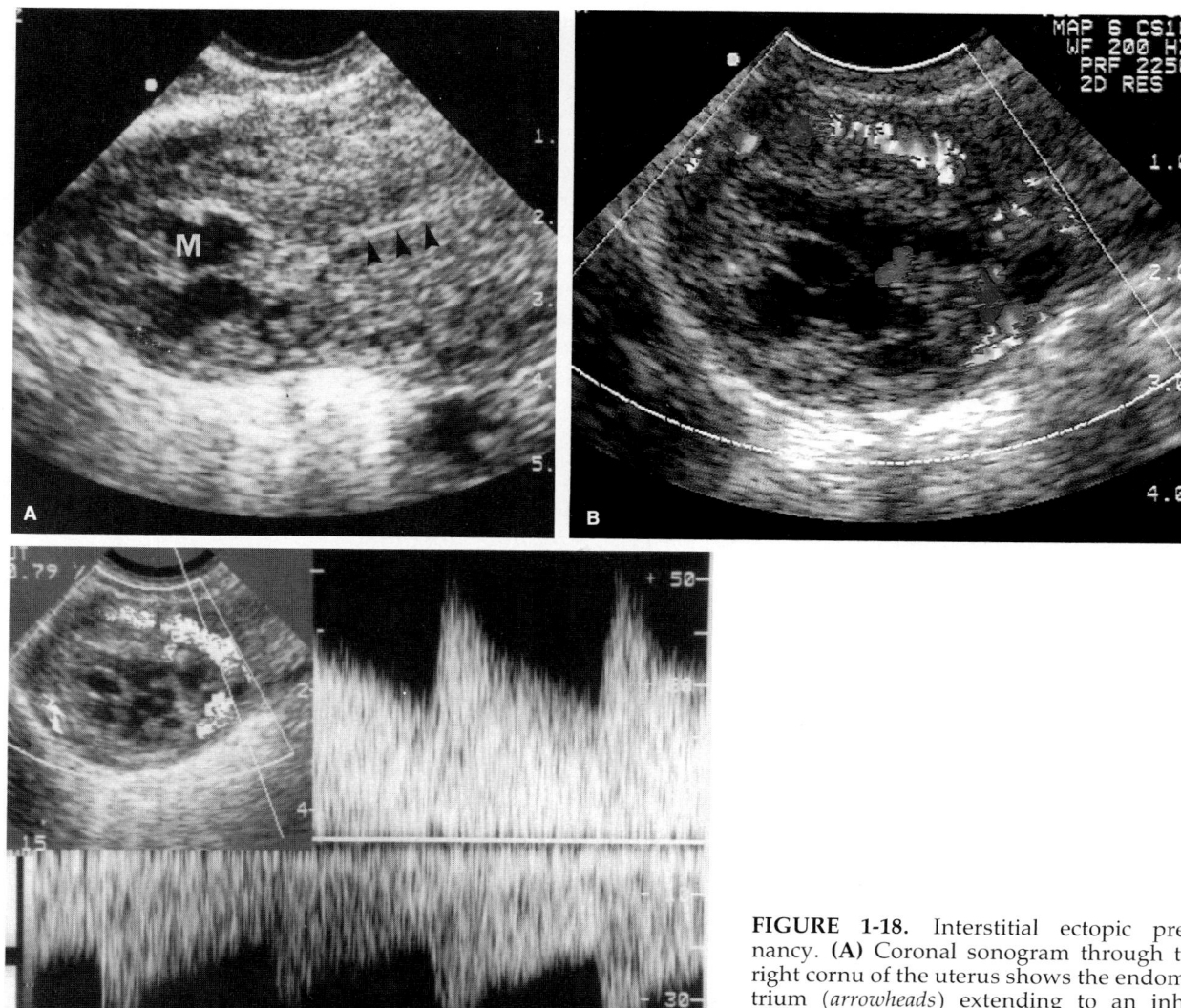

FIGURE 1-18. Interstitial ectopic pregnancy. **(A)** Coronal sonogram through the right cornu of the uterus shows the endometrium (*arrowheads*) extending to an inhomogeneous mass (M). **(B)** Endovaginal color flow Doppler and **(C)** pulsed Doppler demonstrate peritrophoblastic flow.

Interstitial (Cornual) Pregnancy

About 95% of ectopic pregnancies occur in the ampullary or isthmic portions of the fallopian tube.[41] The second most common site is in the intramural portion of the tube (interstitial pregnancy). Ovarian, cervical, and abdominal sites of ectopic pregnancy are extremely rare.

Because of its intramural location, an interstitial ectopic pregnancy ruptures later than other tubal gestations, often causing massive intraperitoneal hemorrhage from dilated uterine vessels. The mortality of interstitial pregnancy is therefore higher than for other tubal ectopic pregnancies. Although not specific, the sonographic diagnosis of an inter-stitial pregnancy is suggested by an eccentric location of the gestational sac surrounded by an incomplete myometrial mantle. If the gestational sac encroaches to within 5 mm of the uterine serosa, an interstitial ectopic pregnancy should be suspected.[36] In our experience, cornual ectopic pregnancies can be differentiated from eccentric intrauterine implantations by absence of the double-decidual ring in a cornual ectopic pregnancy and direct extension of the endometrial canal to the mid-portion of the cornual mass.[41a] This finding may be helpful in making the diagnosis of a cornual ectopic pregnancy, even in the absence of a demonstrable gestational sac in the cornua (see Fig. 1-18).

EARLY PREGNANCY FAILURE

After demonstrating the presence of an intrauterine gestation, the next step in first-trimester diagnosis is determining whether or not the embryo or fetus is alive. The sonographic diagnosis of early pregnancy failure depends on the stage of development.

> *Stage A:* Loss within the first 2 weeks after conception (3–4 weeks of menstrual age; called *subclinical loss*) or loss before the patient has missed a menstrual period. There is often no sonographic evidence of pregnancy at this stage.
> *Stage B:* Loss at 5 to 6 weeks of menstrual age. The sonographic diagnosis of pregnancy failure is usually based on gestational sac findings.
> *Stage C:* Loss at 7 to 8 weeks of menstrual age. The sonographic diagnosis of embryonic demise is usually based on demonstration of an abnormal embryo or gestational sac.
> *Stage D:* Loss at 9 to 12 weeks of menstrual age. The sonographic diagnosis of embryonic demise is usually based on demonstration of an abnormal embryo. Structural embryonic abnormalities (eg, head, heart) can sometimes be demonstrated with ultrasound.

Knowing the frequency and timing of pregnancy loss during normal gestation is integral to evaluating prenatal diagnostic techniques such as EVS. It has long been suspected that preclinical loss rates are high in humans, and in the past decade new data concerning these losses have become available. Cohort studies indicate that many women who show positive β-hCG assays never show clinical evidence of pregnancy. A study by Wilcox and associates[42] showed a 31% rate of pregnancy loss after implantation in normal, healthy volunteers.[5] In this series, 22% of all pregnancies aborted early, resulting in subclinical loss. Cytogenic abnormalities have also been documented in 20% of ostensibly normal in vitro fertilization embryos.[43] All the above cases are consistent with the pivotal studies of Hertig and Rock, who showed high frequencies of morphologic abnormalities in preimplantation embryos.[44,45] Loss rates are influenced by maternal age, smoking, alcohol, and other variables.

In addition to these causes of early pregnancy loss, the corpus luteum fails to support adequately the implanted conceptus. This is known as a *luteal phase defect* and may be a result of a shortened luteal phase with ovulation induction and in vitro fertilization or of luteal dysfunction, which occurs most commonly in obese women and women older than 37 years of age.[46]

Blumenfeld and Ruach found that in a group undergoing ovulation induction and in patients with previous abortions, repetitive hCG administration two times weekly in the 6th and 10th weeks of menstrual age resulted in the rate of miscarriage being significantly decreased from 49% to 17.8% ($P < .01$).[46]

After the gestational sac becomes demonstrable by ultrasound, the diagnosis of early pregnancy failure can be made reliably using sonographic criteria.

Sonographic Diagnosis (Flow Diagrams 1 and 2)

Embryonic Cardiac Activity

The presence of cardiac activity indicates that the embryo or fetus is alive. The predictive value of cardiac activity with respect to the ultimate viability of the pregnancy depends on the menstrual age at the time of examination.[4] After 7 weeks of menstrual age, the pregnancy loss rate is 2% to 2.3%,[47,48] and after 16 weeks, the rate is only 1%.[49] Most pregnancy failure occurs early, either as subclinical loss or in embryos younger than 7 weeks of menstrual age. In a series of 96 patients with embryonic CRL of less than 5 mm (6.5 weeks of menstrual age), EVS demonstration of cardiac activity was associated with a pregnancy loss rate of 24%.[4]

As noted in the section on the embryo and amnion, absence of sonographically demonstrable cardiac activity is not necessarily abnormal. Using transabdominal ultrasound, normal embryos of less than 9 mm CRL may have absent cardiac activity.[28] Using EVS, normal embryos of less than 4 or 5 mm CRL (depending on the series) may have absent cardiac activity.[4,28] The absence of cardiac activity in larger embryos is diagnostic of embryonic demise, assuming that the scan has been performed on modern equipment, using a high-frame rate, and that the frame-averaging mode has been turned off and the focal zone set appropriately (Fig. 1-19).

Gestational Sac Characteristics

In many patients, the embryo cannot be seen at the time of initial sonographic examination, and the diagnosis of embryonic demise cannot be made on the basis of embryonic cardiac activity. In those patients, it may be possible to make the diagnosis

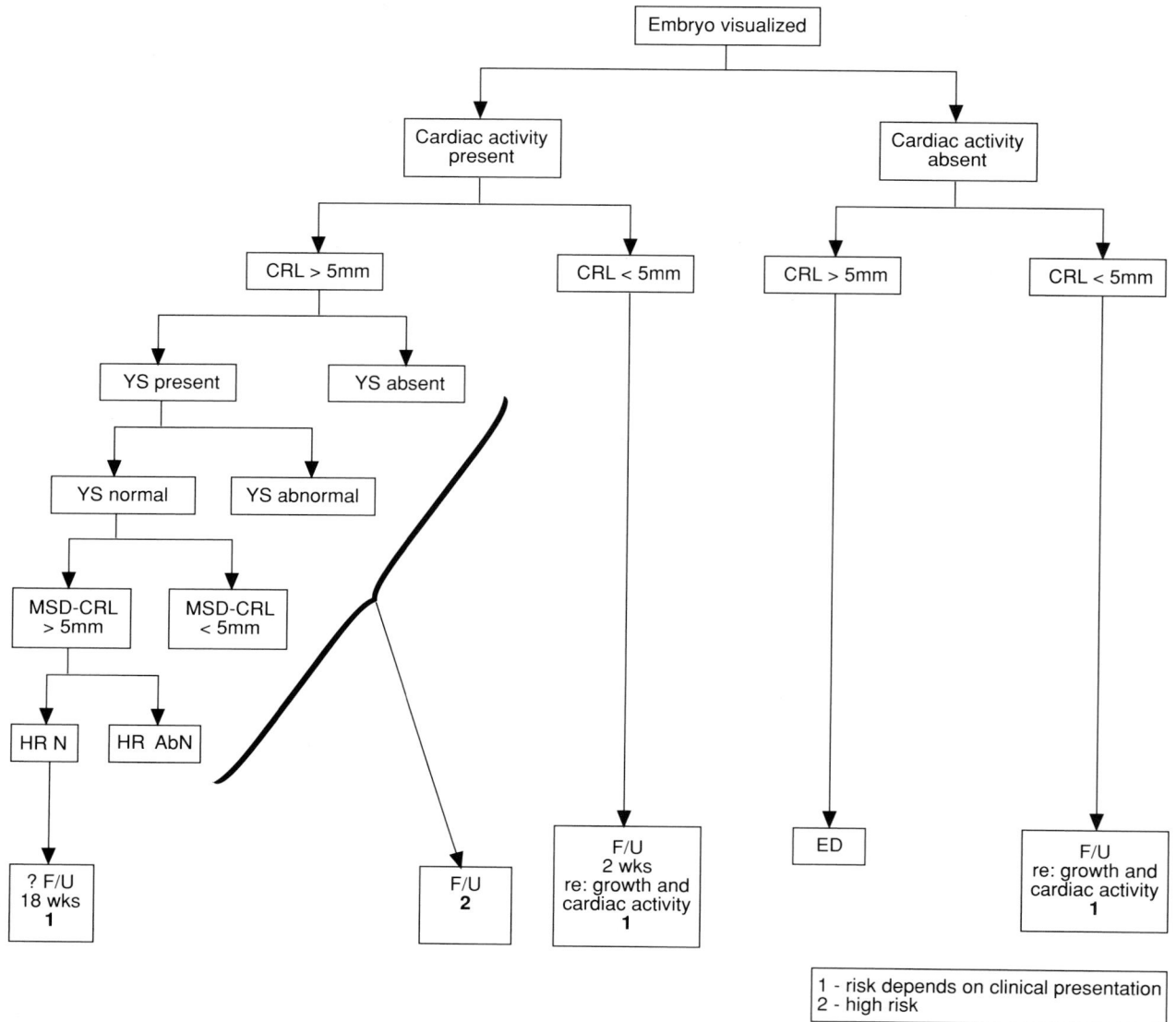

Flow Diagram 1. Early intrauterine pregnancy: EVS decision table. (ED, embryonic demise; CRL, crown-to-rump length; YS, yolk sac; HR, embryonic heart rate; N, normal; AbN, abnormal; MSD, mean gestational sac diameter; F/U, follow-up. The follow-up categories are: 1—risk depends on clinical presentation; 2—high risk requiring close follow-up.)

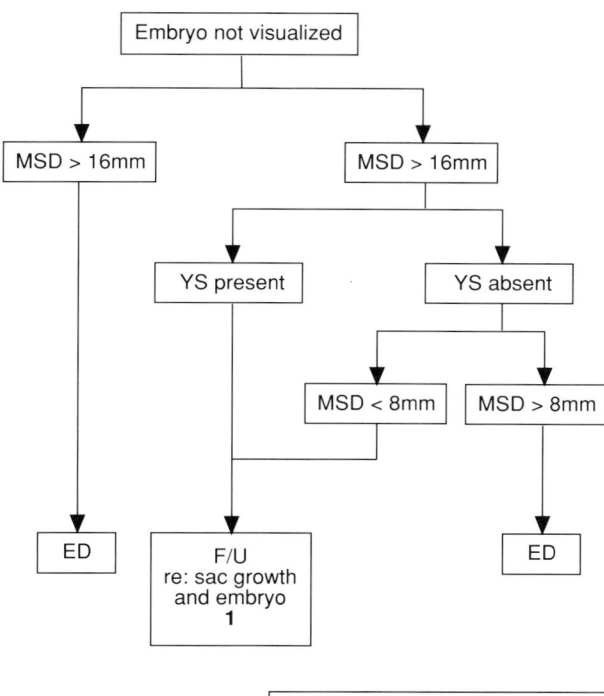

Flow Diagram 2. Early intrauterine pregnancy: EVS decision table. (ED, embryonic demise; MSD, mean gestational sac diameter; YS, yolk sac; F/U, follow-up. The follow-up categories are: 1—risk depends on clinical presentation; 2—high risk requiring close follow-up.)

of pregnancy failure based on gestational sac characteristics.[50]

The most reliable indicator of abnormal outcome based on gestational sac characteristics is abnormal gestational sac size.[3,50] In 1985, Bernard and Cooperberg observed that a sac larger than 2 cm in diameter without an embryo had a poor outcome.[51] In 1986, using transabdominal ultrasound, Nyberg and colleagues defined an abnormally large gestational sac as 25 mm in diameter and lacking an embryo or as 20 mm in diameter and lacking a yolk sac.[50]

These criteria were reevaluated for EVS.[3] Using EVS, if the MSD is 8 mm without a demonstrable yolk sac or 16 mm without a demonstrable embryo, the gestational sac is abnormally large, indicating pregnancy failure. We allow a 1- to 2-mm leeway in the MSD measurements as a margin of error (Fig. 1-20).

We consider other gestational sac criteria to be less reliable in the diagnosis of embryonic demise and use them as ancillary findings. These criteria include: distorted gestational sac shape (Fig. 1-21), thin decidual reaction (less than 2 mm), weak decidual amplitude, absent double-decidual sign, or abnormally low position of the gestational sac within the endometrial cavity.[50]

Normal gestational sac growth is 1.1 mm/day or more. Nyberg and colleagues found that patients

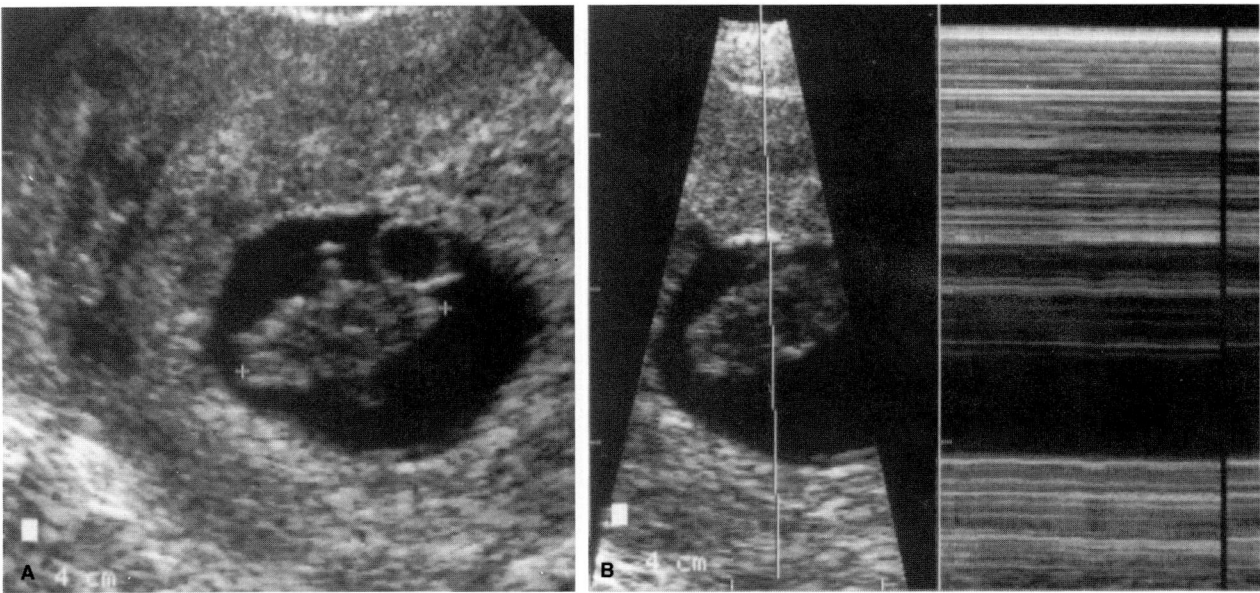

FIGURE 1-19. Embryonic demise: absent cardiac activity. **(A)** Endovaginal sonogram of an embryo measuring 1.42 cm crown-to-rump length (*calipers*) and a yolk sac. **(B)** Absence of cardiac activity on the M-mode tracing.

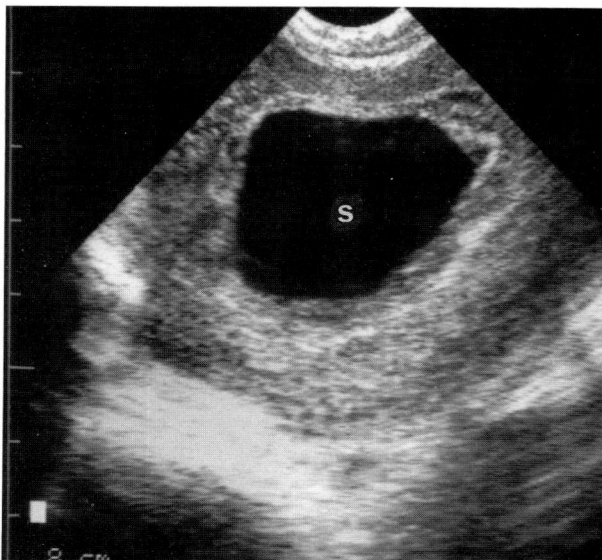

FIGURE 1-20. Early pregnancy failure: abnormal gestational sac size. Coronal endovaginal sonogram shows a gestational sac (s) with a mean diameter of about 3 cm. Neither a yolk sac nor an embryo is identified.

with early pregnancy failure had MSD growth rates of less than 0.7 mm/day.[52] In practice, we use this information as a guideline in planning for follow-up ultrasound examinations in patients in whom a diagnosis cannot be made on initial examination.

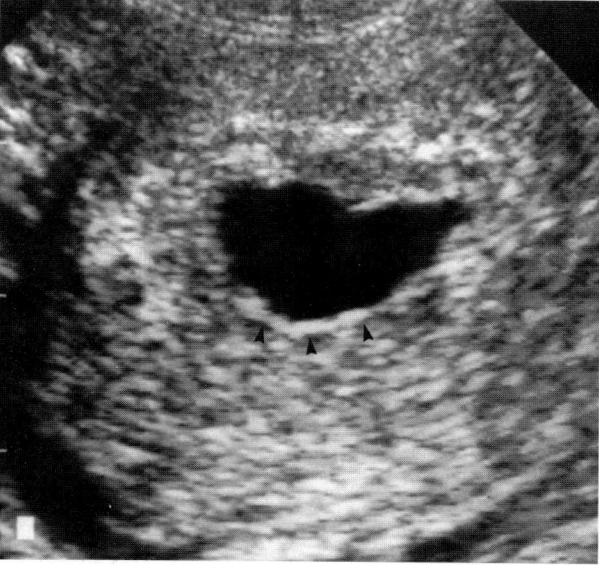

FIGURE 1-21. Early pregnancy failure: distorted gestational sac shape, thin decidual reaction, weak decidual amplitude. Coronal sonogram shows a sac with a grossly irregular shape and a thin decidual reaction (*arrowheads*).

Amnion and Yolk Sac Criteria

Other findings that can be useful in the diagnosis of embryonic demise include a collapsing, irregularly marginated amnion, visualization of the amnion in the absence of a visible embryo, and yolk sac calcification.[53] In general, however, other signs of embryonic demise are present when these findings are positive.

Sonographic Predictors of Abnormal Outcome

Sonographic findings may be used to predict abnormal outcome in the presence of a live embryo or before visualization of the embryo. These findings can be used to identify a high-risk subgroup of embryos that are at risk for embryonic demise or subsequent diagnosis of fetal anomaly and require close follow-up.

Embryonic Bradycardia

Although embryonic cardiac activity indicates that the embryo is alive at the time of examination, a slow heart rate may suggest impending demise. Laboda and associates described a series of five embryos between 5 and 8 weeks of menstrual age with heart rates less than 85 beats/min, all of whom subsequently aborted spontaneously.[54]

Comparison of MSD and CRL

Bromley and colleagues found that in 16 patients between 5.5 and 9 weeks of menstrual age, in whom the MSD was less than 5 mm greater than the CRL (ie, MSD − CRL < 5 mm), 15 of 16 had spontaneous first-trimester abortions[55] (Fig. 1-22).

Yolk Sac Size and Shape

Although the subject is still controversial,[56] in our experience, yolk sac size and shape may be useful as relative predictors of abnormal outcome.[22] Perhaps the most important consideration is that yolk sac abnormalities may predict abnormal outcome in pregnancies that appear completely normal by all other ultrasound criteria.

We found that between 5 and 10 weeks of menstrual age, when the yolk sac diameter is outside the 5% and 95% confidence intervals compared with the MSD (Fig. 1-23), the risk of abnormal outcome increases from about 24% to about 44.4% to 60%.[22] In our experience, yolk sac diameters of ≥5.6 mm between 5 and 10 weeks of menstrual age (Fig. 1-24) are always associated with abnormal outcome (either embryonic demise or fetal anomaly).[22]

A persistently abnormal yolk sac shape is also a predictor of abnormal outcome.[22] Although our

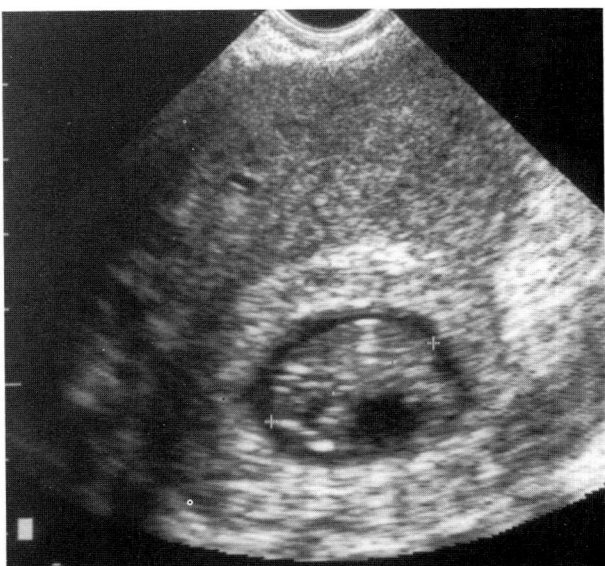

FIGURE 1-22. Predictors of abnormal outcome: MSD − CRL < 5 mm. Coronal sonogram shows a 2.5-cm embryo (*calipers*) within a relatively small gestational sac. The embryo was dead on follow-up examination.

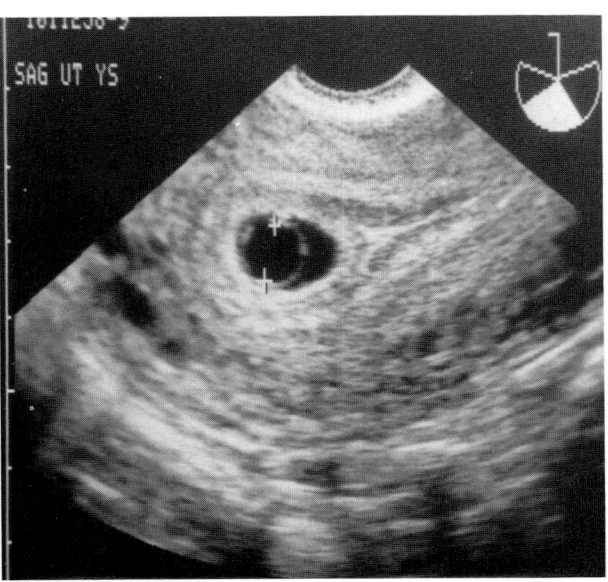

FIGURE 1-24. Large yolk sac. Endovaginal sonogram (sagittal plane) at 5.5 weeks of menstrual age shows an abnormally large yolk sac (*calipers*) with an internal diameter of 7.5 mm.

data are preliminary, when the yolk sac shape is crenated or irregular in contour, outcome appears to depend on the appearances of the yolk sac on follow-up examination in 1 week. In our series, if the yolk sac shape reverted to normal, outcome was always normal. If the yolk sac shape remained abnormal, the embryos were at increased risk for embryonic demise or fetal anomaly (Fig. 1-25).[22]

We use yolk sac data to determine which pregnancies are at increased risk for abnormal outcome. In the absence of other indicators of abnormal outcome, patients with abnormalities of yolk sac size or shape are followed closely in the first trimester. If the embryo survives the first trimester, sonographic follow-up is performed at 18 weeks of menstrual age to exclude a sonographically demonstrable anomaly. Genetic counseling is also offered.

Ratio of β-hCG to Mean Gestational Sac Diameter

Nyberg and colleagues found that 65% of abnormal pregnancies had a disproportionately low serum β-hCG level for gestational sac size.[57]

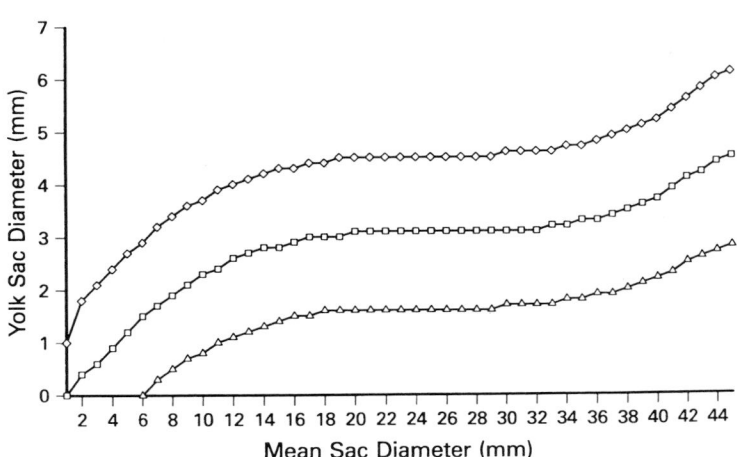

FIGURE 1-23. Normal first-trimester obstetrical data. Yolk sac diameter versus mean gestational sac diameter. □, mean; △, 5% confidence interval; ◇, 95% confidence interval.

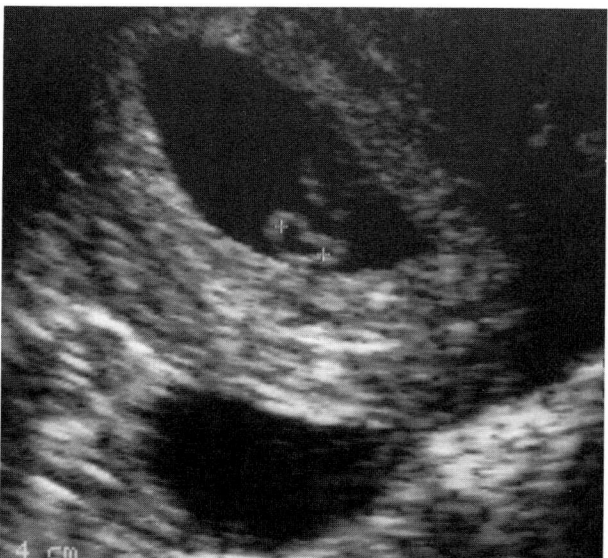

FIGURE 1-25. Irregular yolk sac. Endovaginal sonogram shows an irregular, 3-mm yolk sac (*calipers*).

FETAL ANOMALIES

With EVS, it is possible to image the embryo in its earliest stages of development. Although the embryo can be seen even before the onset of cardiac pulsation,[4] the actual diagnosis of anomalies is limited by the resolution of ultrasound equipment and by the morphologic appearance of a specific anomaly at the time of sonographic examination. In general, the diagnosis of gross anomalies such as cystic hygromas (Fig. 1-26) and large cranial cysts (Fig. 1-27) can be made in the first trimester with either transabdominal ultrasound or EVS.[58] Case reports of first-trimester diagnoses of polydactyly, ectopia cordis,[59] and other less obvious anomalies have been published, but most diagnoses of anomalies are made in the second or third trimesters.

Many severe anomalies may have a normal sonographic appearance in the first trimester. The most dramatic example is anencephaly,[60] which may only become obvious after ossification of the calvarium occurs at 12 weeks of menstrual age. Anencephaly results from failure of closure of the rostral neuropore at 42 days (6 weeks) of menstrual age.[14] At about 8 weeks of menstrual age, a fetal head may be identified in an anencephalic embryo either because the cerebral cortex is normally disproportionately small at this stage or because abnormal neural tissue is present superior to the orbits and skull base.

Similarly, even severe renal anomalies are usually beyond the resolution of available equipment in the first trimester. The kidneys do not reach their adult position until 11 weeks, the bladder is seen in only half of normal fetuses by 12 weeks, and amniotic fluid volume does not depend on fetal renal function until the second trimester.

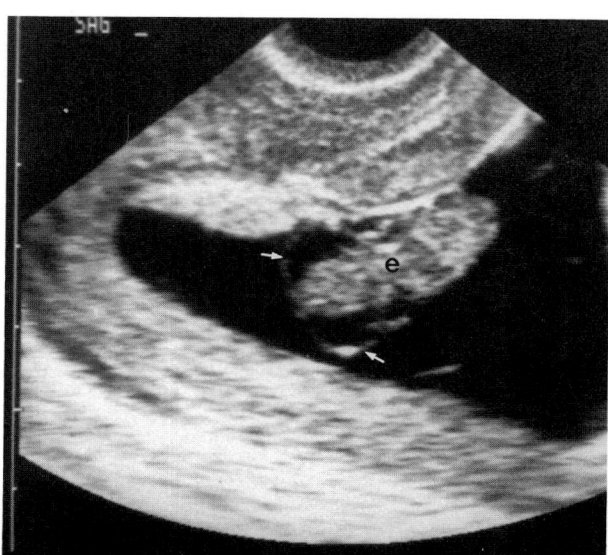

FIGURE 1-26. Cystic hygromas (9.5 weeks of menstrual age). Endovaginal sonogram showing bilateral cystic hygromas (*arrows*) in an embryo (e) with Turner's syndrome.

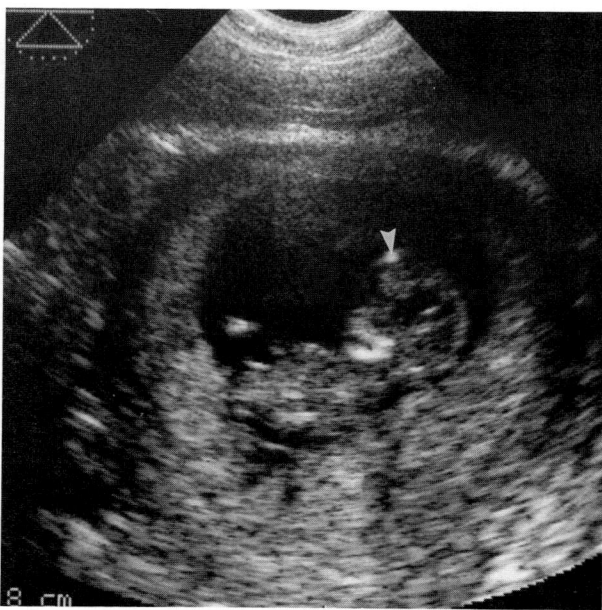

FIGURE 1-27. Encephalocele. Anterior encephalocele (*arrowhead*) at 10.5 weeks of menstrual age.

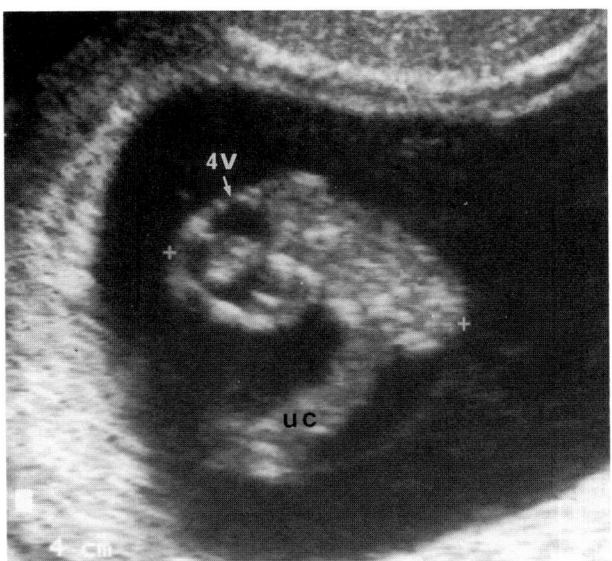

FIGURE 1-28. Normal embryonic intracranial anatomy at 9 weeks of menstrual age. The embryonic rhombencephalon (4V) is well visualized. The umbilical cord (uc) is also shown.

Conversely, in the first trimester, normal embryologic anatomy may mimic the sonographic appearances of fetal anomalies because of developmental stage. The fetal rhombencephalon (Figs. 1-28 and 1-29) appears as a cystic structure in the posterior fossa beginning at 7 weeks of menstrual age and should not be mistaken for an intracranial cyst or hydrocephalus.[61] The telencephalic and mesencephalic vesicles can also be seen at this stage.[62]

Physiologic mid-gut hernia is often demonstrated as a small (6–9 mm) echogenic mass protruding into the umbilical cord at about 8 weeks of menstrual age and is still present in 20% of normal fetuses up to 12 weeks.[63] Small cysts measuring 2 to 7.5 mm are present in the umbilical cord in 0.4% of normal first-trimester pregnancies and are of no clinical significance[64] (see Fig. 1-29).

EXTRACHORIONIC FLUID COLLECTIONS

Subchorionic accumulation of blood is not uncommon in the first trimester and may be associated with vaginal bleeding. In a group of patients presenting with vaginal bleeding between 10 and 20 weeks of menstrual age, identification of a subchorionic hemorrhage was associated with a 50% fetal loss rate.[65]

Subchorionic hemorrhage may be due to abruption of the edge of the chorion frondosum and decidua basalis complex or to marginal sinus rupture.[66] Although the hemorrhage usually abuts or

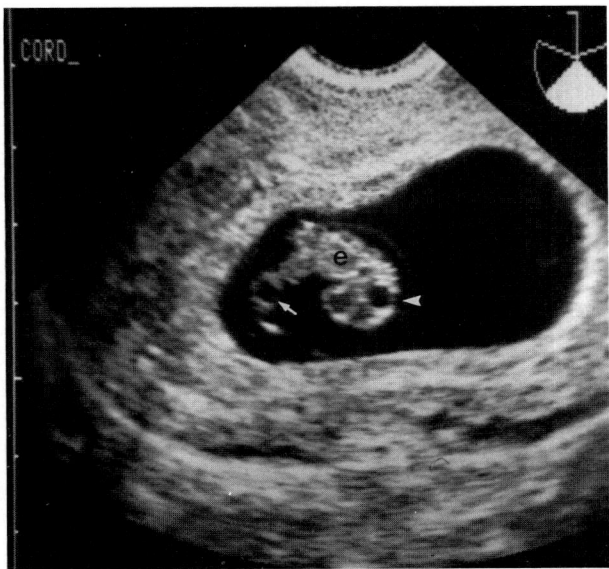

FIGURE 1-29. Umbilical cord cyst. A 2-mm cyst (*arrow*) is present in the umbilical cord of this normal embryo (e) at 9 weeks of menstrual age. A normal fourth ventricle (*arrowhead*) is also shown. A subsequent sonogram at 16.5 weeks showed a normal fetus and disappearance of the cord cyst.

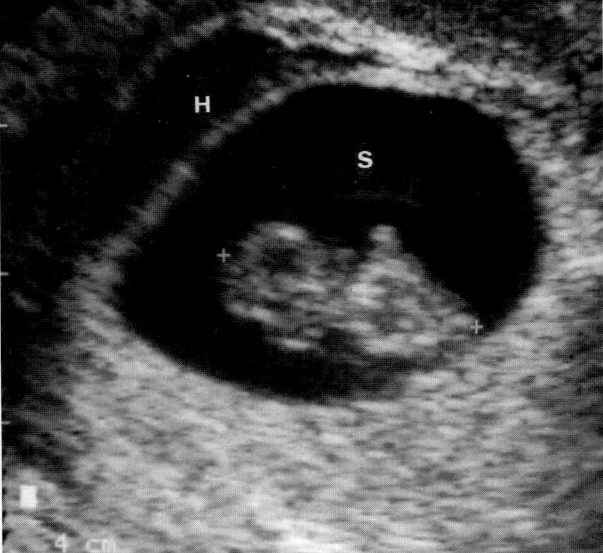

FIGURE 1-30. Subchorionic hemorrhage. Endovaginal sonogram demonstrating a subchorionic hemorrhage (H) within the endometrial canal adjacent to a gestational sac (s) that contains a live embryo with an 18.5-mm crown-to-rump length (8.5–9 weeks of menstrual age).

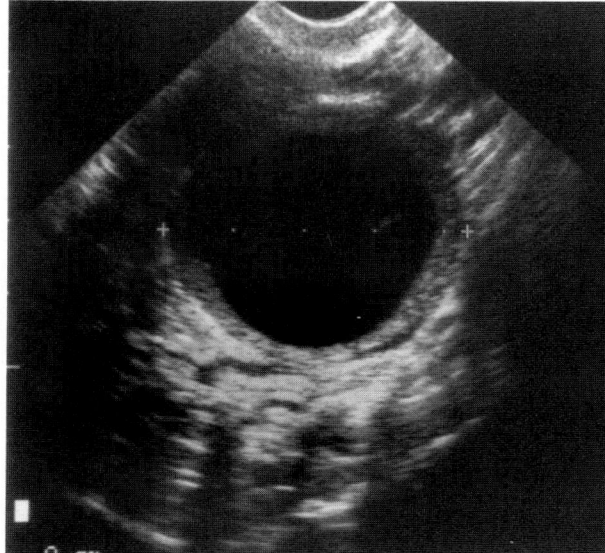

FIGURE 1-31. Corpus luteum cyst of pregnancy. Endovaginal sonogram in the coronal plane through the left adnexa of a patient in early pregnancy showing a 4.5-cm corpus luteum cyst (*calipers*).

isoechoic with the chorionic fluid in 1 to 2 weeks (Figs. 1-4 and 1-30).

FIRST-TRIMESTER MASSES

Ovarian

The most common mass seen in the first trimester of pregnancy is the corpus luteum cyst.[67] The corpus luteum cyst secretes progesterone to support the pregnancy until the placenta can take over its hormonal function.

The corpus luteum forms in the secretory phase of the menstrual cycle and increases in size if a pregnancy occurs. The corpus luteum of pregnancy is usually less than 5 cm in diameter and most commonly appears as a thin-walled, unilocular cyst[67] (Fig. 1-31).

The appearance of the corpus luteum cyst, however, may vary considerably. Corpus luteum cysts may be much larger, occasionally attaining a size of greater than 10 cm. Internal septations and echogenic debris may be present secondary to internal hemorrhage (Fig. 1-32). The cyst wall and septations may be markedly thick.

A hemorrhagic corpus luteum cyst may be impossible to differentiate from a pathologic cyst on the basis of a single ultrasound examination. Corpus luteum cysts usually regress or decrease in size by follow-up sonographic examination at 16 to

elevates the edge of the chorion frondosum and decidua basalis complex, the bulk of the hemorrhage is usually situated between the decidua capsularis and chorion laeve complex and the decidua vera. Acute hemorrhage may be hyperechoic or isoechoic relative to the chorion, and it becomes

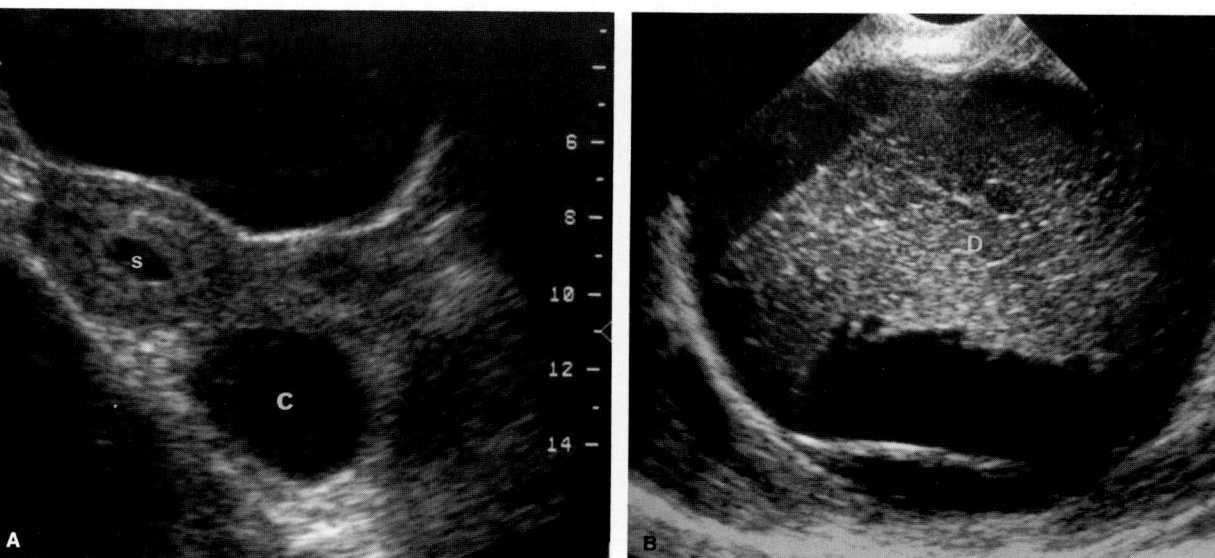

FIGURE 1-32. Hemorrhagic corpus luteum cyst. **(A)** Sagittal transabdominal sonogram shows the uterus with an early gestational sac (s) and a 4-cm corpus luteum cyst (c) in the posterior cul de sac. **(B)** Endovaginal sonogram of the corpus luteum cyst shows internal echogenic material (D) consistent with hemorrhage.

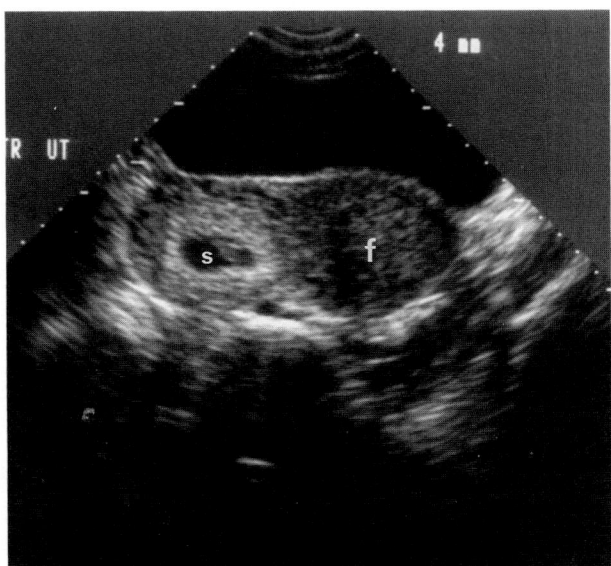

FIGURE 1-33. Uterine fibroid in pregnancy. Coronal transabdominal sonogram shows a hypoechoic fibroid (f) arising from the left lateral aspect of the uterine corpus. A normally positioned intrauterine gestational sac (s) is present.

18 weeks of menstrual age. Cystic masses that persist should be followed. Surgical intervention is often indicated in large cysts that do not regress by the middle of the second trimester. Not all corpus luteum cysts regress, however, and differentiation from a pathologic cyst may be impossible.

Other cystic masses may present for the first time in the first trimester of pregnancy because of displacement by the enlarged uterus. Although

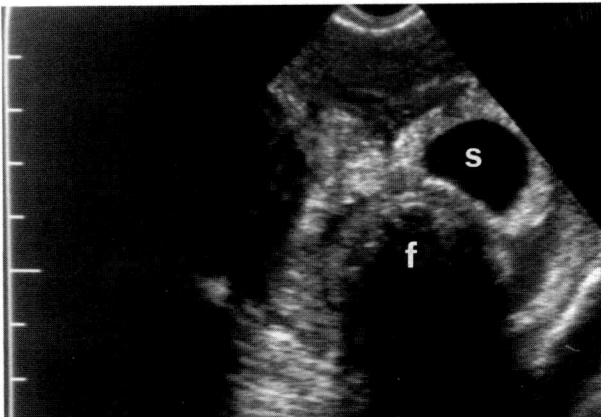

FIGURE 1-34. Uterine fibroid in pregnancy. Endovaginal sonogram in the coronal plane shows a calcified fibroid (f) casting an acoustic shadow. The relation of the fibroid to the gestational sac (s) is clearly demonstrated.

malignant ovarian neoplasm associated with pregnancy is rare,[68] torsion, rupture, and dystocia are not. When elective surgical intervention is indicated, it is usually performed in the second trimester, when the likelihood of inducing premature labor is considered to be lowest. Dermoid cysts may present a characteristic appearance of a cystic mass with focal calcification and layering of fluids of different echogenicities within the cystic area. Other cystic masses may be more difficult to differentiate from corpus luteum cysts. All cysts should be followed carefully to assess change in size.[67]

Uterine

Uterine fibroids are common pelvic masses that are often identified during pregnancy. Most fibroids do not change in size during pregnancy. Some fibroids, however, may enlarge rapidly due to stimulation by estrogen. Infarction and necrosis may occur due to rapid growth. These patients often experience pain.

Sonographically, uterine fibroids appear as solid uterine masses that attenuate sound to a variable degree (Fig. 1-33), may or may not be calcified (Fig. 1-34), and may have focal cystic areas related to necrosis.

Fibroids may be differentiated from focal myometrial contractions by the transient nature of myometrial contractions. A repeat examination 20 to 30 minutes after the initial examination reveals disappearance of a focal myometrial contraction, whereas a fibroid will still be present. Fibroids also may distort the uterine contour (serosal surface), whereas focal myometrial contractions usually do not.

REFERENCES

1. Levi CS, Lyons EA, Dashefsky SM: The first trimester. In Rumack CM, Wilson SR, Charboneau JW (eds): Diagnostic Ultrasound. St. Louis: Mosby Year Book, 1991: 692–722.
2. Dashefsky SM, Lyons EA, Levi CS, et al: Suspected ectopic pregnancy: Endovaginal and transvesical ultrasound. Radiology 1988; 169:181–184.
3. Levi CS, Lyons EA, Lindsay DJ: Early diagnosis of nonviable pregnancy with endovaginal ultrasound. Radiology 1988; 167:383–385.
4. Levi CS, Lyons EA, Zheng XH, et al: Endovaginal ultrasound: Demonstration of cardiac activity in embryos of less than 5.0 mm in crown rump length. Radiology 1990; 176:71–74.
5. Dillon EH, Feycock AL, Taylor KJW: Pseudogestational sacs: Doppler US differentiation from normal

or abnormal intrauterine pregnancies. Radiology 1990; 176:359–364.

6. Taylor KJW, Ramos IM, Feycock AL, et al: Ectopic pregnancy: Duplex Doppler evaluation. Radiology 1989; 173:93–97.

7. Pellerito JS, Taylor KJW, Quedens-Case C, et al: Ectopic pregnancy: Evaluation with endovaginal colour flow imaging. Radiology 1992; 183:407–411.

8. Emerson DS, Cartier MS, Altieri LA, et al: Diagnostic efficacy of endovaginal colour flow imaging in an ectopic pregnancy screening program. Radiology 1992; 183:413–420.

9. Moore KL: The beginning of development: The first week. In Moore KL: The Developing Human: Clinically Oriented Embryology, 4th ed. Philadelphia: WB Saunders, 1988: 13–37.

10. Moore KL: Formation of the bilaminar embryo: The second week. In Moore KL: The Developing Human: Clinically Oriented Embryology, 4th ed. Philadelphia: WB Saunders, 1988: 38–49.

11. Moore KL: Formation of the trilaminar embryo: The third week. In Moore KL: The Developing Human: Clinically Oriented Embryology, 4th ed. Philadelphia: WB Saunders, 1988: 50–64.

12. Moore KL: Formation of basic organs and systems: The fourth to eighth weeks. In Moore KL: The Developing Human: Clinically Oriented Embryology, 4th ed. Philadelphia: WB Saunders, 1988: 65–86.

13. Moore KL: The fetal period: The ninth week to birth. In Moore KL: The Developing Human: Clinically Oriented Embryology, 4th ed. Philadelphia: WB Saunders, 1988: 87–103.

14. Moore KL: The nervous system. In Moore KL: The Developing Human: Clinically Oriented Embryology, 4th ed. Philadelphia: WB Saunders, 1988: 364–401.

15. Ackerman TE, Levi CS, Lyons EA, et al: Decidual cyst: Endovaginal sonographic sign of ectopic pregnancy. Radiology 1993; 189:727–731.

16. Yeh H-C, Goodman JD, Carr L, Rabinowitz JG: Intradecidual sign: A US criterion of early intrauterine pregnancy. Radiology 1986; 161:463–467.

17. Cartier MS, Altieri LA, Emerson DS, et al: Diagnostic efficacy of endovaginal color flow Doppler in an ectopic pregnancy screening program. Radiology 1990; 177(P):117.

18. Nyberg DA, Laing FC, Filly RA, et al: Ultrasonographic differentiation of the gestational sac of early intrauterine pregnancy from the pseudogestational sac of ectopic pregnancy. Radiology 1983; 146:755–759.

19. Bree RL, Edwards ML, Bohm-Velez, et al: Transvaginal sonography in the evaluation of normal early pregnancy: Correlation with HCG level. AJR 1989; 153:75–79.

20. Nyberg DA, Filly RA, Laing FC, et al: Ectopic pregnancy: Diagnosis by sonography correlated with quantitative HCG levels. J Ultrasound Med 1987; 6(3):145–150.

21. Moore KL: The placenta and fetal membranes. In Moore KL: The Developing Human: Clinically Oriented Embryology, 4th ed. Philadelphia: WB Saunders, 1988: 104–130.

22. Lindsay DJ, Lovett IS, Lyons EA, et al: Yolk sac diameter and shape at endovaginal US: Predictors of pregnancy outcome in the first trimester. Radiology 1992; 183:115–118.

23. Nyberg DA, Mack LA, Harvey D, Wang K: Value of the yolk sac in evaluating early pregnancies. J Ultrasound Med 1988; 7(3):129–135.

24. Yeh H-C, Rabinowitz JG: Amniotic sac development: Ultrasound features of early pregnancy. The double bleb sign. Radiology 1988; 166(1):97–103.

25. Levi CS, Lyons EA, Lindsay DJ, Gratton D: The sonographic evaluation of multiple gestation pregnancy. In Fleischer AC, Romero R, Manning FA, Jeanty P, James AE Jr.: The Principles and Practice of Ultrasonography in Obstetrics and Gynecology, 4th ed. Norwalk, CT: Appleton and Lange, 1991: 359–379.

26. Mahony BS, Filly RA, Callen PW: Amnionicity and chorionicity in twin pregnancies: Prediction using ultrasound. Radiology 1985; 155:205–209.

27. Cadkin AV, McAlpin J: Detection of fetal cardiac activity between 41 and 43 days of gestation. J Ultrasound Med 1984; 3(11):499–503.

28. Pennell RG, Needleman L, Pajak T, et al: Prospective comparison of vaginal and abdominal sonography in normal early pregnancy. J Ultrasound Med 1991; 10:63–67.

29. Rempen A: Diagnosis of viability in early pregnancy with vaginal sonography. J Ultrasound Med 1990; 9: 711–716.

30. Howe RS, Isaacson KJ, Albert JL, Coutifaris CB: Embryonic heart rate in early human pregnancy. J Ultrasound Med 1991; 10:367–371.

31. Atrash HK, Friede A, Hogue CJR: Ectopic pregnancy mortality in the United States, 1970–1983. Obstet Gynecol 1987; 70:817–822.

32. Lawson HW, Atrash HK, Saftlas AF, et al: Ectopic pregnancy surveillance, United States, 1970–1985. MMWR CDC Surveillance Summary 1988; 37(5):9–18.

33. Coupet E: Ectopic pregnancy: The surgical epidemic. J Natl Med Assoc 1989; 81:567–572.

34. Hann LE, Bachman DM, McArdle CR: Coexistent intrauterine and ectopic pregnancy: A reevaluation. Radiology 1984; 152:151–154.

35. Rein MS, Di Salvo DN, Friedman AJ: Heterotopic pregnancy associated with in vitro fertilization and embryo transfer: A possible role for routine vaginal ultrasound. Fertil Steril 1989; 51(6):1057–1058.

36. Fleischer AC, Pennell RG, McKee MS, et al: Ectopic pregnancy: Features at transvaginal sonography. Radiology 1990; 174:375–378.

37. Nyberg DA, Hughes MP, Mack LA, Wang KY: Extrauterine findings of ectopic pregnancy at transvaginal US: Importance of echogenic fluid. Radiology 1991; 178:823–826.

38. Timor-Tritsch IE, Yeh MN, Peisner DB, et al: The use of transvaginal ultrasonography in the diagnosis of ectopic pregnancy. Obstet Gynecol 1989; 161: 157–161.

39. Thorsen MK, Lawson TL, Aiman EJ, et al: Diagnosis of ectopic pregnancy: Endovaginal vs transabdominal sonography. AJR 1990; 155:307–310.

40. Mahony BS, Filly RA, Nyberg DA, Callen PW: Sonographic evaluation of ectopic pregnancy. J Ultrasound Med 1985; 4:221–228.

41. Cartwright PS: Ectopic pregnancy. In Jones HW III, Wentz AC, Burnett LC (eds): Novak's Textbook of Gynecology, 11th ed. Baltimore: Williams and Wilkins, 1988: 479–506.

41a. Ackerman TE, Levi CS, Dashefsky SM, et al: Interstitial line: Sonographic finding in interstitial (cornual) ectopic pregnancy. Radiology 1993; 189:83–87.

42. Wilcox AJ, Weinberg CR, O'Connor JF, et al: Incidence of early loss of pregnancy. N Engl J Med 1988; 319(4):189–194.

43. Bateman BG, Felder R, Kolp LA, Burkett B, Nunley WC Jr.: Subclinical pregnancy loss in clomiphene citrate-treated women. Fertil Steril 1992; 57:25–27.

44. Hertig AT, Rock J: A series of potentially abortive ova recovered from fertile women prior to the first missed menstrual period. Am J Obstet Gynecol 1949; 58:968–993.

45. Hertig AT, Rock J, Adams BC, Menkin MC: Thirty-four fertilized human ova, good, bad and indifferent, recovered from 210 women of known fertility: A study of biologic wastage in early human pregnancy. Pediatrics 1959; 23:202–211.

46. Blumenfeld Z, Ruach M: Early pregnancy wastage: The role of repetitive human chorionic gonadotrophin supplementation during the first 8 weeks of gestation. Fertil Steril 1992; 58:19–23.

47. Cashner KA, Christopher CR, Dysert GA: Spontaneous fetal loss after demonstration of a live fetus in the first trimester. Obstet Gynecol 1987; 70:827–830.

48. Wilson RD, Kendrick V, Wittmann BK, McGillivray B: Spontaneous abortion and pregnancy outcome after normal first-trimester ultrasound examination. Obstet Gynecol 1986; 67:352–355.

49. Simpson JL: Incidence and timing of pregnancy losses: Relevance to evaluating safety of early prenatal diagnosis. Am J Med Genet 1990; 35:165–73.

50. Nyberg DA, Laing FC, Filly RA: Threatened abortion: Sonographic distinction of normal and abnormal gestation sacs. Radiology 1986; 158:397–400.

51. Bernard KG, Cooperberg PL: Sonographic differentiation between blighted ovum and early viable pregnancy. AJR 1985; 144:597–602.

52. Nyberg DA, Mack LA, Laing FC, et al: Distinguishing normal from abnormal gestational sac growth in early pregnancy. J Ultrasound Med 1987; 6:23–26.

53. Harris RD, Vincent LM, Askin FB: Yolk sac calcification: A sonographic finding associated with intrauterine embryonic demise in the first trimester. Radiology 1988; 166:109–110.

54. Laboda LA, Estroff JA, Benacerraf BR: First trimester bradycardia: A sign of impending fetal loss. J Ultrasound Med 1989; 8:561–563.

55. Bromley B, Harlow BL, Laboda LA, Benacerraf BR: Small sac size in the first trimester: A predictor of poor fetal outcome. Radiology 1991; 178:375–377.

56. Kurtz AB, Needleman L, Pennell RG, et al: Can detection of the yolk sac in the first trimester be used to predict the outcome of pregnancy? A prospective sonographic study. AJR 1992; 158:843–847.

57. Nyberg DA, Filly RA, Filho DRD, et al: Abnormal pregnancy: Early diagnosis by US and serum chorionic gonadotropin levels. Radiology 1986; 158:393–396.

58. Cullen MT, Green J, Whetham J, et al: Transvaginal ultrasonographic detection of congenital anomalies in the first trimester. Am J Obstet Gynecol 1990; 163: 466–476.

59. Bennett TL, Burlbaw J, Drake CK, Finley BE: Diagnosis of ectopia cordis at 12 weeks gestation using transabdominal ultrasonography with color flow Doppler. J Ultrasound Med 1991; 10:695–696.

60. Goldstein RB, Filly RA: Prenatal diagnosis of anencephaly: Spectrum of sonographic appearances and distinction from the amniotic band syndrome. AJR 1988; 151:547–550.

61. Cyr DR, Mack LA, Nyberg DA, et al: Fetal rhombencephalon: Normal US findings. Radiology 1988; 166: 691–692.

62. Timor-Tritsch IE, Monteagudo A, Warren WB: Transvaginal ultrasonographic definition of the central nervous system in the first and early second trimesters. Am J Obstet Gynecol 1991; 164:497–503.

63. Schmidt W, Yarkoni S, Crelin ES, Hobbins JC: Sonographic visualization of physiologic anterior abdominal wall hernia in the first trimester. Obstet Gynecol 1987; 69:911–915.

64. Skibo LK, Lyons EA, Levi CS: First-trimester umbilical cord cysts. Radiology 1992; 182:719–722.

65. Sauerbrei EE, Pham DH: Placental abruption and subchorionic hemorrhage in the first half of pregnancy: US appearance and clinical outcome. Radiology 1986; 160:109–112.

66. Nyberg DA, Cyr DR, Mack LA, et al: Sonographic spectrum of placental abruption. AJR 1987; 148:161–164.

67. Fleischer AC, Boehm FH, James AE Jr: Sonographic evaluation of pelvic masses and maternal disorders occurring during pregnancy. In Sanders RC, James AE Jr (eds): The Principles and Practice of Ultrasonography in Obstetrics and Gynecology, 3rd ed. Norwalk, CT: Appleton-Century-Crofts, 1985: 435–447.

68. Pennes DR, Bowerman RA, Silver TM: Echogenic adnexal masses associated with first-trimester pregnancy: Sonographic appearance and clinical significance. J Clin Ultrasound 1985; 13:391–396.

John P. McGahan and Manuel Porto:
DIAGNOSTIC OBSTETRICAL ULTRASOUND.
© 1994 J.B. Lippincott Company.

Lyndon M. Hill

Chapter 2

Important Obstetrical Measurements

The sonographic estimations of gestational age, growth rate, and size depend on the ability of ultrasound to give precise measurements of specific fetal dimensions. Although gestational age, size, and maturity usually develop in parallel, they may evolve independently and therefore must be assessed individually.

During the first half of pregnancy, a remarkably constant pattern of fetal development crosses geographic, ethnic, and socioeconomic lines. Fetal growth during this part of pregnancy appears to reflect an inherent genetic drive.[1-3]

Both cross-sectional and longitudinal studies of fetal growth assume a normal population with similar growth trajectories. Physicians use the convention that gestation starts with the first day of the last menstrual period, but this date is frequently unknown or grossly inaccurate. Furthermore, the interval between menstruation and ovulation, which averages about 14 days, may vary by more than a week. The intervals between ovulation, fertilization, and implantation also vary. Hence, certain irreducible sources for error exist in the clinical as well as sonographic assessment of gestational age. For example, the average fetus gains 10 mm in crown-to-rump length (CRL) be-tween 14 and 15 weeks' gestation.[4] This 10-mm difference, however, could be found in two fetuses of the same gestational age merely as a result of the variability in the time of conception. Consequently, the range in any sonographic assessment of gestational age should be reported. The pitfalls of various measurements are presented throughout this chapter rather than in a separate section.

GESTATIONAL SAC

The first sonographic evidence for an intrauterine pregnancy is the identification of a gestational sac, representing primarily the chorionic cavity. The gestational sac can be visualized with transvaginal sonography by as early as 4.5 menstrual weeks. Because the chorionic cavity measures only 1 mm at 4 weeks' gestation, the reported visualization of a gestational sac before 4.5 weeks' gestation reflects an inaccurate assessment of gestational age. The implantation of the blastocyst into the uterine wall results in its eccentric position relative to the endometrial stripe.

The gestational sac increases in mean gestational sac diameter (MSD) by about 1 mm/day (range, 0.71–1.75 mm/day).[5]

An excellent correlation exists between hCG level, menstrual age, and gestational sac size[6,7] as expressed for the First-International Reference Preparation (Table 2-1; Fig. 2-1). Nyberg and colleagues found that hCG determinations, utilizing the Second International Standard, strongly correlate with gestational sac size until a gestational age of 8 weeks, at which time the MSD is about 2.5 cm and an embryo should be easily detected.[8] Because hCG levels rise exponentially with time, a range of hCG levels is observed for any given gestational sac size (Fig. 2-2).

When attempting to correlate hCG level with MSD, it is important to know the laboratory's methodology. The Second International Standard numerically is about half the International Reference Preparation. Table 2-2 outlines the relation of gestational age, hCG level, and transvaginal ultrasound findings.

An average linear measurement of a gestational sac is obtained from three dimensions (length, width, and depth), measured from inner edge to inner edge (Fig. 2-3). The shape of a gestational sac may vary from round to ovoid or tear-drop depending on bladder volume (Fig. 2-4), uterine contractility (Fig. 2-5), or the presence of myomas immediately adjacent to the sac. The empty-bladder transvaginal technique obviates the need for and subsequent distortion of a distended maternal bladder.

The overall accuracy of the gestational sac in estimating embryonic age is about 1 week.[9] Hellman and associates compared MSD with gestational age between 5 and 12 weeks' gestation[10] (Table 2-3). After 6 to 7 weeks' gestation, CRL rather than MSD should be used to date a pregnancy.

A comparison of the MSD to the CRL may provide helpful prognostic information. The small gestational sac syndrome occurs in about 2% of pregnancies scanned between 5.3 and 9.4 weeks' gestation (Figs. 2-6 and 2-7). Dickey and associates found pregnancy loss rates of 80%, 26.5%, and 10.6% when the gestational sac to CRL difference was less than 5 mm, between 5 and 7.9 mm, and more than 8 mm, respectively.[11] This syndrome occurs more often in karyotypically normal fetuses. Meegdes and colleagues reported that chorionic villous vascularization is deficient in cases of embryonic death and blighted ova.[12] Hence, suboptimal oxygen exchange appears to be the cause of embryonic demise, possibly as late as 8 weeks' gestation. These results are consistent with Stern and Coulam's finding that fetal pole size was small in 86% of pregnancies lost after fetal cardiac activity was documented.[13]

TABLE 2-1. Expected hCG Levels for Increasing Mean Gestational Sac Diameter Measurements

Mean Gestational Sac Diameter (mm)	Expected Mean (U/L)	Serum hCG Levels* 95% Prediction Interval (IU/L)
3	710	1050–2800
4	2320	1440–3760
5	3100	1940–4980
6	4090	2580–6530
7	5340	3400–8450
8	6880	4420–10,810
9	8770	5680–13,660
10	11040	7220–17,050
11	13730	9050–21,040
12	16870	11,230–25,640
13	20480	13,750–30,880
14	24560	16,650–36,750
15	29110	19,910–43,220
16	34100	23,530–50,210
17	39460	27,470–57,640
18	45120	31,700–65,380
19	50970	36,130–73,280
20	56900	40,700–81,150
21	62760	45,300–88,790
22	68390	49,810–95,990
23	73640	54,120–102,540
24	78350	58,100–108,230
25	82370	61,640–112,870
26	85560	64,600–116,310
27	87820	66,900–118,420
28	89050	68,460–119,130
29	89230	69,220–118,420
30	88340	69,150–116,310

* Expected mean serum hCG values were calculated from the regression equation in Figure 2-1 and have been rounded off to the nearest 10 IU/L. The 95% prediction intervals (rounded to the nearest 10 IU/L) were calculated from the best-fitting quadratic regression lines obtained from the lower and upper confidence limits, respectively, for the individual predicted values for each original observation in the study.

hCG values expressed for First International Reference Preparation.

(Daya S, Wood S, Ward S, et al: Transvaginal ultrasound scanning in early pregnancy and correlation with human chorionic gonadotropin levels. JCU 1991; 19:139–142.)

CROWN-TO-RUMP LENGTH

The sonographic measurement of CRL was introduced by Robinson in 1973.[14] The advent of transvaginal sonography has permitted the visualiza-

(text continues on p. 31)

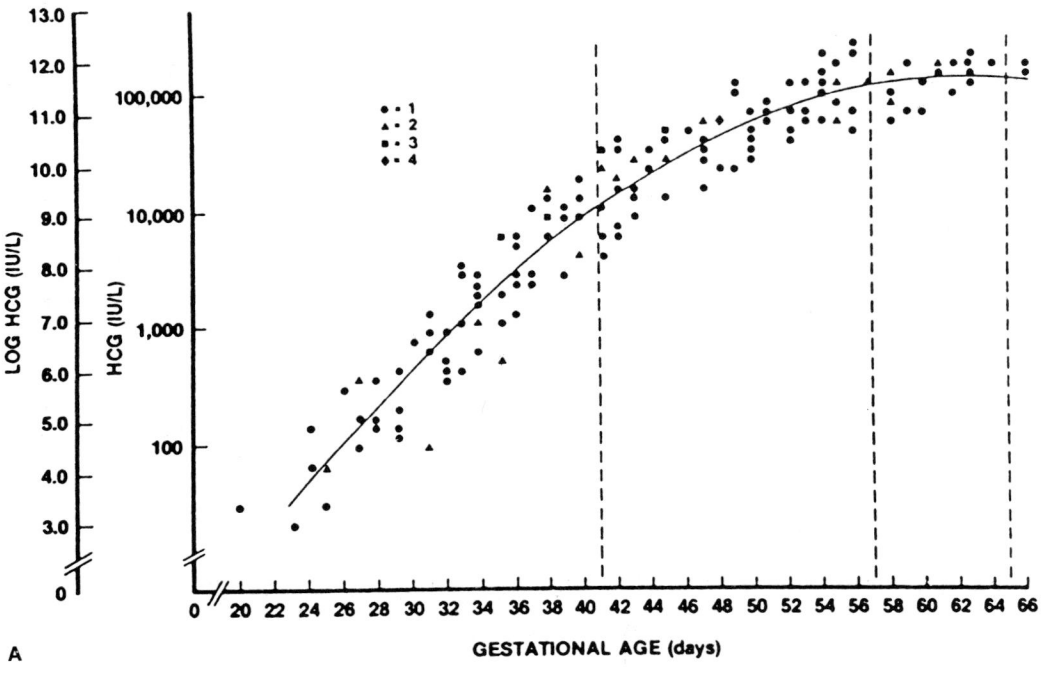

A

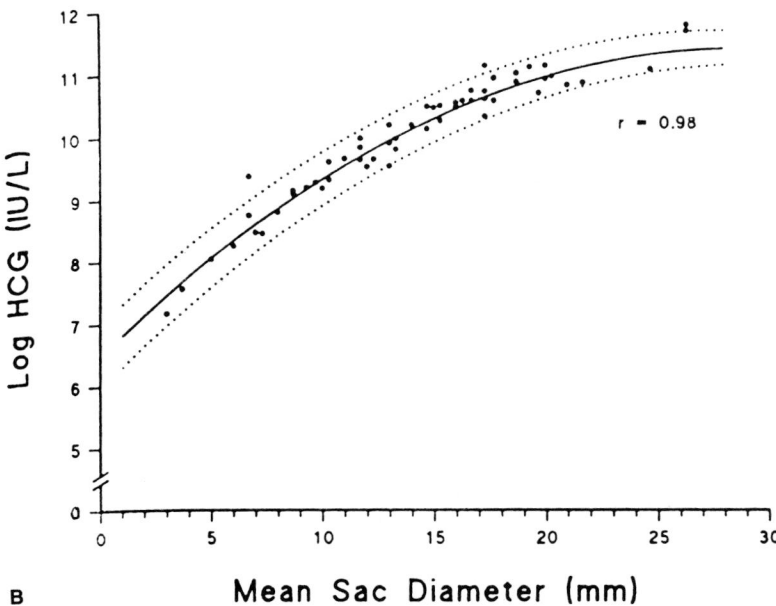

B

FIGURE 2-1. **(A)** hCG increase in normal early pregnancy. Symbols correspond to the indicated number of data points. hCG values are for First International Reference Preparation. (Daya S: Human chorionic gonadotropin increase in normal early pregnancy. Am J Obstet Gynecol 1987; 156:286.) **(B)** hCG increase in normal early pregnancy with respect to mean gestational sac size. (Daya, S, Woods S, Ward S, et al: Transvaginal ultrasound scanning in early pregnancy and correlation with human chorionic gonadotropin levels. JCU 1991; 19:139.)

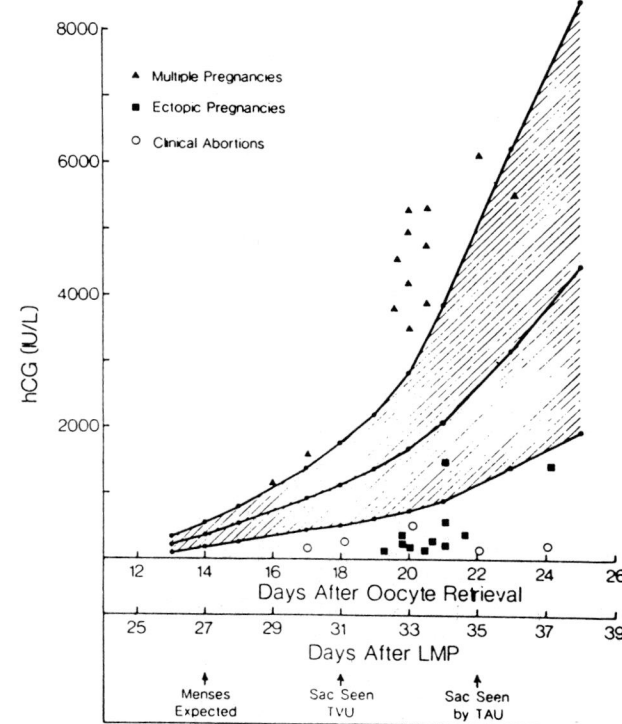

FIGURE 2-2. Range and median hCG with gestational age. TVU, transvaginal ultrasound; TAU, transabdominal ultrasound. hcG values are for First International Reference Preparation. (Hay DL, et al: Aust N Z J Obstet Gynecol 1989; 39:165.)

TABLE 2-2.   Relation of Gestational Age, hCG Level, and Transvaginal Ultrasound Findings

| Ultrasound Findings | Days From Last Menstrual Period | β-hCG mIU/mL | |
		First International Reference Preparation	Second International Standard
Sac	34.8 ± 2.2	1398 ± 155	914 ± 106
Fetal pole	40.3 ± 3.4*	5113 ± 298*	3783 ± 683
Fetal heart motion	46.9 ± 6.0*	17208 ± 3772*	13178 ± 2898*

* $P < .05$ when compared with sac.

(Fossum GT, Davajan V, Kletzky OA: Early detection of pregnancy with transvaginal ultrasound. Fertil Steril 1988; 49:789.)

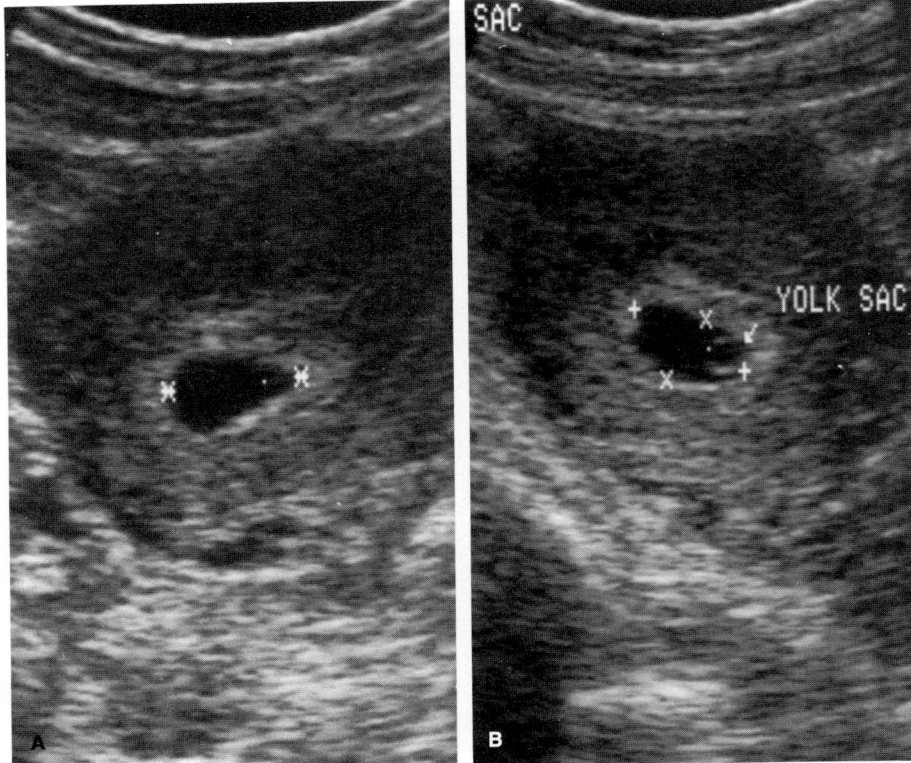

FIGURE 2-3. Gestational sac at 5.4 weeks. **(A)** Transverse. **(B)** Sagittal. The yolk sac is visualized within the gestational sac.

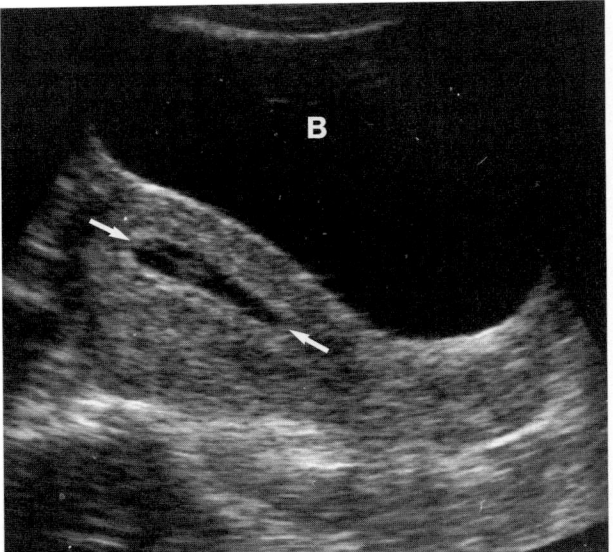

FIGURE 2-4. 8-week-old gestational sac (*arrows*) compressed by a full bladder (B).

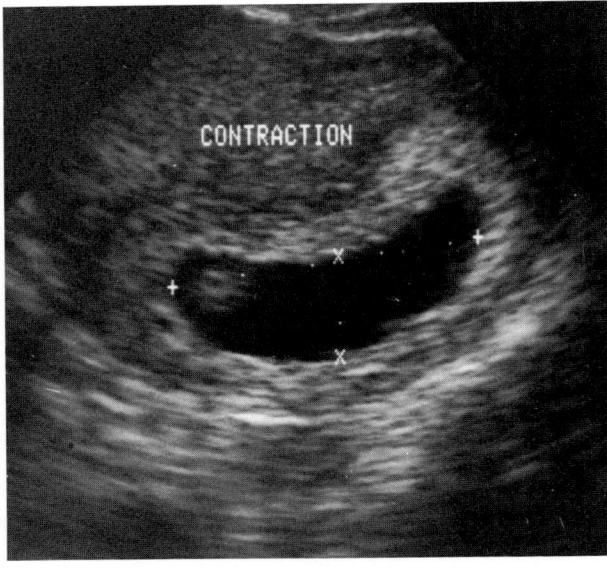

FIGURE 2-5. Transvaginal scan of an ovoid, 9-week-old gestational sac. The effect of the uterine contraction on the contour of the gestational sac can be seen.

TABLE 2-3.   Gestational Sac Measurement Table

Mean Predicted Gestational Sac (cm)	Gestational Age (wk)	Mean Predicted Gestational Sac (cm)	Gestational Age (wk)
1.0	5.0	3.6	8.8
1.1	5.2	3.7	8.9
1.2	5.3	3.8	9.0
1.3	5.5	3.9	9.2
1.4	5.6	4.0	9.3
1.5	5.8	4.1	9.5
1.6	5.9	4.2	9.6
1.7	6.0	4.3	9.7
1.8	6.2	4.4	9.9
1.9	6.3	4.5	10.0
2.0	6.5	4.6	10.2
2.1	6.6	4.7	10.3
2.2	6.8	4.8	10.5
2.3	6.9	4.9	10.6
2.4	7.0	5.0	10.7
2.5	7.2	5.1	10.9
2.6	7.3	5.2	11.0
2.7	7.5	5.3	11.2
2.8	7.6	5.4	11.3
2.9	7.8	5.5	11.5
3.0	7.9	5.6	11.6
3.1	8.0	5.7	11.7
3.2	8.2	5.8	11.9
3.3	8.3	5.9	12.0
3.4	8.5	6.0	12.2
3.5	8.6		

$$\text{Gestational Age (weeks)} = \frac{\text{Gestational Sac (cm)} + 2.543}{0.702}$$

(Hellman LM, Kobayashi M, Fillisti L, et al: Growth and development of the human fetus prior to the twentieth week of gestation. Am J Obstet Gynecol 1969; 103:784.)

tion and measurement of embryonic poles of 2 mm. The embryonic heart begins to pulsate at the beginning of the 6th week of gestation (CRL between 1.5 and 3 mm).[15] Hence, a potentially viable embryo may be seen before cardiac activity has been initiated[16] (Fig. 2-8).

When first seen, the greatest length rather than a true CRL must be measured. Once a gestational age of 8 weeks is obtained, a true CRL can be measured (Fig. 2-9). Because human motor activity begins between 7 and 8 weeks from the last menstrual period, embryonic motion may affect the CRL measurement obtained. The embryo normally rests with a kyphotic curvature of the spine. During periods of motor activity, the fetus straightens, permitting an accurate CRL measurement (Fig. 2-10).

Growth of the CRL is exponential up to 12 weeks of gestational age and linear thereafter. Measurement of the embryonic CRL generally is considered the most accurate method of assessing gestational age[17] (Table 2-4). Hadlock and colleagues found the variability in predicting menstrual age by CRL to be relatively constant at about 8% (2 standard deviations) when expressed as a percentage of the predicted value.[4] For example, the 95% confidence interval would increase from 0.7 weeks at 9 weeks' gestation to 1.1 weeks at 14 weeks' gestation.

The sequential appearance of embryonic structures with transvaginal ultrasonography may be used to date first-trimester pregnancies. The gestational sac is the only visible structure at 4.5 weeks

(text continues on p. 34)

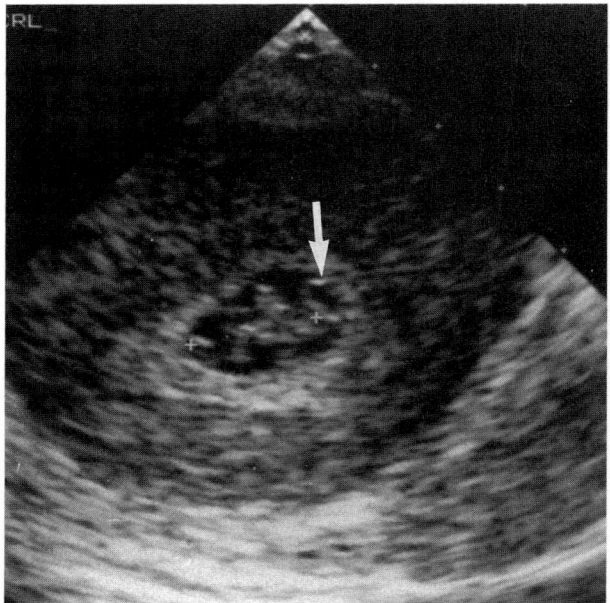

FIGURE 2-6.   Small gestational sac syndrome. There is less than a 5-mm difference between the mean sac diameter and the crown-to-rump length. The *arrow* indicates the yolk sac.

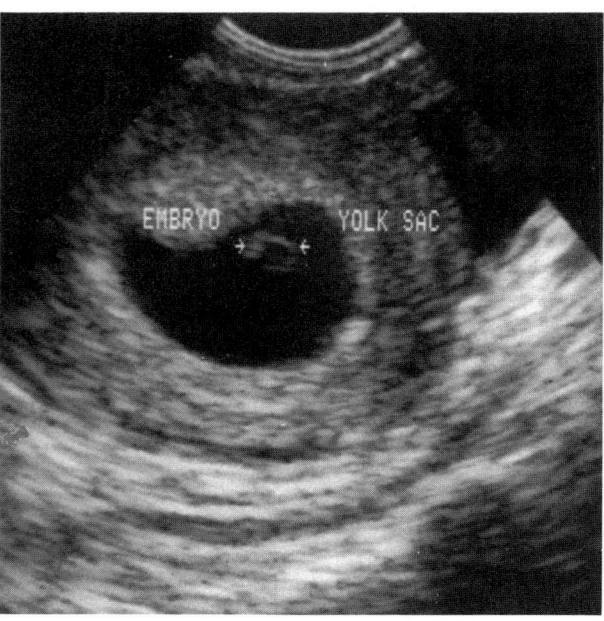

FIGURE 2-8.   A 3-mm embryo without cardiac activity is immediately adjacent to the yolk sac. Cardiac activity was documented 1 week later.

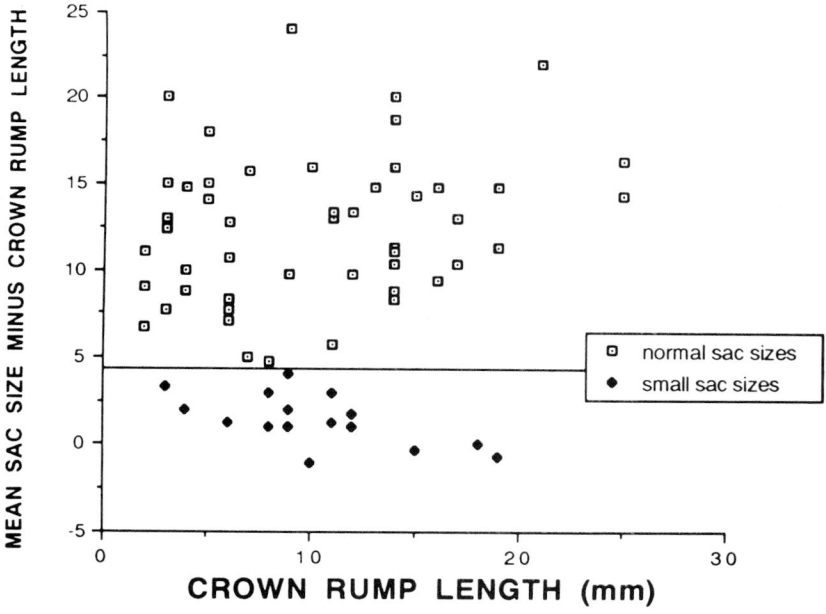

FIGURE 2-7.   Distribution of mean sac diameter minus crown-to-rump length versus crown-to-rump length in patients with small gestational sacs and in those with normal-sized sacs. (Bromley B, et al: Small sac size in the first trimester: A predictor of poor fetal outcome. Radiology 1991; 178:375–377.)

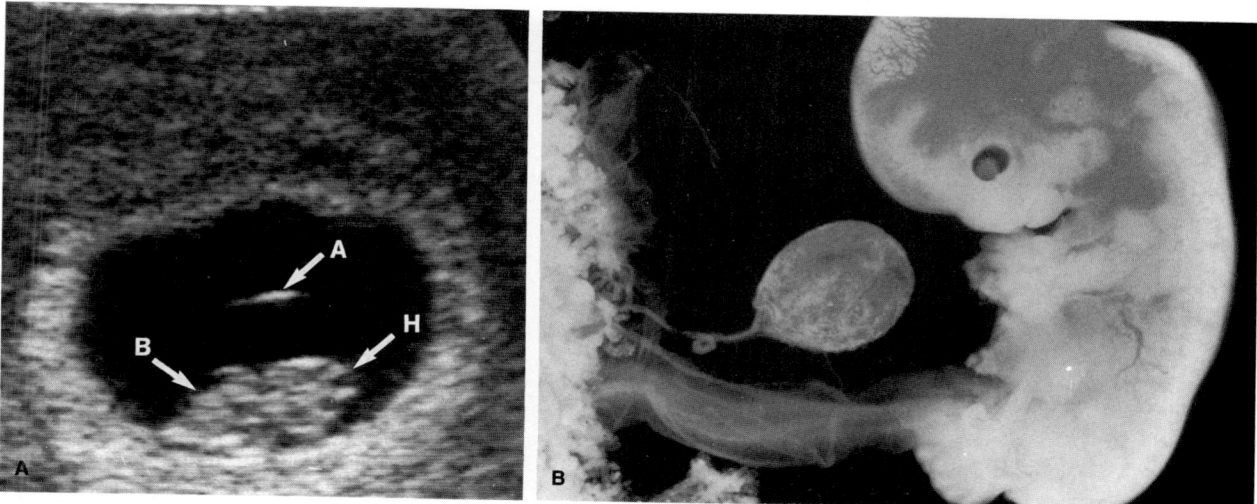

FIGURE 2-9.   Eight menstrual weeks. **(A)** Transabdominal scan. h, head; b, body; a, amnion. **(B)** Photograph taken at the same gestational age.

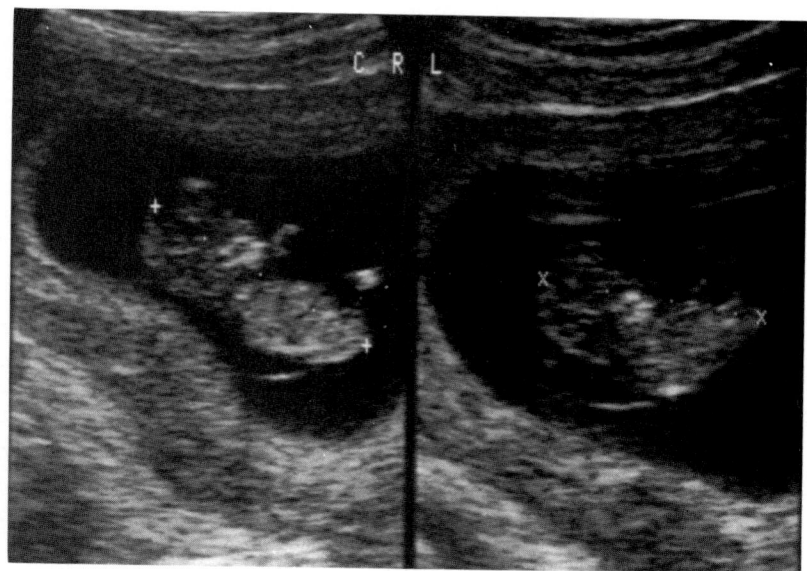

FIGURE 2-10. Accurate crown-to-rump length of 4 cm with fetal straightening **(left)** compared with inaccurate crown-to-rump length of 3.4 cm with fetus in kyphotic position **(right).**

TABLE 2-4.   Predicted Menstrual Age (Weeks) From Crown-to-Rump Length Measurements (cm)

CRL (cm)	MA (wk)	CRL (cm)	MA (wk)	CRL (cm)	MA (wk)	CRL (cm)	MA (wk)	CRL (cm)	MA (wk)	CRL (cm)	MA (wk)
0.2	5.7	2.2	8.9	4.2	11.1	6.2	12.6	8.2	14.2	10.2	16.1
0.3	5.9	2.3	9.0	4.3	11.2	6.3	12.7	8.3	14.2	10.3	16.2
0.4	6.1	2.4	9.1	4.4	11.2	6.4	12.8	8.4	14.3	10.4	16.3
0.5	6.2	2.5	9.2	4.5	11.3	6.5	12.8	8.5	14.4	10.5	16.4
0.6	6.4	2.6	9.4	4.6	11.4	6.6	12.9	8.6	14.5	10.6	16.5
0.7	6.6	2.7	9.5	4.7	11.5	6.7	13.0	8.7	14.6	10.7	16.6
0.8	6.7	2.8	9.6	4.8	11.6	6.8	13.1	8.8	14.7	10.8	16.7
0.9	6.9	2.9	9.7	4.9	11.7	6.9	13.1	8.9	14.8	10.9	16.8
1.0	7.1	3.0	9.9	5.0	11.7	7.0	13.2	9.0	14.9	11.0	16.9
1.1	7.2	3.1	10.0	5.1	11.8	7.1	13.3	9.1	15.0	11.1	17.0
1.2	7.4	3.2	10.1	5.2	11.9	7.2	13.4	9.2	15.1	11.2	17.1
1.3	7.5	3.3	10.2	5.3	12.0	7.3	13.4	9.3	15.2	11.3	17.2
1.4	7.7	3.4	10.3	5.4	12.0	7.4	13.5	9.4	15.3	11.4	17.3
1.5	7.9	3.5	10.4	5.5	12.1	7.5	13.6	9.5	15.3	11.5	17.4
1.6	8.0	3.6	10.5	5.6	12.2	7.6	13.7	9.6	15.4	11.6	17.5
1.7	8.1	3.7	10.6	5.7	12.3	7.7	13.8	9.7	15.5	11.7	17.6
1.8	8.3	3.8	10.7	5.8	12.3	7.8	13.8	9.8	15.6	11.8	17.7
1.9	8.4	3.9	10.8	5.9	12.4	7.9	13.9	9.9	15.7	11.9	17.8
2.0	8.6	4.0	10.9	6.0	12.5	8.0	14.0	10.0	15.9	12.0	17.9
2.1	8.7	4.1	11.0	6.1	12.6	8.1	14.1	10.1	16.0	12.1	18.0

MA, menstrual age. The 95% confidence interval is 8% of the predicted age.

(Hadlock FP, Shah YP, Kanon DJ, et al: Fetal crown-rump length: Re-evaluation of relation to menstrual age (15–18 weeks) with high-resolution real-time ultrasound. Radiology 1992; 182:501–505.)

of menstrual age. At 5 weeks' gestation, the yolk sac is visible. An embryonic pole and cardiac activity are first seen by 6 weeks of menstrual age.[18] In the first trimester, umbilical cord length is about equivalent to CRL (Fig. 2-11).

SECOND AND THIRD TRIMESTERS

Biparietal Diameter

The biparietal diameter (BPD) remains the standard against which other parameters for gestational age assessment are compared[19] (Fig. 2-12; Table 2-5). A reliable BPD can usually be obtained by 13 weeks' gestation. The anatomic landmarks used to ensure the accuracy and reproducibility of this measurement include: (1) a midline falx, (2) the thalami symmetrically positioned on either side of the falx, and (3) visualization of the septum pellucidum at one third the frontooccipital distance from the sinciput. A leading edge–to–lead-ing edge measurement is obtained. The measurement error inherent in caliper placement is 1 to 2 mm.[20] The imaging of a midline echo alone is *not* sufficient to obtain an accurate BPD. Johnson and associates produced variations of the BPD of up to 19 mm by scanning at various angles through the head, even with the midline still imaged.[21]

In a sonographer-oriented routine ultrasound program, Campbell and colleagues found that a BPD obtained before 18 weeks' gestation was better than an optimal menstrual history or a CRL measurement for estimating the date of delivery.[22] Between 18 and 28 weeks' gestation, the BPD was equal to an optimal menstrual history in determining the due date. It was only after 28 weeks' gestation that an optimal patient history became a better predictor of the patient's due date. Because an 18-week ultrasound examination can provide not only an accurate assessment of gestational age but also a complete anatomic survey, routine dating studies primarily should be performed during the second trimester.

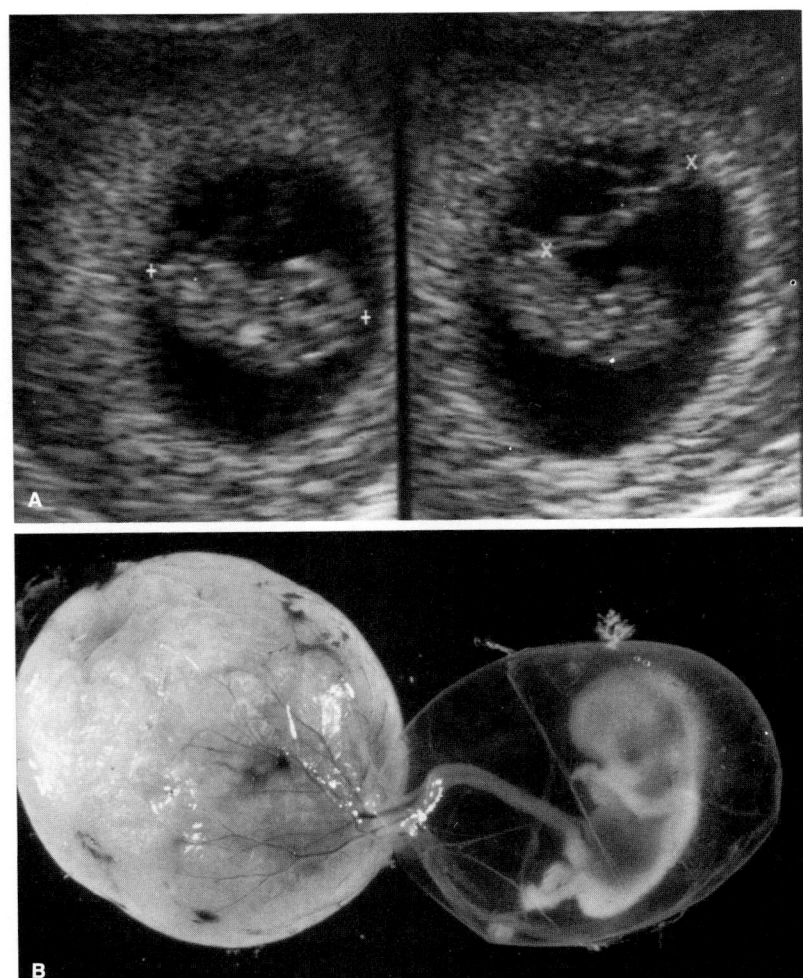

FIGURE 2-11. 9.6 menstrual weeks. **(A)** The crown-to-rump length and cord length are of equivalent size. **(B)** Photograph taken at the same gestational age.

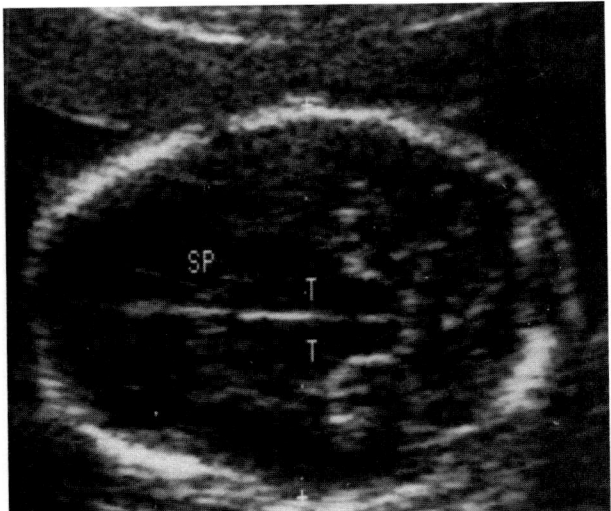

FIGURE 2-12. Biparietal diameter (+ to +) at 18 menstrual weeks. T, thalami; SP, septum pellucidum.

Cephalic Index

An abnormal fetal position or a significant reduction in amniotic fluid can affect the shape of the calvarium and thereby reduce the reliability of the BPD. The *cephalic index* is defined as the outer-to-outer measurement at the level of the BPD divided by the frontooccipital diameter times 100 (Fig. 2-13); an index of less than 74% indicates dolichocephaly (Fig. 2-14), and more than 83% indicates brachycephaly. If the cephalic index is more than 1 standard deviation from the mean, the head circumference should be used rather than the BPD for gestational age assessment.[23]

Although Hadlock and colleagues reported that the cephalic index was constant,[23] Gray and associates found it to vary with gestational age: the highest and lowest mean cephalic indices were observed at 14 and 28 weeks' gestation, respectively.[24]

TABLE 2-5.   Predicted Menstrual Ages*
for Biparietal Diameter Values From 2 to 10 cm

BPD (cm)	Menstrual Age (wk)	BPD (cm)	Menstrual Age (wk)
2.0	12.2	6.1	25.0
2.1	12.5	6.2	25.3
2.2	12.8	6.3	25.7
2.3	13.1	6.4	26.1
2.4	13.3	6.5	26.4
2.5	13.6	6.6	26.8
2.6	13.9	6.7	27.2
2.7	14.2	6.8	27.6
2.8	14.5	6.9	28.0
2.9	14.7	7.0	28.3
3.0	15.0	7.1	28.7
3.1	15.3	7.2	29.1
3.2	15.6	7.3	29.5
3.3	15.9	7.4	29.9
3.4	16.2	7.5	30.4
3.5	16.5	7.6	30.8
3.6	16.8	7.7	31.2
3.7	17.1	7.8	31.6
3.8	17.4	7.9	32.0
3.9	17.7	8.0	32.5
4.0	18.0	8.1	32.9
4.1	18.3	8.2	33.3
4.2	18.6	8.3	33.8
4.3	18.9	8.4	34.2
4.4	19.2	8.5	34.7
4.5	19.5	8.6	35.1
4.6	19.9	8.7	35.6
4.7	20.2	8.8	36.1
4.8	20.5	8.9	36.5
4.9	20.8	9.0	37.0
5.0	21.2	9.1	37.5
5.1	21.5	9.2	38.0
5.2	21.8	9.3	38.5
5.3	22.2	9.4	38.9
5.4	22.5	9.5	39.4
5.5	22.8	9.6	39.9
5.6	23.2	9.7	40.5
5.7	23.5	9.8	41.0
5.8	23.9	9.9	41.5
5.9	24.2	10.0	42.0
6.0	24.6		

* Menstrual age = $6.8954 + 2.6345(BPD) + 0.008771(BPD)^3$; ($r^2 = 98.7\%$).
(Hadlock FP, Deter LR, Harrist RD, Park SK: Fetal biparietal diameter: A critical reevaluation of the relation to menstrual age by means of real-time ultrasound. J Ultrasound Med 1982; 1:97–104.)

Kasby and Poll reported an abnormal cephalic index in one third of 100 consecutive term breech infants.[25] In the presence of premature rupture of the membranes with oligohydramnios, the BPD was found to underestimate gestational age.[26] Al-

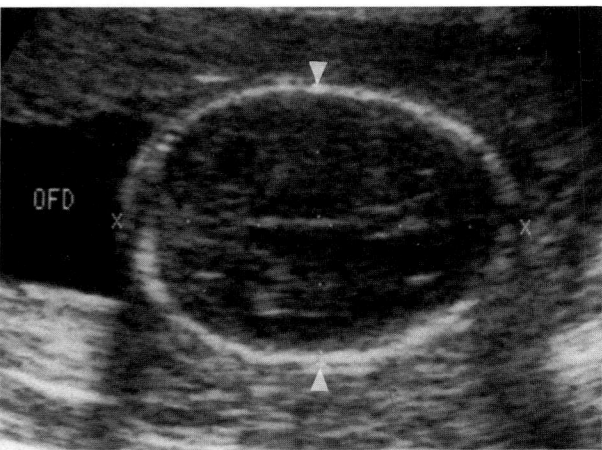

FIGURE 2-13.   The cephalic index: outer-to-outer distance at the level of the biparietal diameter (*arrowheads*), divided by occipital–frontal diameter (OFD; x to x) times 100.

though it is readily acknowledged that dolichocephaly can result in an incorrect estimate of gestational age, molding of the fetal head to the contour of the uterine walls may also cause a reduction in both the BPD and frontooccipital diameter, resulting in a normal cephalic index as well as an erroneous estimation of gestational age. Molding may account for a diminution in cephalic diameters of 0.5 cm or greater.[27]

As gestational age advances, the reliability of the BPD, as well as other fetal measurements, for the assessment of gestational age decreases (Table 2-6). The increase in variation is due to several factors: there are inherent differences between fetal sizes at term, and the late flattening of the BPD curve in the third trimester means that even a

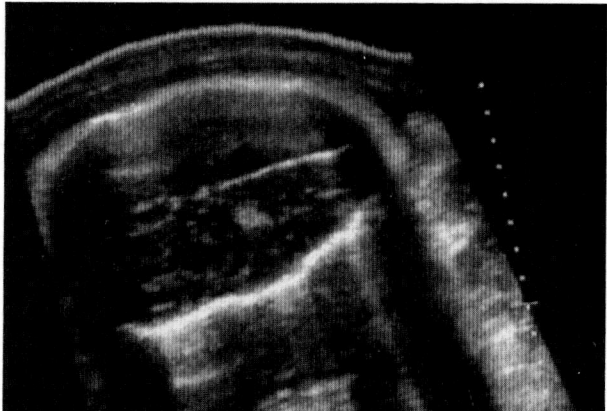

FIGURE 2-14.   Dolichocephaly: cephalic index is 60%.

TABLE 2-6. Variability in Predicting Gestational Age by Different Fetal
Parameters: Estimates of Variability (wk)*

Gestational Age (wk)	Biparietal Diameter[19]	Head Circumference[28]	Abdominal Circumference[30]	Femur Length[36]	Radius[34]	Transverse Cerebellar Diameter[47]
12–18	±0.8	±1.3	±1.9	±1.5	±1.8	±1.0
18–24	±1.4	±1.6	±2.0	±2.1	±2.2	±1.8
24–30	±1.3	±2.3	±2.2	±2.6	±2.8	±2.0
30–36	±2.0	±2.7	±3.0	±3.2	±3.5	±2.4
36–42	±3.6	±3.4	±2.5	±3.8	±4.0	±3.8

* 95% confidence interval

TABLE 2-7. Predicted Menstrual Age* for Head Circumference

Head Circumference (cm)	Menstrual Age (wk)	Head Circumference (cm)	Menstrual Age (wk)
8.0	13.4	22.5	24.4
8.5	13.7	23.0	24.9
9.0	14.0	23.5	25.4
9.5	14.3	24.0	25.9
10.0	14.6	24.5	26.4
10.5	15.0	25.0	26.9
11.0	15.3	25.5	27.5
11.5	15.6	26.0	28.0
12.0	15.9	26.5	28.1
12.5	16.3	27.0	29.2
13.0	16.6	27.5	29.8
13.5	17.0	28.0	30.3
14.0	17.3	28.5	31.0
14.5	17.7	29.0	31.6
15.0	18.1	29.5	32.2
15.5	18.4	30.0	32.8
16.0	18.8	30.5	33.5
16.5	19.2	31.0	34.2
17.0	19.6	31.5	34.9
17.5	20.0	32.0	35.5
18.0	20.4	32.5	36.3
18.5	20.8	33.0	37.0
19.0	21.2	33.5	37.7
19.5	21.6	34.0	38.5
20.0	22.1	34.5	39.2
20.5	22.5	35.0	40.0
21.0	23.0	35.5	40.8
21.5	23.4	36.0	41.6
22.0	23.9		

* Menstrual age = $8.8 + 0.55$ (head circumference) + 2.8×10^{-4} (head circumference)^3; $r^2 = 97.9\%$; 1 SD = 1.18 weeks.

(Hadlock FP, Deter LR, Harrist RB, Park SK: Fetal head circumference: Relation to menstrual age. AJR 1982; 138:649–653.)

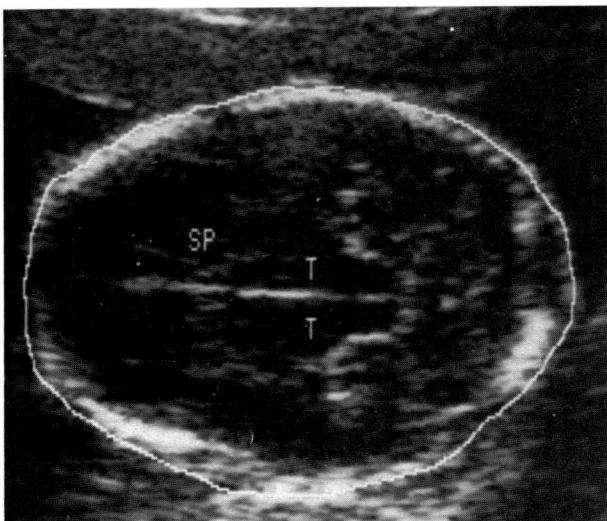

FIGURE 2-15. Head circumference at 18 menstrual weeks. T, thalami; sp, septum pellucidum.

small increase in the BPD is associated with a large increase in gestational age.

Head Circumference

Because of the variations in head shape, measurement of the head circumference has become an integral part of assessing gestational age in the second and third trimesters (Table 2-7; Fig. 2-15). The variability inherent in estimating fetal age from the head circumference is generally greater than that seen with the BPD (see Table 2-6).[28]

The head circumference can also be used to monitor fetal growth between two examinations and to compare the effects of growth disturbances (eg, macrosomia and growth retardation) on different fetal body parts (head circumference/abdominal circumference ratio). In addition, the head circumference is an integral part of several fetal weight estimate formulas.

Abdominal Circumference

The sonographic measurement of the abdominal circumference at the level of the stomach and umbilical vein was initially described by Campbell and Wilkin to estimate fetal weight.[29] Hadlock and colleagues[30] (Table 2-8) and others[31,32] used the abdominal circumference to estimate gestational age. Greater variability is seen when predicting gestational age using the abdominal circumference than using the BPD, except during the interval of 36 to 42 weeks' gestation, when the abdominal circum-

ference is slightly more accurate than the BPD (see Table 2-6).

As with head circumference, specific anatomic landmarks must be visible to obtain an accurate abdominal circumference measurement. These include:

- A circular abdominal circumference
- A 90-degree transaxial view of the spine
- Ability to visualize the stomach within the left mid-abdomen
- An umbilical portion of the left portal vein that is equidistant from the two lateral sides of the body and not contiguous with the anterior abdominal wall (Fig. 2-16)

Because the umbilical vein cannot be visualized with the spine at 12 o'clock (Fig. 2-17), an abdominal circumference measurement should not be taken with the fetus in this position. If the abdominal circumference is elliptical (Fig. 2-18) rather than circular, the error in either weight estimation or gestational age assessment can be substantial.[33]

Fetal Extremities

Any of the fetal long bones may be used to assess gestational age[34–36] (Table 2-9). Because the femur is the longest and most easily imaged long bone, it is most frequently measured to assess gestational age.

Potential sources for error in the measurement of the femur length include the type of transducer used (sector, linear, or curvilinear) and the angle of inclination with which the ultrasound beam strikes the femur. The femur length charts were derived from femur measurements perpendicular to the transducer beam.[35–37] Hence, to control for the effect of angling, the femur should be measured in this manner.[38] Unfortunately, lateral measurements are inherently less accurate due to beam broadening and dynamic range considerations.[39] A femur measured in the axial plane (Fig. 2-19) is significantly shorter than one measured in the lateral plane (Fig. 2-20), resulting in up to a 2.6-week difference in gestational age prediction.[40,41]

The normal diaphysis of the femur has a curved medial border and a straight lateral border[42] (see Fig. 2-20). Only the osseous part of the femoral shaft is measured. A number of studies found the femur length to be superior to the BPD in assessing gestational age.[1,43,44] As with other fetal parameters, the standard deviation of the gestational age estimate increases with age (see Table 2-6). The

TABLE 2-8.   Predicted Menstrual Age*
for Abdominal Circumference Values

Abdominal Circumference (cm)	Menstrual Age (wk)	Abdominal Circumference (cm)	Menstrual Age (wk)
10.0	15.6	23.5	27.7
10.5	16.1	24.0	28.2
11.0	16.5	24.5	28.7
11.5	16.9	25.0	29.2
12.0	17.3	25.5	29.7
12.5	17.8	26.0	30.1
13.0	18.2	26.5	30.6
13.5	18.6	27.0	31.1
14.0	19.1	27.5	31.6
14.5	19.5	28.0	32.1
15.0	20.0	28.5	32.6
15.5	20.4	29.0	33.1
16.0	20.8	29.5	33.6
16.5	21.3	30.0	34.1
17.0	21.7	30.5	34.6
17.5	22.2	31.0	35.1
18.0	22.6	31.5	35.6
18.5	23.1	32.0	36.1
19.0	23.6	32.5	36.6
19.5	24.0	33.0	37.1
20.0	24.5	33.5	37.6
20.5	24.9	34.0	38.1
21.0	25.4	34.5	38.7
21.5	25.9	35.0	39.2
22.0	26.3	35.5	39.7
22.5	26.8	36.0	40.2
23.0	27.3	36.5	40.8

* Menstrual age $= 7.6070 + 0.7645 \, (AC) + 0.00393 \, (AC)^2$; $r^2 = 97.8\%$; 1 $SD = 1.2$ weeks.

(Hadlock FP, Deter LR, Harrist RB, Park SK: Fetal abdominal circumference as a predictor of menstrual age. AJR 1982; 139:367–370.)

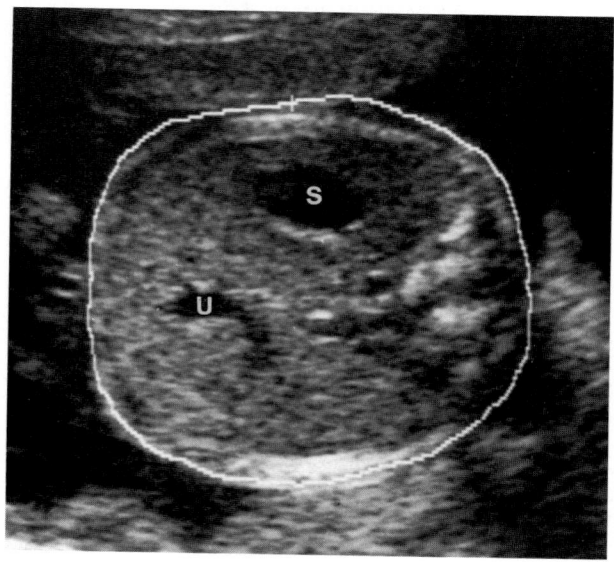

FIGURE 2-16.   Abdominal circumference at the level of the fetal stomach (s) and umbilical vein (u).

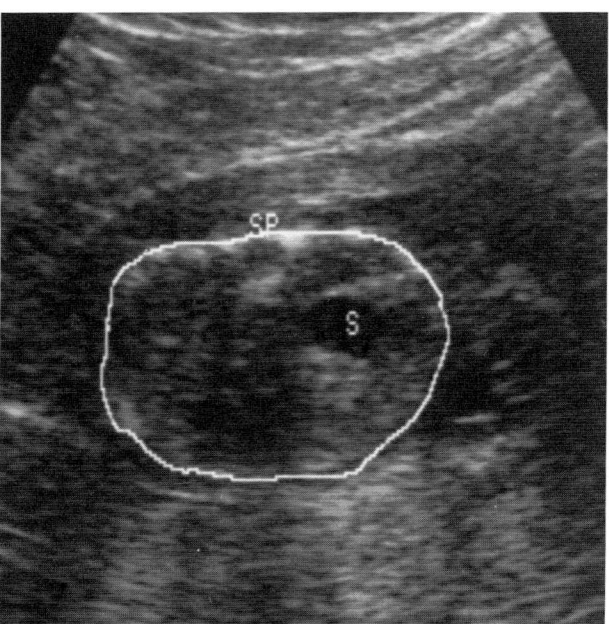

FIGURE 2-17. Although the stomach is visualized, this is an incorrect abdominal circumference because the spine is at 12 o'clock and the umbilical vein cannot be visualized. s, stomach; sp, spine.

coefficient of determination and variability associated with the measurement of the humerus, radius, ulna, tibia, and fibula is comparable to that associated with measurement of the femur (Fig. 2-21).

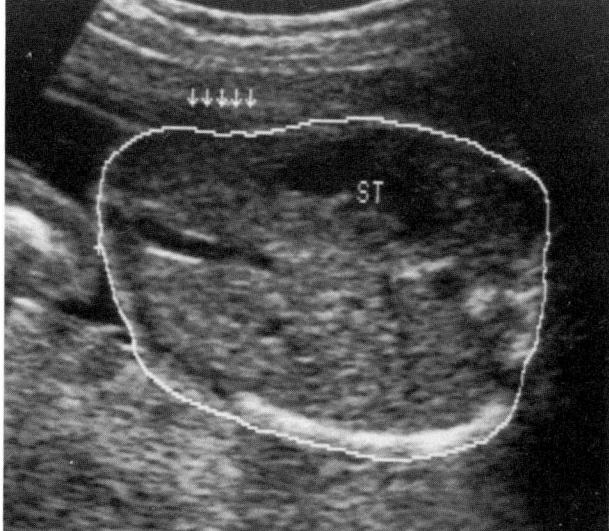

FIGURE 2-18. An elliptical abdominal circumference may be produced when too much pressure (↓) is placed on the fetus with the transducer. st, stomach.

Composite Assessment of Gestational Age

In a normal fetus, any of the standard fetal parameters (BPD, head and abdominal circumference, fetal length) may be larger than or smaller than the mean value anticipated for gestational age (ie, a 75th percentile head circumference and a 25th percentile abdominal circumference). A composite assessment of gestational age using all four parameters gives a lower systematic random error than any single parameter.[43,45,46] For example, the overall variability is increased by 33% (1.02–1.36 weeks) when the BPD is used alone in contrast to the composite assessment of gestational age.[43]

The sonographer must determine that a specific measurement is not affected by a pathologic process or growth disturbance before incorporating it into the composite assessment of gestational age. In macrosomal fetuses of diabetic and nondiabetic women, Hill and colleagues found that the head circumference and abdominal circumference significantly overestimated gestational age, while the femur length and transverse cerebellar diameter were both able to predict gestational age accurately.[47]

Another problem associated with using a composite assessment of gestational age relates to the use of a measurement that is disproportionately small or large. Body proportionality (cephalic index and the femur length/BPD, femur length/abdominal circumference, and head circumference/abdominal circumference ratios) should be assessed before incorporating a particular parameter into the composite. For example, the femur length would not be used to assess gestational age in a dwarf, and the BPD and head circumference would not be used to determine gestational age in a fetus affected by microcephaly.

Hill and colleagues did not find a point of diminishing returns by adding up to five fetal parameters in the determination of gestational age; that is, the error inherent in measuring several distinctly different structures did not significantly affect variability.[1] Furthermore, by obtaining all four measurements (BPD, head circumference, abdominal circumference, and fetal or other long bone length), the sonographer is more likely to detect not only abnormalities of fetal growth but also certain congenital anomalies.

The accuracy in estimating gestational age from fetal size decreases as the fetus matures. The use of multiple parameters to assess gestational age results in a 2 standard deviation variability of about 7%. Hence, the variability at 20 weeks' ges-

TABLE 2-9. Gestational Ages as Obtained From the Long Bones (in Weeks + Days)

Bone Length (mm)	Femur Percentile			Humerus Percentile			Ulna Percentile			Tibia Percentile		
	5th	50th	95th	5th	50th	95th	5th	50th	95th	5th	50th	95th
10	10 + 3	12 + 4	14 + 6	9 + 6	12 + 4	15 + 2	10 + 1	13 + 1	16 + 1	10 + 4	13 + 3	16 + 2
11	10 + 5	12 + 6	15 + 1	10 + 1	12 + 6	15 + 4	10 + 4	13 + 4	16 + 4	10 + 6	13 + 5	16 + 4
12	11 + 1	13 + 2	15 + 4	10 + 3	13 + 1	15 + 6	10 + 6	13 + 6	16 + 6	11 + 1	14 + 1	17
13	11 + 3	13 + 4	15 + 6	10 + 6	13 + 4	16 + 1	11 + 1	14 + 1	17 + 2	11 + 4	14 + 3	17 + 2
14	11 + 5	13 + 6	16 + 1	11 + 1	13 + 6	16 + 4	11 + 4	14 + 4	17 + 5	11 + 6	14 + 6	17 + 5
15	12	14 + 1	16 + 3	11 + 3	14 + 1	16 + 6	11 + 6	15	18	12 + 1	15 + 1	18
16	12 + 3	14 + 4	16 + 6	11 + 6	14 + 4	17 + 2	12 + 2	15 + 3	18 + 3	12 + 4	15 + 4	18 + 3
17	12 + 5	14 + 6	17 + 1	12 + 1	14 + 6	17 + 4	12 + 5	15 + 5	18 + 6	13	15 + 6	18 + 6
18	13	15 + 1	17 + 3	12 + 4	15 + 1	18	13 + 1	16 + 1	19 + 1	13 + 2	16 + 1	19 + 1
19	13 + 3	15 + 4	17 + 6	12 + 6	15 + 4	18 + 2	13 + 4	16 + 4	19 + 4	13 + 5	16 + 4	19 + 4
20	13 + 5	15 + 6	18 + 1	13 + 1	15 + 6	18 + 5	13 + 6	16 + 6	20	14 + 1	17	19 + 6
21	14 + 1	16 + 2	18 + 4	13 + 4	16 + 2	19 + 1	14 + 2	17 + 2	20 + 3	14 + 4	17 + 3	20 + 2
22	14 + 3	16 + 4	18 + 6	13 + 6	16 + 5	19 + 3	14 + 5	17 + 5	20 + 6	14 + 6	17 + 6	20 + 5
23	14 + 5	16 + 6	19 + 1	14 + 2	17 + 1	19 + 6	15 + 1	18 + 1	21 + 1	15 + 1	18 + 1	21 + 1
24	15 + 1	17 + 2	19 + 4	14 + 5	17 + 3	20 + 1	15 + 4	18 + 4	21 + 4	15 + 4	18 + 4	21 + 3
25	15 + 3	17 + 4	19 + 6	15 + 1	17 + 6	20 + 4	16	19	22 + 1	16	18 + 6	21 + 6
26	15 + 6	18	20 + 1	15 + 4	18 + 1	21	16 + 3	19 + 3	22 + 4	16 + 3	19 + 2	22 + 1
27	16 + 1	18 + 2	20 + 4	15 + 6	18 + 4	21 + 3	16 + 6	19 + 6	22 + 6	16 + 6	19 + 5	22 + 4
28	16 + 4	18 + 5	20 + 6	16 + 2	19	21 + 6	17 + 2	20 + 2	23 + 3	17 + 1	20 + 1	23
29	16 + 6	19	21 + 1	16 + 5	19 + 3	22 + 1	17 + 5	20 + 6	23 + 6	17 + 4	20 + 4	23 + 4
30	17 + 1	19 + 3	21 + 4	17 + 1	19 + 6	22 + 4	18 + 1	21 + 1	24 + 2	18 + 1	21	23 + 6
31	17 + 4	19 + 6	22	17 + 4	20 + 2	23	18 + 4	21 + 5	24 + 6	18 + 4	21 + 3	24 + 2
32	17 + 6	20 + 1	22 + 2	18	20 + 5	23 + 4	19 + 1	22 + 1	25 + 1	18 + 6	21 + 6	24 + 5
33	18 + 2	20 + 4	22 + 5	18 + 3	21 + 1	23 + 6	19 + 4	22 + 5	25 + 5	18 + 6	21 + 6	24 + 5
34	18 + 5	20 + 6	23 + 1	18 + 6	21 + 4	24 + 2	20 + 1	23 + 1	26 + 1	19 + 2	22 + 1	25 + 1
35	19	21 + 1	23 + 3	19 + 2	22	24 + 6	20 + 4	34 + 4	26 + 5	19 + 5	22 + 4	25 + 4
36	19 + 3	21 + 4	23 + 6	19 + 5	22 + 4	25 + 1	21 + 1	24 + 1	27 + 1	20 + 1	23 + 1	26
37	19 + 6	22	24 + 1	20 + 1	22 + 6	25 + 5	21 + 4	24 + 4	27 + 5	20 + 4	23 + 4	26 + 3
38	20 + 1	22 + 3	24 + 4	20 + 4	23 + 3	26 + 1	22 + 1	25 + 1	28 + 1	21	23 + 6	26 + 6
39	20 + 4	22 + 5	24 + 6	21 + 1	23 + 6	26 + 4	22 + 4	25 + 4	28 + 5	21 + 4	24 + 3	27 + 2
40	20 + 6	23 + 1	25 + 2	21 + 4	24 + 2	27 + 1	23 + 1	26 + 1	29 + 1	21 + 6	24 + 6	27 + 5
41	21 + 2	23 + 4	25 + 5	22	24 + 6	27 + 4	23 + 4	26 + 5	29 + 5	22 + 3	25 + 2	28 + 1
42	21 + 5	23 + 6	26 + 1	22 + 4	25 + 2	28	24 + 1	27 + 1	30 + 2	22 + 6	25 + 5	28 + 4
43	22 + 1	24 + 2	26 + 4	23	25 + 5	28 + 4	24 + 5	27 + 5	30 + 6	23 + 2	26 + 1	29 + 1
44	22 + 4	24 + 5	26 + 6	23 + 4	26 + 1	29	25 + 1	28 + 2	31 + 2	23 + 5	26 + 4	29 + 4
45	22 + 6	25	27 + 1	24	26 + 5	29 + 4	25 + 6	28 + 6	31 + 6	24 + 1	27 + 1	30
46	23 + 1	25 + 3	27 + 4	24 + 4	27 + 1	30	26 + 2	29 + 3	32 + 3	24 + 4	27 + 4	30 + 4
47	23 + 4	25 + 6	28	25	27 + 5	30 + 4	26 + 6	29 + 6	33	25 + 1	28	30 + 6
48	24	26 + 1	28 + 3	25 + 4	28 + 1	31	27 + 3	30 + 4	33 + 4	25 + 4	28 + 4	31 + 3
49	24 + 3	26 + 4	28 + 6	26	28 + 6	31 + 4	28	31 + 1	34 + 1	26 + 1	29	31 + 6
50	24 + 6	27	29 + 1	26 + 4	29 + 2	32	28 + 4	31 + 4	34 + 5	26 + 4	29 + 3	32 + 2
51	25 + 1	27 + 3	29 + 4	27 + 1	29 + 6	32 + 4	29 + 1	32 + 1	35 + 2	27	29 + 6	32 + 6
52	25 + 4	27 + 6	30	27 + 4	30 + 2	33 + 1	29 + 5	32 + 6	35 + 6	27 + 4	30 + 3	33 + 2
53	26	28 + 1	30 + 3	28 + 1	30 + 6	33 + 4	30 + 2	33 + 3	36 + 3	28	30 + 6	33 + 6
54	26 + 3	28 + 4	30 + 6	28 + 5	31 + 3	34 + 1	30 + 6	34	37	28 + 4	31 + 3	34 + 2
55	26 + 6	29 + 1	31 + 2	29 + 1	32	34 + 5	31 + 4	34 + 4	37 + 5	29	31 + 6	34 + 6
56	27 + 2	29 + 4	31 + 5	29 + 6	32 + 4	35 + 2	32 + 1	35 + 1	38 + 2	29 + 4	32 + 3	35 + 2
57	27 + 5	29 + 6	32 + 1	30 + 2	33 + 1	35 + 6	32 + 6	35 + 6	38 + 6	30	32 + 6	35 + 6
58	28 + 1	30 + 2	32 + 4	30 + 6	33 + 4	36 + 3	33 + 3	36 + 3	39 + 4	30 + 4	33 + 3	36 + 2
										31	33 + 6	36 + 6

(continued)

TABLE 2-9. *(Continued)*

Bone Length (mm)	Femur Percentile			Humerus Percentile			Ulna Percentile			Tibia Percentile		
	5th	50th	95th	5th	50th	95th	5th	50th	95th	5th	50th	95th
59	28 + 4	30 + 5	32 + 6	31 + 3	34 + 1	36 + 6	34	37 + 1	40 + 1	31 + 4	34 + 3	37 + 2
60	28 + 6	31 + 1	33 + 2	32	34 + 6	37 + 4	34 + 4	37 + 5	40 + 6	32	34 + 6	37 + 6
61	29 + 3	31 + 4	33 + 6	32 + 4	35 + 2	38 + 1	35 + 2	38 + 2	41 + 3	32 + 4	35 + 3	38 + 2
62	29 + 6	32	34 + 1	33 + 1	35 + 6	38 + 5	35 + 6	39	42	33	35 + 6	38 + 6
63	30 + 1	32 + 3	34 + 4	33 + 6	36 + 4	39 + 2	36 + 4	39 + 4	42 + 5	33 + 4	36 + 4	39 + 3
64	30 + 5	32 + 6	35 + 1	34 + 3	37 + 1	39 + 6	37 + 1	40 + 2	43 + 2	34 + 1	37	39 + 6
65	31 + 1	33 + 2	35 + 4	35	37 + 5	40 + 4				34 + 4	37 + 4	40 + 3
66	31 + 4	33 + 5	35 + 6	35 + 4	38 + 2	41 + 1				35 + 1	38	41
67	32	34 + 1	36 + 3	36 + 1	38 + 6	41 + 5				35 + 5	38 + 4	41 + 4
68	32 + 3	34 + 4	36 + 6	36 + 6	39 + 4	42 + 2				36 + 1	39 + 1	42
69	32 + 6	35	37 + 1	37 + 3	40 + 1	42 + 6				36 + 6	39 + 5	42 + 4
70	33 + 2	35 + 4	37 + 5									
71	33 + 5	35 + 6	38 + 1									
72	34 + 1	36 + 3	38 + 4									
73	34 + 4	36 + 6	39									
74	35 + 1	37 + 2	39 + 4									
75	35 + 4	37 + 5	39 + 6									
76	36	38 + 1	40 + 3									
77	36 + 3	38 + 4	40 + 6									
78	36 + 6	39 + 1	41 + 2									
79	37 + 2	39 + 4	41 + 5									
80	37 + 6	40	42 + 1									

(Jeanty P, Rodesch F, Delbeke D, Dumont JE: Estimation of gestational age from measurements of fetal long bones. J Ultrasound Med 1984; 3:75–79.)

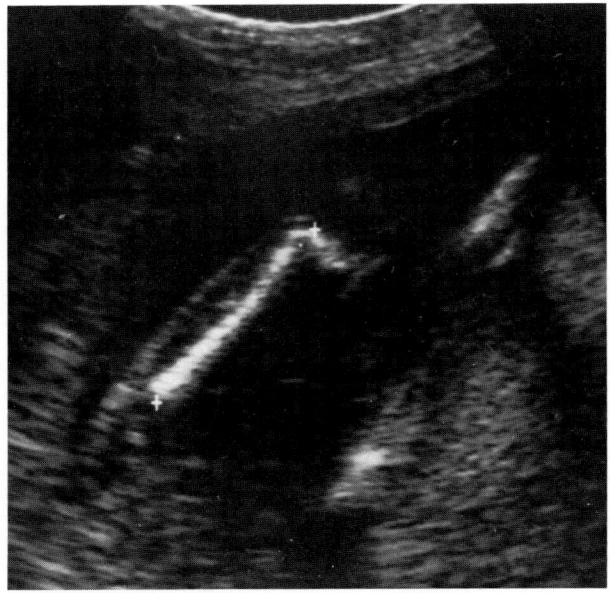

FIGURE 2-19. An inappropriately measured femur length.

tation is about 1.4 weeks and that at 30 weeks' gestation, about 2.1 weeks.[48]

Alternative Parameters to Assess Gestational Age

Because the fetal period is a time of active growth and maturation, normograms can be established for a wide range of fetal parameters against gestational age. A particular parameter's ability to be measured, however, does not indicate that it will be particularly efficacious for gestational age assessment. Although these secondary parameters may be helpful in selected cases, they are not recommended for routine use.

Embryonic trunk circumference,[49] orbital diameter,[50] clavicle length,[51] fractional spine length,[52] thigh circumference,[53] and foot length[54] are but a few of the fetal parameters that have been correlated with gestational age (Fig. 2-22). Clavicle length is obtained as the maximal length of the

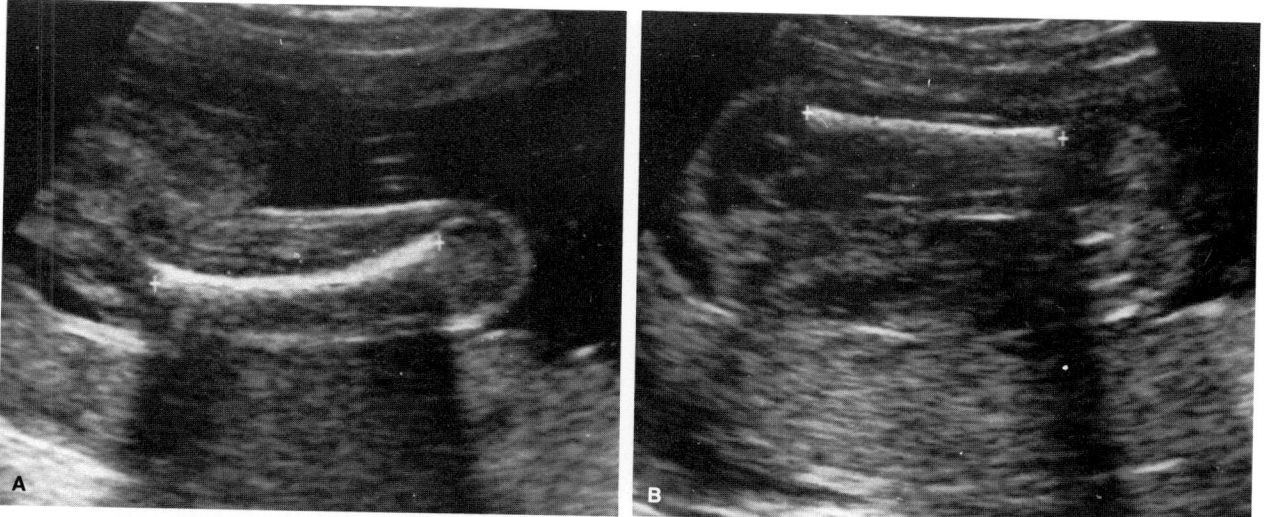

FIGURE 2-20. Femur length. **(A)** Curved medial border. **(B)** Straight lateral border. The markers outline the appropriate length of the femur.

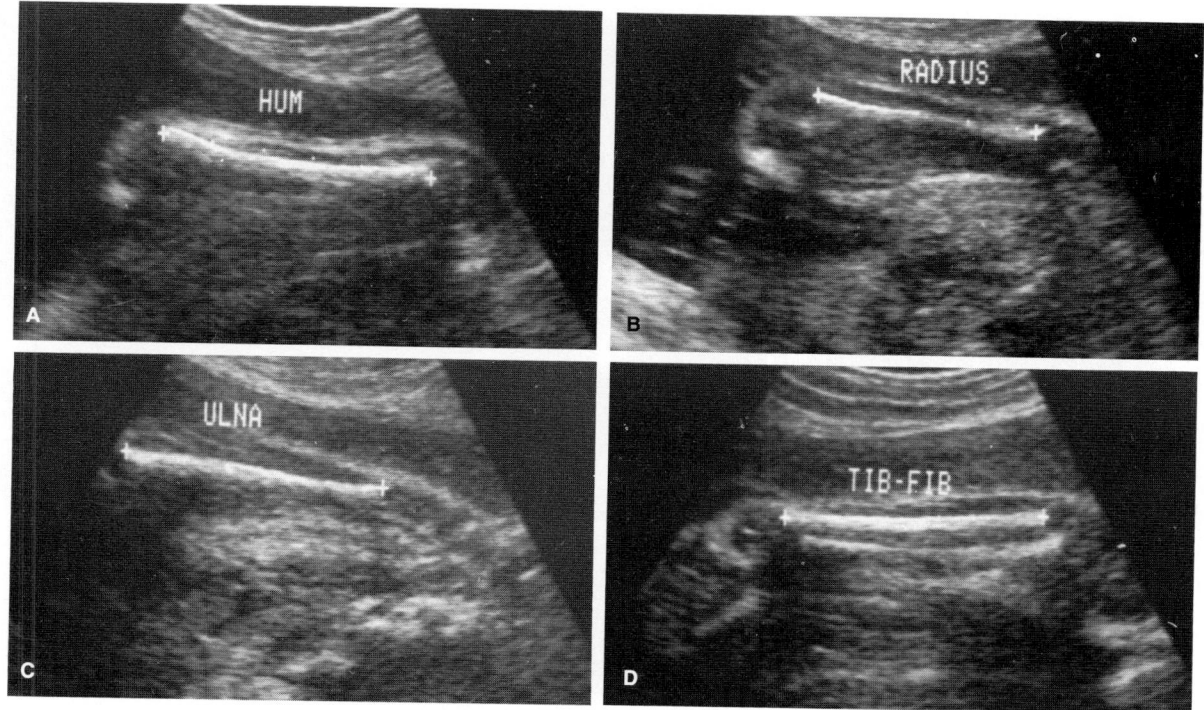

FIGURE 2-21. Measurements of additional long bones. **(A)** Humerus. **(B)** Radius. **(C)** Ulna. **(D)** Tibia and fibula.

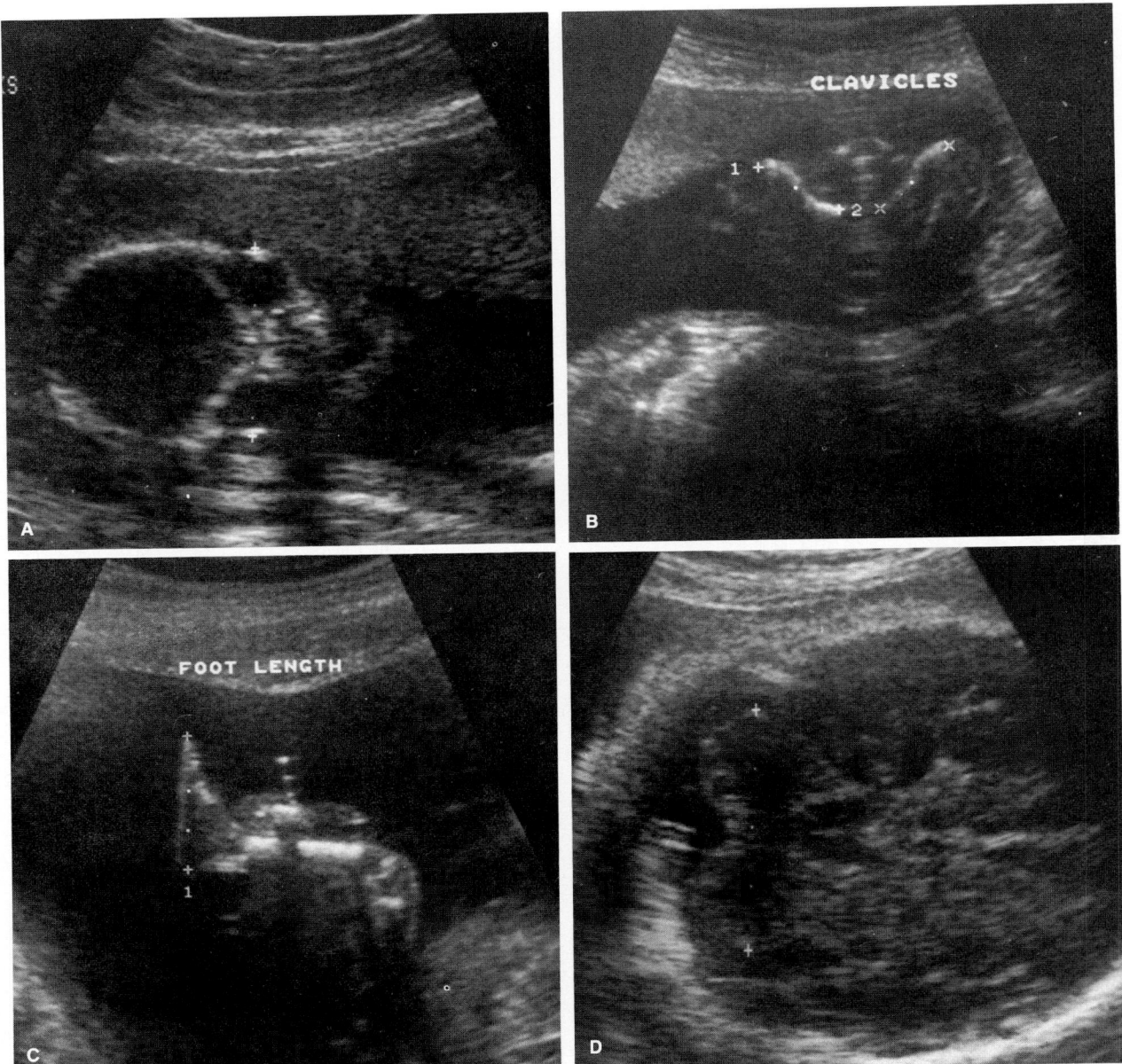

FIGURE 2-22. Alternative parameters to assess gestational age. **(A)** Coronal scan to obtain orbital diameter (19 weeks). **(B)** Transverse scan of the upper thorax to obtain clavicle length (20 weeks). **(C)** Foot length obtained by measurement from the sole to the toes (20 weeks). **(D)** Scan through the posterior fossa to obtain a transverse cerebellar diameter (32 weeks).

TABLE 2-10. Gestational Age for Clavicular Length

Clavicle Length (mm)	Gestational Age (weeks + days) Percentile		
	5th	*50th*	*95th*
11	8 + 3	13 + 6	17 + 2
12	9 + 1	14 + 4	18 + 1
13	10 + 0	14 + 3	19 + 6
14	11 + 6	15 + 2	20 + 5
15	12 + 5	16 + 1	21 + 4
16	12 + 3	18 + 0	21 + 3
17	13 + 2	18 + 5	22 + 2
18	14 + 1	19 + 4	23 + 0
19	16 + 0	19 + 3	24 + 6
20	16 + 6	20 + 2	25 + 5
21	17 + 4	21 + 2	26 + 4
22	17 + 3	22 + 6	26 + 2
23	18 + 2	23 + 5	27 + 1
24	19 + 1	24 + 4	28 + 0
25	21 + 0	24 + 3	29 + 6
26	21 + 5	25 + 1	30 + 5
27	22 + 4	26 + 0	30 + 3
28	22 + 3	27 + 6	31 + 2
29	23 + 2	28 + 5	32 + 1
30	24 + 0	29 + 4	34 + 0
31	25 + 6	29 + 2	34 + 6
32	26 + 5	30 + 1	35 + 4
33	27 + 4	31 + 0	35 + 3
34	27 + 3	32 + 6	36 + 2
35	28 + 1	33 + 5	37 + 1
36	29 + 0	33 + 3	39 + 0
37	30 + 6	34 + 2	39 + 5
38	31 + 5	35 + 1	40 + 4
39	32 + 4	37 + 0	40 + 3
40	32 + 2	37 + 6	41 + 2
41	33 + 1	38 + 4	42 + 0
42	35 + 0	38 + 3	43 + 6
43	35 + 6	39 + 2	44 + 5
44	36 + 5	40 + 1	45 + 4
45	36 + 3	41 + 6	45 + 3

(Yarkoni S, Schmidt W, Jeanty P, et al: Clavicular measurement: A new biometric parameter for fetal evaluation. J Ultrasound Med 1987; 4:467.)

clavicle on transverse scans of the upper fetal chest[51] (Table 2-10). Thigh circumference is obtained on a transverse axis at the junction of the upper and middle third of the thigh, where there is a change in the profile of the femur[53] (Table 2-11). Foot length is the maximal length of the foot from the sole to the toes[54] (Table 2-12; see Fig. 2-22C).

Between 14 and 20 weeks' gestation, the transverse cerebellar diameter (see Fig. 2-22D), in millimeters, is roughly equivalent to the gestational age, in weeks[47] (Table 2-13). The estimated variability associated with determining gestational age from the transverse cerebellar diameter is about equivalent to the standard fetal biometric measurements outlined previously[47] (see Table 2-6). The primary reason for viewing the cerebellum and cisterna magna, however, is for the detection of central nervous system malformations.[55,56]

Fetal Growth

In the third trimester, the accuracy of sonographic gestational age assessment is improved by obtaining serial measurements at sufficiently spaced intervals to account for the inherent error of measurement (ie, more than 2 weeks). If the gesta-

TABLE 2-11. Thigh Circumference Growth Curve

Menstrual Age (wk)	Thigh Circumference (cm)		
	*Lower Limit**	*Predicted Value†*	*Upper Limit‡*
22	5.9	7.1	8.4
23	6.3	7.7	9.1
24	6.8	8.3	9.8
25	7.3	8.9	10.4
26	7.8	9.5	11.1
27	8.3	10.0	11.8
28	8.7	10.6	12.5
29	9.2	11.2	13.2
30	9.7	11.8	13.9
31	10.2	12.4	14.6
32	10.7	13.0	15.2
33	11.1	13.5	15.9
34	11.6	14.1	16.6
35	12.1	14.7	17.3
36	12.6	15.3	18.0
37	13.1	15.9	18.7
38	13.5	16.4	19.4
39	14.0	17.0	20.0
40	14.5	17.6	20.7

* Lower Limit = predicted value − 0.1768(predicted value)

† Predicted Value = 5.6893 + 0.58257 (MA)

‡ Upper Limit = predicted value + 0.1768(predicted value)

2 SD = 17.68%

(Deter RL, Warda A, Rossavik IV, et al: Fetal thigh circumference: A critical evaluation of its relationship to menstrual age. J Clin Ultrasound 1986; 14:105–110.)

TABLE 2-12. Comparison of Mean Postpartum and Ultrasonographic Foot Length With Streeter's Pathologic Data (1920)

Gestation Week	Streeter's Data (mm)	Ultrasonographic Foot Length (mm)	Postpartum Foot Length (mm)
11	7	8	
12	9	9	
13	11	10	
14	14	16	
15	17	16	
16	20	21	
17	23	24	
18	27	27	
19	31	28	
20	33	33	33
21	35	35	
22	40	38	
23	42	42	
24	45	44	
25	48	47	48
26	50	51	
27	53	54	52
28	55	58	
29	57	57	57
30	59	61	60
31	61	62	60
32	63	63	66
33	65	67	68
34	68	68	71
35	71	71	72
36	74	74	74
37	77	75	78
38	79	78	78
39	81	78	80
40	83	82	81
41			82
42			82
43			84

(Mercer BM, Sklar S, Shariatmadar A, et al: Fetal foot length as a predictor of gestational age. Am J Obstet Gynecol 1987; 156:350.)

tional age estimate at the second examination agrees with the first, the confidence interval of the sonographic evaluation of gestational age is reduced.[46] For example, if a pregnancy has been dated at 34 weeks' gestation by last menstrual period, but the composite assessment of gestational age by sonography is 30 weeks, a second examination should be performed in 2 to 3 weeks. If the second ultrasound examination agrees with the first, fetal growth has been normal, indicating that the patient's dating by last menstrual period was

incorrect. When serial examinations do not agree, the clinician cannot rely on the ultrasound examination to accurately assess gestational age. Although anatomic landmarks (discussed later) may provide additional information with respect to a gestational age *range,* management should be based on assessment of fetal well-being and the detection of signs suggesting impaired fetal growth.

Anatomic Landmarks

The maturation, as well as the growth, of specific fetal organ systems were evaluated previously. In the third trimester, the small and large intestine are readily identified, and the latter can be measured.[57] The presence of colonic haustra is associated with a gestational age of more than 30 weeks. The addition of colonic diameter (Fig. 2-23) to the presence of haustra has a stronger correlation with gestational age in the third trimester than either the BPD or the femur length.

TABLE 2-13. Predicted Gestational Ages for Transverse Cerebellar Diameters of 14 to 56 mm

Cerebellum (mm)	Gestational Age (wk)	Cerebellum (mm)	Gestational Age (wk)
14	15.2	35	29.4
15	15.8	36	30.0
16	16.5	37	30.6
17	17.2	38	31.2
18	17.9	39	31.8
19	18.6	40	32.3
20	19.3	41	32.8
21	20.0	42	33.4
22	20.7	43	33.9
23	21.4	44	34.4
24	22.1	45	34.8
25	22.8	46	35.3
26	23.5	47	35.7
27	24.2	48	36.1
28	24.9	49	36.5
29	25.5	50	36.8
30	26.2	51	37.2
31	26.9	52	37.5
32	27.5	54	38.0
33	28.1	55	38.3
34	28.8	56	38.5

(Hill LM, Guzick D, Fries J, et al: The transverse cerebellar diameter in estimating gestational age in the large for gestational age fetus. Obstet Gynecol 1990; 75:981–985.)

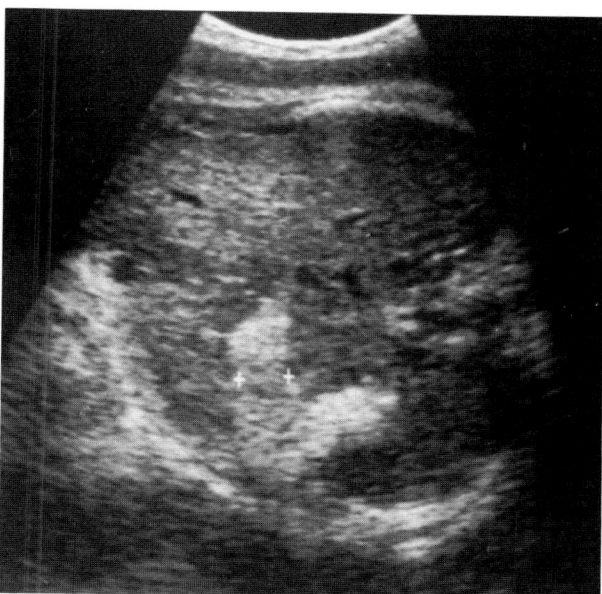

FIGURE 2-23. Large bowel diameter. Meconium is visualized within the colon (*graticules*).

In the normally growing fetus, the distal femoral (Fig. 2-24) and proximal tibial (Fig. 2-25) epiphyseal ossification centers may be seen sonographically within a relatively narrow gestational age range. The distal femoral epiphysis is 1 to 2 mm (measured axially) in 72% of fetuses at 33 weeks' gestation and is 3 mm by 37 weeks' gestation in 84% of fetuses (see Figure 2-25). The proximal tibial epiphysis is not seen before 34 weeks' gestation and attains a size of 3 mm after a gestational age of 38 weeks in 94% of fetuses[58] (see Figure 2-25).

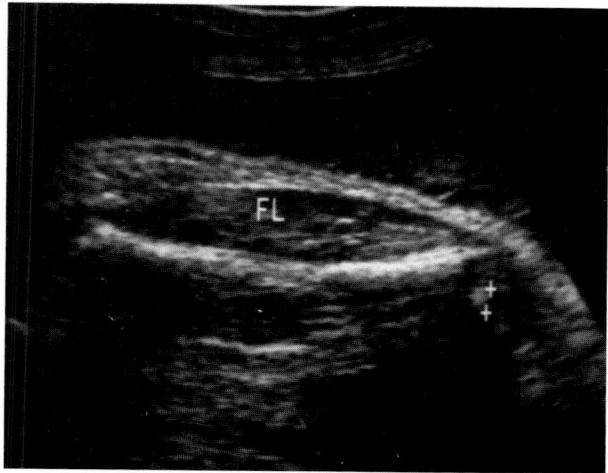

FIGURE 2-24. The *graticules* outline the distal femoral epiphysis. fl, femur length.

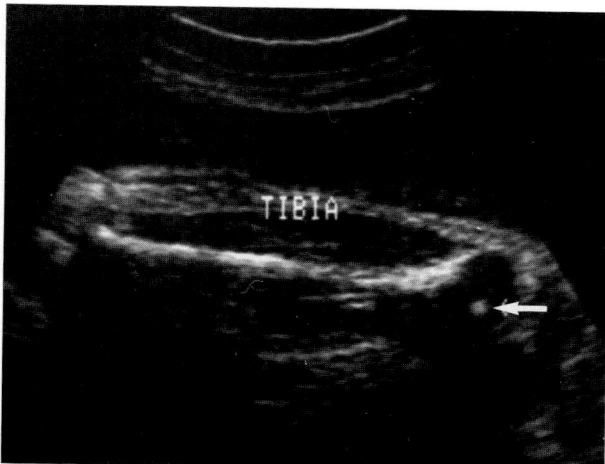

FIGURE 2-25. The proximal tibial epiphysis (*arrow*) at 41 weeks' menstrual age.

ure 2-25). A proximal humeral epiphysis of 1 mm is associated with a 0.69 probability that the gestational age is 40 weeks.[59]

The prediction of gestational age based on fetal organ maturation is less affected by biologic variability than fetal biometry.

CONCLUSION

This chapter reviewed the most reliable sonographic measurements used for gestational age assessment. Technique is important in obtaining appropriate images; however, the subsequent assignment of gestational age is an interpretation based on not only biometry but also maternal history, an evaluation of the fetal environment, and a careful fetal anatomic survey. It cannot be emphasized too strongly that antepartum factors contribute an important independent parameter that may significantly impact the eventual assignment of gestational age. In specific cases, a second ultrasound examination in 2 to 3 weeks may be required to assess the rate of fetal growth and thus further refine the sonographic prediction of gestational age.

REFERENCES

1. Hill LM, Guzick D, Hixson J, et al: Composite assessment of gestational age: A comparison of institutionally derived and published regression equations. Am J Obstet Gynecol 1992; 166:551–555.
2. Hadlock FP, Harrist RB, Shah YP, et al: Sonographic fetal growth standards: Are current data applicable

to a racially mixed population? J Ultrasound Med 1990; 9:157–160.

3. Liggins GC: The drive to fetal growth. In Beard RW, Nathanielz PW (eds): Fetal Physiology and Medicine. Philadelphia: WB Saunders, 1976: 254–270.

4. Hadlock FP, Shah YP, Kanon DJ, et al: Fetal crown-rump length: Re-evaluation of relation to menstrual age (15–18 weeks) with high-resolution real-time ultrasound. Radiology 1992; 182:501–505.

5. Nyberg DA, Mack LA, Laing FC, Patten RM: Distinguishing normal from abnormal gestational sac growth in early pregnancy. J Ultrasound Med 1987; 6:23–27.

6. Daya S: Human chorionic gonadotropin increase in normal early pregnancy. Am J Obstet Gynecol 1987; 156:286–290.

7. Daya S, Woods S, Ward S, et al: Transvaginal ultrasound scanning in early pregnancy and correlation with human chorionic gonadotropin levels. JCU 1991; 19:139–142.

8. Nyberg DA, Filly RA, Filho DLD, et al: Abnormal pregnancy: Early diagnosis by ultrasound and serum chorionic gonadotropin levels. Radiology 1986; 158:393–396.

9. Jouppila PC: Length and depth of the uterus and the diameter of the gestational sac in normal gravidas during early pregnancy. Acta Obstet Gynecol Scand 1971; 50(suppl 15):29–31.

10. Hellman LM, Kobayashi M, Fillisti L, Lavenhar M: Growth and development of the human fetus prior to the twentieth week of gestation. Am J Obstet Gynecol 1969; 103:789–800.

11. Dickey RP, Olar TX, Taylor SN, et al: Relationship of small gestational sac crown-rump length differences to abortion and abortus karyotypes. Obstet Gynecol 1992; 79:554–557.

12. Meegdes BH, Ingenhoes R, Peeters LL, Exalto N: Early pregnancy wastage: Relationship between chorionic vascularization and embryonic development. Fertil Steril 1988; 49:216–220.

13. Stern JJ, Coulam CB: Mechanism of recurrent spontaneous abortion. I. Ultrasonographic findings. Am J Obstet Gynecol 1992; 166:1844–1852.

14. Robinson HP: Sonar measurement of fetal crown-rump length as means of assessing maturity in first-trimester pregnancy. Br Med J 1973; 4:28–31.

15. Fossum GT, Davajan V, Kletzky OA: Early detection of pregnancy with transvaginal ultrasound. Fertil Steril 1988; 49:788–791.

16. Levi CS, Lyons EA, Zheng XH, et al: Endovaginal ultrasound: Demonstration of cardiac activity in embryos of less than 5.0 mm in crown-rump length. Radiology 1990; 176:71–74.

17. Pedersen JF: Fetal crown-rump length measurement by ultrasound in normal pregnancy. Br J Obstet Gynaecol 1982; 89:929–930.

18. Warren WB, Timor-Tritsch I, Peisner DB, et al: Dating the early pregnancy by sequential appearance of embryonic structures. Am J Obstet Gynecol 1989; 161:747–753.

19. Hadlock FP, Deter LR, Harrist RD, Park SK: Fetal biparietal diameter: A critical reevaluation of the relation to menstrual age by means of real-time ultrasound. J Ultrasound Med 1982; 1:97–104.

20. Davison JM, Lind T, Farr V, Whittingham TA: The limitations of ultrasonic cephalometry. J Obstet Gynaecol Br Commonwealth 1973; 80:769–775.

21. Johnson ML, Dunne MG, Mack LA, Rashbaum CL: Evaluation of fetal intracranial anatomy by static and real-time ultrasound. JCU 1980; 8:311–18.

22. Campbell S, Warsof SL, Little D, Cooper DJ: Routine ultrasound screening for the prediction of gestational age. Obstet Gynecol 1985; 65:613–620.

23. Hadlock FP, Deter RL, Carpenter RJ, Park SK: Estimating fetal age: Effect of head shape on BPD. AJR 1981; 137:83–85.

24. Gray DL, Songster GS, Parvin CA, Crane JP: Cephalic index: A gestational age-dependent biometric parameter. Obstet Gynecol 1989; 74:600–603.

25. Kasby CB, Poll V: The breech head and its ultrasound significance. Br J Obstet Gynaecol 1982; 89:106–110.

26. Wolfson RN, Zador I, Halvorsen P, et al: Biparietal diameter in premature rupture of membranes: Errors in estimating gestational age. JCU 1983; 11:371–374.

27. Hill LM, Breckle R, Gehrking WC: The variable effects of oligohydramnios on the biparietal diameter and the cephalic index. J Ultrasound Med 1984; 3:93–95.

28. Hadlock FP, Deter RL, Harrist RB, Park SK: Fetal head circumference: Relation to menstrual age. AJR 1982; 138:649–653.

29. Campbell S, Wilkin D: Ultrasonic measurement of fetal abdominal circumference in the estimation of fetal weight. Br J Obstet Gynaecol 1975; 82:689–697.

30. Hadlock FP, Deter RL, Harrist RB, Park SK: Fetal abdominal circumference as a predictor of menstrual age. AJR 1982; 139:367–370.

31. Hoffbauer H, Arabin PB, Baumann ML: Control of fetal development with multiple ultrasonic body measures. Contrib Gynecol Obstet 1979; 6:147–156.

32. Tamura RK, Sabbagha RE: Percentile ranks of sonar fetal abdominal circumference measurement. Am J Obstet Gynecol 1980; 138:475–479.

33. Rossavik IK, Deter RL: The effect of abdominal profile shape changes on the estimation of fetal weight. JCU 1984; 12:57–59.

34. Hill LM, Guzick D, Thomas ML, Fries JK: Fetal radius length: A critical evaluation of race as a factor in gestational age assessment. Am J Obstet Gynecol 1989; 161:193–199.

35. Hadlock FP, Harrist RB, Deter RL, Park SK: Fetal femur length as a predictor of menstrual age: Sonographically measured. AJR 1982; 138: 875–878.

36. Jeanty P, Rodesch F, Delbeke D, Dumont JE: Estimation of gestational age from measurements of fetal long bones. J Ultrasound Med 1984; 3:75–79.

37. O'Brien GD, Queenan JT, Campbell S: Assessment of gestational age in the second trimester by real-time ultrasound measurement of the femur length. Am J Obstet Gynecol 1981; 139:540–545.

38. Lessoway VA, Schulzer M, Wittmann BL: Sonographic measurement of the fetal femur: Factors affecting accuracy. JCU 1990; 18:471–476.

39. Wells PNT: Biomedical Ultrasonics. New York: Academic Press, 1977: 150–155.

40. Abramowicz J, Jaffe R: Comparison between lateral and axial ultrasonic measurements of the fetal femur. Am J Obstet Gynecol 1988; 159:921–922.

41. Pretorius DH, Nelson TR, Manco-Johnson M: Fetal age estimation by ultrasound: The impact of measurement errors. Radiology 1984; 152:763–766.

42. Abrams SL, Filly RA: Curvature of the fetal femur: A normal sonographic finding. Radiology 1989; 6:203–207.

43. Hadlock FP, Deter RL, Harrist RB, Park SK: Estimating fetal age: Computer-assisted analysis of multiple fetal growth parameters. Radiology 1984; 152:497–501.

44. Yagel S, Adoni A, Oman S, et al: A statistical examination of the accuracy of combining femoral length and biparietal diameter as an index of fetal gestational age. Br J Obstet Gynaecol 1986; 93:109–115.

45. Ott WJ: Accurate gestational dating. Obstet Gynecol 1985; 66:311–315.

46. Rose BI, Lamb EJ: Multiple simultaneous predictors of gestational age: An application of Bayes' theorem. Am J Perinatol 1988; 5:44–50.

47. Hill LM, Guzick D, Fries J, et al: The transverse cerebellar diameter in estimating gestational age in the large for gestational age fetus. Obstet Gynecol 1990; 75:981–985.

48. Hadlock FP: Sonographic estimation of fetal age and weight. Radiol Clin North Am 1990; 28:39–50.

49. Reece EA, Scioscia AL, Green J, et al: Embryonic trunk circumference: A new biometric parameter for estimation of gestational age. Am J Obstet Gynecol 1987; 156:713–715.

50. Mayden SL, Tortora M, Berkowitz RL, et al: Orbital diameters: A new parameter for prenatal diagnosis and dating. Am J Obstet Gynecol 1982; 144:289–297.

51. Yarkoni S, Schmidt W, Jeanty P, et al: Clavicular measurement: A new biometric parameter for fetal evaluation. J Ultrasound Med 1985; 4:467–470.

52. Li DF, Woo JS: Fractional spine length: A new parameter for assessing fetal growth. J Ultrasound Med 1986; 5:379–583.

53. Deter RL, Warda A, Rossavik IK, et al: Fetal thigh circumference: A critical evaluation of its relationship to menstrual age. J Clin Ultrasound 1986; 14:105–110.

54. Mercer BM, Sklar S, Shariatmadar A, et al: Fetal foot length as a predictor of gestational age. Am J Obstet Gynecol 1987; 156:350–355.

55. Hill LM, Martin JG, Fries J, Hixson J: The role of the transcerebellar view in the detection of fetal central nervous system anomaly. Am J Obstet Gynecol 1991; 164:1220–1224.

56. Filly RA, Cardoza JD, Goldstein RB, Berkovitch AJ: Detection of fetal central nervous system anomalies: A practical level of effort for a routine sonogram. Radiology 1989; 172:403–408.

57. Goldstein I, Lockwood C, Hobbins JC: Ultrasound assessment of fetal intestinal development in the evaluation of gestational age. Obstet Gynecol 1987; 70:682–686.

58. Goldstein I, Lockwood C, Belanger K, Hobbins J: Ultrasonographic assessment of gestational age with the distal femoral and proximal tibial ossification centers in the third trimester. Am J Obstet Gynecol 1988; 158:127–130.

59. Goldstein I, Reece EA, O'Connor TZ, Hobbins JC: Estimating gestational age in the term pregnancy with a model based on multiple indices of fetal maturity. Am J Obstet Gynecol 1989; 161:1235–1238.

John P. McGahan and Manuel Porto:
DIAGNOSTIC OBSTETRICAL ULTRASOUND.
© 1994 J.B. Lippincott Company.

Dru E. Carlson

Chapter 3

Large-for-Date Pregnancies

A maternal fundal height that measures 3 cm or more greater than the estimated gestational age at last menses or at a previous ultrasound warrants a detailed sonographic evaluation of fetal size, anatomy, and amniotic fluid volume as soon as possible.[1] Occasionally, the body habitus of an obese woman confounds the practitioner's ability to measure accurately the fundal height, but since this quick physical measurement is routinely performed at each prenatal office visit, it is often the first clue that either the fetal size, number, structure, or environment is abnormal. A list of the possible causes of large-for-date pregnancies can be found in in Table 3-1.[2]

INACCURATE DATING

The most common explanation of a large-for-date pregnancy is inaccurate dating. Often vaginal bleeding that occurs early in pregnancy may be mistaken for a normal period. It has been estimated that in 20% to 40% of all pregnancies, the true menstrual age is uncertain.[3] Ultrasound may be helpful in documenting menstrual age, and this

may include taking a variety of measurements (see Chapter 2.) In the first trimester of pregnancy, this includes the crown-to-rump length. Later measurements may include the biparietal diameter (BPD), head circumference, abdominal circumference, and femur length. Thus, an ultrasound examination done in the first to early second trimesters of pregnancy may help to alleviate confusion in a large number of pregnancies thought to be large-for-date pregnancies.

MULTIPLE PREGNANCIES

Sonography may be helpful in determining whether the pregnancy is single or multiple.[4] A patient presenting with a large-for-date pregnancy may in fact have a twin pregnancy. Especially in monochorionic pregnancies, however, there is a higher incidence of congenital anomalies that also may contribute to the large-for-date pregnancy. Thus, one twin may have a congenital anomaly that may be a source of polyhydramnios and thus another cause for the pregnancy being larger than expected (Fig. 3-1).

TABLE 3-1. Possible Causes of Large-for-Date Pregnancies

Inaccurate dating
Multiple pregnancies
Hydatidiform mole
Diabetes mellitus
Macrosomia
Polyhydramnios
  Idiopathic
  Fetal abnormality
Pregnancy and a mass

MOLAR PREGNANCY

Hydatidiform mole is rare, occurring in about 1 in 15,000 to 20,000 pregnancies. The classic ultrasound appearance of a molar pregnancy includes a uterus that is filled entirely with a homogeneous vesicular tissue without accompanying fetal parts (Fig. 3-2). Molar pregnancy may have accompany-

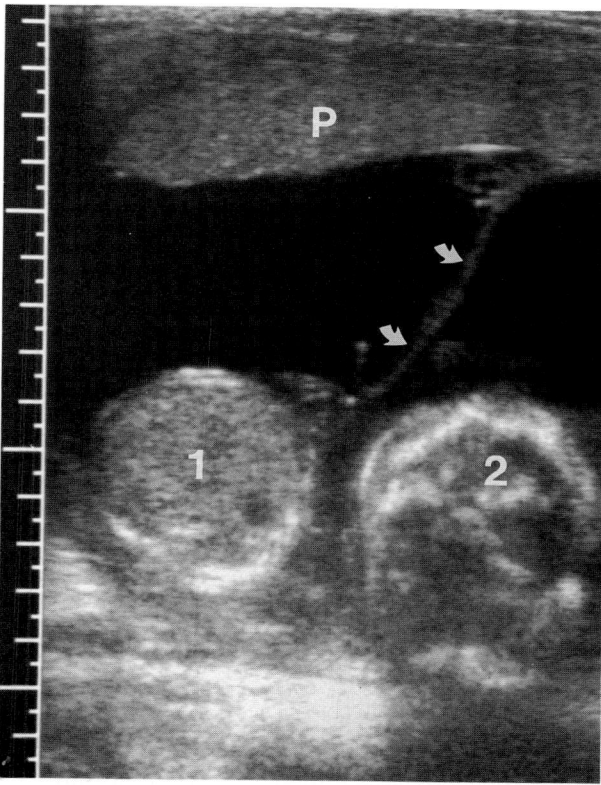

FIGURE 3-1. Twins plus polyhydramnios. Two causes of large-for-dates. The twins (1 and 2) are separated by membranes (*arrow*), and both sacs have polyhydramnios. P, placenta. (Courtesy of John P. McGahan, MD, Sacramento, CA.)

ing thecal luteal cysts that are bilateral. Hydatidiform mole and its variations are discussed in Chapter 6.

MATERNAL OBESITY

One cannot begin a discussion of the evaluation of the large-for-date pregnancy without discussing the quandary of obesity. The risk of diabetes is increased seven times in a *morbidly obese* woman, defined as a woman with a prepregnancy body weight of more than 135% the ideal. Perinatal loss is increased 30% due to diabetes, hypertension, and macrosomic fetuses with traumatic deliveries.[5] Many physicians believe that if the blood glucose level is well controlled in insulin-dependent diabetic mothers, there is no risk of a macrosomic fetus. Unfortunately, this is not always true. In one study, 43% of insulin-dependent diabetics gave birth to macrosomic infants even when they were considered well controlled.[6] The key clue was a large amount of weight gain in the third trimester, which correlated with a higher hemoglobin A1 level. Thus, one should always be suspicious of macrosomia in all diabetic pregnancies and perform frequent ultrasound assessments to monitor growth.

A patient with poorly controlled diabetes that is lacking any vasculopathy has been shown in longitudinal studies to be the ideal candidate for a macrosomic infant, again with the most fetal weight gain occurring in the third trimester. Apparently, early fetal growth is not profoundly affected by diabetic control.[7]

In the ultrasound evaluation of these difficult-to-image patients, several scanning tips are helpful in trying to assess fetal size:

1. Use the umbilicus as a window to the fetus. Put a large amount of imaging gel into the umbilicus, and then insert a sector transducer or vaginal probe. This eliminates several centimeters of adipose, and manipulation of the angle of the probe often produces a relatively clear picture.
2. To obtain a good BPD in the vertex-positioned fetus, place the sheathed vaginal probe transducer just slightly into the vaginal introitus. This results in the head becoming well outlined and easier to measure. The biggest concern is underestimating the weight of the fetus and having an unexpected macrosomic baby with the risk of shoulder

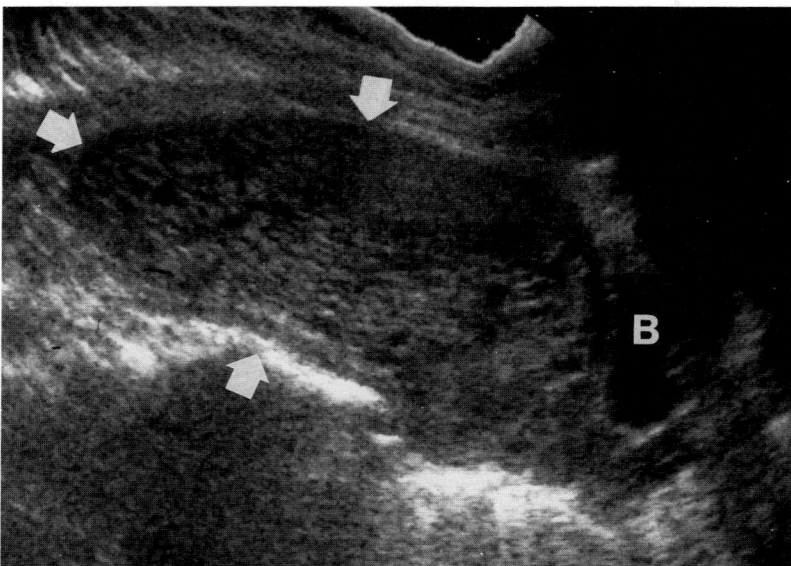

FIGURE 3-2. Hydatidiform mole. Longitudinal scan of the uterus showing absence of fetal parts and fairly classic appearance of hydatidiform mole (*arrows*). B, bladder. (McGahan JP, Osborn A: Sonographic evaluation of the large-for-dates pregnancy. Perinat Neonat 1985; 9:45–52.)

dystocia. Getting the clearest image is the best help in estimating weight.

3. Having an assistant elevate the abdominal pannus occasionally allows an improved image. Regardless, it is important to inform the patient that the quality of ultrasound imaging and exact estimation of weight are highly dependent on the distance from the probe to the fetus.

The examiner should be aware that many fetal anomalies besides macrosomia are associated with insulin-dependent diabetic mothers. These include brain malformations (such as holoprosencephaly), cardiac lesions, and incomplete development of the lower pelvis (caudal regression). A disturbing study from Italy showed that strict maternal control does not exclude accelerated fetal cardiac growth and abnormal development of cardiac function even though cardiac structure may be normal.[8] Therefore, careful attention to the size of the fetal heart may be warranted throughout gestation.

FETAL MACROSOMIA

Various methods exist for estimating accurately the size of the overweight fetus, but there is no one excellent way to precisely predict macrosomia. The problem lies in the fact that the best ultrasound estimation can differ from the actual weight by 10% or more. This is an acceptable variance in the average-weight fetus, but in the macrosomic fetus,

it may amount to several hundred grams of potentially damaging error. Watson calculated that to achieve a 90% confidence that a newborn will actually weigh more than 4000 g, one must estimate the fetal weight by ultrasound at 4750 g.[9]

First, the physician should always look at the parents when assessing a fetus with macrocephaly or large hands or feet. Often the abnormality is not a syndrome but an expression of a familial propensity. Next, the physician should be aware of several genetic syndromes that are associated with large-for-date newborns and search for related anomalies (Table 3-2). Some of these syndromes are listed next.

Beckwith-Wiedemann syndrome is a sporadic abnormality that is seen with macroglossia and occasionally an umbilical hernia, which may appear on ultrasound as a small omphalocele. The unusual fissures of the ears are not easily appreciated at prenatal examination. The diagnosis is confirmed by adrenocortical cytomegaly, often with pancreatic hyperplasia that is manifested by severe neonatal hypoglycemia. Adrenal cysts and nephromegaly have been described as aiding in the ultrasound diagnosis of this disease.[10]

Marshall-Smith syndrome is a sporadic disease characterized by markedly accelerated skeletal maturation that results in a long, relatively thin newborn.[11] An overestimation of weight occurs because the head and femur are so much larger than anticipated. Occasionally, these fetuses demonstrate an absent corpus callosum or an omphalocele. Unfortunately, these are mentally retarded and poorly thriving newborns.

TABLE 3-2. Macrosomic Syndromes*

Syndrome	Bone Maturation	Macrocephaly
Beckwith-Wiedemann	Not accelerated	Yes + omphalocele
Marshall-Smith	Marked acceleration	Yes + occasional absent corpus callosum
Weaver's	Marked acceleration	No + camptodactyly (finger flexions)
Sotos'	Not accelerated	Marked + big hands and feet
Ruvalcaba-Myhre-Smith's	Not accelerated	Marked

* These are possible causes of large-for-date pregnancies for which ultrasound may be useful.

Weaver's syndrome also shows accelerated bone maturation but has the added problem of camptodactyly of the hands and foot deformities such as talipe equinovarus that can be seen on ultrasound.[12]

Sotos' syndrome is associated with profound macrocephaly, with the head circumference at least 4.5 standard deviations above the mean and usually mild dilation of the cerebral ventricles.[13] There is no consistent pattern of brain malformation. The hands and feet are also large for gestational age. Mental retardation is present in up to 80% of these children.

Ruvalcaba-Myhre-Smith syndrome also presents with profound macrocephaly, but the cerebral ventricles are always normal in size.[14] The newborn has macrosomia and poor tone, but normal adult stature is seen. Unusual pigmentation of the skin is seen in early childhood. Polyhydramnios is seen on ultrasound, probably due to the poor fetal tone.

The suspicion of macrosomia starts with the third-trimester examination of an enlarged fundal height and should always include a careful interview with the patient to elicit a history of other large babies, diabetes in this or other pregnancies, current amount of weight gain, and any specific genetic diseases in the family. The ultrasound examination should always be performed with attempts to see the fetus through various maternal "windows." Finally, the physician should accept the limited ability to estimate an accurate fetal weight in the large-for-date newborn. This limitation also should be understood by the patient and her family.

POLYHYDRAMNIOS

The ultrasound evaluation of a large-for-date pregnancy should always include an accurate measurement of the amniotic fluid volume. Over the last 10 years, there have been several attempts to clarify the most accurate ultrasound method for defining clinically significant polyhydramnios. A single largest vertical pocket of more 8 cm has been proposed and endorsed by many authors.[15,16] Others think that the qualitative impression of polyhydramnios is adequate.[17] In 1990, we compared these concepts with the four-quadrant technique of measuring fluid: the *amniotic fluid index* (AFI).[18] This technique involves holding the transducer perpendicular to the floor and dividing the maternal uterus into four quadrants. The linea nigra and umbilicus serve as longitudinal and vertical markers of the measuring pockets. These are then added together to give the AFI, which is normally 13 ± 5 cm[19] (Fig. 3-3). Because 2 standard deviations above the average 13 cm is 23 cm, we used 24 cm as the lower limit of clinically significant poly-

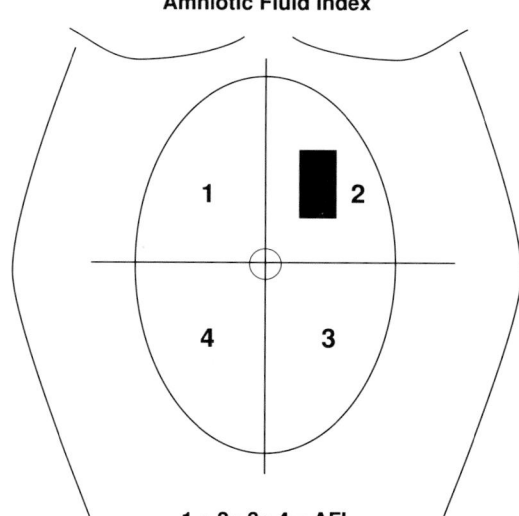

Amniotic Fluid Index

1 + 2+ 3+ 4 = AFI

FIGURE 3-3. Amniotic fluid index (AFI) is calculated by adding the largest vertical pocket of amniotic fluid in the four quadrants of the pregnant uterus.

hydramnios. One hundred and twelve nondiabetic women were referred with the descriptive diagnosis of polyhydramnios made by experienced ultrasonographers. There was poor correlation between these descriptions and fetal outcome. Forty-nine of the 112 met the definition of polyhydramnios (AFI of at least 24 cm). This allowed the inclusion of all fetuses with structural or chromosomal abnormalities. Interestingly, seven patients had an AFI of less than 24 cm but the classic definition of polyhydramnios of one fluid pocket that was at least 8 cm. None of these patients had poor fetal outcome or polyhydramnios diagnosed at delivery. Since this study, several other authors have endorsed this method of measurement.[20–22]

Just as in a macrosomic fetus, a critical question is whether the patient is diabetic. Gestational diabetes that is poorly controlled or undetected can be associated with increased amniotic fluid. A diabetic screening test should be employed whenever polyhydramnios is diagnosed, with or without an anatomic lesion in the fetus.

When the examiner determines that the AFI is at least 24 cm, a detailed look at the fetal anatomy is warranted. Over 100 fetal anomalies can be associated with polyhydramnios. Experience shows that certain areas of the fetus are crucial to include in this examination; these are listed in Table 3-3.

A systematic, calculated examination of the fetus with polyhydramnios allows the examiner to identify the structural abnormalities commonly associated with this condition. The examiner should start at the fetal head and work caudally down the fetal body, asking and answering the questions presented next and highlighted in Table 3-4. (These specific abnormalities are not detailed here but are presented in other chapters throughout this book.)

TABLE 3-3. Targeted Ultrasound

Brain
Anencephaly
Hydrocephaly
Encephalocele
Tumors
Lissencephaly

Chest
Cystic adenomatoid malformations of the lung
Pulmonary sequestration
Diaphragmatic hernia

Mouth
Cleft lip
Cleft palate
Micrognathia
Epignathus
Macroglossia

Heart
Congestive heart failure
Arrhythmia
Complex heart malformations

Neck
Goiter
Teratoma
Hemangioma
Tracheal atresia

Abdomen
Esophageal atresia
Omphalocele
Duodenal atresia
Bowel obstructions

---

* Polyhydramnios is often accompanied by associated fetal malformations, which may be localized to areas in the fetus as examined on a targeted ultrasound.

Head

1. Is a structural *brain malformation* causing poor swallowing and thus increased fluid? This can be seen with fetal *hydrocephalus*, holoprosencephaly, anencephaly, intracranial teratomas, and other brain malformations (Fig. 3-4). Carefully measure the ventricular atrium, which should be no larger than 1 cm. The choroid plexus should fill the lateral ventricle. If the edge is dangling, this is suspicious for hydrocephalus. Examine the midline. The falx should be straight. If it disappears on the frontal part of the brain, be concerned about holoprosencephaly. If it is pushed to one side, look for intracranial tumors or *intraventricular hemorrhage*. The septum pellucidum should be easily visualized at the level of the biparietal diameter. If not, look higher in the brain and see whether it has moved toward the center, implying an absent corpus callosum. Make sure that the cerebellum is symmetric and that the cisterna magna is less than 1 cm. *Dandy-Walker malformations* are easily missed but have been seen with polyhydramnios. (These abnormalities are covered in more detail in Chapter 8.)

TABLE 3-4. Seven Questions to be Asked When Examining a Fetus With Polyhydramnios

Area	Question	Malformation	Ultrasound Clues
1. Head	Brain malformation?	Hydrocephaly	Atrium > 1 cm
		Holoprosencephaly	No normal midline
		Anencephaly	No BPD, no cranium above orbits
		Intracranial tumor	Midline shifted
2. Neck and Mouth	Obstruction?	Goiter	Hyperextended neck
		Teratoma or hemangioma	Soft-tissue mass
		Cleft palate	Micrognathia, large echolucency mouth
		Median facial cleft	Hypertelorism or cleft lip
		Choanal atresia	Diagnosis of exclusion
3. Heart	Failure?	Arrhythmia	M-mode
		Complex lesions	Abnormal heart ultrasound
		Teratoma or hemangioma	Soft tissue masses in other body sites
		Severe anemia	Cardiomegaly or tricuspid regurgitation
		Viral infection	Cardiomyopathy or "bright" heart walls
		Arteriovenous malformation	Cystic vascular brain lesion
4. Chest	Compression?	Cystic adenomatoid malformation	Echogenic leading to cystic lung mass or displaced heart
		Pulmonary sequestration	Doppler flow abnormal, echogenic mass
		Diaphragmatic hernia	Complex mass in chest, no stomach below diaphragm, heart displaced
5. Esophagus	Stomach?	Tracheoesophageal fistula	No stomach, VATER association, fetal vomiting
6. Upper Gastrointestinal Tract	Obstruction?	Duodenal atresia	"Double-bubble" sign
		Small intestine atresias or stenosis	Multiple lucencies in abdomen, fetal vomiting
		Meconium ileus	"Bright" plug of meconium, multiple lucencies
7. Neurologic Examination	Poor tone?	Arthrogryposis multiforme	Hands, feet, legs, or arms do not move normally
		Neu-Laxova	+ Micrognathia
		Cerebral-ocular-facial syndrome	+ Hypotelorism and micrognathia
		Aneuploidy	+ Clenched hands and/or multiple anomalies
		Pena-Shokeir	+ Micrognathia small chest
		Multiple pterygium	+ Bands at joints

Neck and Mouth

2. Is there possible *obstruction* of the esophagus? This can be seen with *choanal atresia, cleft palate, median facial cleft, goiter,* and *teratoma.* The U-shaped cleft soft palate is usually associated with micrognathia. *Goiter* and *neck teratomas* cause a hyperextended head. Epignathus or oral teratomas are seen as large diffusive masses arising out of the mouth. *Medionasal facial cleft* is seen as a bony extension of a cleft lip with marked hypertelorism and split nose, and the outline of the bony defect is easily demarcated.

Heart

3. Is there *heart failure?* There can be pathologic *increased output* by the fetal heart caused by a vascular lesion, such as a *hemangioma,* or *arterial venous malformation* of other parts of the body, or a condition resulting in *severe anemia,*

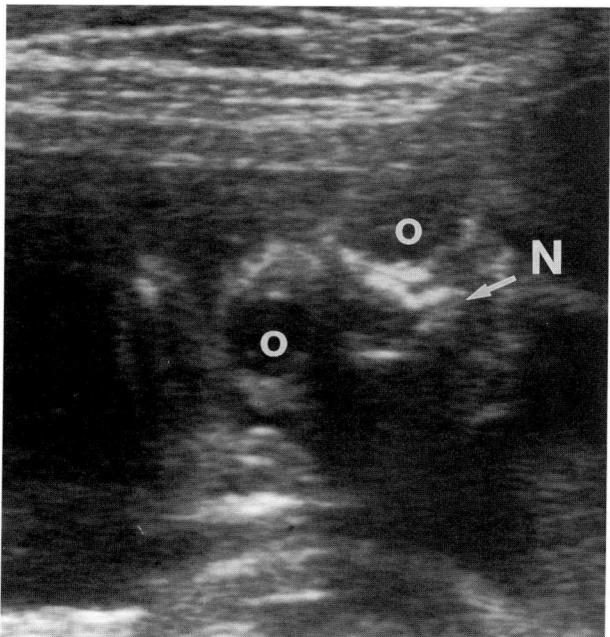

FIGURE 3-4. Anencephaly. Coronal ultrasound through the face showing the nose (N) and prominent orbits (O) and no bony calvarium or brain tissue above the orbits. Note that the bony orbits are close to the side wall of the uterus, which would not occur if brain tissue were present. There was mild polyhydramnios. (Courtesy of John P. McGahan, MD, Sacramento, CA.)

such as *isoimmunization*, or fetal *viral infection*. Severe anemia usually causes an increase in the biventricular outer dimension of the heart, as measured by M-mode echocardiography. Tricuspid regurgitation is a common feature of failure. Viral infections, such as coxsackievirus, can cause a large and dense heart with bright lesions in the ventricular walls. Decreased output can also result in cardiac failure originating from *fetal arrhythmia* (heart block or supraventricular tachycardia) or complex cardiac malformations. Arrhythmias are best appreciated by M-mode echocardiography. *Complex cardiac malformations* should be evaluated by a more complete ultrasound examination, as explained in Chapter 12.

Chest

4. Is a lesion in the fetal chest causing *compression* or *diversion* of blood? This can be seen with *cystic adenomatoid malformations of the lung* (CAML), *pulmonary sequestration*, and *diaphragmatic hernia*. CAML can be appreciated as an echogenic area in the chest with or

without small or large cysts within it (depending on the type; Fig. 3-5). Pulmonary sequestration can be seen as an echogenic mass separate from the normal lung lobulations. It often has a separate Doppler flow signature from the rest of the pulmonary tree. Diaphragmatic hernia should be considered when visualizing a complex thoracic mass with no demonstrable subdiaphragmatic stomach. A longitudinal view often helps to outline the normal diaphragm, and the examiner should carefully watch the fetus breathe and the diaphragm move normally. All three conditions can be associated with displacement of the heart.

Esophagus

5. Is the fetal stomach identified? If not, *esophageal atresia* or *tracheoesophageal fistula* should be considered. It can be normal to not visualize a recently emptied stomach for as long as 2 hours. If there is polyhydramnios and the examiner cannot demonstrate a normal stomach, the fetus should be considered to have esophageal atresia or tracheoesophageal fistula until proved otherwise. Careful observation of the fetal

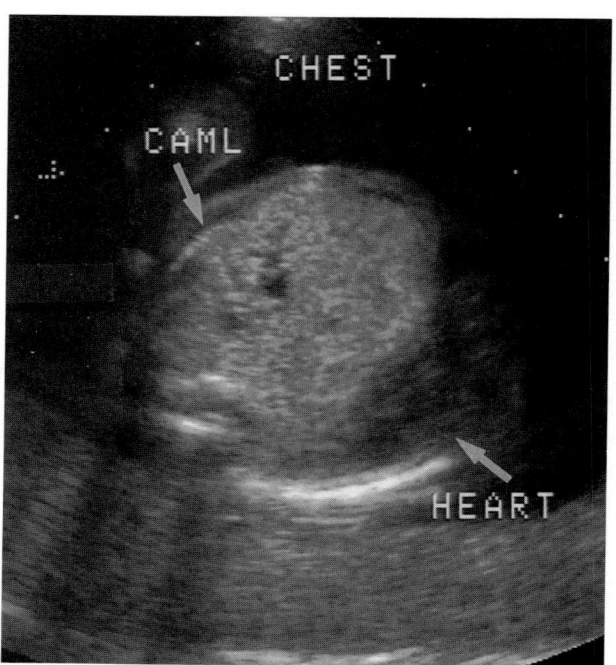

FIGURE 3-5. Cystic adenomatoid malformation. Cross section through fetal chest, with echogenic mass within the left hemithorax representing a cystic adenomatoid malformation of lung (CAML). Note the heart pushed to the right side of the chest.

VATER Association

Features

V → Vertebral defects
VSD/cardiac defects

A → Anal atresia

TE → Tracheoesophageal fistula

R → Radial dysplasia
Renal anomaly

FIGURE 3-6. VATER association comprises several typical features, three or more of which are needed for diagnosis. Many of these may be difficult to recognize prenatally.

abdomen over time can be helpful. Occasionally, dilation of the esophageal pouch can be seen in the upper chest. When in doubt, there are two reasons always to raise concern for this lesion: (1) the association between Down's syndrome and esophageal atresia, and (2) the potential complications of pulmonary aspiration that result from feeding a newborn with a tracheoesophageal fistula. The VATER association should be considered in chromosomally normal fetuses with an absent stomach bubble. The various anomalies that are described with this association are seen in Figure 3-6.

Upper Gastrointestinal Tract

6. Is an obstruction distal to the stomach causing fetal regurgitation? This is seen with *duodenal atresia* ("double-bubble" sign) or *small intestine obstruction*, which result in multiple, circular, fluid-filled loops of bowel. One third of all cases of duodenal atresia are associated with Down's syndrome[20] (Fig. 3-7). The most frequent type of duodenal atresia results from the presents of a membrane. There can also be a ring of pancreas *(annular pancreas)* encircling the duodenum.[23] The ultrasound clue is two cystic structures at the level of the stomach with a small connection (see Fig. 3-7). It is critical to hold the transducer perpendicular to the spine. A potential pitfall involves having the ultrasound plane of section through the normal stomach in such a way that the proximal and distal stomach presents as two cystic structures, thus giving

the false diagnosis of duodenal atresia. Small bowel obstructions are associated with polyhydramnios. The lumen of the small bowel should never exceed 7 mm; if it does, true obstruction is diagnosed. The more distal the obstruction, the less likely is the presence of polyhydramnios. A *meconium ileus* associated with cystic fibrosis must be excluded in any obstruction with a hyperechoic mass of meconium and multiple loops of dilated bowel (Fig. 3-8). The fastest method to diagnose cystic fibrosis is by amniocentesis or karyotype, with cells for cystic fibrosis screening. Initially, screen the parents for the commercially available mutations to focus the laboratory's attention on the appropriate defect in the fetus (Table 3-5). Prenatal knowledge of this disease is imperative to good neonatal care.

Neurologic Examination

7. Is an abnormality in the neurologic function of the fetus (but not an appreciated intracranial lesion) causing poor movement and swallowing? This may be associated with *arthrogryposis multiforme, Neu-Laxova,* and sometimes *aneuploidy.* This important observation centers on the evaluation of the overall tone of the fetus. Is it moving normally? The examiner should see clearly the hands open and shut. Are the feet strangely postured and fixed, or do they turn and flex easily? Is there normal movement of the fetal mouth, with easily observed sucking, opening, and shutting? One way to determine the difference between fetal regurgitation secondary to obstruction and a neurologic movement disorder is to place a color flow Doppler over the mouth of the fetus. With the color flow Doppler set at a sensitivity used to visualize the cord, projectile vomiting can be seen as movement of amniotic fluid out of the fetal mouth. A vomiting fetus with a bowel obstruction demonstrates repeated bouts of explosive fluid eruptions from its open mouth and protruding tongue (Fig. 3-9). A neurologically abnormal fetus either never opens or never closes its mouth in a normal manner. While looking at the movement of the fetal mouth, the examiner also should measure the mandible of the fetus.[24] Micrognathia is often observed with neurologically abnormal fetuses who have never moved their mouths normally.

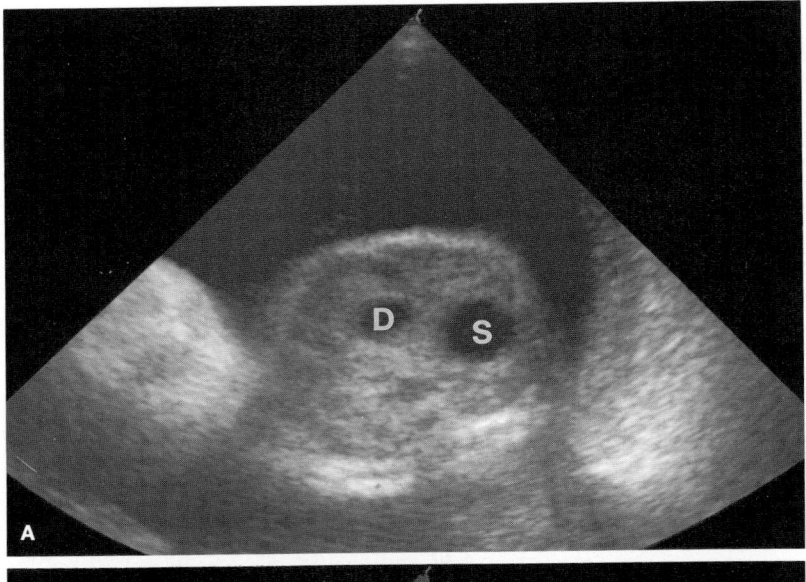

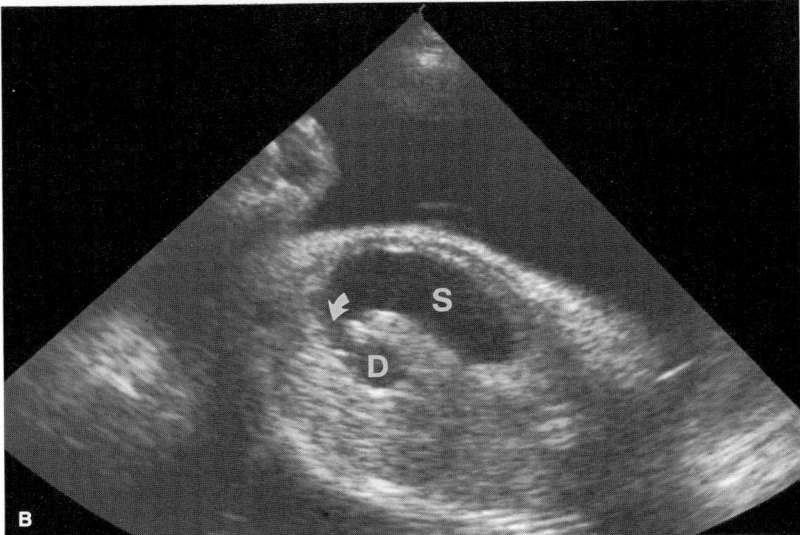

FIGURE 3-7. Duodenal atresia. **(A)** Transverse scan through the fetal abdomen demonstrates classic findings of "double bubble," indicative of dilated stomach (S) and duodenum (D). **(B)** Oblique scan demonstrates the more proximal cystic structure representing the stomach (S), which communicates (*arrow*) with the more distal dilated duodenum (D). (Courtesy of John P. McGahan, MD, Sacramento, CA.)

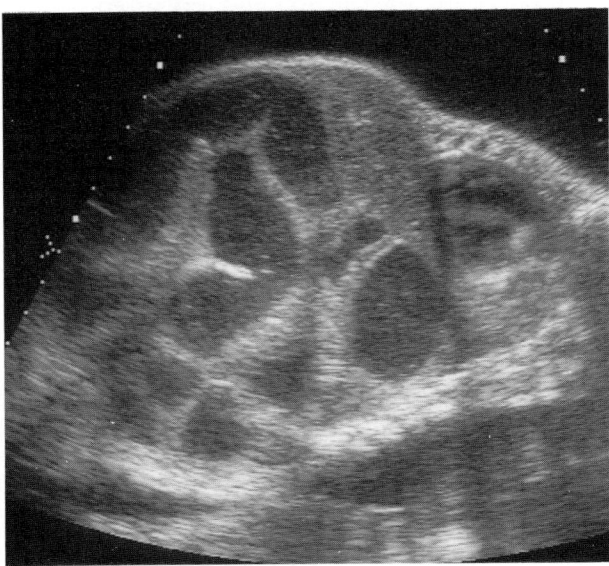

FIGURE 3-8. Meconium ileus. Longitudinal view of meconium ileus and massively dilated loops of bowel. Note the bright plug of meconium in center of abdomen. Chest to the right is normally formed but appears small secondary to enlarged abdominal circumference.

TABLE 3-5. Mutations Known to be Associated With Cystic Fibrosis

Mutation	Frequency (%)
ΔF508	73
G551D	2.4
G542X	2.2
W1282X	1.6
R553X	1.1
N1303K	1.1
R560T	1
1717G-A	0.6
621 + 1	0.6
Δ1507	0.4
R117H	0.4
S549N	0.1

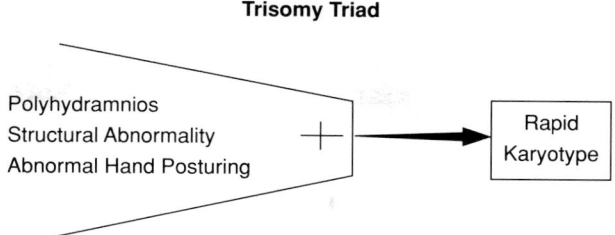

FIGURE 3-10. When the pregnancy is accompanied by polyhydramnios, fetal structural abnormalities in the hand should be scanned to check for abnormal posturing, which is another clue for abnormal fetal karyotype.

Should all patients with polyhydramnios be offered invasive genetic evaluation? If a fetus displays the triad of polyhydramnios, a structural abnormality, and abnormal hand posturing, the parents should be offered fetal karyotyping to rule out aneuploidy (Fig. 3-10). In a study of 49 patients with polyhydramnios, 6 fetuses demonstrated this triad, and all had trisomic karyotypes.[25] Three had trisomy 18, one had trisomy 13, and two had trisomy 21. The fetuses with trisomy 18 or 13 demonstrated classic clenched hands. Fetuses with trisomy 18 or 13 often have overlapping bones in their hands that never open and shut normally, but their arms still move and thus there is the ap-

pearance of bright spots on the ultrasound screen (Fig. 3-11). (This is different from movement disorder problems, such as arthrogryposis multiforme, which display a lack of the ability to move the arms and legs as well as the hands.) In addition, fetuses with trisomy 13 can have polydactyly and other anomalies. The anomalies seen in the fetuses in this study included ventricular septal defect, hydrocephalus with cleft lip and palate, and diaphragmatic hernia. The fetuses with trisomy 21 showed gastrointestinal atresia that accounted for the polyhydramnios. In addition, these fetuses with trisomy 21 and polyhydramnios had wide-open hands with sluggish closure of the fingers. Fetuses with this triad should have a rapid karyotype offered in the form of an invasive procedure such as umbilical blood sampling or placental biopsy. In the instances of normal fetal hand movement in which an anatomic lesion is seen, the fami-

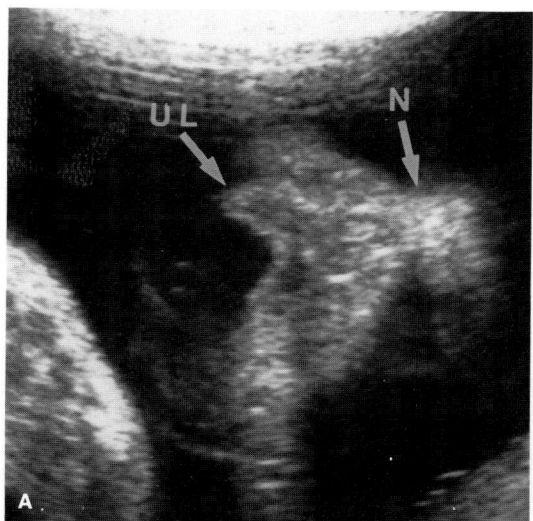

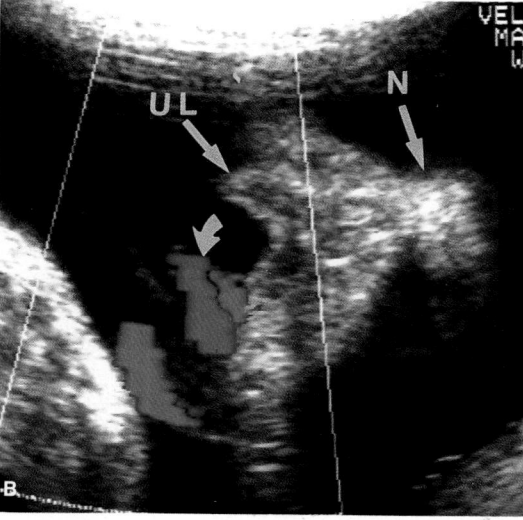

FIGURE 3-9. Fetal regurgitation. **(A)** Fetal face with mouth open and with explosive regurgitation secondary to bowel obstruction. **(B)** Fetal face with color flow Doppler demonstrating amniotic fluid exuding from mouth (*arrow*). N, nose; UL, upper lip.

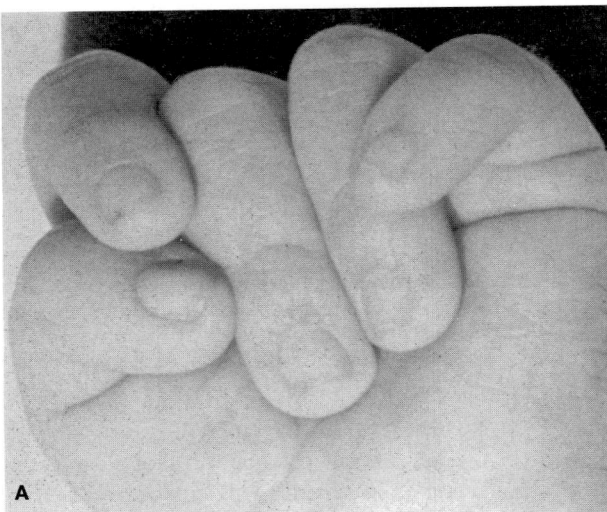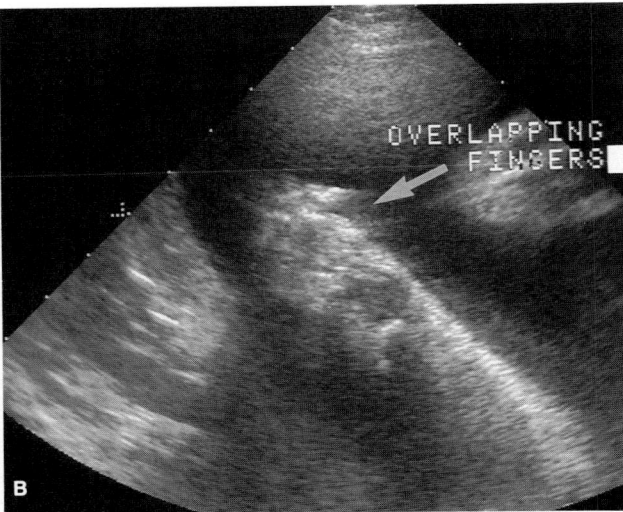

FIGURE 3-11.   Trisomy 18. **(A)** Typical overlapping fingers of trisomy 18. **(B)** Ultrasound showing bright spots of overlapping fingers in fetus with trisomy 18.

lies should still be offered karyotyping, although the urgency of the result can be tempered by the gestational age of the fetus. All fetuses with a structural abnormality should have chromosomal evaluation offered regardless of the amniotic fluid status.[26]

The controversy arises as to whether every patient who has polyhydramnios but no obvious anatomic abnormality in the fetus should be offered genetic karyotyping. The confidence of the ultrasonographer is paramount in this situation. If there is no lesion and the hands are moving normally, there is apparently little quantifiable increased risk for trisomy. The examination, however, must include the seven concerns listed previously and should stress echocardiography of the heart, excellent evaluation of the fetal brain, documented normal movement of the hands, and documented normal stomach and abdomen. If there is any uncertainty as to whether these structures have been adequately evaluated, the practitioner should error on the side of offering genetic amniocentesis.[27] Fetuses with Down's syndrome typically do not have polyhydramnios unless there is a physical abnormality that predisposes toward that condition, such as a bowel obstruction or a brain abnormality. The fetus with a lethal trisomy usually has obvious hand clenching and several anatomic abnormalities (see Fig. 3-11). If the examiner faithfully and carefully answers the seven questions listed previously, he or she will not miss the opportunity to diagnose a chromosomally abnormal fetus.

In addition, the thorough sonographer should always follow these two rules of accurate ultrasound diagnosis, particularly when faced with the challenge of polyhydramnios:

1. If a fetal structure is not seen to be clearly normal, it is abnormal until proved otherwise. Request another examiner to attempt to visualize the areas of interest you cannot. Sometimes maternal adipose, fetal position, or the increased distance from the probe to the fetus because of polyhydramnios makes clear visualization impossible.
2. If a fetal structure appears to be abnormal, it is. If possible, this presumed abnormality should be confirmed by a second examiner.

PREGNANCY AND A MASS

It has been estimated that close to 40% of all women have a uterine myoma sometime during their lives. Most fibroids are small and do not interfere with pregnancy. Some fibroids, however, may become large during pregnancy and undergo necrosis degeneration (Fig. 3-12). Also, fibroids present in the lower uterine segment may cause significant dystocia during labor. Thus, when the uterus is larger than expected, an ultrasound examination should be performed. This is helpful in documenting causes such as uterine fibroids.

Corpus luteal cysts are common during the first trimester of pregnancy. Usually, these enlarge to 5

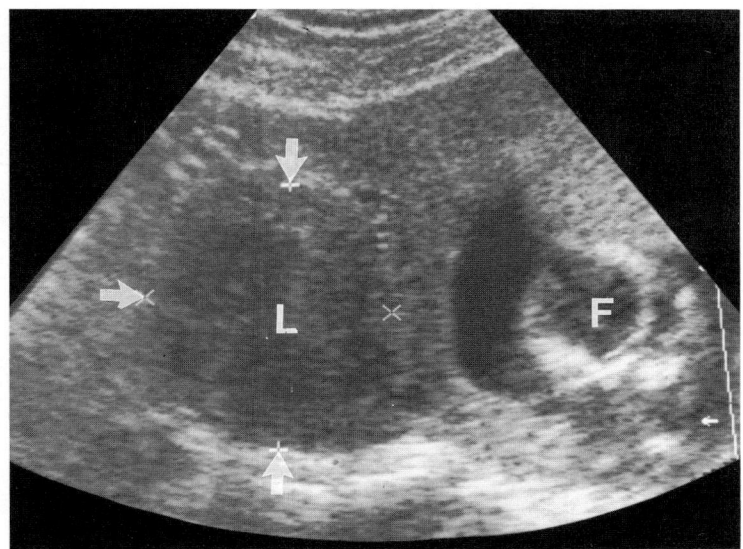

FIGURE 3-12. Pregnancy with leiomyoma. Transverse scan of the pregnant uterus demonstrates the fetus (F) and a uterine leiomyoma (L) located within the fundus of the uterus. This is another cause of large-for-dates. (Courtesy of John P. McGahan, MD, Sacramento, CA.)

to 6 cm and then spontaneously regress. Other ovarian or paraovarian masses, however, such as endometriosis or even ovarian tumors, may accompany pregnancy. Sonography may be helpful in detecting such abnormalities.[2,28]

REFERENCES

1. Jimenez JM, Tyson JE, Reisch JS: Clinical measures of gestational age in normal pregnancies. Obstet Gynecol 1983; 61:348.
2. McGahan JP, Osborn A: Sonographic evaluation of the large-for-dates pregnancy. Perinat Neonat 1985; 9:45–52.
3. Bowie JD, Andreotti RF: Estimating gestational age in utero. Radiol Clin North Am 1980; 20:325–334.
4. Levi S: Ultrasonic assessment of high rate of human multiple pregnancy in the first trimester. JCU 1976; 14:3–5.
5. Abrams B, Parker J: Overweight and pregnancy complications. Int J Obes 1988; 12:193.
6. Berk MA, Mimouni F, Miodovnik M, et al: Macrosomia in infants of insulin-dependent diabetic mothers. Pediatrics 1989; 83:1029.
7. Reece EA, Smikle C, O'Connor TZ, et al: A longitudinal study comparing growth in diabetic pregnancies with growth in normal gestations: 1. The fetal weight. Obstet Gynecol Surv 1990; 45:160.
8. Desmedt EJ, Henry OA, Beischer N: Polyhydramnios and associated maternal and fetal complications in singleton pregnancies. Br J Obstet Gynecol 1990; 97:1115.
9. Watson WJ, Seeds JW: Sonographic diagnosis of macrosomia. In Divon MY (ed): Abnormal Fetal Growth. New York: Elsevier, 1991: 233.
10. Wieacker P, Wilhelm C, Greiner P, Schillinger H: Prenatal diagnosis of Wiedemann-Beckwith syndrome. J Perinat Med 1989; 17:351.
11. Charon A, Gillerot Y, Van Maldergem LO, et al: The Marshall-Smith syndrome. Eur J Pediatr 1990; 150:54.
12. Ardinger HH, Hanson JW, Harrod MJ, et al: Further delineation of Weaver syndrome. J Pediatr 1986; 108:228.
13. Cole TR, Hughes HE: Sotos syndrome. J Med Genet 1990; 27:571.
14. DiLiberti JH: Correlation of skeletal muscle biopsy with phenotype in the familial macrocephaly syndromes. J Med Genet 1992; 29:46.
15. Schifrin BS, Guntres V, Gergely RC, et al: The role of real-time scanning in antenatal fetal surveillance. Am J Obstet Gynecol 1981; 140:525.
16. Ellis JW: Disorders of the umbilical cord, placenta, membranes and amniotic fluid. Curr Prob Obstet Gynecol 1981; 4:18.
17. Landy HJ, Isada NB, Larsen JW: Genetic implications of idiopathic hydramnios. Am J Obstet Gynecol 1987; 157:114.
18. Carlson DE, Platt LD, Medearis AL, Horenstein JM: Quantifiable polyhydramnios: Diagnosis and management. Obstet Gynecol 1990; 75:989.
19. Phelan JP, Smith CV, Broussard P, Small M: Amniotic fluid volume assessment with the four-quadrant technique at 36-42 weeks gestation. J Reprod Med 1987; 32:540.
20. Hoskins IA, McGovern PG, Ordorica SA, et al: Amniotic fluid index: Correlation with amniotic fluid volume. Am J Perinat 1992; 9:315.
21. Magann EF, Nolan TE, Hess LW, et al: Measurement of amniotic fluid volume: Accuracy of ultrasonography techniques. Am J Obstet Gynecol 1992; 167(6):1533.

22. Brady K, Polzin WJ, Kopelman JUN, Read JA: Risk of chromosomal abnormalities in patients with idiopathic polyhydramnios. Obstet Gynecol 1992; 79(2):234.

23. Aubrespy P, Derlon S, Seriat-Gautier B: Congenital duodenal obstruction: A review of 82 cases. Prog Pediatr Surg 1978; 11:109.

24. Otto CE, Platt LD: The fetal mandible measurement: An objective determination of fetal jaw size. Ultrasound Obstet Gynecol 1991; 1:12.

25. Carlson DE, Platt LD, Medearis AL: The ultrasound triad of fetal hydramnios, abnormal hand posturing and any other anomaly predict autosomal trisomy. Obstet Gynecol 1992; 72:731.

26. Platt LD, DeVore GR, Lopez E, et al: Role of amniocentesis in ultrasound-detected fetal malformations. Obstet Gynecol 1986; 68:153.

27. Stoll CG, Alembik Y, Dott B: Study of 156 cases of polyhydramnios and congenital malformations in a series of 118,265 consecutive births. Am J Obstet Gynecol 1991; 165(3):586.

28. McGahan JP, Phillips HE, Oi RH: Coexistent endometriomas in pregnancy: Sonographic appearance. JCU 1982; 10:180–182.

John P. McGahan and Manuel Porto:
DIAGNOSTIC OBSTETRICAL ULTRASOUND.
© 1994 J.B. Lippincott Company.

Michael Y. Divon   Itai Bar-Hava

Chapter 4

Fetal Surveillance: An Overview

The past 20 years have seen numerous advances in technology that have allowed the clinician indirect access to the fetus. The use of electronic fetal monitoring equipment allows for fetal heart rate (FHR) testing in the form of the nonstress test (NST) or the contraction stress test (CST). With the advent of real-time sonographic equipment, imaging of the fetus has become possible, allowing assessment of fetal biophysical activities in the form of the biophysical profile.

Common indications for antepartum fetal testing include: history of unexplained fetal death, decreased fetal movements, maternal chronic hypertension, preeclampsia, maternal diabetes mellitus, chronic renal disease, cyanotic heart disease, Rh or other isoimmunization, hemoglobinopathies, immunologic disorders, oligohydramnios or polyhydramnios, intrauterine growth retardation (IUGR), multiple gestation, postdate pregnancy, and premature rupture of the membranes.

CONTROL OF FETAL HEART RATE AND PHYSIOLOGY OF BIOPHYSICAL ACTIVITIES

Several investigators have suggested that late decelerations are the earliest sign of fetal hypoxia and that this response occurs before changes in fetal blood pH, FHR baseline, variability, or reactivity. Similarly, late decelerations appear before accelerations disappear. Fetal pH is normal when late decelerations are first detected, and FHR accelerations disappear only after further hypoxemia occurs.[1,2] The sensitivity of a specific area in the central nervous system to hypoxia is unknown. A gradual hypoxia concept has been proposed: the biophysical activities that appear first in fetal development are relatively more resistant to hypoxia than activities controlled by central nervous system areas, which mature later and require more oxygen for growth.[3] According to this concept, severe fetal asphyxia is associated with cessation of all biophysical activities, while milder hypoxia initially would result in the loss of FHR reactivity and fetal breathing movements (Table 4-1).

Hypoxia is not the only factor that modifies fetal biophysical activities. Drugs that depress central nervous system activity affect all the variables listed previously except late decelerations. Fetal breathing is stimulated by hyperglycemia and is significantly decreased a few days before spontaneous labor.[4]

FHR decelerations commonly are seen with hypertonic uterine contractions, supine hypotension, oligohydramnios, and other conditions resulting in excessive pressure or occlusion of the umbilical cord.

TABLE 4-1. Fetal Central Nervous System Centers

Center	Activity		
Cortex	Fetal tone		↑
Cortex, nuclei	Fetal movements		
Ventral surface of 4th ventricle	Fetal breathing movements	Embryogenesis	Hypoxia
Posterior hypothalamus, medulla	Nonstress test	↓	

Because the FHR reactivity center matures at about 26 to 28 weeks of gestation, extreme prematurity should be considered when evaluating FHR responses to hypoxia. Several studies have demonstrated that some healthy fetuses may have minimal FHR accelerations even before 26 weeks' gestation. After 33 weeks' gestation, however, FHR reactivity is not significantly different than in the term fetus.

The presence of normal biophysical activities indicates an intact, functioning, and nonhypoxic central nervous system. The absence of a given activity, however, commonly presents a clinical dilemma. This may represent benign conditions, such as physiologic fetal quiet sleep and prematurity, or it may be a manifestation of congenital anomalies or central nervous system depression induced by maternal medication. The challenge exists in distinguishing the absence of a biophysical activity due to quiet sleep from that attributable to fetal asphyxia. Recent studies have shown that human fetal activity is strongly correlated to behavioral states. Fetal breathing movements, gross fetal body movements, and FHR reactivity occur in episodes lasting 20 to 60 minutes every 60 to 90 minutes. Thus, the most common cause of an absent fetal biophysical activity is a period of fetal quiet sleep.

NONSTRESS TEST

The NST is based on the premise that a healthy (nonasphyxiated) fetus demonstrates fetal movements at varying intervals and that these movements are associated with a reflex increase in the FHR. The technique is as follows:

1. The patient is placed in semi-Fowler's or lateral recumbent position.
2. Blood pressure measurements are taken every 10 minutes.
3. With the use of an event marker, any fetal movement is marked on the tracing.

4. Good-quality FHR and uterine activity are monitored for 20 to 40 minutes.

The following set of criteria for interpretation is one of several used successfully at various fetal testing centers:

Reactive NST:
- Normal FHR baseline (110–160 beats/min)
- At least two FHR accelerations in 20 minutes (*accelerations* defined as an increase of at least 15 beats/min above the baseline lasting at least 15 seconds), associated with fetal movements

Nonreactive NST:
- No FHR accelerations noted
- Baseline FHR outside or within the normal range

Uncertain reactivity:
- Fewer than two FHR accelerations in a 20-minute period
- FHR baseline abnormalities (eg, bradycardia, tachycardia, late or variable decelerations)

A reactive NST is associated with fetal survival for 1 week in 98% of cases. A nonreactive NST is associated with poor fetal outcome in only 20% of cases (ie, high false-positive rate).

The main advantage of the NST over other fetal testing modalities is its simplicity. Other benefits are that it is brief (20–40 minutes), is relatively inexpensive, lacks contraindications, is easy to interpret, and is available as an office or outpatient procedure.

The NST is an extremely useful screening technique in the management of high-risk pregnancies. Its high false-positive rate (ie, nonreactive NST in a nonasphyxiated fetus), however, necessitates additional testing before intervention. Additionally, false-negative tests (ie, reactive NST with poor fetal outcome) detected in some diabetic, postdate, and IUGR fetuses probably warrants twice-weekly testing in these patients.

OXYGEN CHALLENGE OR CONTRACTION STRESS TEST

The oxygen challenge test (OCT), or CST, is based on the premise that placental perfusion is normally decreased during uterine contractions. A decrease in fetal PO_2 accompanies, but lags behind, the uterine contraction. A healthy (well-oxygenated) fetus is unaffected by this decrease in PO_2; however, if fetal PO_2 is below normal, the additional decrease caused by contractions may result in fetal hypoxia and FHR late decelerations. The technique is as follows:

1. The patient is placed in semi-Fowler's or left lateral tilt position.
2. Blood pressure is measured every 10 minutes.
3. At least a 10-minute tracing of baseline FHR and uterine contractions is obtained.
4. When three spontaneous uterine contractions are detected during the baseline recording, the test is complete. Otherwise, oxytocin administration (or nipple stimulation) is begun until three uterine contractions occur in 10 minutes.
5. If late decelerations occur with each contraction, the test is positive before obtaining three contractions in a 10-minute period.
6. After the establishment of three contractions per 10 minutes, the oxytocin is discontinued, and the patient is monitored until uterine contractions have ceased.

This test is interpreted as follows:

Negative OCT: normal baseline FHR with absence of late decelerations

Positive OCT: persistent late decelerations (with at least half of uterine contractions)

Suspicious OCT: intermittent late decelerations, variable decelerations, or abnormal baseline FHR (less than 110 beats/min or more than 160 beats/min)

Hyperstimulation OCT: late decelerations or abnormal baseline FHR associated with excessive uterine activity (ie, duration of contractions more than 90 seconds or frequency of contractions more than 5 in 10 minutes)

Unsatisfactory OCT: poor-quality FHR tracing or inability to stimulate three contractions per 10 minutes

A negative OCT is highly indicative of good fetal health (1 week survival in about 99% of cases). A positive OCT is associated with poor fetal outcome in about half of cases. A positive-reactive test (late decelerations in the presence of accelerations) is prognostically better than a positive test with decreased baseline FHR variability.

Relative contraindications to the OCT are the following:

- Risk for preterm delivery (eg, patients with incompetent cervix, premature rupture of membranes, twins, polyhydramnios)

TABLE 4-2. Biophysical Profile Scoring: Techniques and Interpretation

Biophysical Profile	Normal (Score = 2)	Abnormal (Score = 0)
FBM	At least one episode of 30 seconds duration in 30 minutes	Absent FBM or no episode of >30 seconds in 30 minutes
Gross body movements	At least three discrete body or limb movements in 30 minutes (episodes of active continuous movements considered a single movement)	Two or fewer episodes of body or limb movements in 30 minutes
Fetal tone	At least one episode of active extension with return to flexion of fetal limbs, spine, or trunk. Opening and closing of hand considered normal tone.	Slow extension with return to partial flexion, movement of limb in full extension, or absent fetal movements
Reactive FHR	At least two episodes of FHR accelerations of >15 beats/min and of at least 15 seconds' duration associated with fetal movement in 30 minutes	Less than two episodes of acceleration of FHR or acceleration of <15 beats/min in 30 minutes
Qualitative AFV	At least one pocket of AF that measures at least 2 cm in two perpendicular planes	No AF pocket of 2 cm in two perpendicular planes

FBM, fetal breathing movements; FHR, fetal heart rate; AFV, amniotic fluid volume; AF, amniotic fluid.

TABLE 4-3.   Biophysical Profile Scoring: Management Protocol

Score	Interpretation	Management
10	Normal infant, low risk for chronic asphyxia	Repeat testing at weekly intervals. Repeat twice weekly in patients with diabetes, IUGR, and >41 weeks' gestation.
8	Normal infant, low risk for chronic asphyxia	Repeat testing at weekly intervals. Repeat testing twice weekly in patients with diabetes, IUGR, and >41 weeks' gestation. Oligohydramnios may be an indication for delivery, depending on gestational age.
6	Suspect chronic asphyxia	Repeat testing in 4–6 hours. Delivery is recommended if oligohydramnios is present >36 weeks.
4	Suspect chronic asphyxia	If >36 weeks with favorable cervix, delivery is recommended. If <36 weeks and L/S ≤2, repeat test in 24 hours. If repeat score ≥4, delivery is recommended.
0–2	Strong suspicion of chronic asphyxia	Extend testing time to 120 minutes. If persistent score <4, delivery is recommended regardless of gestational age.

L/S, amniotic fluid lecithin : sphinogmyelin; IUGR, intrauterine growth retardation.

- Placenta previa
- Previous classic cesarean section

FETAL BIOPHYSICAL PROFILE

Various fetal biophysical activities can be evaluated with the use of real-time sonography. These include gross body movements, breathing movements, and tone. Real-time sonography also allows for evaluation of the intrauterine environment for variables such as the amount of amniotic fluid and blood flow. An acute insult to the fetus may result in decreased fetal body and breathing movements, a nonreactive NST, and decreased fetal tone. If the insult is sustained (ie, chronic asphyxia), oligohydramnios may develop.[5,6]

Observation of multiple fetal biophysical activities has been suggested as a clinical tool to differentiate the asphyxiated fetus from the sleeping fetus[7] (Table 4-2). Table 4-3 delineates a management protocol.[7] There are no known contraindications to fetal biophysical testing. The NST is the primary test commonly used in most centers. Biophysical profile scoring or the OCT/CST is used as a backup test for a nonreactive NST. Increasing the frequency of NST to twice weekly resulted in a corrected stillbirth rate of 1.9/1000 after a reactive test. Thus, it is recommended that an NST be performed twice a week on all postdate, diabetic, and IUGR patients.

Patient management is often dictated by the amount of amniotic fluid (postdate and IUGR patients). The detection of fetal anomalies combined with the ability to evaluate the amount of amniotic fluid are frequently stated as advantages of the biophysical profile over additional FHR testing in the form of OCT/CST.

REFERENCES

1. Martin CB, De Haan J, Van der Wildt B, et al: Mechanisms of late decelerations in the fetal heart rate: A study with autonomic blocking agents in fetal lamb. Eur J Obstet Gynaecol Reprod Biol 1979; 9:361–373.
2. Murata Y, Martin CB Jr, Ikenoue T, et al: Fetal heart rate accelerations and late decelerations during the course of intrauterine death in chronically catheterized rhesus monkeys. Am J Obstet Gynecol 1982; 144:218–223.
3. Vintzileous, AM, Campbell WA, Ingardia CJ, et al: The fetal biophysical profile and its predictive value. Obstet Gynecol 1983; 62:271.
4. Patrick J, Campbell K, Carmichael L, et al: Patterns of human fetal breathing during the last 10 weeks of pregnancy. Obstet Gynecol 1980; 56:24–30.
5. Ott WJ: The current status of intrapartum fetal monitoring. Obstet Gynecol Surv 1976; 31:339–364.
6. Manning FA, Morrison I, Harman CR, et al: Fetal assessment based on fetal biophysical profile scoring: Experience in 19,221 referred high-risk pregnancies. II. An analysis of false-negative fetal deaths. Am J Obstet Gynecol 1987; 157:880–884.
7. Brar HS, Platt LD, Devore GR: Antepartum fetal surveillance: The biophysical profile. Clin Obstet Gynecol 1987; 30:936–947.

John P. McGahan and Manuel Porto:
DIAGNOSTIC OBSTETRICAL ULTRASOUND.
© 1994 J.B. Lippincott Company.

Michael Y. Divon   Raphael Boldes   John P. McGahan

Chapter 5

Assessment of Intrauterine Growth Retardation

RISK

Intrauterine growth retardation (IUGR) is associated with an increased incidence of neonatal mortality and morbidity.[1] Relative to infants with normal growth, IUGR is associated with a higher incidence of perinatal mortality, low Apgar scores, perinatal asphyxia, hypothermia, polycythemia, hypocalcemia, pulmonary hemorrhage, and impaired immune function.[2] Because interference with fetal growth may also influence brain development, one may expect to detect an association between fetal growth retardation and subsequent neurologic handicap. The purpose of this chapter is to review ultrasound methods of assessment of abnormal fetal growth, to present conclusions regarding these methods, and to present methods of logical assessment of these high-risk pregnancies.

DEFINITION AND CLASSIFICATION

Intrauterine growth is determined by comparing the actual size of the newborn to an expected norm for gestational age. Because birthweight is the most accessible and reliable measure of the newborn, it is the most commonly used indicator of fetal growth.

Fetal size and fetal growth, however, are often confused in clinical practice. *IUGR* denotes a pathologic process stemming from growth restriction. In contrast, *small for gestational age* (SGA) identifies the infant whose birthweight is below an arbitrary percentile for gestational age. The 10th percentile is most widely used for this purpose. Using birthweight criteria as the gold standard for intrauterine growth, however, presents a few problems.[3] SGA fetuses thus fall into three categories (Table 5-1). Most SGA fetuses are otherwise normal. These fetuses are not at risk for the sequelae of IUGR. The second group includes fetuses who are growth retarded owing to factors intrinsic to the fetus; this group often is classified as *symmetric growth-retarded fetuses* (Table 5-2). These fetuses have an insult that is fixed at the time of detection and in most cases is irreversible. This group includes those with chromosomal abnormalities, structural defects, or an early intrauterine insult from infection or drugs. They usually have a fixed defect that will not benefit from early delivery. The

TABLE 5-1. Classification of Small-for-Gestational-Age Fetuses

Type	Description
I	Constitutionally small fetuses (not at risk for intrauterine growth retardation)
II	Growth retarded (intrinsic to fetus)
III	Growth retarded (extrinsic to fetus)

third group includes those fetuses affected by extrinsic abnormalities such as maternal hypertension, placental infarct, or placental insufficiency; they often are classified as *asymmetric growth-retarded fetuses*. These fetuses, in theory, will benefit from detection and therapy, such as early delivery, to allow them to escape from a "hostile" environment. There may be an overlap between the second and third groups, which is explained in the next section in more detail.

SYMMETRIC VERSUS ASYMMETRIC

Growth and symmetry are affected by the nature and severity of the underlying growth restrictive process as well as by its timing and duration. In 1963, Gruenwald identified two distinct patterns of diminished growth: symmetric and asymmetric.[4] Early-phase growth disturbance (typically first-trimester and early second-trimester) often culminates in symmetric growth retardation. Because growth in this phase is primarily due to cell hyperplasia, restriction of growth results in a lower cell count. Thus, the newborn is symmetrically small (ie, concomitant decrease in the size of the head, trunk, length, and all other body organs). This pattern is often seen in growth disturbance associated

TABLE 5-2. Causes of IUGR

Intrinsic Factors
Chromosomal abnormalities
Congenital structural defects
Infection
Drugs and medications

Extrinsic Factors
Maternal disease
Placental abnormalities
Uterine anomalies

with chromosomal anomalies, congenital malformations, and transplacental infections (see Table 5-2). In the asymmetric type, the growth rate of the trunk is smaller than that of other organs. This is caused by relative depletion of the actively growing liver combined with decreased subcutaneous fat deposition. Third-trimester growth abnormalities, such as those seen with extrinsic factors, restrict growth during the hypertrophic growth phase (see Table 5-2). Due to preferential perfusion of the brain, the asymmetrically growth-retarded newborn may be identified by an abnormally increased head circumference (HC)/abdominal circumference (AC) ratio.

These symmetric and asymmetric patterns may merge and become indistinguishable. A maternal vascular disease beginning early in pregnancy may cause symmetric growth retardation. Likewise, an asymmetrically growth-retarded fetus may become symmetric once brain sparring or linear growth is no longer maintained. This phenomenon has been identified as *late flattening of the biparietal diameter (BPD)* and is associated with increased neonatal morbidity. It is commonly believed that placental insufficiency results in asymmetric growth retardation, whereas chromosomal abnormalities are associated with symmetric IUGR. Recent data presented by Nicolaides and colleagues indicate, however, that some fetal genetic diseases may be associated with severe asymmetric growth.[5] Thus, there may be considerable overlap between symmetric and asymmetric IUGR.

CLINICAL DIAGNOSIS

Screening for IUGR by serial fundal height and maternal weight gain assessment should be performed routinely during prenatal care. Decreased fundal height may be associated with IUGR in as many as half of IUGR pregnancies.[6] Clinical risk assessment does not, however, appear adequately and consistently to predict IUGR (Table 5-3). Fur-

TABLE 5-3. Risk Factors for IUGR

Decreased fundal height
Previous delivery of growth-retarded infant
Cigarette smoking
Poor maternal weight gain
Prepregnancy maternal underweight
Maternal low birthweight
Lack of prenatal care

TABLE 5-4.   Criteria Proposed for the Sonographic Diagnosis of IUGR

General Description	Specific Application
Small BPD	BPD < 5th percentile
	BPD < 25th percentile
	BPD < 10th percentile, third trimester
	BPD < 10th percentile, GA 18–21 wk
	BPD ≤ 87 mm, GA > 34 wk
Slow rate of BPD growth on serial scans	> 1 SD below mean
	> 2 SD below mean
Advanced placental grade	Grade 3
Elevated FL/AC	> 23.5%
	> 24%
Small BPD and advanced placental grade	BPD ≤ 87 mm; grade 3
Decreased AFV	No pocket > 1 cm
	Subjective oligohydramnios
Low TIUV	> 1 SD below mean
	> 1.5 SD below mean
	< 10th percentile, GA based on LMP
	< 10th percentile, GA based on BPD
Low EFW	> 1.5 SD below mean
Elevated HC/AC	> 95th percentile
	> 2 SD above mean for *all* exams

BPD, biparietal diameter; FL/AC, fetal length/abdominal circumference ratio; AFV, amniotic fluid volume; TIUV, total intrauterine volume; EFW, estimated fetal weight; HC/AC, head circumference/abdominal circumference ratio; GA, gestational age; LMP, last menstrual period.

(Benson CB, Doubilet PM, Saltzman DH: Intrauterine growth retardation: Predictive value of US criteria for antenatal diagnosis. Radiology 1986; 160:415–417.)

ther evaluation by sonographic assessment should be offered to patients with risk factors and a high index of suspicion for development of this disease.

ULTRASOUND ASSESSMENT

Ultrasound is the only direct method available for assessing fetal size. It also provides for an assessment of factors associated with IUGR, such as fetal anomalies, oligohydramnios, and increased placental impedance. A thorough evaluation should include a detailed study of fetal, umbilical, and placental structural abnormalities. Measurement of the BPD, HC, AC, femur length (FL), and amniotic fluid volume as well as other measurements have been used to predict IUGR[7,8] (Table 5-4). Morphometric ratios such as the HC/AC ratio and the FL/AC ratio, as well as a sonographic estimate of fetal weight, can then be derived from these measurements. Sensitivities, specificities, and positive and negative predictive values from a number of studies, as summarized by Benson, are presented in Table 5-5.[7,8]

Umbilical arterial Doppler velocity studies provide data regarding placental impedance and may

be useful in patients who are at increased risk of IUGR.[9] A number of different criteria have been proposed for diagnosis of IUGR using Doppler (Table 5-6). The sensitivity, specificity, and positive and negative predictive value for some of these Doppler measurements, as summarized by Benson, are presented in Table 5-7.[9]

Biparietal Diameter

Several studies have evaluated the ability of both single and serial BPD measurements to identify IUGR.[10] The results vary widely, and these measurements may not identify asymmetric IUGR. Therefore, their main utility is in identifying the symmetrically small fetus.

Femur Length

A strong positive correlation between fetal FL and neonatal crown-to-heel length has been demonstrated.[11] The experience with this measurement as an independent predictor of IUGR is limited. O'Brien and Queenan showed that FL helps differentiate between symmetric and asymmetric patterns of growth retardation.[12] Overall, both the

TABLE 5-5.   Value of Sonographic Criteria in Detecting IUGR

Criterion	Sensitivity (%)	Specificity* (%)	Predictive Value* Positive (%)	Negative (%)
Advanced placental grade	62	64	16	94
Elevated FL/AC	34–49	78–83	18–20	92–93
Low TIUV	57–80	72–76	21–24	92–97
Small BPD	24–88	62–94	21–44	92–98
Small BPD and advanced placental grade	59	86	32	95
Slow rate of BPD growth	75	84	35	97
Low EFW	89	88	45	99
Decreased AFV	24	98	55	92
Elevated HC/AC	82	94	62	98

* A range of values is given for a criterion when different studies apply that criterion in two or more ways.
For abbreviations, see Table 5-4.
(Benson CB, Doubilet PM, Saltzman DH: Intrauterine growth retardation: Predictive value of US criteria for antenatal diagnosis. Radiology 1986; 160:415–417.)

size of the fetal head and length of the femur are affected late in most cases of IUGR; therefore, these measurements are relatively insensitive and are seldom used as independent predictors of IUGR.

Abdominal Circumference

Measurement of the fetal AC is commonly used for identification of the growth-retarded fetus. This measurement reflects the size of the liver (which correlates with the degree of fetal malnutrition) as well as the volume of subcutaneous fat. In addition, the AC is decreased in both symmetric and asymmetric growth retardation. Therefore, it is not surprising that sonographic measurements of the AC predict growth retardation more accurately than either the BPD or the FL. In a large study of 3616 sonographically dated pregnancies, Warsof and colleagues showed that AC measurements predict IUGR with a sensitivity of 61%, specificity of 95%, true-positive rate of 86%, and true-negative rate of 83%.[13] Similarly, other investigators reported relatively high positive predictive values for this measurement (range, 84%–100%).[14-16] Accurate pregnancy dating is essential for the interpretation of AC measurements. Uncertainty about gestational age occurs frequently, however, and makes the differentiation between the appropriate-for-gestational-age and the growth-retarded fetus difficult. Because growth of the fetal abdomen is linear from 15 weeks of gestation onward, determi-

nation of the rate of growth offers a gestational age–independent parameter for identifying the IUGR fetus. Divon and colleagues found a significant difference in the rate of growth of the fetal AC between IUGR fetuses and fetuses that were appropriate for gestational age.[17] They found that an increase in fetal AC of less than 10 mm per 14 days has a sensitivity of 85% in identifying the IUGR fetus, especially when gestational age is uncertain.

Morphometric Ratios

The comparison of growth in some body organs relative to others has led to the development of a number of sonographically derived morphometric ratios. These ratios are useful in the diagnosis of asymmetric IUGR, in which the AC is smaller than expected when compared with either the size of the head or the length of the femur. Consequently, abnormally elevated FL/AC or HC/AC ratios aid in the identification of the asymmetrically growth-retarded fetus. Kurjak and colleagues correctly identified 80% of growth-retarded fetuses with the use of the HC/AC ratio.[15] In contrast, Divon and colleagues applied this ratio to a population of IUGR fetuses of mixed causes and reported a relatively low sensitivity of 36%, with specificity of 90%, positive predictive value of 67%, and negative predictive value of 72%.[18]

Hadlock and colleagues reported on the use of the FL/AC ratio as a gestational age–independent index of fetal growth.[16] From 21 weeks' gestation

TABLE 5-6. Criteria Proposed for Diagnosis of IUGR Using Doppler

I. Arterial waveform criteria
  A. Umbilical artery
      S/D ratio > 95th percentile*
      S/D ratio > 3
      S/D ratio > 2 SD above mean
      S/D ratio > 1 SD above mean
      S/D ratio − regression with GA
      PI > 2 SD above mean*
      PI > 3 SD above mean
      PoI > 2 SD above mean
      ImI > 2 SD above mean
      Relative flow rate index > 1 SD above mean
      Decay time > 1 SD above mean
      Absent or reversed diastolic flow*
  B. Uterine arcuate artery
      S/D ratio > 95th percentile*
      D/S ratio < 5th percentile*
      RI > 2 SD above mean (≥ 0.58)*
      Frequency index profile > 2 SD above mean*
  C. Fetal descending thoracic aorta
      Absent diastolic flow*
      PI > 2 SD above mean
  D. Fetal internal carotid artery
      PI > 2 SD below mean*
  E. Combined umbilical and uterine arcuate arteries
      Umbilical artery S/D > 95th percentile *and* uterine arcuate artery D/S < 5th percentile*
      Umbilical artery S/D > 95th percentile *or* uterine arcuate artery D/S < 5th percentile*
II. Volume blood flow criteria
  A. Umbilical vein
      < 10th percentile*
      Two successive readings < 10th percentile*
      Total flow deficit

* Criteria for which sensitivity and specificity can be determined from the literature. Many of the standard deviations, means, and percentiles refer to values adjusted for gestational age.

SD, standard deviation; S/D, systolic/diastolic ratio; PI, pulsatility index; PoI, Pourcelot index; ImI, impedance index; D/S, diastolic/systolic ratio; RI, resistance index.

(Benson CB, Doubilet PM: Doppler criteria for intrauterine growth retardation: Predictive values. J Ultrasound Med 1988; 7:655–659.)

to term, the normally grown fetus has an FL/AC of about 22% (± 2% standard deviation). An FL/AC of more than 23.5% was associated with a sensitivity of 60% and a specificity of 90% for identification of the growth retarded fetus. Similarly, Divon and colleagues reported a sensitivity of 55% for the same cut-off value and concluded that this parameter is useful in differentiating between the fetus demonstrating appropriate growth and the growth-retarded fetus when gestational age is uncertain.[17]

Birthweight

The most commonly used definition of IUGR is a birthweight less than the 10th percentile for gestational age. Therefore, it is reasonable to use sonographic estimation of fetal weight to diagnose IUGR in the antenatal period. Various equations that incorporate different variables (ie, BPD, HC, AC, and FL) have been proposed in an attempt to accurately estimate the fetal weight.[19] In general, these estimates are associated with a mean absolute error of about 7% to 10%. Several investigators evaluated the ability of fetal weight estimates to identify the fetus with growth retardation. Divon and colleagues estimated fetal weight using Hadlock's formula based on BPD and AC and reported a sensitivity and specificity of 87%, positive predictive value of 78%, and negative predictive value of 92% for estimated fetal weight less than the 10th percentile for gestational age.[18] Compared with other indices used to detect IUGR, such as HC/AC, FL/AC, amniotic fluid volume, and Doppler velocimetry, the best predictor appeared to be an estimated fetal weight of less than the 10th percentile.

Amniotic Fluid

Decreased amniotic fluid (oligohydramnios) has long been recognized as a complication of fetal growth retardation. This is probably caused by decreased urination secondary to decreased renal perfusion reflecting redistribution of blood flow from nonvital to vital organs. Manning and associates used real-time sonography to qualitatively assess amniotic fluid volume in 120 pregnancies in which fetal growth retardation was suspected.[20] Defining oligohydramnios as the largest vertical pocket of fluid measuring less than 1 cm, they reported a sensitivity of 84%, specificity of 97%, positive predictive value of 90%, and negative predictive value of 95%. Other investigators, however, did not confirm these results. Divon and colleagues evaluated 127 patients referred with a clinical suspicion of IUGR.[18] Oligohydramnios was defined by the vertical dimension of the largest pocket of fluid measuring less than 2 cm. They reported a sensitivity of only 16% and a specificity of 98%. The low sensitivity and high specificity of amniotic fluid volume as an indicator of IUGR have also been reported by others.[21–23]

The presence of oligohydramnios assumes increased importance when gestational age is questionable. If oligohydramnios is present in the absence of ruptured membranes, congenital anom-

TABLE 5-7. Doppler Criteria for IUGR: Performance Characteristics*

Criterion	Sensitivity (%)	Specificity (%)	Predictive Values + (%)	Predictive Values − (%)
I. Vessels studied by at least two groups				
A. Uterine arcuate artery				
RI ≥ 0.58	67	64	17	94
S/D ratio > 95th percentile	34	88	24	92
D/S ratio < 5th percentile	60	80	25	95
FIP > 2 SD above mean	57	89	37	95
B. Umbilical vein				
Flow < 10th percentile	71	79	28	96
Low flow on two successive readings	73	89	42	97
C. Umbilical artery				
S/D ratio > 95th percentile	68	85	34	96
S/D ratio > 3	78	83	34	97
Absent or reversed diastolic flow	37	93	39	93
PI > 2 SD above mean	93	91	54	99
D. Umbilical artery and uterine artery				
One or both abnormal	80	29	11	93
Both abnormal	36	97	57	93
II. Vessels studied by one group				
A. Fetal internal carotid artery				
B. Fetal aorta PI > 2 SD below mean	89	95	66	99
Absent diastolic flow	45	100	100	94

RI, resistive index; S/D, systolic/diastolic ratio; D/S, diastolic/systolic ratio; PI, pulsatility index; FIP, frequency index profile.
(Benson CB, Doubilet PM: Doppler criteria for intrauterine growth retardation: Predictive values. J Ultrasound Med 1988; 7:655–659.)

alies, or post-date fetuses, then IUGR is the most likely explanation. In such patients, the presence of oligohydramnios can be considered a gestational age–independent predictor of IUGR.

Other Measurements

Reece and associates reported that the growth of the *fetal cerebellum* is unaffected by IUGR.[24] They measured the transverse cerebellar diameter in 19 IUGR fetuses with good dates. This measurement was consistently predictive of gestational age, whereas most of the other sonographic measurements were smaller than expected. The authors suggested that this sonographic measurement can serve as a reliable predictor of gestational age in growth-retarded fetuses. In a subsequent study, Lee and associates studied 19 IUGR fetuses and concluded that the transverse cerebellar diameter is a useful predictor of gestational age in fetuses with asymmetric growth retardation.[25] They ad-

vised caution, however, when using this measurement to predict gestational age in symmetrically growth-retarded fetuses.

A variety of other suggestions for diagnosing IUGR have been reported in recent years. These include *placental grading, thigh and calf circumferences,* and *thoracic to abdominal circumference ratios.* Although some of these concepts appear promising, they must be confirmed by additional studies.

DOPPLER VELOCIMETRY

Normal fetal growth is determined by multiple maternal and fetal variables. Continuous blood flow on either side of the placenta and adequate fetal perfusion are obviously an absolute necessity. Indeed, fetal growth retardation is associated with various abnormalities of the uteroplacental, umbilical, and fetal circulations.[26,27]

Uterine Artery

On the maternal side, some evidence suggests that changes in the uterine artery velocity waveforms (arcuate arteries) may be detected as early as the second trimester in some pregnancies that eventually develop IUGR, preeclampsia, or fetal death.[28] Other investigators also reported that in some cases of IUGR, abnormal uterine perfusion may be the first sign of a developing disease process.[29,30] In contrast, Newnham and colleagues evaluated uteroplacental blood flow at 14, 18, 24, 28, and 34 weeks of gestation and reported that abnormal waveforms were significantly correlated with the future development of fetal hypoxia but were not predictive of subsequent development of IUGR.[31] Both Chambers and colleagues[14] and Jacobson and associates[32] concluded that Doppler studies of the uteroplacental perfusion are of limited clinical value owing to their poor sensitivity and high false-positive rate.

Umbilical Artery and Descending Aorta

On the fetal side, many studies reported a significant decrease in end-diastolic flow of the umbilical artery and the descending aorta of the growth-retarded fetus.[27] These studies indicate that some forms of IUGR may result from *placental insufficiency,* with increased placental impedance reflecting a decrease in the number of intraplacental arterial channels.[33,34] A decreased pulsatility index in the internal carotid arteries reported in some of these fetuses reflects enhanced perfusion of the brain and probably indicates redistribution of blood flow, resulting in the brain-sparring effect.[35]

Trudinger and associates recently reported on 2178 high-risk pregnant patients in whom umbilical artery velocity waveforms were evaluated.[36] The incidence of IUGR (birthweight less than the 10th percentile) in this population was 27%; half of these IUGR fetuses had an abnormal (more than the 95th percentile) umbilical arterial systolic/diastolic (S/D) ratio. Based on their large study population, these authors concluded that "in high risk pregnancy Doppler umbilical artery flow velocity waveforms predict the most compromised fetuses in terms of growth retardation and requirement for neonatal intensive care."

The combined use of Doppler velocity with real-time ultrasound for the diagnosis of IUGR was reported by Divon and colleagues.[18] These authors concluded that neither sonographic nor Doppler tests were uniformly successful in identifying the growth-retarded infant. Overall, the best predic-

TABLE 5-8.   Umbilical Artery Flow Systolic/Diastolic Ratio*

Weeks	Mean	Upper Limit
24	3.5	4.25
25	3.4	4.1
26	3.3	3.9
27	3.2	3.75
28	3.1	3.7
29	3.0	3.6
30	2.9	3.5
31	2.85	3.45
32	2.8	3.4
33	2.7	3.3
34	2.6	3.15
35	2.55	3.1
36	2.45	3.0
37	2.4	2.9
38	2.35	2.8
39	2.3	2.65
40	2.2	2.5

* This table represents a composite of graphs found in a number of references.

Courtesy of James D. Bowie, MD, Duke University Medical Center, Durham, NC.

(Adapted from Hertzberg BS: Intrauterine growth retardation. In Rifkin MD, Charboneau JW, Laing FC [eds]: Syllabus Special Course: Ultrasound 1991. The Radiological Society of North America, December 1991: 147–158.)

tion was offered by sonographic estimates of fetal weight, which correctly identified 39 of 45 IUGR infants. An S/D ratio greater than 3 was seen in 49% of the IUGR fetuses. Similar results were reported by other authors.[14,37] Upper limits of umbilical arterial Doppler waveform utilizing S/D ratios throughout pregnancy are adapted from Hertzberg and presented in Table 5-8.[3] Reviewing other studies, however, it becomes obvious that a normal umbilical artery velocity waveform does not always guarantee ideal fetal outcome.[38]

Extreme forms of increased placental impedance are sometimes coupled with absent or reversed diastolic velocities (Figs. 5-1 and 5-2). This situation is clearly abnormal and is often associated with an abnormal karyotype, maternal hypertension, or severe fetal growth retardation.[39] Several studies described the ominous outcome found in fetuses with extremely abnormal umbilical artery velocity waveforms.[40–42] Due to high mortality rates of 50% to 90%, some authors suggest that an aggressive management protocol is justified.[43,44] Guidelines for the clinical management of the fetus with markedly diminished umbilical artery end-

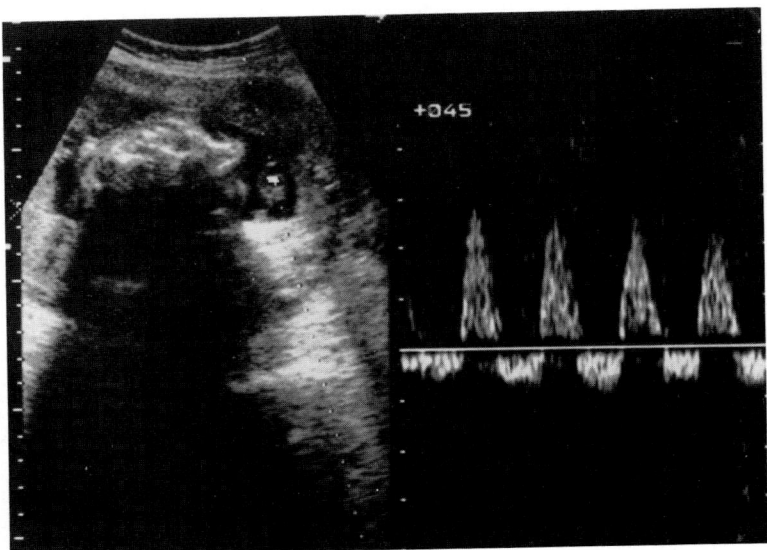

FIGURE 5-1. Reversed end-diastolic flow in a patient with decreased fetal movement and severe growth retardation at 30 weeks' gestation.

diastolic flow were suggested by Divon and colleagues.[45] Fifty-one fetuses with an S/D ratio of more than 2 standard deviations above the mean for gestational age were managed conservatively with intensive daily fetal monitoring (fetuses with congenital or chromosomal anomalies were excluded). Their results suggest that immediate delivery of the fetus with diminished end-diastolic flow may not be mandatory. These authors concluded that the combined use of fetal biophysical

testing with commonly used maternal and fetal indications for delivery results in acceptable fetal outcome and prolongation of gestational age.

It is possible to conclude from these studies that umbilical artery velocimetry is a rational test to perform when IUGR is suspected. It is useful in both establishing the diagnosis and determining the intensity of subsequent fetal surveillance. Its utility in screening the general population for IUGR, however, appears limited.

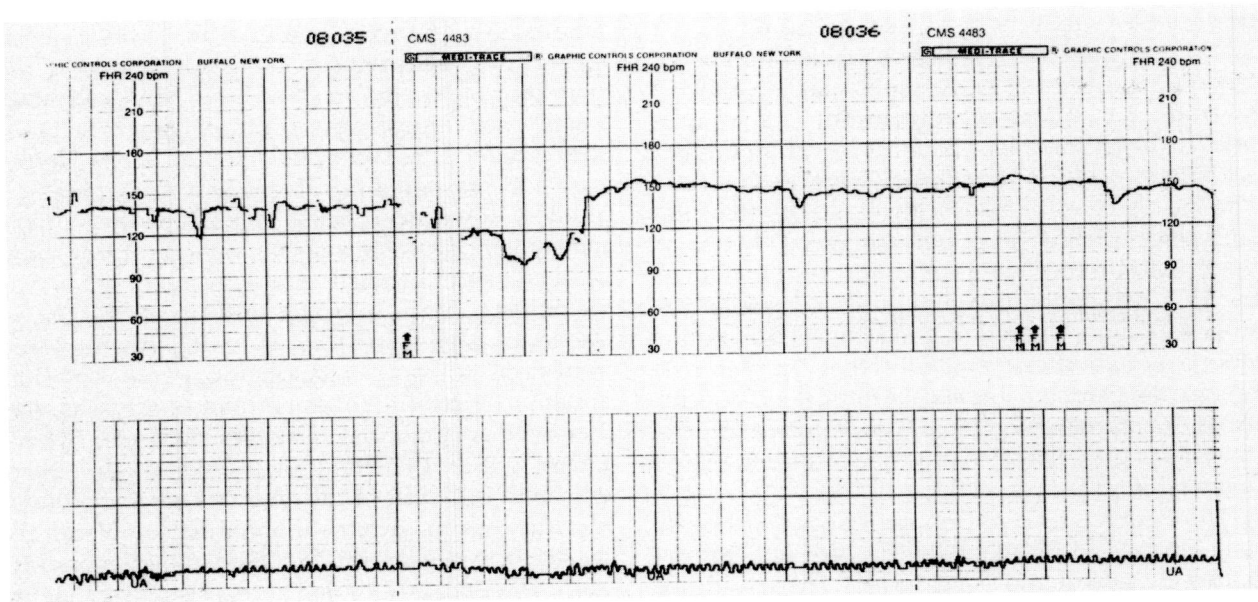

FIGURE 5-2. A nonreactive non-stress test with fetal heart rate decelerations obtained on the same fetus as in Figure 5-1.

TABLE 5-9.   Proposed Approach to Detect IUGR: Menstrual Age Established

I. Establish menstrual age
   A. Reliable history (in vitro fertilization)
   B. Ultrasound
      CRL in first trimester
      BPD + FL < 20 wk
      HC + FL > 20 wk (less reliable)
II. Compare menstrual age with abdominal circumference using lower 10th percentile (−1.28 SD (see Tables 5-11 and 5-12).
III. Compare menstrual age with weight using Shepard's formula and 5th percentile (see Table 5-13).

CRL, crown-to-rump length; BPD, biparietal diameter; FL, femur length; HC, head circumference.

(Adapted from Hertzberg BS: Intrauterine growth retardation. In Rifkin MD, Charboneau JW, Laing FC [eds]: Syllabus Special Course: Ultrasound 1991. The Radiological Society of North America, December, 1991: 147–158.)

ULTRASOUND ASSESSMENT: TWO APPROACHES

Two logical methods have been proposed for evaluating IUGR. One method was proposed by Hertzberg,[3] and the other is a multiparametric scoring system adapted from Benson.[7,8]

As proposed by Hertzberg, one of two approaches may be taken when evaluating IUGR, depending on whether maternal age can be reliably assessed[3] (Tables 5-9 and 5-10). Both these ap-

TABLE 5-10.   Proposed Approach to Detect IUGR: Menstrual Age Cannot Reliably Be Established

I. If menstrual age cannot be established, use age-independent ratios such as:
      FL/AC ratio
II. After initial ultrasound, repeat ultrasound every 2–3 wk to check for:
      Lag in growth of AC
      Lack of increase in fetal weight
III. Use other tests of fetal well-being, such as Doppler examination, biophysical profile, nonstress test, and contraction stress test.

FL, femur length; AC, abdominal circumference; HC, head circumference.

(Adapted from Hertzberg BS: Intrauterine growth retardation. In Rifkin MD, Charboneau JW, Laing FC [eds]: Syllabus Special Course: Ultrasound 1991. The Radiological Society of North America, December, 1991: 147–158.)

proaches are aimed at identifying the SGA fetus. If the menstrual age can be reliably obtained, the first approach, outlined in Table 5-9, can be followed. On the other hand, when the menstrual age cannot be reliably obtained, the second approach, outlined in Table 5-10, should be followed.

Both these approaches need further evaluation and testing by large population groups and other examiners to further assess their accuracy.

Method I: Established Menstrual Age[3]

Reliable menstrual age is obtained with convincing clinical history (eg, in vitro fertilization, artificial insemination, or accurate menstrual history consistent with early pelvic examination) or by an early ultrasound examination. Early ultrasound examination may be used to establish menstrual age in the first trimester by obtaining a crown-to-rump length. During the second trimester, a combination of the BPD and FL can be used before 20 weeks. After 20 weeks, a combination of the HC and the FL may be used; however, the accuracy of sonographic determination of gestational age decreases as the pregnancy advances. Once the menstrual age of the pregnancy is obtained, that menstrual age can be compared with the AC or fetal weight. The 10th percentile (ie, −1.28 standard deviations) below the mean may be used as the threshold interpretation for an abnormal AC measurement. If the AC falls below this cut-off level, the fetus is considered to be an SGA fetus (Tables 5-9, 5-11, and 5-12).

Alternatively, the menstrual age can be compared with the fetal weight using one of several formulas. Either the 5th or the 10th percentile estimate of the fetal weight can be used as the means for defining SGA. A comparison of measurements of the 5th percentile fetal weight with various gestational ages is presented in Table 5-13. The menstrual age compared with fetal weight using other formulas can be used.[19] About 75% of SGA fetuses can be detected using the 5% cut-off for weight and Shepard's formula for a 40% positive predictive value in a fairly low-risk population.[3]

Method I: Menstrual Age Not Reliably Estimated[3]

If menstrual age cannot be reliably estimated, diagnosis of IUGR becomes very difficult. In this situation, alternative methods outlined in Table 5-10 may be used. Ratios, such as femur length to ab-

(text continues on p. 79)

TABLE 5-11. Abdominal Circumference Compared With Gestational Age

AC (mm)	Estimated Gestational Age (wk)																			
	22	23	24	25	26	27	28	29	30	31	32	33	34	35	36	37	38	39	40	41
175	0.00	-0.89	-1.64	-2.33	-2.97	-3.52	-4.06	-4.57	-5.14	-5.67	-6.53	-7.12	-7.54	-7.89	-8.05	-8.53	-9.19	-9.42	-10.28	-11.24
178	0.24	-0.67	-1.43	-2.13	-2.77	-3.33	-3.88	-4.40	-4.97	-5.50	-6.35	-6.94	-7.37	-7.72	-7.89	-8.37	-9.03	-9.26	-10.11	-11.06
180	0.40	-0.52	-1.29	-2.00	-2.65	-3.21	-3.76	-4.29	-4.86	-5.39	-6.24	-6.82	-7.26	-7.61	-7.79	-8.26	-8.92	-9.16	-10.00	-10.94
182	0.56	-0.37	-1.14	-1.87	-2.52	-3.09	-3.65	-4.17	-4.74	-5.28	-6.12	-6.71	-7.14	-7.50	-7.68	-8.16	-8.81	-9.05	-9.89	-10.82
184	0.72	-0.22	-1.00	-1.73	-2.39	-2.97	-3.53	-4.06	-4.63	-5.17	-6.00	-6.59	-7.03	-7.39	-7.58	-8.05	-8.70	-8.95	-9.78	-10.71
186	0.88	-0.07	-0.86	-1.60	-2.26	-2.85	-3.41	-3.94	-4.51	-5.06	-5.88	-6.47	-6.91	-7.28	-7.47	-7.95	-8.59	-8.84	-9.67	-10.59
188	1.04	0.07	-0.71	-1.47	-2.13	-2.73	-3.29	-3.83	-4.40	-4.94	-5.76	-6.35	-6.80	-7.17	-7.37	-7.84	-8.49	-8.74	-9.56	-10.47
190	1.20	0.22	-0.57	-1.33	-2.00	-2.61	-3.18	-3.71	-4.29	-4.83	-5.65	-6.24	-6.69	-7.06	-7.26	-7.74	-8.38	-8.63	-9.44	-10.35
192	1.36	0.37	-0.43	-1.20	-1.87	-2.48	-3.06	-3.60	-4.17	-4.72	-5.53	-6.12	-6.57	-6.94	-7.16	-7.63	-8.27	-8.53	-9.33	-10.24
194	1.52	0.52	-0.29	-1.07	-1.74	-2.36	-2.94	-3.49	-4.06	-4.61	-5.41	-6.00	-6.46	-6.83	-7.05	-7.53	-8.16	-8.42	-9.22	-10.12
196	1.68	0.67	-0.14	-0.93	-1.61	-2.24	-2.82	-3.37	-3.94	-4.50	-5.29	-5.88	-6.34	-6.72	-6.95	-7.42	-8.05	-8.32	-9.11	-10.00
198	1.84	0.81	0.00	-0.80	-1.48	-2.12	-2.71	-3.26	-3.83	-4.39	-5.18	-5.76	-6.23	-6.61	-6.84	-7.32	-7.95	-8.21	-9.00	-9.88
200	2.00	0.96	0.15	-0.67	-1.35	-2.00	-2.59	-3.14	-3.71	-4.28	-5.06	-5.65	-6.11	-6.50	-6.74	-7.21	-7.84	-8.11	-8.89	-9.76
202	2.16	1.11	0.30	-0.53	-1.23	-1.88	-2.47	-3.03	-3.60	-4.17	-4.94	-5.53	-6.00	-6.39	-6.63	-7.11	-7.73	-8.00	-8.78	-9.65
204	2.32	1.26	0.44	-0.40	-1.10	-1.76	-2.35	-2.91	-3.49	-4.06	-4.82	-5.41	-5.89	-6.28	-6.53	-7.00	-7.62	-7.89	-8.67	-9.53
206	2.48	1.41	0.59	-0.27	-0.97	-1.64	-2.24	-2.80	-3.37	-3.94	-4.71	-5.29	-5.77	-6.17	-6.42	-6.89	-7.51	-7.79	-8.56	-9.41
208	2.64	1.56	0.74	-0.13	-0.84	-1.52	-2.12	-2.69	-3.26	-3.83	-4.59	-5.18	-5.66	-6.06	-6.32	-6.79	-7.41	-7.68	-8.44	-9.29
210	2.80	1.70	0.89	0.00	-0.71	-1.39	-2.00	-2.57	-3.14	-3.72	-4.47	-5.06	-5.54	-5.94	-6.21	-6.68	-7.30	-7.58	-8.33	-9.18
212	2.96	1.85	1.04	0.13	-0.58	-1.27	-1.88	-2.46	-3.03	-3.61	-4.35	-4.94	-5.43	-5.83	-6.11	-6.58	-7.19	-7.47	-8.22	-9.06
214	3.12	2.00	1.19	0.27	-0.45	-1.15	-1.76	-2.34	-2.91	-3.50	-4.24	-4.82	-5.31	-5.72	-6.00	-6.47	-7.08	-7.37	-8.11	-8.94
216	3.28	2.15	1.33	0.40	-0.32	-1.03	-1.65	-2.23	-2.80	-3.39	-4.12	-4.71	-5.20	-5.61	-5.89	-6.37	-6.97	-7.26	-8.00	-8.82
218	3.44	2.30	1.48	0.53	-0.19	-0.91	-1.53	-2.11	-2.69	-3.28	-4.00	-4.59	-5.09	-5.50	-5.79	-6.26	-6.86	-7.16	-7.89	-8.71
220	3.60	2.44	1.63	0.67	-0.06	-0.79	-1.41	-2.00	-2.57	-3.17	-3.88	-4.47	-4.97	-5.39	-5.68	-6.16	-6.76	-7.05	-7.78	-8.59
222	3.76	2.59	1.78	0.80	0.07	-0.67	-1.29	-1.89	-2.46	-3.06	-3.76	-4.35	-4.86	-5.28	-5.58	-6.05	-6.65	-6.95	-7.67	-8.47
224	3.92	2.74	1.93	0.93	0.20	-0.55	-1.18	-1.77	-2.34	-2.94	-3.65	-4.24	-4.74	-5.17	-5.47	-5.95	-6.54	-6.84	-7.56	-8.35
226	4.08	2.89	2.07	1.07	0.33	-0.42	-1.06	-1.66	-2.23	-2.83	-3.53	-4.12	-4.63	-5.06	-5.37	-5.84	-6.43	-6.74	-7.44	-8.24
228	4.24	3.04	2.22	1.20	0.47	-0.30	-0.94	-1.54	-2.11	-2.72	-3.41	-4.00	-4.51	-4.94	-5.26	-5.74	-6.32	-6.63	-7.33	-8.12
230	4.40	3.19	2.37	1.33	0.60	-0.18	-0.82	-1.43	-2.00	-2.61	-3.29	-3.88	-4.40	-4.83	-5.16	-5.63	-6.22	-6.53	-7.22	-8.00
232	4.56	3.33	2.52	1.47	0.73	-0.06	-0.71	-1.31	-1.89	-2.50	-3.18	-3.76	-4.29	-4.72	-5.05	-5.53	-6.11	-6.42	-7.11	-7.88
234	4.72	3.48	2.67	1.60	0.87	0.07	-0.59	-1.20	-1.77	-2.39	-3.06	-3.65	-4.17	-4.61	-4.95	-5.42	-6.00	-6.32	-7.00	-7.76
236	4.88	3.63	2.81	1.73	1.00	0.20	-0.47	-1.09	-1.66	-2.28	-2.94	-3.53	-4.06	-4.50	-4.84	-5.32	-5.89	-6.21	-6.89	-7.65
238	5.04	3.78	2.96	1.87	1.13	0.33	-0.35	-0.97	-1.54	-2.17	-2.82	-3.41	-3.94	-4.39	-4.74	-5.21	-5.78	-6.11	-6.78	-7.53
240	5.20	3.93	3.11	2.00	1.27	0.47	-0.24	-0.86	-1.43	-2.06	-2.71	-3.29	-3.83	-4.28	-4.63	-5.11	-5.68	-6.00	-6.67	-7.41
242	5.36	4.07	3.26	2.13	1.40	0.60	-0.12	-0.74	-1.31	-1.94	-2.59	-3.18	-3.71	-4.17	-4.53	-5.00	-5.57	-5.89	-6.56	-7.29
244	5.52	4.22	3.41	2.27	1.53	0.73	0.00	-0.63	-1.20	-1.83	-2.47	-3.06	-3.60	-4.06	-4.42	-4.89	-5.46	-5.79	-6.44	-7.18
246	5.68	4.37	3.56	2.40	1.67	0.87	0.13	-0.51	-1.09	-1.72	-2.35	-2.94	-3.49	-3.94	-4.32	-4.79	-5.35	-5.68	-6.33	-7.06
248	5.84	4.52	3.70	2.53	1.80	1.00	0.25	-0.40	-0.97	-1.61	-2.24	-2.82	-3.37	-3.83	-4.21	-4.68	-5.24	-5.58	-6.22	-6.94
250	6.00	4.67	3.85	2.67	1.93	1.13	0.38	-0.29	-0.86	-1.50	-2.12	-2.71	-3.26	-3.72	-4.11	-4.58	-5.14	-5.47	-6.11	-6.82
252	6.16	4.81	4.00	2.80	2.07	1.27	0.50	-0.17	-0.74	-1.39	-2.00	-2.59	-3.14	-3.61	-4.00	-4.47	-5.03	-5.37	-6.00	-6.71
254	6.32	4.96	4.15	2.93	2.20	1.40	0.63	-0.06	-0.63	-1.28	-1.88	-2.47	-3.03	-3.50	-3.89	-4.37	-4.92	-5.26	-5.89	-6.59

256	-6.47	-5.78	-5.16	-4.81	-4.26	-3.79	-3.39	-2.91	-2.35	-1.76	-1.17	-0.51	0.06	0.75	1.53	2.33	3.07	4.30	5.11	6.48
258	-6.35	-5.67	-5.05	-4.70	-4.16	-3.68	-3.28	-2.80	-2.24	-1.65	-1.06	-0.40	0.18	0.88	1.67	2.47	3.20	4.44	5.26	6.64
260	-6.24	-5.56	-4.95	-4.59	-4.05	-3.58	-3.17	-2.69	-2.12	-1.53	-0.94	-0.29	0.30	1.00	1.80	2.60	3.33	4.59	5.41	6.80
262	-6.12	-5.44	-4.84	-4.49	-3.95	-3.47	-3.06	-2.57	-2.00	-1.41	-0.83	-0.17	0.42	1.13	1.93	2.73	3.47	4.74	5.56	6.96
264	-6.00	-5.33	-4.74	-4.38	-3.84	-3.37	-2.94	-2.46	-1.88	-1.29	-0.72	-0.06	0.55	1.25	2.07	2.87	3.60	4.89	5.70	7.12
266	-5.88	-5.22	-4.63	-4.27	-3.74	-3.26	-2.83	-2.34	-1.76	-1.18	-0.61	0.06	0.67	1.38	2.20	3.00	3.73	5.04	5.85	7.28
268	-5.76	-5.11	-4.53	-4.16	-3.63	-3.16	-2.72	-2.23	-1.65	-1.06	-0.50	0.17	0.79	1.50	2.33	3.13	3.87	5.19	6.00	7.44
270	-5.65	-5.00	-4.42	-4.05	-3.53	-3.05	-2.61	-2.11	-1.53	-0.94	-0.39	0.29	0.91	1.63	2.47	3.27	4.00	5.33	6.15	7.60
272	-5.53	-4.89	-4.32	-3.95	-3.42	-2.95	-2.50	-2.00	-1.41	-0.82	-0.28	0.40	1.03	1.75	2.60	3.40	4.13	5.48	6.30	7.76
274	-5.41	-4.78	-4.21	-3.84	-3.32	-2.84	-2.39	-1.89	-1.29	-0.71	-0.17	0.51	1.15	1.88	2.73	3.53	4.27	5.63	6.44	7.92
276	-5.29	-4.67	-4.11	-3.73	-3.21	-2.74	-2.28	-1.77	-1.18	-0.59	-0.06	0.63	1.27	2.00	2.87	3.67	4.40	5.78	6.59	8.08
278	-5.18	-4.56	-4.00	-3.62	-3.11	-2.63	-2.17	-1.66	-1.06	-0.47	0.04	0.74	1.39	2.13	3.00	3.80	4.53	5.93	6.74	8.24
280	-5.06	-4.44	-3.89	-3.51	-3.00	-2.53	-2.06	-1.54	-0.94	-0.35	0.13	0.86	1.52	2.25	3.13	3.93	4.67	6.07	6.89	8.40
282	-4.94	-4.33	-3.79	-3.41	-2.89	-2.42	-1.94	-1.43	-0.82	-0.24	0.22	0.97	1.64	2.38	3.27	4.07	4.80	6.22	7.04	8.56
284	-4.82	-4.22	-3.68	-3.30	-2.79	-2.32	-1.83	-1.31	-0.71	-0.12	0.31	1.09	1.76	2.50	3.40	4.20	4.93	6.37	7.19	8.72
286	-4.71	-4.11	-3.58	-3.19	-2.68	-2.21	-1.72	-1.20	-0.59	0.00	0.40	1.20	1.88	2.63	3.53	4.33	5.07	6.52	7.33	8.88
288	-4.59	-4.00	-3.47	-3.08	-2.58	-2.11	-1.61	-1.09	-0.47	0.11	0.49	1.31	2.00	2.75	3.67	4.47	5.20	6.67	7.48	9.04
290	-4.47	-3.89	-3.37	-2.97	-2.47	-2.00	-1.50	-0.97	-0.35	0.21	0.58	1.43	2.12	2.88	3.80	4.60	5.33	6.81	7.63	9.20
292	-4.35	-3.78	-3.26	-2.86	-2.37	-1.89	-1.39	-0.86	-0.24	0.32	0.67	1.54	2.24	3.00	3.93	4.73	5.47	6.96	7.78	9.36
294	-4.24	-3.67	-3.16	-2.76	-2.26	-1.79	-1.28	-0.74	-0.12	0.42	0.76	1.66	2.36	3.13	4.07	4.87	5.60	7.11	7.93	9.52
296	-4.12	-3.56	-3.05	-2.65	-2.16	-1.68	-1.17	-0.63	0.00	0.53	0.84	1.77	2.48	3.25	4.20	5.00	5.73	7.26	8.07	9.68
298	-4.00	-3.44	-2.95	-2.54	-2.05	-1.58	-1.06	-0.51	0.10	0.63	0.93	1.89	2.61	3.38	4.33	5.13	5.87	7.41	8.22	9.84
300	-3.88	-3.33	-2.84	-2.43	-1.95	-1.47	-0.94	-0.40	0.21	0.74	1.02	2.00	2.73	3.50	4.47	5.27	6.00	7.56	8.37	10.00
302	-3.76	-3.22	-2.74	-2.32	-1.84	-1.37	-0.83	-0.29	0.31	0.84	1.11	2.11	2.85	3.63	4.60	5.40	6.13	7.70	8.52	10.16
304	-3.65	-3.11	-2.63	-2.22	-1.74	-1.26	-0.72	-0.17	0.41	0.95	1.20	2.23	2.97	3.75	4.73	5.53	6.27	7.85	8.67	10.32
306	-3.53	-3.00	-2.53	-2.11	-1.63	-1.16	-0.61	-0.06	0.51	1.05	1.29	2.34	3.09	3.88	4.87	5.67	6.40	8.00	8.81	10.48
308	-3.41	-2.89	-2.42	-2.00	-1.53	-1.05	-0.50	0.05	0.62	1.16	1.38	2.46	3.21	4.00	5.00	5.80	6.53	8.15	8.96	10.64
310	-3.29	-2.78	-2.32	-1.89	-1.42	-0.95	-0.39	0.15	0.72	1.26	1.47	2.57	3.33	4.13	5.13	5.93	6.67	8.30	9.11	10.80
312	-3.18	-2.67	-2.21	-1.78	-1.32	-0.84	-0.28	0.26	0.82	1.37	1.56	2.69	3.45	4.25	5.27	6.07	6.80	8.44	9.26	10.96
314	-3.06	-2.56	-2.11	-1.68	-1.21	-0.74	-0.17	0.36	0.92	1.47	1.64	2.80	3.58	4.38	5.40	6.20	6.93	8.59	9.41	11.12
316	-2.94	-2.44	-2.00	-1.57	-1.11	-0.63	-0.06	0.46	1.03	1.58	1.73	2.91	3.70	4.50	5.53	6.33	7.07	8.74	9.56	11.28
318	-2.82	-2.33	-1.89	-1.46	-1.00	-0.53	0.05	0.56	1.13	1.68	1.82	3.03	3.82	4.63	5.67	6.47	7.20	8.89	9.70	11.44
320	-2.71	-2.22	-1.79	-1.35	-0.89	-0.42	0.15	0.67	1.23	1.79	1.91	3.14	3.94	4.75	5.80	6.60	7.33	9.04	9.85	11.60
322	-2.59	-2.11	-1.68	-1.24	-0.79	-0.32	0.26	0.77	1.33	1.89	2.00	3.26	4.06	4.88	5.93	6.73	7.47	9.19	10.0	11.76
324	-2.47	-2.00	-1.58	-1.14	-0.68	-0.21	0.36	0.87	1.44	2.00	2.09	3.37	4.18	5.00	6.07	6.87	7.60	9.33	10.15	11.92
326	-2.35	-1.89	-1.47	-1.03	-0.58	-0.11	0.46	0.97	1.54	2.11	2.18	3.49	4.30	5.13	6.20	7.00	7.73	9.48	10.30	12.08
328	-2.24	-1.78	-1.37	-0.92	-0.47	0.00	0.56	1.08	1.64	2.21	2.27	3.60	4.42	5.25	6.33	7.13	7.87	9.63	10.44	12.24
330	-2.12	-1.67	-1.26	-0.81	-0.37	0.11	0.67	1.18	1.74	2.32	2.36	3.71	4.55	5.38	6.47	7.27	8.00	9.78	10.59	12.40
332	-2.00	-1.56	-1.16	-0.70	-0.26	0.22	0.77	1.28	1.85	2.42	2.44	3.83	4.67	5.50	6.60	7.40	8.13	9.93	10.74	12.56
334	-1.88	-1.44	-1.05	-0.59	-0.16	0.32	0.87	1.38	1.95	2.53	2.53	3.94	4.79	5.63	6.73	7.53	8.27	10.07	10.89	12.72
336	-1.76	-1.33	-0.95	-0.49	-0.05	0.43	0.97	1.49	2.05	2.63	2.62	4.06	4.91	5.75	6.87	7.67	8.40	10.22	11.04	12.88
338	-1.65	-1.22	-0.84	-0.38	0.06	0.54	1.08	1.59	2.15	2.74	2.71	4.17	5.03	5.88	7.00	7.80	8.53	10.37	11.19	13.04
340	-1.53	-1.11	-0.74	-0.27	0.17	0.65	1.18	1.69	2.26	2.84	2.80	4.29	5.15	6.00	7.13	7.93	8.67	10.52	11.33	13.20
342	-1.41	-1.00	-0.63	-0.16	0.28	0.76	1.28	1.79	2.36	2.95	2.89	4.40	5.27	6.13	7.27	8.07	8.80	10.67	11.48	13.36
344	-1.29	-0.89	-0.53	-0.05	0.39	0.86	1.38	1.90	2.46	3.05	2.98	4.51	5.39	6.25	7.40	8.20	8.93	10.81	11.63	13.52
346	-1.18	-0.78	-0.42	0.06	0.50	0.97	1.49	2.00	2.56	3.16	3.07	4.63	5.52	6.38	7.53	8.33	9.07	10.96	11.78	13.68

continued

TABLE 5-11. *(Continued)*

AC (mm)	Estimated Gestational Age (wk)																			
	22	23	24	25	26	27	28	29	30	31	32	33	34	35	36	37	38	39	40	41
348	13.84	11.93	11.11	9.20	8.47	7.67	6.50	5.64	4.74	3.16	3.26	2.67	2.10	1.59	1.08	0.61	0.18	-0.32	-0.67	-1.06
350	14.00	12.07	11.26	9.33	8.60	7.80	6.63	5.76	4.86	3.24	3.37	2.77	2.21	1.69	1.19	0.72	0.29	-0.21	-0.56	-0.94
352	14.16	12.22	11.41	9.47	8.73	7.93	6.75	5.88	4.97	3.33	3.47	2.87	2.31	1.79	1.30	0.83	0.41	-0.11	-0.44	-0.82
354	14.32	12.37	11.56	9.60	8.87	8.07	6.88	6.00	5.09	3.42	3.58	2.97	2.41	1.90	1.41	0.94	0.53	0.00	-0.33	-0.71
356	14.48	12.52	11.70	9.73	9.00	8.20	7.00	6.12	5.20	3.51	3.68	3.08	2.51	2.00	1.51	1.06	0.65	0.13	-0.22	-0.59
358	14.64	12.67	11.85	9.87	9.13	8.33	7.13	6.24	5.31	3.60	3.79	3.18	2.62	2.10	1.62	1.17	0.76	0.27	-0.11	-0.47
360	14.80	12.81	12.00	10.00	9.27	8.47	7.25	6.36	5.43	3.69	3.89	3.28	2.72	2.21	1.73	1.28	0.88	0.40	0.00	-0.35
362	14.96	12.96	12.15	10.13	9.40	8.60	7.38	6.48	5.54	3.78	4.00	3.38	2.82	2.31	1.84	1.39	1.00	0.53	0.14	-0.24
364	15.12	13.11	12.30	10.27	9.53	8.73	7.50	6.61	5.66	3.87	4.11	3.49	2.92	2.41	1.95	1.50	1.12	0.67	0.29	-0.12
366	15.28	13.26	12.44	10.40	9.67	8.87	7.63	6.73	5.77	3.96	4.21	3.59	3.03	2.51	2.05	1.61	1.24	0.80	0.43	0.00
368	15.44	13.41	12.59	10.53	9.80	9.00	7.75	6.85	5.89	4.04	4.32	3.69	3.13	2.62	2.16	1.72	1.35	0.93	0.57	0.15
370	15.60	13.56	12.74	10.67	9.93	9.13	7.88	6.97	6.00	4.13	4.42	3.79	3.23	2.72	2.27	1.83	1.47	1.07	0.71	0.31
372	15.76	13.70	12.89	10.80	10.07	9.27	8.00	7.09	6.11	4.22	4.53	3.90	3.33	2.82	2.38	1.94	1.59	1.20	0.86	0.46
374	15.92	13.85	13.04	10.93	10.20	9.40	8.13	7.21	6.23	4.31	4.63	4.00	3.44	2.92	2.49	2.06	1.71	1.33	1.00	0.62
376	16.08	14.00	13.19	11.07	10.33	9.53	8.25	7.33	6.34	4.40	4.74	4.10	3.54	3.03	2.59	2.17	1.82	1.47	1.14	0.77
378	16.24	14.15	13.33	11.20	10.47	9.67	8.38	7.45	6.46	4.49	4.84	4.21	3.64	3.13	2.70	2.28	1.94	1.60	1.29	0.92
380	16.40	14.30	13.48	11.33	10.60	9.80	8.50	7.58	6.57	4.58	4.95	4.31	3.74	3.23	2.81	2.39	2.06	1.73	1.43	1.08
382	16.56	14.44	13.63	11.47	10.73	9.93	8.63	7.70	6.69	4.67	5.05	4.41	3.85	3.33	2.92	2.50	2.18	1.87	1.57	123
384	16.72	14.59	13.78	11.60	10.87	10.07	8.75	7.82	6.80	4.76	5.16	4.51	3.95	3.44	3.03	2.61	2.29	2.00	1.71	1.38
386	16.88	14.74	13.93	11.73	11.00	10.20	8.88	7.94	6.91	4.84	5.26	4.62	4.05	3.54	3.14	2.72	2.41	2.13	1.86	1.54
388	17.04	14.89	14.07	11.87	11.13	10.33	9.00	8.06	7.03	4.93	5.37	4.72	4.15	3.64	3.24	2.83	2.53	2.27	2.00	1.69
390	17.20	15.04	14.22	12.00	11.27	10.47	9.13	8.18	7.14	5.02	5.47	4.82	4.26	3.74	3.35	2.94	2.65	2.40	2.14	1.85

This table was generated with a computer program. To use the table, choose the column containing the measured AC on the left and the column containing the estimated gestational age (in menstrual weeks) at the top. The value at the interception of these two columns is the number of SDs the measured AC is above or below (−) the mean AC for gestational age.

(Courtesy of Louis Humphrey and James D. Bowie, MD, Duke University Medical Center, Durham, NC. With permission of Hertzberg BS: Intrauterine growth retardation. In Rifkin MD, Charboneau JW, Laing FC [eds]: Syllabus Special Course: Ultrasound 1991. The Radiological Society of North America, December 1991:147–158.)

TABLE 5-12. Converting Between Percentiles and Standard Deviations

Percentiles	SDs
25th	(−)0.68
20th	(−)0.84
15th	(−)1.04
10th	(−)1.28
5th	(−)1.64
2.28th	(−)2.0

(Courtesy of James D. Bowie, MD, Duke University Medical Center, Durham, NC. Hertzberg BS: Intrauterine growth retardation. In Rifkin MD, Charboneau JW, Laing FC [eds]: Syllabus Special Course: Ultrasound 1991. The Radiological Society of North America, December, 1991: 147–158.)

TABLE 5-14. IUGR Score*

Component	Score
Maternal blood pressure	0 if normal 6.8 if elevated
Amniotic fluid volume	0 if normal or elevated 9.1 if borderline or mild oligohydramnios 14.8 if moderate or severe oligohydramnios
Estimated fetal weight	−13.1 × age-standardized estimated fetal weight (expressed in SD below mean)
Constant	39.2

SD, standard deviation.

* The IUGR score is a total of four component scores.

(Benson CB, Boswell SB, Brown DL, et al: Improved prediction of intrauterine growth retardation with use of multiple parameters. Radiology 1988; 168:7–12.)

dominal circumference, may be helpful to detect asymmetric growth. Use of other ratios is less reliable. Head circumference to abdominal circumference ratio, which varies through gestational age, is only helpful when the gestational age is known. Other alternatives include a repeat ultrasound examination every 2 to 3 weeks to check for lag of growth of the abdominal circumference or lack of increase of fetal weight. Unfortunately, the lower limits of expected lag of growth or weight increase are poorly documented in the literature. Finally, fetuses that are considered at risk for IUGR may be further evaluated with other examinations, such as Doppler, biophysical profile, non-stress testing, or

TABLE 5-13. Shepard's Formula: Weight Versus Gestational Age*

Gestational Age (wk)	Percentile			Gestational Age (wk)	Percentile		
	5th	50th	95th		5th	50th	95th
9	44	45	46	25	650	871	1,172
10	46	48	51	26	745	1,000	1,347
11	50	54	59	27	847	1,139	1,536
12	57	63	71	28	957	1,288	1,740
13	67	77	90	29	1,074	1,448	1,958
14	81	96	116	30	1,199	1,618	2,189
15	100	122	151	31	1,331	1,798	2,434
16	125	155	196	32	1,468	1,984	2,688
17	155	197	253	33	1,608	2,176	2,950
18	192	247	322	34	1,750	2,369	3,213
19	237	307	404	35	1,888	2,557	3,469
20	288	377	499	36	2,017	2,734	3,711
21	346	456	607	37	2,131	2,890	3,925
22	411	545	728	38	2,221	3,016	4,100
23	484	644	862	39	2,276	3,099	4,225
24	563	753	1,010	40	2,287	3,131	4,290

* Values are weight (in grams).

(Jeanty P, Cantraine F, Romero R, et al: A longitudinal study of fetal weight growth. J Ultrasound Med 1984; 3:321–328.)

TABLE 5-15. IUGR Probability Based on the IUGR Score

Fetuses	IUGR Score	Probability of IUGR (%)
All (n = 356)	<50	3
	50–60	13
	>60	74
With no dating by early US (n = 222)	<50	2
	50–60	19
	>60	67
With dating by early US (n = 134)	<60	3
	≥60	86

(Benson CB, Belville JS, Lentini JF, et al: Intrauterine growth retardation: Diagnosis based on multiple parameters—A prospective study. Radiology 1990; 177:499–502.)

contraction stress testing. These are discussed in more detail in Chapter 4.

Method II: Multiparameter Approach[7,8]

To increase the predictive value of a positive test, a scoring system that has a range from 0 to 100 was developed to diagnose IUGR. This scoring system was based on three parameters: estimated fetal weight, amniotic fluid volume, and maternal blood pressure status.[7,8] The IUGR score and the various components of the score are listed in Table 5-14. This is a combined score based on the three parameters plus a constant of 39.2.

The maternal blood pressure is scored as 0 if the patient is normotensive and 6.8 if she has elevated blood pressure. Amniotic fluid volume is scored as 0 if there is

TABLE 5-16. Critical Values for Estimated Fetal Weight (g) for Diagnosing or Excluding Growth Retardation by Means of an IUGR Score

GA	Status of Maternal Blood Pressure and Amniotic Fluid Volume*					
	Nl BP Nl/Poly	*Nl BP M–M Olig*	*Nl BP Sev Olig*	*Htn Nl/Poly*	*Htn M–M Olig*	*Htn Sev Olig*
26	516–660	646–826	743–950	610–780	763–976	878–1123
27	597–761	745–949	855–1090	704–898	878–1119	1009–1285
28	693–877	859–1087	982–1244	813–1030	1008–1276	1153–1460
29	803–1008	988–1239	1124–1410	937–1176	1152–1446	1312–1646
30	931–1155	1132–1405	1281–1589	1078–1337	1311–1627	1483–1840
31	1075–1317	1293–1584	1452–1779	1234–1512	1484–1819	1667–2042
32	1235–1493	1468–1774	1635–1976	1405–1698	1670–2018	1860–2248
33	1411–1682	1656–1973	1830–2180	1590–1895	1865–2223	2061–2456
34	1600–1880	1853–2177	2031–2386	1785–2098	2067–2429	2266–2662
35	1798–2083	2055–2382	2236–2590	1987–2302	2272–2633	2471–2863
36	1997–2285	2257–2583	2437–2789	2189–2504	2474–2830	2671–3056
37	2192–2479	2452–2774	2631–2976	2383–2696	2666–3016	2861–3236
38	2371–2658	2631–2949	2807–3147	2563–2872	2843–3186	3034–3400
39	2526–2812	2785–3101	2961–3296	2717–3025	2996–3335	3185–3545
40	2645–2933	2906–3223	3083–3419	2838–3147	3118–3458	3307–3668
41	2717–3013	2985–3310	3166–3511	2915–3232	3202–3551	3396–3766
42	2736–3045	3016–3356	3205–3567	2942–3274	3243–3609	3447–3836

* For each pair, estimated weight less than the lower value corresponds to an IUGR score above 60 and thus allows confident diagnosis of IUGR (positive predictive value = 74%). Estimated weight greater than the upper value corresponds to an IUGR score below 50 and thus virtually excludes IUGR (negative predictive value = 97%). Estimated weight between the two values is indeterminate for IUGR (probability of IUGR = 13%).

GA, gestational age; Nl BP, normal blood pressure; Htn, hypertension; Nl, normal fluid; Poly, polyhydramnios; M–M, mild to moderate; Olig, oligohydramnios; Sev, severe.

(Benson CB, Belville JS, Lentini JF, et al: Intrauterine growth retardation: Diagnosis based on multiple parameters—A prospective study. Radiology 1990; 177:499–502.)

normal or increased amniotic fluid, 9.1 for mild to moderate oligohydramnios, and 14.8 for severe oligohydramnios. The fetal weight score equals the number of standard deviations the estimated fetal weight falls below the mean for gestation age times 13.1. Finally, the constant value of 39.2 is added to give the IUGR score a range of 0 to 100.[7]

The IUGR score can then be converted into a probability of IUGR (Table 5-15). A score above 60 is associated with a high probability of IUGR, and a score below 50 virtually excludes IUGR (see Table 5-15). Furthermore, Table 5-16 lists two values of fetal weight, taking into account the effects of maternal blood pressure and fetal amniotic fluid volume. If the estimated weight is greater than the value to the right, the total IUGR score would be less than 50, and the probability of IUGR would be less than 3%. Alternatively, if the fetal weight is below the value to the left, the IUGR score would be greater than 60, thus giving a very high probability (74%) of IUGR. As can be identified in Table 5-15, the probability of correctly identifying IUGR based on the scoring system can improve when early dating of the pregnancy is obtained.

CONCLUSION

Intrauterine growth retardation is a common clinical dilemma in both obstetrics and neonatology. Despite extensive research in this field, many questions remain unanswered. Further investigation should improve our understanding of its definition, diagnosis, pathophysiology, and treatment. This chapter reviews the literature and provides some practical guidelines for the diagnosis and management of this condition.

REFERENCES

1. Starfield B, Shapiro S, McCormick M, et al: Mortality and morbidity in infants with intrauterine growth retardation. Pediatrics 1982; 101:978.
2. Heinonen K, Hakulinen A, Jokela V: Survival of the smallest: Time trends and determinants of mortality in a very preterm population during the 1980's. Lancet 1988; 8604:204.
3. Hertzberg BS: Intrauterine growth retardation. In Rifkin MD, Charboneau JW, Laing FC (eds): Syllabus Special Course: Ultrasound 1991. The Radiological Society of North America, December 1991: 147–158.
4. Gruenwald P: Chronic fetal distress and placental insufficiency. Biol Neonate 1963; 5:215.
5. Nicolaides KH, Snijders RJM, Noble P: Cordocentesis in the study of growth retarded fetuses. In Divon

MY (ed): Abnormal Fetal Growth. New York: Elsevier Science, 1991.
6. Rosenberg K, Grant JM, Aitchison T: Measurement of fundal height as screening test for fetal growth retardation. Br J Obstet Gynaecol 1981; 88:115.
7. Benson CB, Belville JS, Lentini JF, Doubilet PM: Intrauterine growth retardation: Diagnosis based on multiple parameters—A prospective study. Radiology 1990; 177:499–502.
8. Benson CB, Boswell SB, Brown DL, et al: Improved prediction of intrauterine growth retardation with use of multiple parameters. Radiology 1988; 168:7–12.
9. Benson CB, Doubilet PM: Doppler criteria for intrauterine growth retardation: Predictive values. J Ultrasound Med 1988; 7:655–659.
10. Guidetti DA, Divon MY: Sonographic detection of the IUGR fetus. In Divon MY (ed): Abnormal Fetal Growth. New York: Elsevier Science, 1991.
11. Ott WJ: Fetal femur length, neonatal crown-heel length and screening for intrauterine growth retardation. Obstet Gynecol 1985; 65:460.
12. O'Brien GP, Queenan JT: Ultrasound fetal femur length in relation to intrauterine growth retardation. Am J Obstet Gynecol 1982; 144:35.
13. Warsof SL, Cooper DJ, Little D, Campbell S: Routine ultrasound screening for antenatal detection of intrauterine growth retardation. Obstet Gynecol 1986; 67:33.
14. Chambers SE, Haskins PR, Haddad NG, et al: A comparison of fetal abdominal circumference measurements and Doppler ultrasound in the prediction of small for dates babies and fetal compromise. Br J Obstet Gynecol 1989; 96:803.
15. Kurjak A, Kirkinen P, Latin V: Biometric and dynamic ultrasound assessment of small for dates infants: Report of 260 cases. Obstet Gynecol 1980; 56:281.
16. Hadlock FP, Deter RL, Harris RB, et al: A date independent predictor of intrauterine growth retardation: Femur length/abdominal circumference ratio. AJR 1983; 141:979.
17. Divon MY, Chamberlain PF, Sipos L, et al: Identification of the small for gestational age fetus with the use of gestational age independent indices of fetal growth. Am J Obstet Gynecol 1986; 155:1197.
18. Divon MY, Guidetti DA, Braverman JJ, et al: Intrauterine growth retardation: A prospective study of the diagnostic value of real time sonography combined with umbilical artery flow velocimetry. Obstet Gynecol 1988; 72:611.
19. Hadlock FP, Deter RL, Harris RB, et al: A date-independent predictor of intrauterine growth retardation: Femur length: abdominal circumference ratio. AJR 1983; 141:979.
20. Manning FA, Hill LM, Platt LD: Qualitative amniotic fluid volume determination by ultrasound: Antepartum detection of intrauterine growth retardation. Am J Obstet Gynecol 1981; 129:255.
21. Patterson RM, Prihoda TJ, Pouliot MR: Sonographic

amniotic fluid measurement and fetal growth retardation: An appraisal. Am J Obstet Gynecol 1987; 157:1406.

22. Chamberlain PR, Manning FA, Morrison I, et al: Ultrasound evaluation of amniotic fluid volume. I. The relationship of marginal and decreased amniotic fluid volumes to perinatal outcomes. Am J Obstet Gynecol 1984; 150:245.

23. Philipson EN, Sokol RJ, Williams T: Oligohydramnios: Clinical association and predictive values for intrauterine growth retardation. Am J Obstet Gynecol 1983; 146:271.

24. Reece EA, Goldstein I, Pilu G, Hobbins JC: Fetal cerebellar growth unaffected by intrauterine growth retardation: A new parameter for prenatal diagnosis. Am J Obstet Gynecol 1987; 157:632.

25. Lee W, Barton S, Comstock CH, et al: Transverse cerebellar diameter: A useful predictor of gestational age for fetuses asymmetric growth retardation. Am J Obstet Gynecol 1991; 165:1044.

26. Fleischer A, Guidetti D, Sublemuller P: Umbilical artery velocity waveforms in the intrauterine growth retarded fetus. Clin Obstet Gynecol 1989; 32:660.

27. Divon MY, Hsu HW: Maternal and fetal velocity waveforms in IUGR. Clin Obstet Gynecol 1992; 35:156.

28. Bewely S, Chard T, Grudzinskas G, et al: Early prediction of uteroplacental complications of pregnancy using Doppler ultrasound, placental function tests and combination testing. Ultrasound Obstet Gynecol 1992; 2:333.

29. Cohen-Overbeek TE, Pearce JM, Campbell S: The antenatal assessment of uteroplacental and fetoplacental blood flow using Doppler ultrasound. Ultrasound Med Biol 1985; 11:329.

30. Trudinger BJ, Giles WB, Cook C: Flow velocity waveforms in the maternal uteroplacental and fetal umbilical placental circulations. Am J Obstet Gynecol 1985; 152:155.

31. Newnham JP, Patterson LL, James IR, et al: An evaluation of the efficacy of Doppler flow velocity waveform analysis as a screening test in pregnancy. Am J Obstet Gynecol 1990; 162:403.

32. Jacobson SL, Imhof R, Manning N, et al: The value of Doppler assessment of the uteroplacental circulation in predicting preeclampsia or intrauterine growth retardation. Am J Obstet Gynecol 1990; 162:110.

33. Giles WB, Trudinger BJ, Baird P: Fetal umbilical artery flow velocity waveforms and placental resistance: Pathological correlation. Br J Obstet Gynaecol 1985; 92:30.

34. Fox RY, Pavlova Z, Benirschke K, et al: The correlation of arterial lesions with umbilical artery Doppler velocity in the placentas of small-for-dates pregnancies. Obstet Gynecol 1990; 75:578.

35. Wladmiroff JW, Wijngaard JAGW, Degani S, et al: Cerebral and umbilical arterial blood flow velocity waveforms in normal and growth retarded pregnancies. Obstet Gynecol 1987; 69:705.

36. Trudinger BJ, Cook CM, Giles WB, et al: Fetal umbilical artery velocity waveforms and subsequent neonatal outcome. Br J Obstet Gynaecol 1991; 98:378.

37. Kay HH, Carrol BB, Dahmus M, Killam AP: Sonographic measurements with umbilical artery Doppler analysis in suspected intrauterine growth retardation. J Reprod Med 1991; 36:65.

38. Drogtrop AP, Bruinse HW, Reuwer PJH: Normal umbilical artery Doppler sonography does not exclude fetal distress. Acta Obstet Gynecol Scand 1990; 69:351.

39. Rochelson B: The clinical significance of absent end diastolic velocity in the umbilical artery waveforms. Clin Obstet Gynecol 1989; 32:692.

40. Arabin B, Siebert M, Jimenez E, Saling E: Obstetrical characteristics of a loss of end diastolic velocities in the fetal aorta and/or umbilical artery using Doppler ultrasound. Gynecol Obstet Invest 1988; 25:173.

41. Brar HS, Platt LD: Antepartum improvement of abnormal umbilical velocimetry: Does it occur? Am J Obstet Gynecol 1989; 160:36.

42. Reed KL, Anderson CF, Shenker L: Changes in intracardial Doppler blood flow velocities in fetuses with absent umbilical artery diastolic flow. Am J Obstet Gynecol 1987; 157:774.

43. Brar HS, Platt LD: Reverse end diastolic flow velocity on umbilical artery velocity in high risk pregnancies: An ominous finding with adverse pregnancy outcome. Am J Obstet Gynecol 1988; 159:559.

44. Schulman H: The clinical implications of Doppler ultrasound analysis of the uterine and umbilical arteries. Am J Obstet Gynecol 1987; 156:899.

45. Divon MY, Girz BA, Liblich L, Langer O: Clinical management of the fetus with markedly diminished umbilical artery end-diastolic flow. Am J Obstet Gynecol 1989; 161:1523.

John P. McGahan and Manuel Porto:
DIAGNOSTIC OBSTETRICAL ULTRASOUND.
© 1994 J.B. Lippincott Company.

Beverly A. Spirt   Lawrence P. Gordon

Chapter 6

The Placenta and Cervix

PLACENTA

A systematic evaluation of the placenta is an important part of every obstetrical ultrasound examination. The texture, location, size, and shape should be assessed as well as the appearance of the retroplacental area (Table 6-1). A thorough understanding of normal placental anatomy and its variations, as well as the pathologic processes that occur, is necessary to correctly interpret the findings at sonography.

Early Development

The gestational sac is first visible with the transvaginal probe at about 4 to 4.5 weeks menstrual age (Fig. 6-1). It is surrounded by a hyperechoic rim that is composed of fetal vessels within immature villi. These villi are surrounded by maternal blood within the lacunar space. As the villi develop, the lacunar space becomes the intervillous space. At about 5 weeks, the villi that are opposite the implantation site begin to regress, and the as-

sociated intervillous space is obliterated, leaving a smooth surface, the *chorion laeve*. The remaining villi, the *chorion frondosum*, develop into the placenta. By 8 to 10 weeks, the early placenta may be identified at sonography (Fig. 6-2).

At this stage, the amniotic sac has not yet reached the size of the chorionic cavity, and the amniotic membrane may be visualized at sonography. Fusion of the amnion and chorion usually occurs at about 12 weeks menstrual age, although rarely they may remain separate throughout gestation (Fig. 6-3).

Fetal blood is supplied to the placenta through the two umbilical arteries that branch within the chorion. Similarly, fetal veins course within the chorion, draining blood from the villi into the single umbilical vein (Fig. 6-4A). Thus, vessels may be seen within the fetal surface of the placenta, particularly in the region of the umbilical cord insertion where they are of larger caliber (Fig. 6-4B). Maternal blood is supplied to the intervillous space by spiral arterioles, which are usually too small to distinguish sonographically. Draining veins along the

TABLE 6-1.   Checklist for Placental Ultrasound

- Location
- Size
- Shape
- Texture
- Retroplacental area

base of the placenta, which may be seen at sonography, return the blood from the intervillous space to the maternal circulation (Fig. 6-4B,C).

The umbilical cord usually inserts eccentrically into the placenta.[1] In less than 2% of cases, the cord inserts into the membranes instead of the placenta (*velamentous insertion;* see Chapter 7). In this situation, the fetal vessels course unprotected between the amnion and the chorion before reaching the placenta, thus risking damage during labor and delivery.

Texture

The relatively hyperechoic granular texture of the placenta results from echoes produced by the branching villi, which are bathed in maternal blood. The placenta maintains a fairly constant

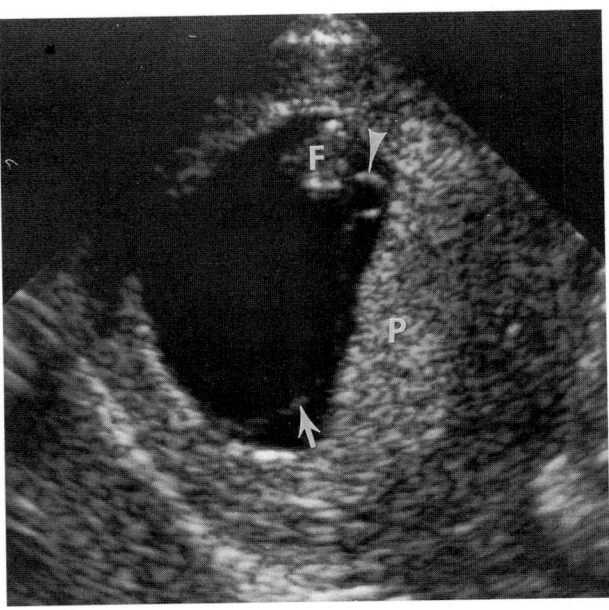

FIGURE 6-2.   Early placenta. Transvaginal scan at 10.3 weeks shows placenta (P) with typical diffuse granular echotexture. The amniotic membrane (*arrow*) is seen. Note yolk sac (*arrowhead*) between amnion and placenta. F, fetus.

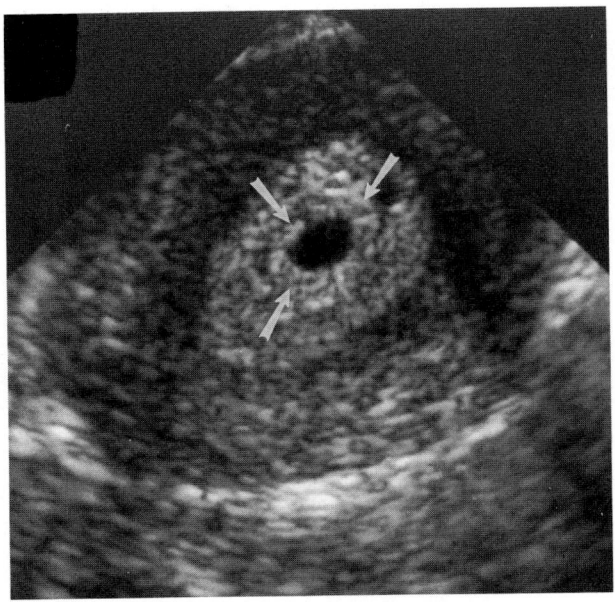

FIGURE 6-1.   Early gestational sac. Transvaginal scan at 4 weeks shows hyperechoic rim of villi (*arrows*) at the periphery of the gestational sac. (Spirt BA, Gordon LP: The placenta. In Rumack CM, Wilson SR, Charbonneau JW [eds]: Diagnostic Ultrasound. St. Louis: Mosby Year Book, 1991: 935–953.)

echotexture throughout the gestational period, with a few exceptions. The most notable exception is calcium deposition, which is commonly visualized in the third trimester (Fig. 6-5). Placental calcification is a physiologic process that occurs throughout pregnancy; it is microscopic in the first two trimesters and becomes macroscopic thereafter. Calcification may be found along the basal plate, in the septa, and in fibrin collections in the subchorionic and intervillous spaces. Chemical, radiographic, and sonographic studies have shown that placental calcification increases exponentially with increasing gestational age and has no clinical significance.[2–5]

The placenta commonly contains anechoic or hypoechoic lesions that are not clinically significant (Table 6-2). Subchorionic fibrin deposition, intervillous thrombosis, and perivillous fibrin deposition are common macroscopic lesions that result from the interactions of the maternal and fetal circulations. All these lesions contain varying amounts of fibrin, which is hypoechoic, and blood (Fig. 6-6).

Most areas of the placenta are densely packed with villi. However, this is not true of the subchorionic space, an area in which blood tends to pool and eddy. At delivery, plaques of laminated subchorionic fibrin are found in about 20% of placentas from uneventful pregnancies.[1] These correlate

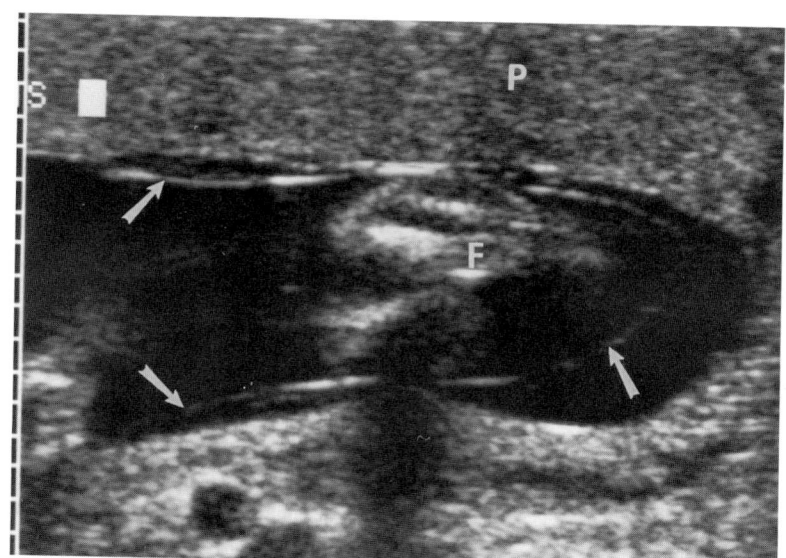

FIGURE 6-3. Nonfusion of amnion and chorion. At 21 weeks, the amniotic membrane (*arrows*) was visualized around the entire circumference of the amniotic cavity. At delivery, the amnion and chorion were separate. F, fetus; P, placenta.

FIGURE 6-4. Placental anatomy. **(A)** The placental circulation. U, umbilical cord; *arrow*, umbilical artery branching in chorion; *arrowhead*, umbilical vein in chorion; SA, spiral arteriole; V, maternal draining veins. (Spirt BA, Kogan EH: Sonography of the placenta. Semin Ultrasound 1980; 1:293–310.) **(B)** Anterior placenta at 29.6 weeks. The placenta (P) maintains the typical granular echotexture. Vessels are seen along the fetal surface, particularly adjacent to the umbilical cord insertion (*arrow*). Note retroplacental draining veins (*arrowheads*). F, fetus. **(C)** Posterior placenta (P) at 22 weeks shows the usual echotexture of the placenta. Note draining retroplacental veins (*arrowheads*).

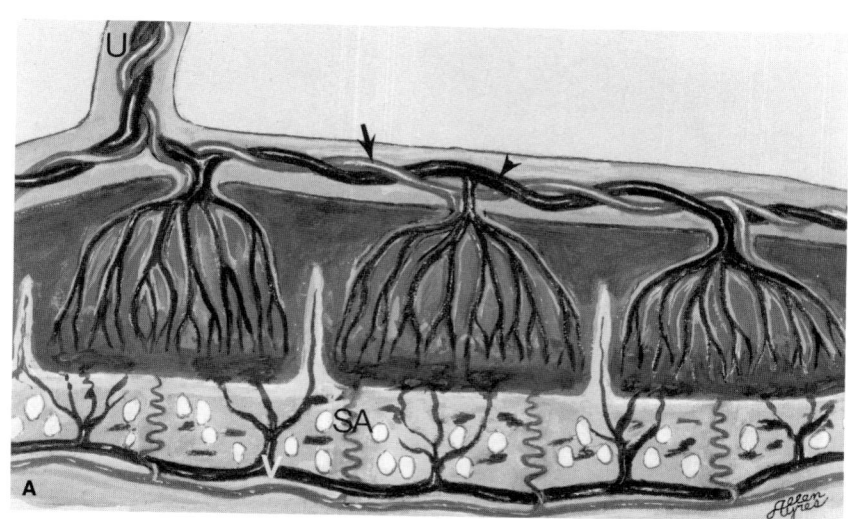

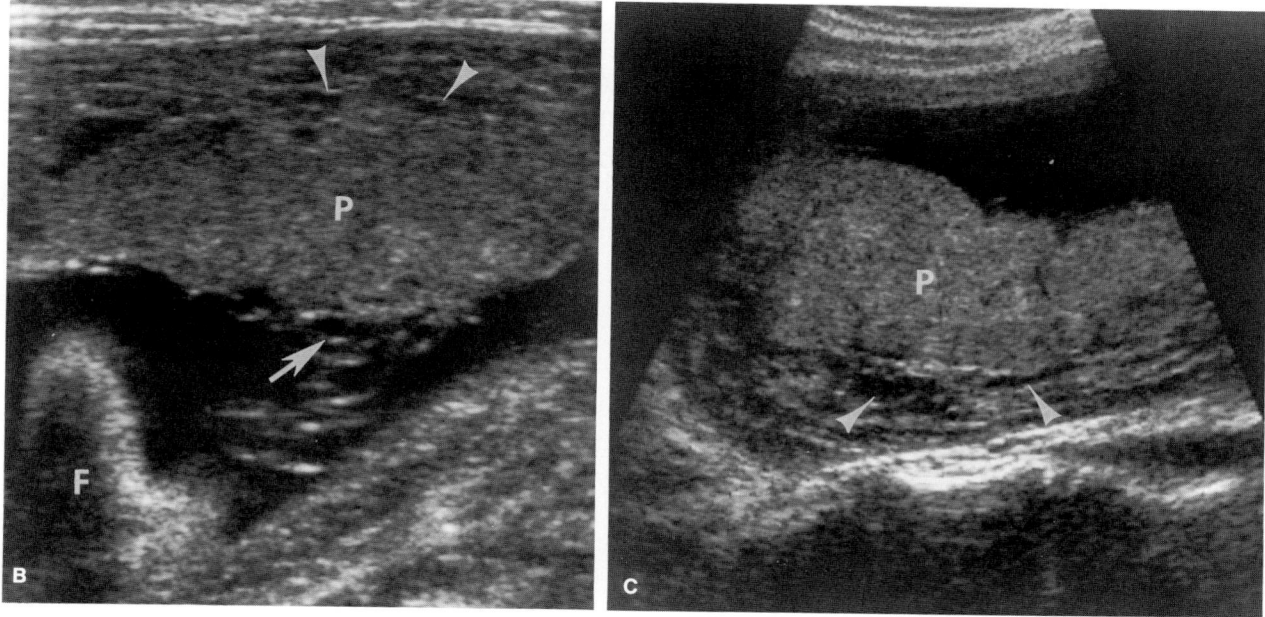

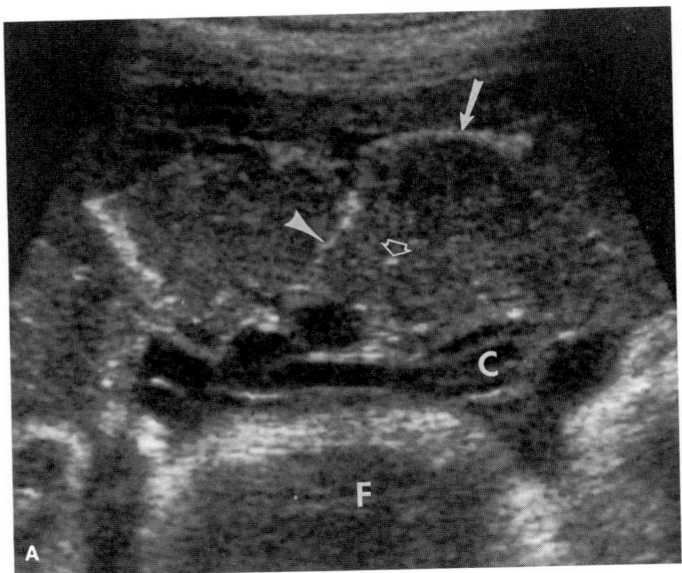

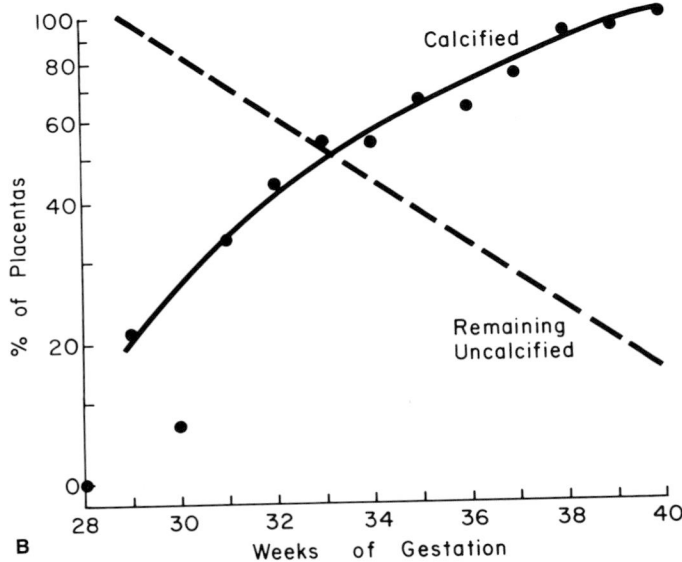

FIGURE 6-5. Placental calcification. **(A)** Anterior placenta at 39 weeks has calcification in the basal plate (*arrow*), along the intraplacental septa (*arrowhead*), and within the parenchyma (*open arrow*). F, fetus; C, umbilical cord. **(B)** Placental calcification versus gestational age. (Spirt BA, Cohen WN, Weinstein HM: The incidence of placental calcification in normal pregnancies. Radiology 1982; 142:707–711.)

TABLE 6-2. Common Anechoic and Hypoechoic Lesions in the Placenta

Lesion	Cause	Microscopic Description	Clinical Significance
Subchorionic fibrin deposition	Pooling of blood in the subchorionic space	Laminated subchorionic fibrin; fresh blood may be present	None
Intervillous thrombosis	Fetal hemorrhage into intervillous space	Laminated fibrin; fetal and maternal erythrocytes	None (theoretically could lead to isoimmunization)
Perivillous fibrin deposition	Pooling of blood in the intervillous space	Fibrotic villi surrounded by nonlaminated fibrin; fresh blood may be present	None
Maternal "lake"	Probable precursor of perivillous fibrin deposition or of intervillous thrombosis (see above)	Empty space	None
Septal cyst	Obstructed septal venous drainage	Small (5–10 mm) cyst in septum	None

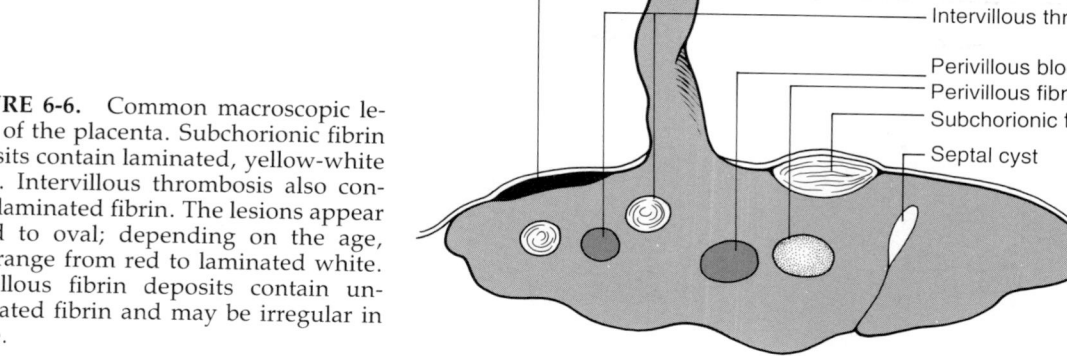

FIGURE 6-6. Common macroscopic lesions of the placenta. Subchorionic fibrin deposits contain laminated, yellow-white fibrin. Intervillous thrombosis also contains laminated fibrin. The lesions appear round to oval; depending on the age, they range from red to laminated white. Perivillous fibrin deposits contain unlaminated fibrin and may be irregular in shape.

with anechoic or hypoechoic subchorionic lesions seen at sonography,[6] in which slow flow may be visible (Fig. 6-7). These lesions can be found as early as 12 weeks menstrual age. They may be prominent (Fig. 6-8), but usually decrease in size as fibrin is laid down.

Pooling and stasis of blood also occurs in the intervillous space, producing anechoic or hypoechoic intraplacental lesions at sonography that may contain slow flow. These correlate with perivillous fibrin deposition at term[7] and are of no clinical significance. Perivillous fibrin deposition is found in 25% of placentas from uncomplicated term pregnancies.[1] Often, a hyperechoic rim is seen around these lesions at sonography, representing compression of the villi bordering the lesion.

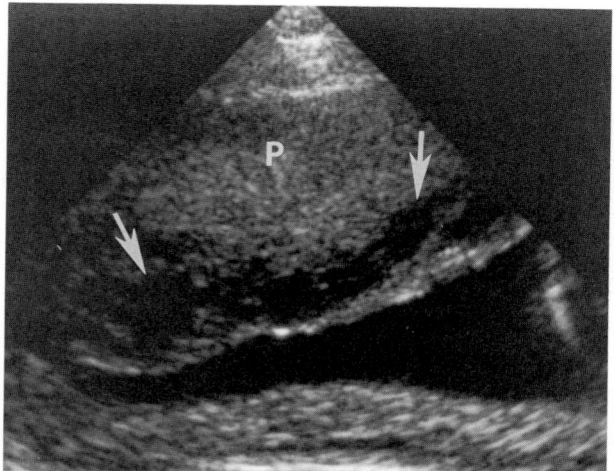

FIGURE 6-7. Subchorionic fibrin deposition. Anterior placenta (P) at 17 weeks shows prominent hypoechoic subchorionic lesion (*arrows*), which correlated with subchorionic fibrin deposition at delivery.

Up to 40% of term placentas from uncomplicated pregnancies contain intervillous thromboses,[8] which result from fetal hemorrhage into the intervillous space.[9] At sonography, these also appear as anechoic or hypoechoic intraplacental lesions,[10] which sometimes contain flow. Laminated fibrin and fetal red cells are found in these lesions at delivery. Intervillous thromboses are not thought to be clinically significant. However, since these are a site of fetal bleeding into the maternal circulation, it is conceivable that such lesions could lead to isoimmunization.

Up to 19% of term placentas from uncomplicated pregnancies contain septal cysts that measure 5 to 10 mm in diameter and appear anechoic at sonography[11] (Fig. 6-9). They occur in the subchorionic region at the apex of placental septa, which are decidua-containing folds of the basal plate formed during the third month of gestation. The septa divide the maternal surface into 15 to 20 lobules; neither the septa, the lobules, nor the cysts have any physiologic significance.

Septal cysts, perivillous fibrin deposition, and intervillous thromboses are sonographically indistinguishable from each other. Sometimes at delivery, a blood-filled space is found to correlate with an anechoic lesion seen at sonography; presumably this represents a stage in the evolution of either perivillous fibrin deposition or intervillous thrombosis (Fig. 6-10).

Infarcts

Ironically, the one common macroscopic lesion that is most likely to have clinical significance, the infarct, cannot be identified at sonography unless it is complicated by hemorrhage.[11] This is probably due to the fact that infarcts contain necrotic villi,

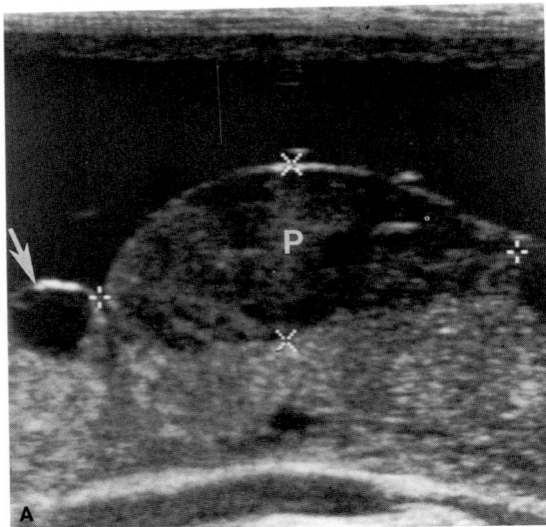
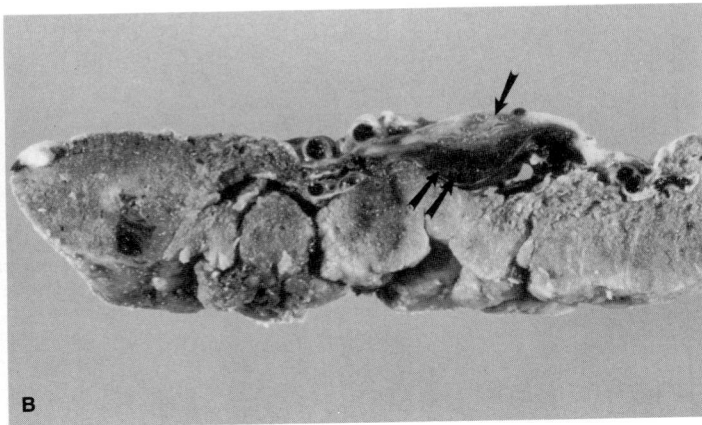

FIGURE 6-8. Subchorionic fibrin deposition. **(A)** Sagittal scan of posterior placenta (P) at 29 weeks shows prominent 4- × 9-cm hypoechoic subchorionic lesion, which contained areas of slow flow within (*cursors*). A vessel is seen adjacent to the lesion (*arrow*). **(B)** Corresponding slice of term placenta shows the lesion is composed of laminated fibrin (*arrow*) and blood (*double arrow*).

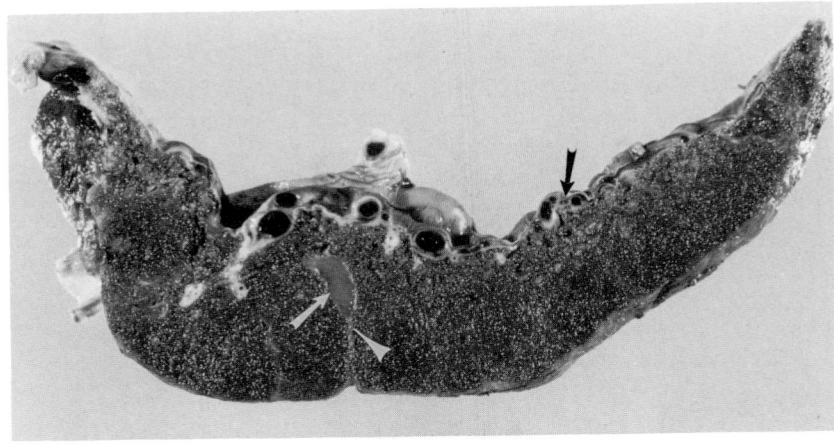

FIGURE 6-9. Cross section of term placenta shows septal cyst (*arrow*) in apex of septum (*arrowhead.*) *Black arrow* indicates fetal surface. (Spirt BA, Gordon LP: The placenta. In Rumack CM, Wilson SR, Charbonneau JW [eds]: Diagnostic Ultrasound. St. Louis: Mosby Year Book, 1991: 935–953.)

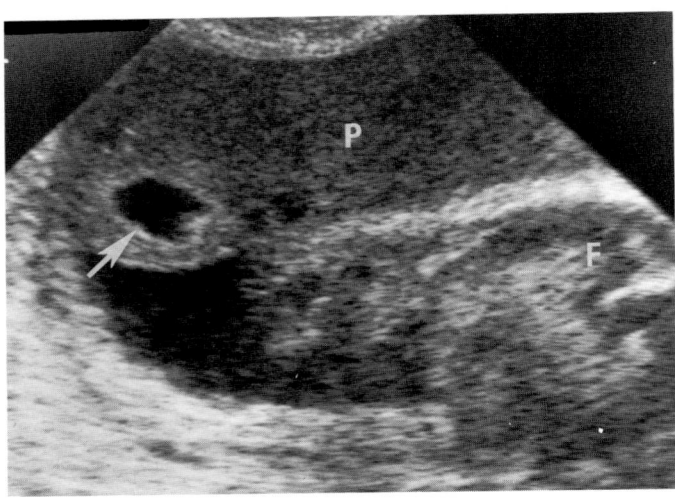

FIGURE 6-10. "Maternal lakes." Anterior placenta at 35 weeks shows anechoic intraplacental lesion (*arrow*). Note apparent rim of compressed villi around lesion. At delivery, the lesion contained blood, which fell out on sectioning. This placenta contained several areas of perivillous fibrin deposition. It is likely that in this patient, the "lake" represented a stage in the evolution of perivillous fibrin deposition. P, placenta; F, fetus. (Spirt BA, Gordon LP: The placenta. In Rumack CM, Wilson SR, Charbonneau JW [eds]: Diagnostic Ultrasound. St. Louis: Mosby Year Book, 1991: 935–953.)

TABLE 6-3.   Abnormal Intraplacental Lesions

Lesion	Incidence	Sonographic Appearance	Clinical Significance
Hydatidiform mole	0.07% in U.S. and Europe, 0.2% in Japan[8]	Multiple anechoic lesions of varying sizes	Premalignant (choriocarcinoma)
Partial mole	?	Enlarged placenta containing multiple anechoic lesions of varying sizes	May develop persistent trophoblastic disease; usually associated with triploidy
Chorioangioma	1% (small lesions)[1]	Solid, well-circumscribed intraplacental mass in which vessels may be distinguished	Small: none Large: fetal hydrops
Teratoma	Rare	Complex solid mass located between amnion and chorion, either on fetal surface of the placenta or adjacent to it	None
Metastases from maternal neoplasms	?	Multiple solid intraplacental nodules of varying sizes	Transplacental spread to fetus (two documented cases of transplacental spread of melanoma)

while the anechoic and hypoechoic lesions described above contain blood, fibrin, or fluid.

Infarcts are a result of disruption of the maternal blood supply to the placenta, due either to an underlying maternal vascular disorder or to retroplacental hematoma. One fourth of term placentas from uncomplicated pregnancies have small, macroscopically visible infarcts that have no clinical significance. Extensive infarction involving greater than 10% of the villi, however, has been associated with intrauterine growth retardation, fetal hypoxia, and fetal demise.[8] In this situation, it is actually the underlying maternal vascular disorder, and not the loss of villi, that is the cause of the problem.

Abnormal Intraplacental Lesions

Abnormal intraplacental lesions that may be seen at sonography include trophoblastic disease (partial and complete hydatidiform mole) and primary and secondary nontrophoblastic neoplasms (Table 6-3).

Partial Hydatidiform Mole

An enlarged placenta containing multiple diffuse anechoic lesions is abnormal and usually represents a partial hydatidiform mole (Fig. 6-11). In this entity, normal villi are interspersed with hydropic villi in the presence of a fetus that is usually abnormal. Most partial moles are triploid.[12] Triploid pregnancies often end in spontaneous abortion. Those that continue past the first trimester frequently present with symptoms of preeclampsia at about 18 weeks menstrual age.

Triploid as well as nontriploid partial moles have been found to develop persistent trophoblastic disease requiring chemotherapy.[13–16] Thus, it is important to follow the serum β-hCG levels in all patients with partial hydatidiform mole.

Complete Hydatidiform Mole

An enlarged uterus filled with solid material containing multiple anechoic lesions (vesicles) of varying sizes, in the absence of a fetus, is seen at sonography with complete hydatidiform mole (Fig. 6-12). The gross appearance of this entity has classically been likened to a bunch of grapes. The vesicles represent dilated, hydropic villi that enlarge with advancing gestational age; no normal placental tissue is found. The smaller vesicles that are present early in gestation may be difficult to distinguish at transabdominal sonography. Transvaginal examination is useful in this situation. Paternal chromosomes and maternal mitochondrial DNA are present in hydatidiform moles.[8] Moles are thought to result from abnormal fertilization of an empty ovum by a single sperm with a duplicated haploid genome (46,XX karyotype) or, less commonly, dispermy (46,XY).[17,18] A coexistent fetus may be found along with a hydatidiform mole in the case of multiple fertilization in which one ovum was empty. In this situation, a normal placenta and fetus should be visualized along with the mole (Fig. 6-13).

Hydatidiform mole cannot always be definitively classified on the basis of gross and microscopic morphology alone. Analysis of DNA content by flow cytometry may increase the accuracy

(text continues on p. 92)

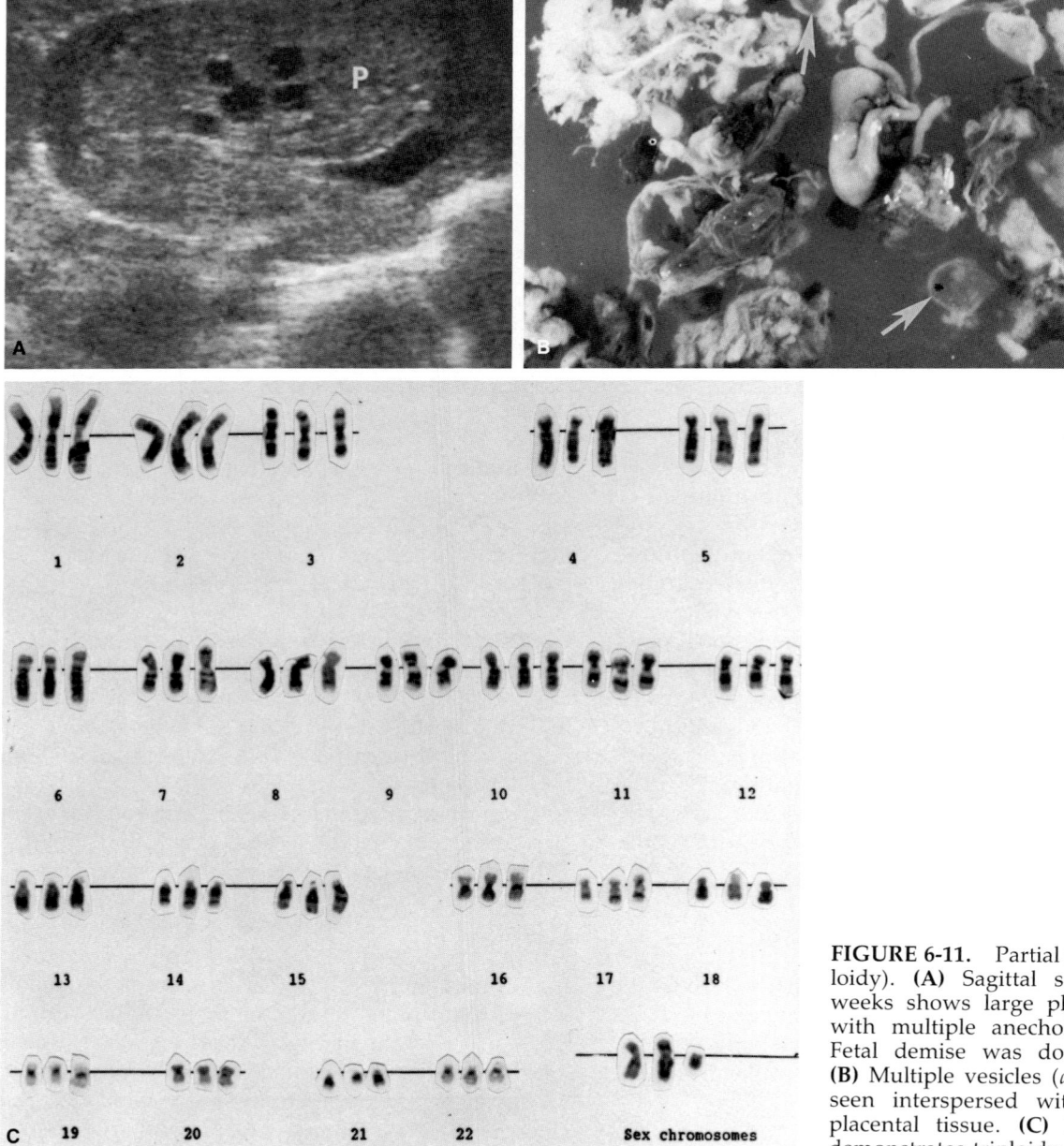

FIGURE 6-11. Partial mole (triploidy). **(A)** Sagittal scan at 15 weeks shows large placenta (P) with multiple anechoic lesions. Fetal demise was documented. **(B)** Multiple vesicles (*arrows*) are seen interspersed with normal placental tissue. **(C)** Karyotype demonstrates triploidy.

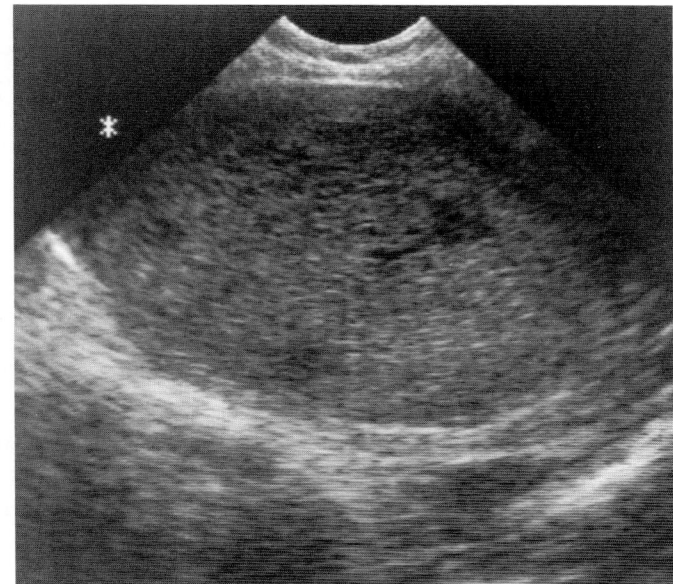

FIGURE 6-12. Hydatidiform mole. Sagittal scan shows enlarged uterus filled with solid material containing multiple small anechoic lesions throughout. This is the typical appearance of a hydatidiform mole. (Spirt BA, Gordon LP: Practical aspects of placental evaluation. Semin Roentgenol 1991; 26:32–49.)

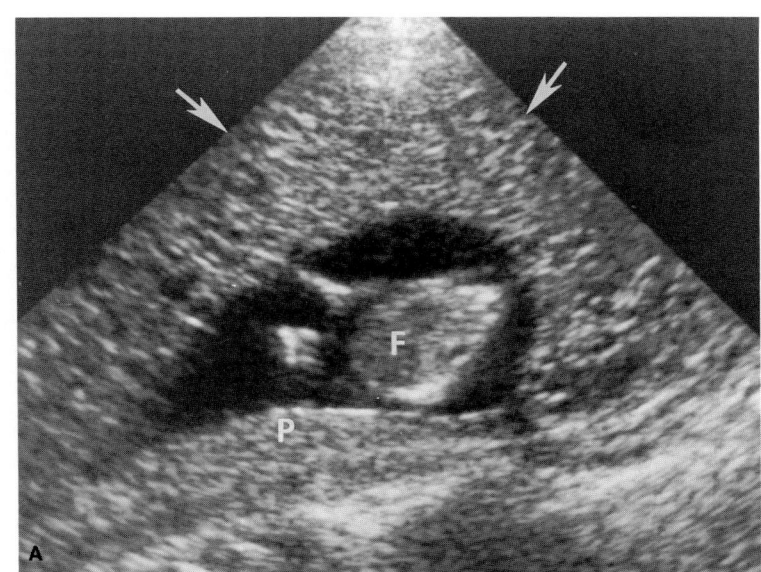

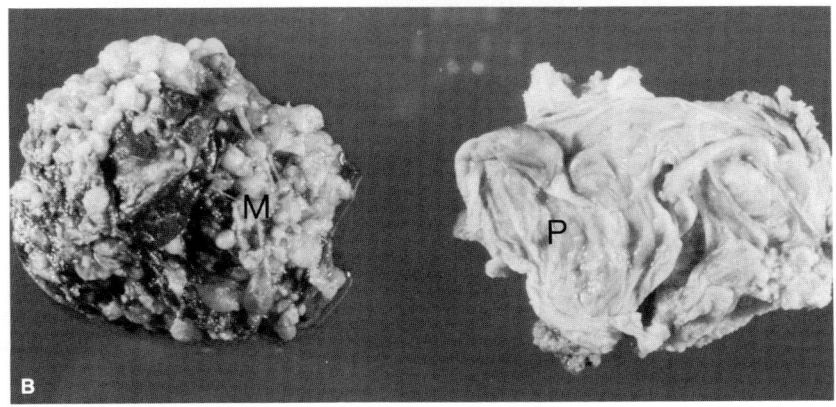

FIGURE 6-13. Hydatidiform mole with coexistent fetus. **(A)** Sector scan at 13 weeks shows large anterior mass (*arrows*) containing multiple anechoic vesicles of varying sizes, along with fetus (F) and separate posterior placenta (P). (Courtesy of Medical Imaging Department, Crouse Irving Memorial Hospital, Syracuse, NY. Spirt BA, Gordon LP: Imaging of the placenta. In Taveras JM, Ferrucci JT [eds]: Radiology: Diagnosis—Imaging—Intervention. Philadelphia: JB Lippincott, 1992.) **(B)** At delivery, a hydatidiform mole (M) was found separate from the placenta (P) and fetus. (Spirt BA, Gordon LP: Practical aspects of placental evaluation. Semin Roentgenol 1991; 26:32–49.)

of the diagnosis.[19] Moles are associated with high serum levels of β-hCG, sometimes resulting in multiple bilateral theca lutein cysts of the ovaries. Persistent trophoblastic disease (choriocarcinoma and invasive mole) occurs in about 10% of patients. Therefore, serum β-hCG levels should be followed closely in all patients with any form of hydatidiform mole.

Primary Nontrophoblastic Tumors

Chorioangioma and teratoma are the only known primary nontrophoblastic tumors of the placenta. Small chorioangiomas are relatively common, occurring in about 1% of systematically sectioned placentas, and have no clinical consequence.[1] Large chorioangiomas are uncommon and may cause significant vascular shunting, leading to fetal cardiac failure and hydrops. Polyhydramnios has been associated with large chorioangiomas, presumably due to fetal cardiac complications.

Large chorioangiomas usually protrude from the fetal surface of the placenta, but a few occur on the maternal surface. They are often surrounded by a distinct fibrous capsule, or a pseudocapsule of compressed villi.[8] At sonography, a well-marginated mass is visualized, usually subchorionic in location (Figs. 6-14 and 6-15). Doppler signals may be obtained from within the mass. It is important to obtain serial sonograms to monitor the fetus for the development of cardiac complications and hydrops.

Placental teratomas are rare. They always lie between the amnion and chorion, either on the fetal surface of the placenta or, less commonly, in the membranes adjacent to the margin of the placenta.[1] They are of no clinical significance.

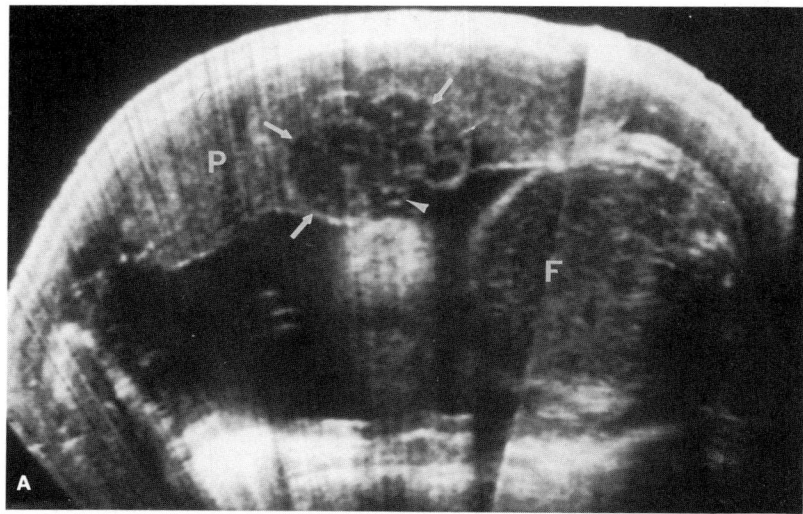

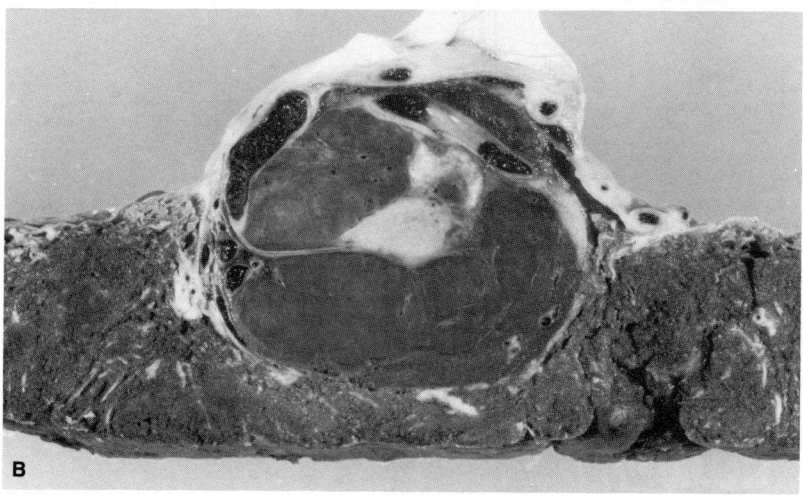

FIGURE 6-14. Chorioangioma. **(A)** Transverse static image at 24 weeks shows complex mass (*arrows*) beneath umbilical cord insertion (*arrowhead*). P, placenta; F, fetus. **(B)** Cross section of placenta shows large subchorionic chorioangioma beneath umbilical cord insertion. Note vessels of varying size within the mass. (Spirt BA, Gordon LP, Cohen WN, et al: Antenatal diagnosis of chorioangioma of the placenta. AJR 1980; 135:1273–1275.)

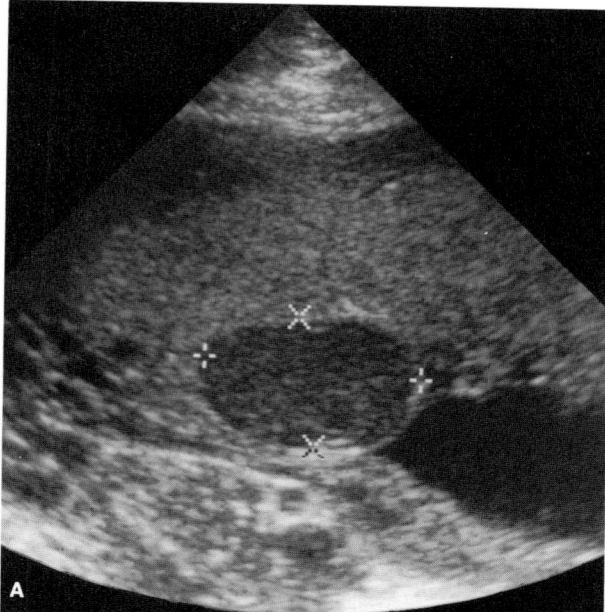

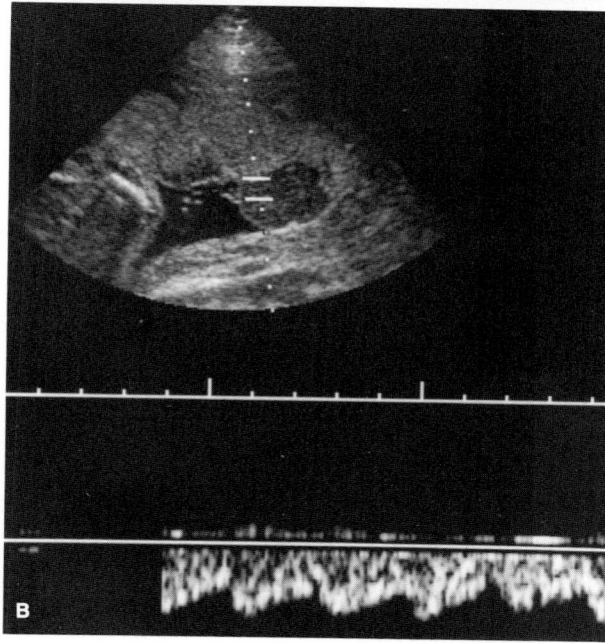

FIGURE 6-15. Chorioangioma. **(A)** Sector scan showing well-circumscribed mass (*cursors*) bulging from the fetal surface of the placenta. **(B)** Doppler cursor placed within the mass demonstrates vascularity of the lesion. (Courtesy of John P. McGahan, MD, Sacramento, CA.)

Size and Shape

The placenta is a fetal organ; its size is proportionate to the size of the fetus.[1,8,20] The fact that a small placenta is associated with a small-for-dates infant does not imply a cause-and-effect relationship.

TABLE 6-4.   Conditions Associated With Small Placentas

- Toxemia
- Maternal hypertension
- Chromosomal abnormalities
- Severe maternal diabetes
- Chronic infection

Small placentas do occur in association with toxemia and maternal hypertension, chromosomal abnormalities, severe maternal diabetes, and chronic infection[21] (Table 6-4).

Placental enlargement is associated with blood group incompatibilities (Fig. 6-16), maternal diabetes, maternal anemia, triploidy, fetal neoplasms, and multiple gestations[1,21] (Table 6-5). Placental size is usually visually assessed. Although some investigators consider the upper limit of normal placental thickness to be 4 cm,[22] we have seen normal placentas greater than 4 cm thick.

The pattern of regression of the chorionic villi

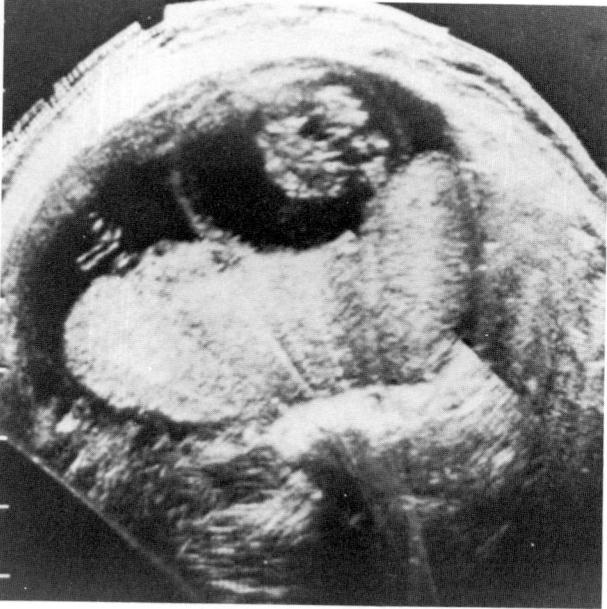

FIGURE 6-16. Rh incompatibility. Transverse static image at 28 weeks shows large placenta. Note marked fetal ascites. (Courtesy of Dr. Edward Bell, Syracuse, NY. Spirt BA, Gordon LP: Sonography of the placenta. In Fleischer AC, Romero R, Manning FA, et al [eds]: The Principles and Practice of Ultrasonography in Obstetrics and Gynecology, 4th ed. Norwalk, CT: Appleton & Lange, 1991: 133–157.)

TABLE 6-5. Conditions Associated With Placental Enlargement

- Blood group incompatibilities
- Maternal diabetes
- Maternal anemia
- Fetal neoplasm
- Triploidy

determines the shape of the placenta. Usually, the placenta is a single mass that is round to oval. However, in 5% to 8% of cases an accessory (succenturiate) lobe is found, connected by vessels to the main mass of the placenta (Fig. 6-17). This abnormality is important to recognize at sonography because of the associated complications, including vasa previa and retained placenta.

Placental and Retroplacental Relationships

Examination of the retroplacental myometrium and decidua is an integral part of the sonographic examination of the placenta. The retroplacental myometrium and decidua appear relatively hypoechoic compared with the placenta. A number of conditions may either mimic or cause a retroplacental mass (Table 6-6).

Placenta Creta

Absence of the normal retroplacental stripe may indicate a focal or diffuse defect of the decidua, which causes the placenta to abnormally adhere to or invade the myometrium (*placenta creta*[23,24]; (Fig. 6-18, Table 6-7). An increased number of intraplacental "lakes" may be seen at sonography.[25,26]

In this condition, the placenta fails to separate at delivery, usually necessitating a hysterectomy.

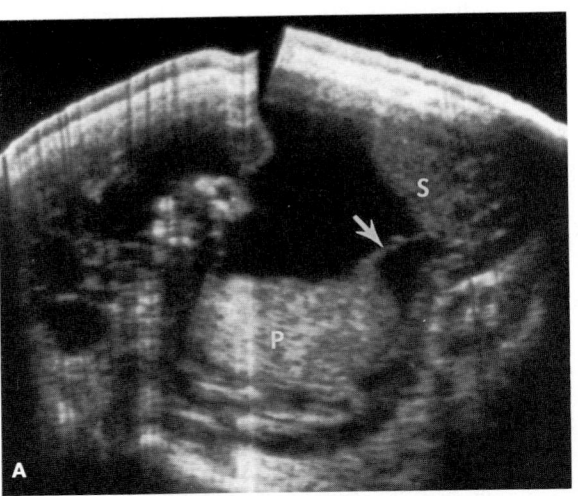

FIGURE 6-17. Succenturiate lobe. **(A)** Transverse scan at 28 weeks shows posterior placenta (P) with left succenturiate lobe (S). *Arrow* indicates membranes elevated over an anechoic space representing a subchorionic hematoma, confirmed at delivery. **(B)** Small succenturiate lobe (S) is connected to the main placenta (P) by vessels. (Spirt BA, Kagan EH, Gordon LP, et al: Antepartum diagnosis of a succenturiate placenta: Sonographic and pathologic correlation. JCU 1981; 9:139–140.)

TABLE 6-6.   Causes of Retroplacental Masses

- Contractions
- Myomas
- Retroplacental hematomas
- Abruptio placenta

TABLE 6-7.   Classification of Placenta Creta

- Placenta accreta: adherent to myometrium
- Placenta increta: invades myometrium
- Placenta percreta: extends through uterine wall

Placenta creta is associated with placenta previa in more than 30% of cases. It occurs with increased frequency in cases of prior cesarean section, multiparity, prior manual removal of a placenta, and uterine scars of other causes. Rupture of the uterus may occur in the antepartum period.[8]

Contractions
Contractions that are imperceptible to the mother occur throughout pregnancy. These contractions cause transient changes in shape of the placenta and retroplacental myometrium, particularly during the latter part of the first trimester and the early part of the second trimester (Fig. 6-19). They may be distinguished from retroplacental myomas and hematomas by rescanning after an interval of 20 minutes to 1 hour to document a change in appearance. Contractions are responsible for many false diagnoses of early placenta previa (discussed later).

Retroplacental Myomas
Retroplacental myomas (Fig. 6-20) are usually well circumscribed and may demonstrate Doppler flow

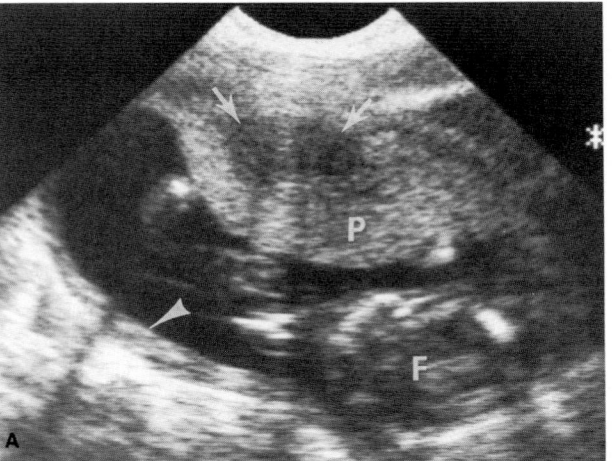

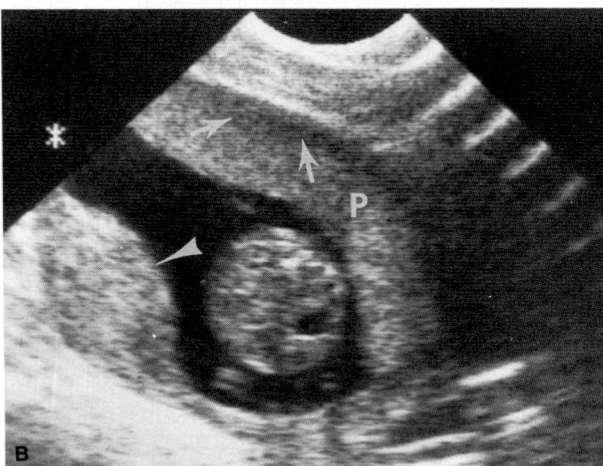

FIGURE 6-19. Contraction. **(A)** Sagittal scan at 16 weeks shows a contraction involving the anterior placenta (P). The retroplacental myometrium shows a hypoechoic pseudomass (*arrows*). The myometrium of the posterior wall of the uterus appears smooth and thin (*arrowhead*). F, fetus. **(B)** Twenty minutes later, the anterior placenta (P) appears smooth, and the retroplacental myometrium is uniform and thin (*arrows*). Note the contraction, which now involves the posterior myometrium (*arrowhead*). (Spirt BA, Gordon LP: The placenta. In Rumack CM, Wilson SR, Charbonneau JW [eds]: Diagnostic Ultrasound. St. Louis: Mosby Year Book, 1991: 935–953.)

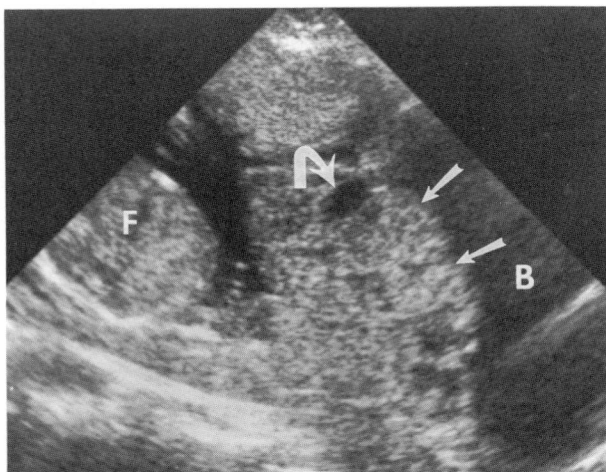

FIGURE 6-18. Placenta percreta. Sagittal scan in patient with antepartum bleeding shows absence of the retroplacental myometrium; the placenta had invaded through the myometrium to the bladder wall (*arrows*). Note the prominent "lake" in the placenta (*curved arrow*). B, maternal bladder; F, fetus. (Courtesy of Medical Imaging Department, Crouse Irving Memorial Hospital, Syracuse, NY.)

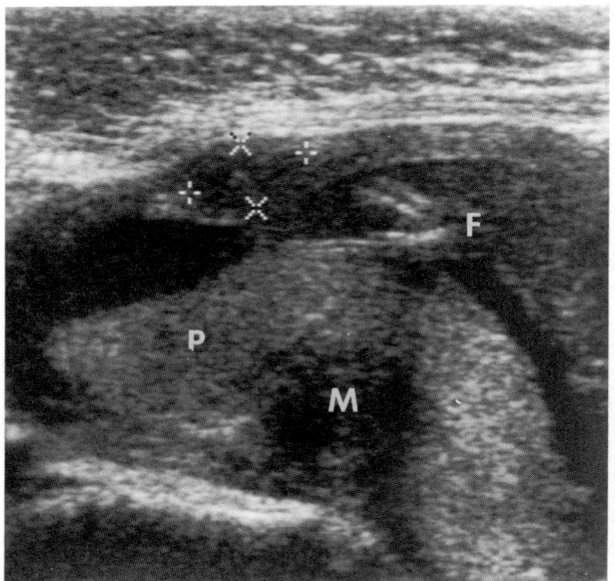

FIGURE 6-20. Retroplacental myoma. Sagittal scan at 16 weeks shows retroplacental myoma (M), which did not change with time. An anterior myoma (*cursors*) is seen as well. P, placenta; F, fetus.

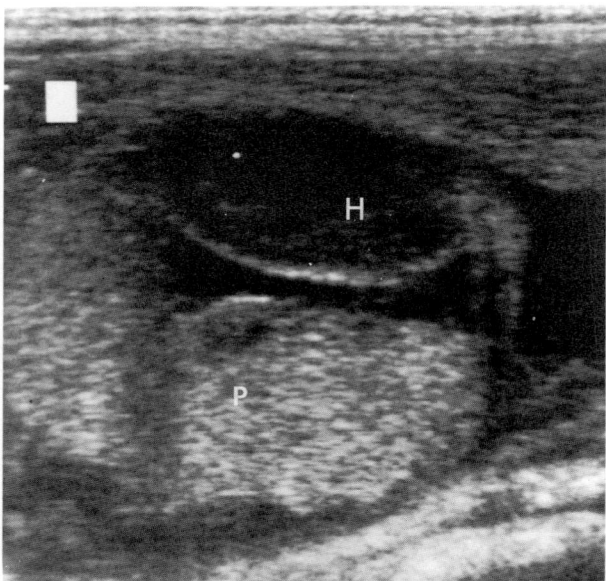

FIGURE 6-21. Subchorionic hematoma. Sagittal linear scan at 27 weeks in patient with vaginal bleeding shows anterior hypoechoic subchorionic collection (H) adjacent to posterofundal placenta (P). Follow-up examination at 30 weeks showed decrease in size of the hematoma. (Spirt BA, Gordon LP: The placenta. In Rumack CM, Wilson SR, Charbonneau JW [eds]: Diagnostic Ultrasound. St. Louis: Mosby Year Book, 1991: 935–953.)

within. The presence of multiple myomas helps to confirm the diagnosis. These lesions usually appear relatively hypoechoic, although large myomas often have a complex echotexture as a result of degeneration and/or hemorrhage.

Chronic Retroplacental and Submembranous Hematomas

Ultrasound examination is useful in the evaluation of antepartum hemorrhage (Table 6-8). Small retroplacental hematomas may occur with or without vaginal bleeding in the first two trimesters and can be difficult to distinguish from retroplacental myomas. Diffuse intravascular coagulopathy sometimes occurs as a result of tissue injury.[27]

Submembranous hematomas are found either adjacent to or at a distance from the placenta (Fig.

6-21). These should be followed to ensure that they decrease in size. There is no increased risk of miscarriage with a small subchorionic hematoma.[28,29]

Abruptio Placenta

Abruptio placenta is an acute event in which separation of the placenta causes severe vaginal bleeding, pain, and hypovolemic shock. It may be due to a number of causes (Table 6-9). Disseminated intravascular coagulopathy may occur as well. Because this is an emergency situation, antepartum sonography is not always performed. In those patients who are sufficiently stable to have an ultra-

TABLE 6-8. Common Causes of Antepartum Hemorrhage

- Normal examination (external bleeding only)
- Retroplacental or submembranous hematoma
- Placenta previa
- Placenta creta
- Abruptio placenta

TABLE 6-9. Causes of Abruptio Placenta

- Preeclampsia
- Cocaine abuse
- Trauma
- Anomalous uterus
- Idiopathic

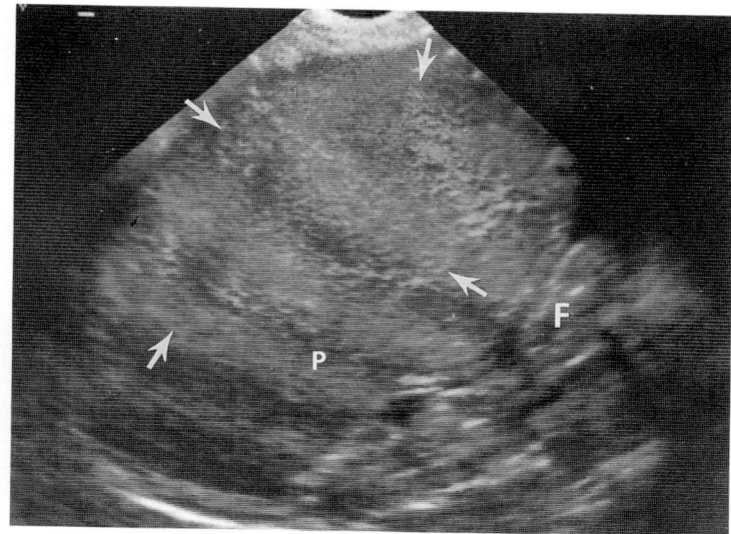

FIGURE 6-22. Abruptio placenta. Transverse scan at 35 weeks shows large hyperechoic retroplacental hematoma (*arrows*). P, placenta; F, fetus. The patient was hypotensive, with acute vaginal bleeding. At cesarean section, a 75% abruption was found. (Courtesy of Department of Medical Imaging, Crouse-Irving Memorial Hospital, Syracuse, NY.)

sound examination, an apparently thickened placenta is visualized with an echogenic collection in the retroplacental area (Fig. 6-22).

Placenta Previa

Placenta previa, in which the placenta covers part or all of the internal os (Fig. 6-23), occurs in less

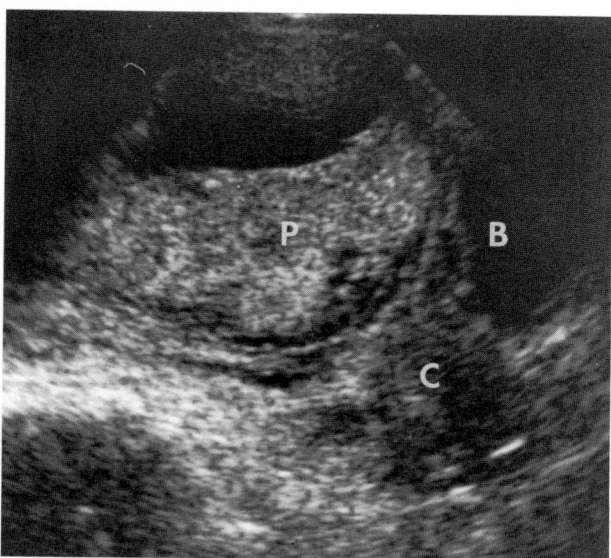

FIGURE 6-23. Placenta previa. Midline sagittal scan at 28 weeks shows posterior placenta (P) completely covering the cervix (C). B, maternal bladder. (Spirt BA, Gordon LP: Practical aspects of placental evaluation. Semin Roentgenol 1991; 26:32–49.)

than 1% of deliveries and necessitates a cesarean section. It is more common in pregnancies in older mothers and in women who smoke.[30]

Placenta previa is often misdiagnosed at sonography due to overfilling of the urinary bladder (Fig. 6-24) or contractions (Fig. 6-25; Table 6-10). Therefore, in the case of suspected placenta previa, it is important to rescan the patient after voiding and/or after a period of at least 20 to 30 minutes to confirm the diagnosis.[31]

Failure to diagnose placenta previa may occur for several reasons (Table 6-11). Although the main mass of the placenta may not be close to the endocervical canal, an accessory or succenturiate lobe of the placenta may cover the canal and thus result in placenta previa. Velamentous cord insertion may result in vase previa, in which the umbilical cord crosses the endocervical canal. This may be a catastrophic event if not recognized (see Chapter 7). Finally, in the late second or third trimester it may be difficult to visualize the internal os of the cervix owing to shadowing by the fetal head. Translabial sonography is useful in these situations to identify placenta previa or vasa previa, as discussed below.

CERVIX

Sonographic evaluation of the cervix is important in the identification of placenta previa and in the evaluation and management of cervical incompetence and premature labor. The endocervical canal, which is continuous with the uterine cavity at

TABLE 6-10. False Diagnosis of Placenta Previa

- Bladder effect
- Contractions

the internal os, is normally about 3 cm in length.[33] When evaluating the cervix with the transabdominal approach, it is important to scan with an empty maternal bladder because an overfull bladder artificially elongates the cervix.[34] Contractions (dis-

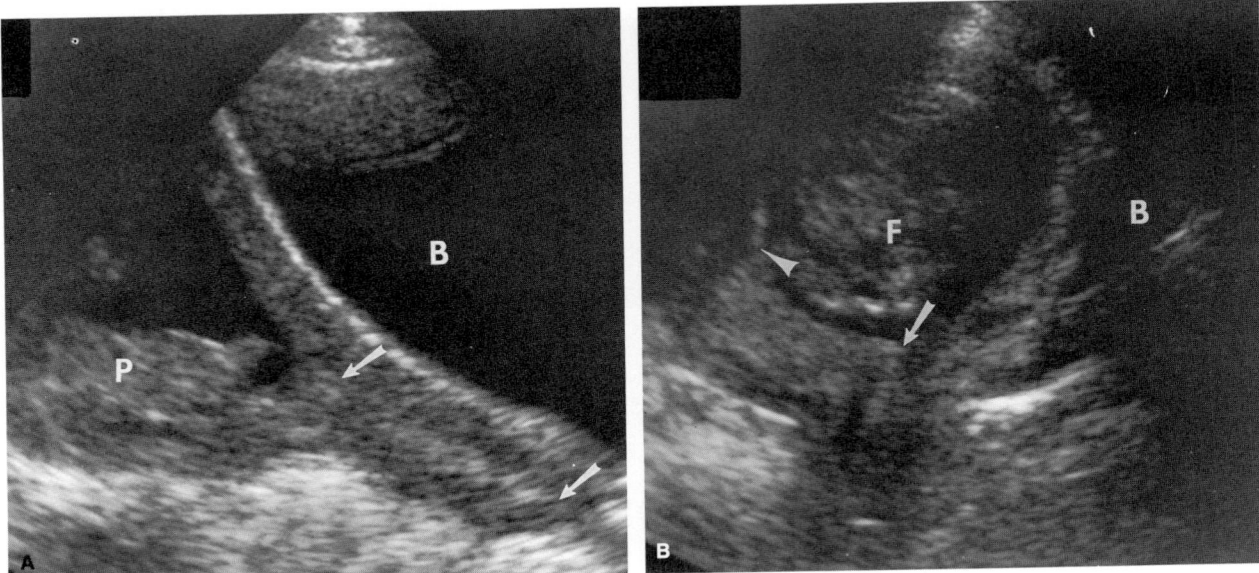

FIGURE 6-24. Bladder effect. **(A)** Midline sagittal scan at 18 weeks shows the edge of the posterior placenta (P) extending over the area of the cervix. The cervix appears abnormally long (*arrows*). B, maternal bladder. **(B)** Postvoid scan shows the placental edge (*arrowhead*) is well away from the internal cervical os (*arrow*). Note the normal vertical orientation of the cervix, as depicted in Fig. 6-26*A*. B, maternal bladder; F, fetus.

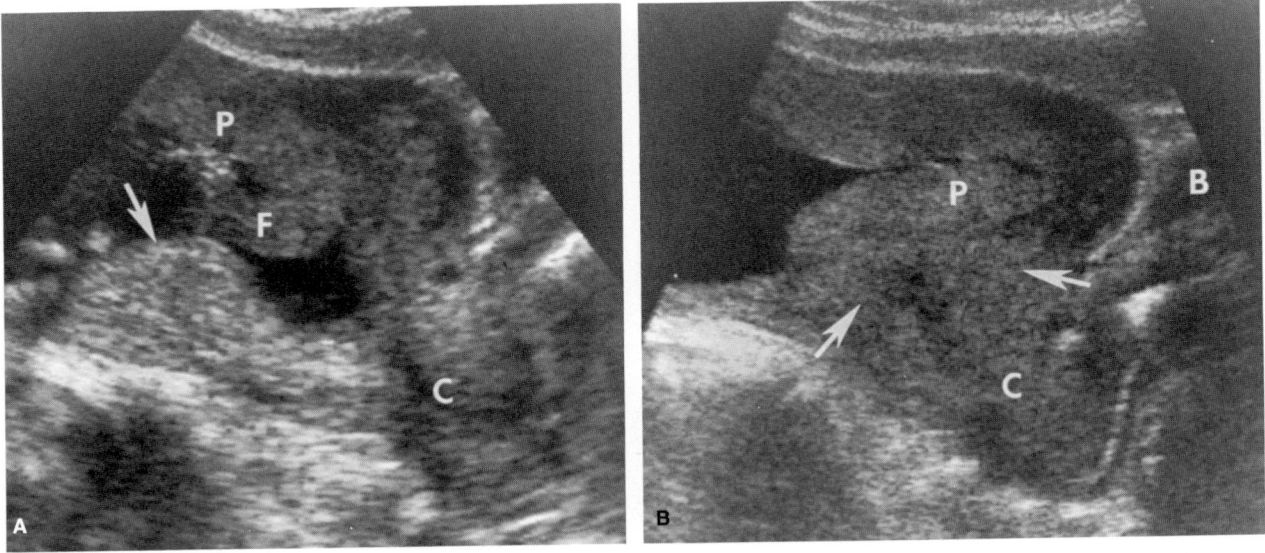

FIGURE 6-25. Contraction mimicking placenta previa. **(A)** Midline sagittal scan at 17 weeks shows the anterior placenta (P) extending over the cervix (C). Note the thickened appearance of the proximal cervix (*arrows*). B, maternal bladder. **(B)** Eighteen minutes later, the appearance has changed. The anterior placenta (P) is well away from the cervix (C). The contraction now involves the posterior wall of the uterus (*arrow*), above the area of the cervix. F, fetus.

TABLE 6-11.   Reasons for Missed Diagnosis of Placenta Previa

• Fetal parts obscuring lower uterine segment
• Succenturiate lobe
• Velamentous cord insertion

cussed earlier) may make it difficult to accurately evaluate the endocervical canal as well. With the transabdominal approach, the cervix is often obscured by fetal parts towards the third trimester. Maternal obesity may also make it difficult to visualize the cervix transabdominally.

Translabial (transperineal) sonography is useful to image the cervix and the lower uterine segment when the transabdominal approach does not succeed.[35,36] The procedure is performed with the bladder empty. The transducer, covered by a gel-filled sterile glove, is placed between the labia minora at the vaginal introitus (Figs. 6-26 and 6-27). In situations in which the fetal parts obscure the cervical os, the translabial approach may be used to exclude placenta previa (Fig. 6-28).

Cervical incompetence, resulting in recurrent spontaneous abortions, is usually due to previous trauma such as termination of pregnancy or surgery.[37] The sonographic appearance may include abnormal shortening of the cervix (Fig. 6-29), mild dilation of the endocervical canal, or bulging and actual protrusion of the amniotic membranes (Fig. 6-30). Sonographic evaluation of the cervix is useful to monitor the effectiveness of cerclage[38] and to evaluate cervical dilation and effacement in cases of preterm labor.

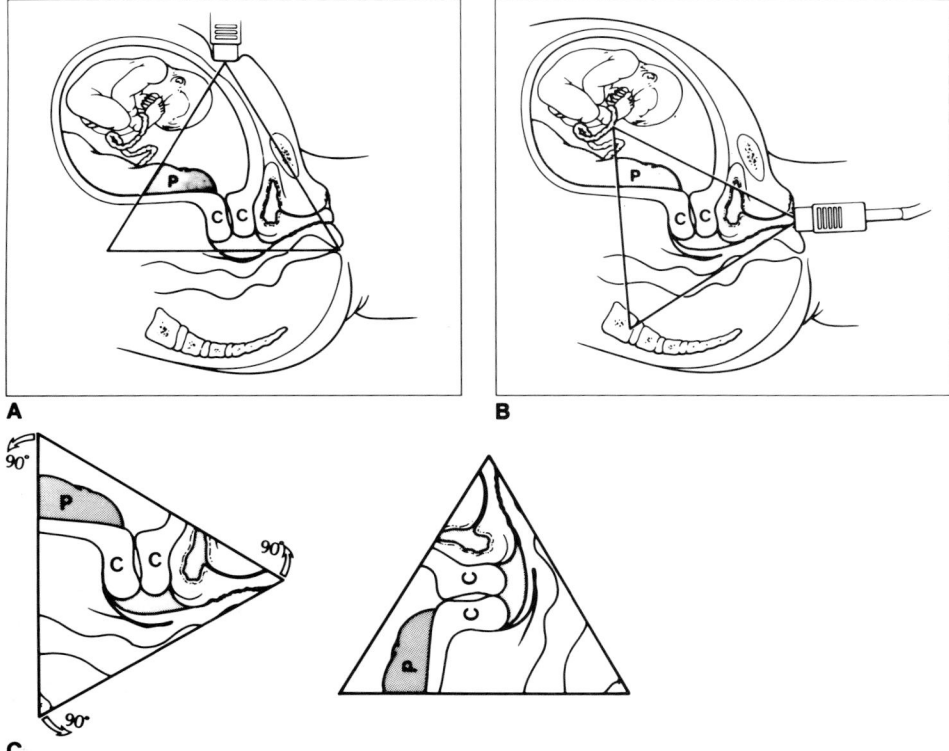

FIGURE 6-26.   Translabial scanning. **(A)** Schematic diagram of transabdominal scan plane shows vertically oriented cervix (C). **(B)** Schematic drawing of translabial scan plane. **(C)** Rotating the transabdominal image about 90 degrees provides an image similar to that seen with translabial scanning. The cervix (C) is oriented horizontally and the placenta (P), vertically. (Hertzberg BS, Bowie JD, Carroll BA, et al: Diagnosis of placenta previa during the third trimester: Role of transperineal sonography. AJR 1992; 159:83–87.)

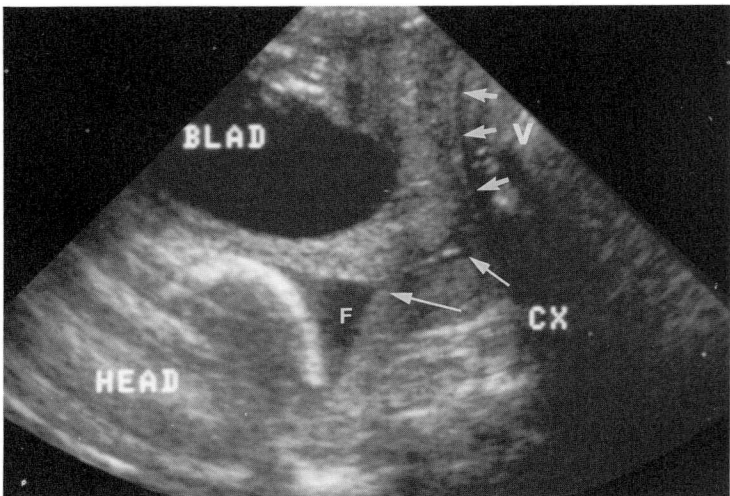

FIGURE 6-27. Normal translabial scan of cervix (CX), which is oriented horizontally. The vagina (V) is oriented vertically. F, amniotic fluid. The fetal head had obscured visualization of the cervical os when the transabdominal approach was used. (Courtesy of Marvin Courtwright, RDMS, UC Davis Medical Center, Sacramento, CA.)

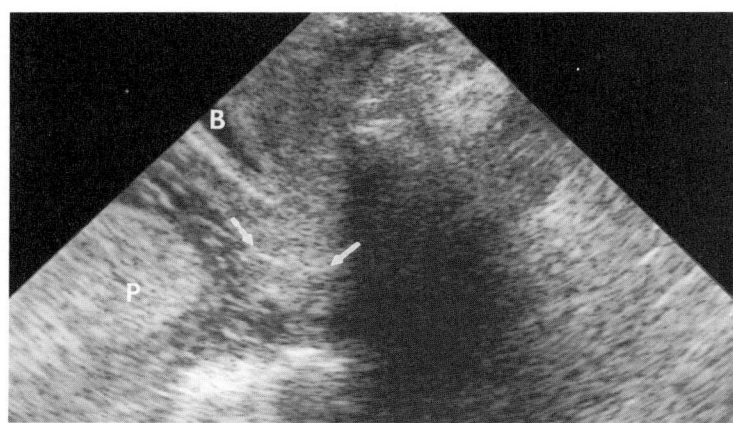

FIGURE 6-28. Placenta previa. Sagittal translabial scan shows posterior placenta (P) overlying the cervix (*arrows* indicate endocervical canal). B, maternal bladder. (Courtesy of Marvin Courtwright, RDMS, UC Davis Medical Center, Sacramento, CA.)

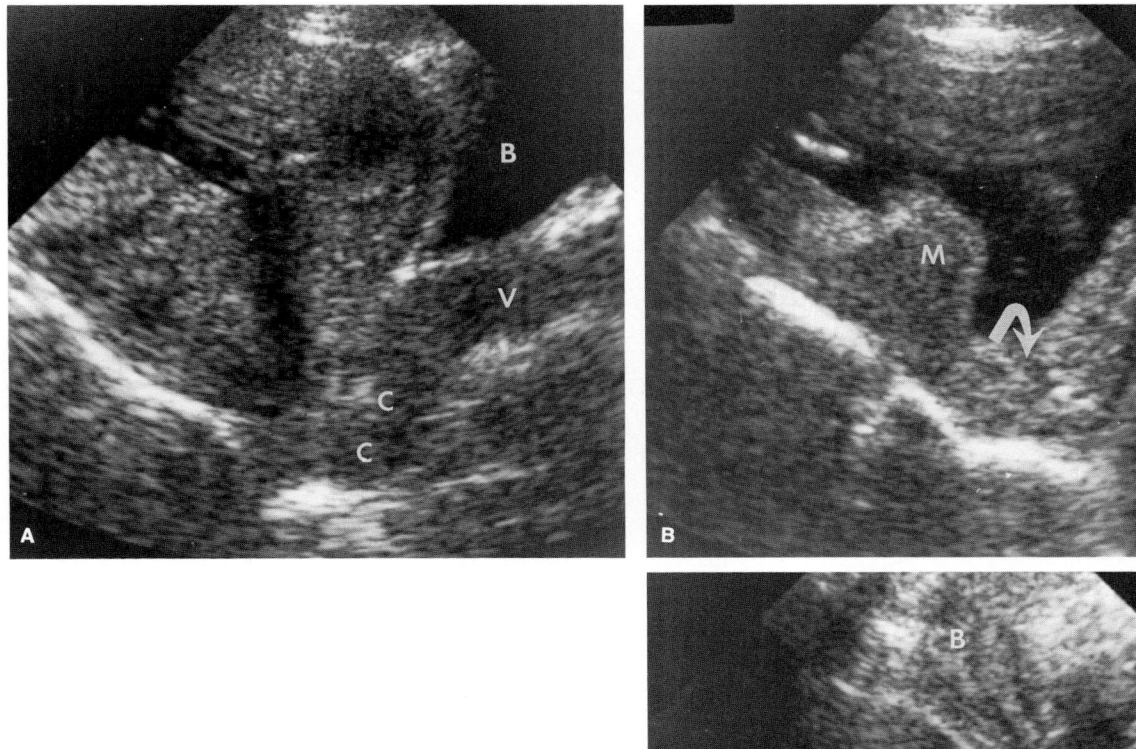

FIGURE 6-29. Cervical incompetence due to prior surgery for diethylstilbestrol exposure. **(A)** Sagittal transabdominal scan at 14 weeks shows prominent contraction involving the lower segment of the uterus. The length of the cervix (C) is difficult to evaluate. V, vagina; B, maternal bladder. **(B)** Half an hour later, the appearance has changed. The contraction now involves the posterior myometrium (M). There appears to be fluid in the endocervical canal (*curved arrow*). **(C)** Translabial scan shows the endocervical canal to measure only 1 cm (*arrows*). Despite cerclage, the patient miscarried within the week. B, empty maternal bladder.

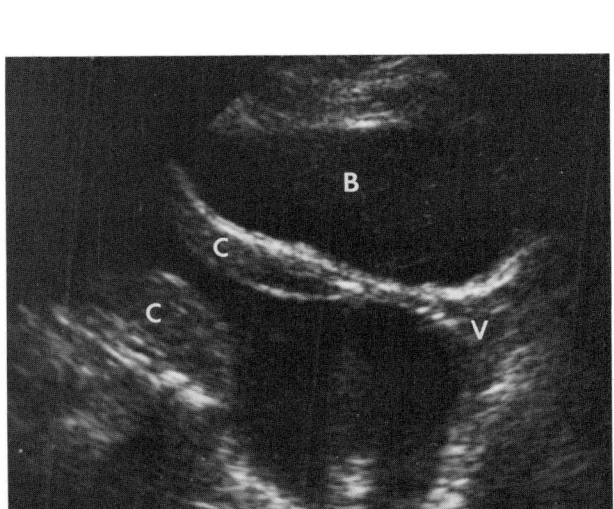

FIGURE 6-30. Cervical incompetence. Transabdominal scan at 16 weeks shows the amniotic sac protruding through the open cervix (C) into the vagina (V). The patient miscarried several hours after the examination. B, maternal bladder.

REFERENCES

1. Fox H: Pathology of the Placenta. Philadelphia: WB Saunders, 1978.
2. Jeacock MK: Calcium content of the human placenta. Am J Obstet Gynecol 1963; 87:34–40.
3. Wentworth P: Macroscopic placental calcification and its clinical significance. J Obstet Gynaecol Br Commonw 1965; 72:215–222.
4. Tindall VR, Scott JS: Placental calcification: A study of 3,025 singleton and multiple pregnancies. J Obstet Gynaecol Br Commonw 1965; 72:356–373.
5. Spirt BA, Cohen WN, Weinstein HM: The incidence of placental calcification in normal pregnancies. Radiology 1982; 142:707–711.
6. Spirt BA, Kagan EH, Rozanski RM: Sonolucent areas in the placenta: Sonographic and pathologic correlation. AJR 1978; 131:961–965.
7. Spirt BA, Gordon LP: Sonography of the placenta. In Fleischer AC, Romero R, Manning FA, et al (eds): The Principles and Practice of Ultrasonography in Obstetrics and Gynecology, 4th ed. Norwalk, CT: Appleton & Lange, 1991: 133–157.
8. Fox H: General pathology of the placenta. In Fox H (ed): Haines and Taylor Obstetrical and Gynaecological Pathology, 3rd ed. Edinburgh: Churchill Livingstone, 1987: 972–1000.
9. Kaplan C, Blanc WA, Elias J: Identification of erythrocytes in intervillous thrombi: A study using immunoperoxidase identification of hemoglobins. Hum Pathol 1982; 113:554–557.
10. Spirt BA, Gordon LP, Kagan EH: Intervillous thrombosis: Sonographic and pathologic correlation. Radiology 1983; 147:197–200.
11. Harris RD, Simpson WA, Pet LR, et al: Placental hypoechoic/anechoic areas and infarction: Sonographic-pathologic correlation. Radiology 1990; 176:75–80.
12. Szulman AE, Surti U: The syndromes of hydatidiform mole. I. Cytogenetic and morphologic correlations. Am J Obstet Gynecol 1978; 131:665–671.
13. Szulman AE, Wong LC, Hsu C: Residual trophoblastic disease in association with partial hydatidiform mole. Obstet Gynecol 1981; 57: 392–394.
14. Szulman AE, Surti U: The clinicopathologic profile of the partial hydatidiform mole. Obstet Gynecol 1982; 59:597–602.
15. Heifetz SA, Czaja J: In situ choriocarcinoma arising in partial hydatidiform mole: Implications for the risk of persistent trophoblastic disease. Pediatr Pathol 1992; 12:601–611.
16. Gardner HA, Lage JM: Choriocarcinoma following a partial hydatidiform mole: A case report. Hum Pathol 1992; 23:468–471.
17. Elston CW: Gestational trophoblastic disease. In Fox H (ed): Haines and Taylor Obstetrical and Gynaecological Pathology, 3rd ed. Edinburgh: Churchill Livingstone, 1987: 1045–1078.
18. Mazur MT, Kurman RJ: Gestational trophoblastic disease. In Kurman RJ (ed): Blaustein's Pathology of the Female Genital Tract, 3rd ed. New York: Springer-Verlag, 1987: 835–875.
19. Conran RM, Hitchcock CL, Popek EJ, et al: Diagnostic considerations in molar gestations. Hum Pathol 1993; 24:41–48.
20. Gruenwald P: The supply line of the fetus: Definitions relating to fetal growth. In Gruenwald P (ed): The Placenta and Its Maternal Supply Line. Lancaster: Medical and Technical Publishing, 1975.
21. Perrin EVDK, Sander CH. Introduction: How to examine the placenta and why. In Perrin EVDK (ed): Pathology of the Placenta. New York: Churchill Livingstone, 1984: 11–12.
22. Hoddick WK, Mahony BS, Callen PW, et al: Placental thickness. J Ultrasound Med 1984; 4:479–482.
23. Pasto ME, Kurtz AB, Rifkin MD, et al: Ultrasonographic findings in placenta increta. J Ultrasound Med 1983; 2:155–159.
24. deMendonca LK: Sonographic diagnosis of placenta accreta: Presentation of six cases. J Ultrasound Med 1988; 7:211–215.
25. Hoffman-Tretin JC, Koenigsberg M, Rabin A, et al: Placenta accreta: Additional sonographic observations. J Ultrasound Med 1992; 11:20–34.
26. Finberg HJ, Williams JW: Placenta accreta: Prospective sonographic diagnosis in patients with placenta previa and prior caesarean section. J Ultrasound Med 1992; 11:333–343.
27. Spirt BA, Kagan EH, Aubry RH: Clinically silent retroplacental hematoma: Sonographic and pathologic correlation. J Clin Ultrasound 1981; 9:203–205.
28. Stabile I, Campbell S, Grudzinskas JG: Threatened miscarriage and intrauterine hematomas: Sonographic and biochemical studies. J Ultrasound Med 1989; 8:289–292.
29. Pedersen JF, Mantoni M: Prevalence and significance of subchorionic hemorrhage in threatened abortion: A sonographic study. AJR 1990; 154:535–537.
30. Naeye RL: Functionally important disorders of the placenta, umbilical cord, and fetal membranes. Hum Pathol 1987; 18:680–691.
31. Artis AA, Bowie JD, Rosenberg ER, et al: The fallacy of placental migration: Effect of sonographic techniques. AJR 1985; 144:799–801.
32. Hertzberg BS, Bowie JD, Carroll BA, et al: Diagnosis of placenta previa during the third trimester: Role of transperineal sonography. AJR 1992; 159:83–87.
33. Mahony BS, Nyberg DA, Luthy DA, et al: Translabial ultrasound of the third-trimester uterine cervix: Correlation with digital examination. J Ultrasound Med 1990; 9:717–723.
34. Hertzberg BS, Bowie JD, Weber TM, et al: Sonography of the cervix during the third trimester of pregnancy: Value of the transperineal approach. AJR 1991; 157:73–76.
35. Singer A: Anatomy of the cervix and physiological

changes of the epithelium. In Fox H (ed): Haines and Taylor Obstetrical and Gynaecological Pathology, 3rd ed. Edinburgh: Churchill Livingstone, 1987: 217–236.

36. Bowie JD, Andreotti RF, Rosenberg ER: Ultrasound appearance of the uterine cervix in pregnancy: The vertical cervix. AJR 1983; 140:737–740.

37. Rushton DI: Pathology of abortion. In Fox H (ed): Haines and Taylor Obstetrical and Gynaecological Pathology, 3rd ed. Edinburgh: Churchill Livingstone, 1987: 1117–1148.

38. Rana J, Davis SE, Harrigan JT: Improving the outcome of cervical cerclage by sonographic follow-up. J Ultrasound Med 1990; 9:275–278.

John P. McGahan and Manuel Porto:
DIAGNOSTIC OBSTETRICAL ULTRASOUND.
© 1994 J.B. Lippincott Company.

Harris J. Finberg

Chapter 7

Umbilical Cord and Amniotic Membranes

UMBILICAL CORD

The umbilical cord is usually given little attention during an obstetrical sonogram, but as the lifeline of the fetus, it is of critical importance. Abnormalities that can have significant impact on fetal well-being may relate to the fetal umbilical origin, the placental insertion, the number of blood vessels contained, the length and spiraling of the cord, and the occurrence of a variety of focal cord lesions.

This chapter also reviews the amniotic membranes and a number of strands, sheets, and shelves that may project into the amniotic cavity.

Normal Anatomy and Embryology

The umbilical cord normally has two arteries and a single vein. Within the fetus, the umbilical arteries arise from the hypogastric arteries and carry deoxygenated blood from the fetus to the placenta. The umbilical vein proceeds in a cephalic midline direction from the umbilicus into the left branch of the portal vein and then into the ductus venosus, bringing oxygenated blood back from the placenta.

The blood vessels of the cord are surrounded by Wharton's jelly, a watery gel, which provides turgor and resistance to compressibility. The cord is covered by amniotic epithelium, which is firmly adherent to the connective tissue. Unlike the amnion, which is loosely applied against the chorion of the gestational cavity, the amnion of the cord cannot be elevated or stripped away.

The cord vessels normally spiral around each other, with the helical pattern usually well established before the end of the first trimester, although occasionally not appearing well coiled until after 20 weeks. It is widely accepted, however, that both the spiraling of the vessels and the overall length of the umbilical cord are directly related to fetal activity.[1] The normal cord averages about 60 cm in length with 40 coils. Restriction of fetal activity, whether due to inadequate amniotic space, intrinsic fetal abnormality, insufficiency of the maternal–placental unit, or physical tethering of the fetus, may result in a cord that is shorter and that has few or absent helical turns.[2]

The embryology of the umbilical cord, fetal gut, and amnion are interrelated.[2] About 2 weeks after fertilization (Fig. 7-1A), an embryonic disk is present that curves around the small, developing amniotic sac, which faces the portion of the chorion that will differentiate into the placenta. The primary yolk sac is present on the opposite surface of the embryo. These structures are surrounded by extraembryonic mesoderm, which fills the remainder of the gestational sac. By the third week this mesoderm has formed a cavity, except in one area, where a bridge of tissue, called the *connecting stalk,* attaches the embryo, amnion, and yolk sac to the outer rind of chorion. This stalk becomes the umbilical cord (see Fig. 7-1B).

As the connecting stalk is developing, a series of coordinated events are also progressing (see Fig. 7-1C):

- The amniotic cavity undergoes rapid enlargement, growing around the edges of the embryo, eventually filling the extraembryonic cavity, and fusing to the surface of the connecting stalk, enveloping the entire embryo.
- The embryo rotates so that the primary yolk sac ends up facing the connecting stalk and developing placenta.
- The embryonic disk begins to flex and fold around the primary yolk sac, which is largely incorporated into the fetus to become the primitive gut. This is accomplished by the growth and fusion of cephalic, caudal, and paired lateral body folds, creating a cylindrical fetus.
- An outpouching of the primary yolk sac grows down into the connecting stalk forming the secondary yolk sac, which bulges into extraembryonic coelom outside the amnion. This is recognized as the structure called the yolk sac on sonograms performed between 5 and 11 weeks of gestation. It remains connected to the fetus by a thin tubular structure within the developing umbilical cord, referred to as the *omphalomesenteric duct.* After 10 weeks of gestation, as the yolk sac shrinks, this duct usually involutes. (The fetal end persists in about 2% of people, remaining as a Meckel's diverticulum on the antimesenteric surface of the distal ileum.)
- An additional, smaller outpouching develops from the caudal end of the primitive gut where the bladder is differentiating. This diverticulum, called the *allantois,* also extends into the developing umbilical cord, and its blood vessels become the umbilical arteries and vein. The allantois is also referred to as the *urachus.* Its persistence may cause a variety of midline abnormalities between bladder and umbilicus as well as cystic remnants in the cord.

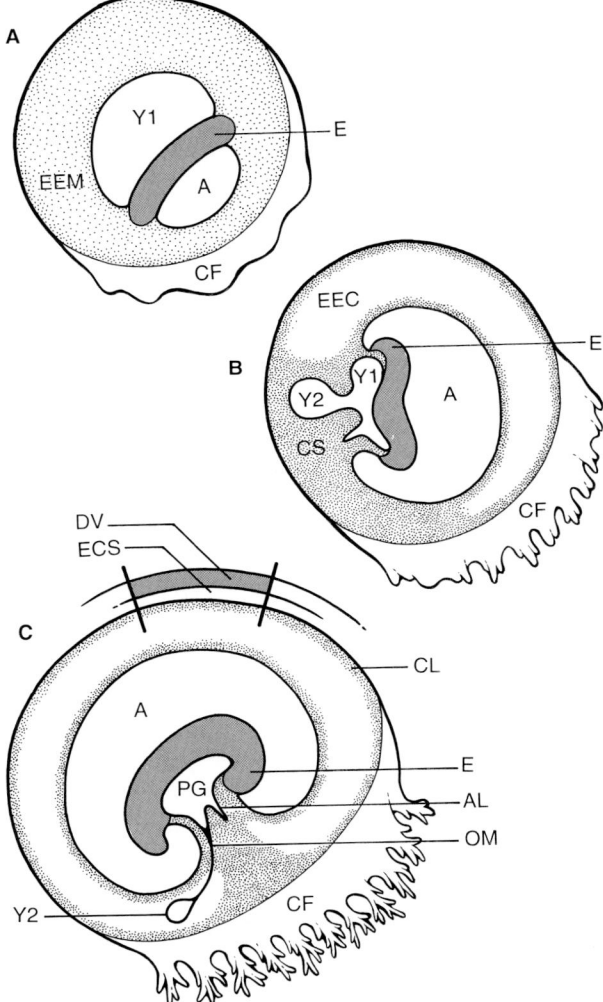

FIGURE 7-1. Development of the umbilical cord and membranes. **(A)** Thirteen days. **(B)** Twenty-one days. **(C)** Twenty-eight days. A, amniotic cavity; AL, allantois; CF, chorion frondosum; CL, chorion laeve; CS, connecting stalk; DV, decidua vera (along endometrium); E, embryo; ECS, extrachorionic space (endometrial cavity); EEC, extraembryonic coelom; EEM, extraembryonic mesoderm; OM, omphalomesenteric duct; PG, primary gut; Y1, primary yolk sac; Y2, secondary yolk sac.

Pitfalls in Evaluating the Umbilical Cord

I. Difficulty in determining the number of cord vessels (eg, due to early gestational stage or obese maternal body habitus). When there are an unusually large number of twists in the cord (tightly coiled), scans can be confusing, and a single artery cord may be mistakenly thought to have a normal three-vessel complement (Fig. 7-2). Useful views include:

   A. Axial to cord

   B. Longitudinal to cord

   C. Axial to fetal abdomen at umbilicus or dome of bladder to see unilateral or bilateral umbilical arteries (Fig. 7-3)

   D. Transvaginal

II. A single umbilical artery (SUA) may be found at one end of the cord with the normal complement of vessels at the other (Fig. 7-4). It is suggested that if the fetal origin has two umbilical arteries, the risk of associated anomalies remains low, like those with a usual three-vessel cord.

   A. In all cases with a single-artery cord segment detected, the fetus should be scanned at the umbilicus to count umbilical arteries there.

   B. A detailed fetal anatomic survey that includes cardiac evaluation should be considered, even in cases with segmental presence of an SUA.

III. A small omphalocele with herniated intestine can simulate a solid mass of the cord, such as hemangioma (Fig. 7-5).

   A. Axial views of the cord origin should be obtained at the umbilicus to seek

continuity of tissue of echointensity similar to that of intestine herniating from the fetal abdomen into the base of the cord.

IV. Focal thickening of Wharton's jelly is not infrequently present with omphaloceles, particularly when they are large (Fig. 7-6). This observation does not appear to have significance beyond that of the omphalocele itself.

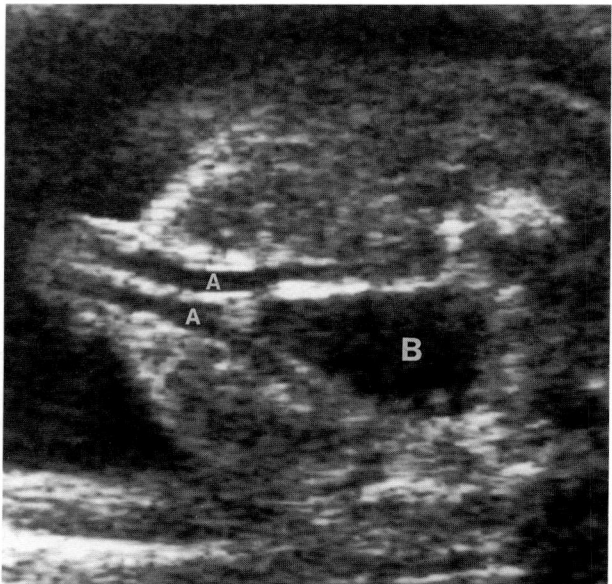

FIGURE 7-3.   The two umbilical arteries (A) enter the fetal abdomen at the umbilicus. They course caudally, separating to straddle the bladder (B) and joining with the hypogastric arteries.

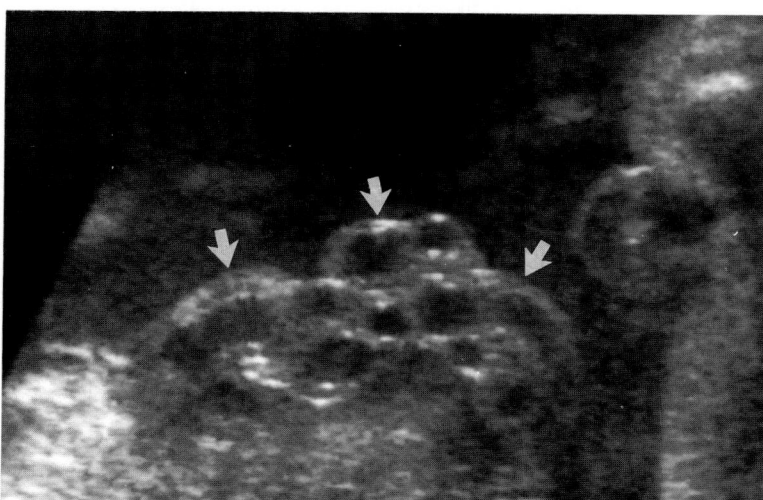

FIGURE 7-2. A single-artery umbilical cord with a large number of vascular coils has developed secondary twists of the whole cord contours, making it difficult to count the vessels accurately (*arrows*). Views at the umbilicus confirmed the presence of only one artery.

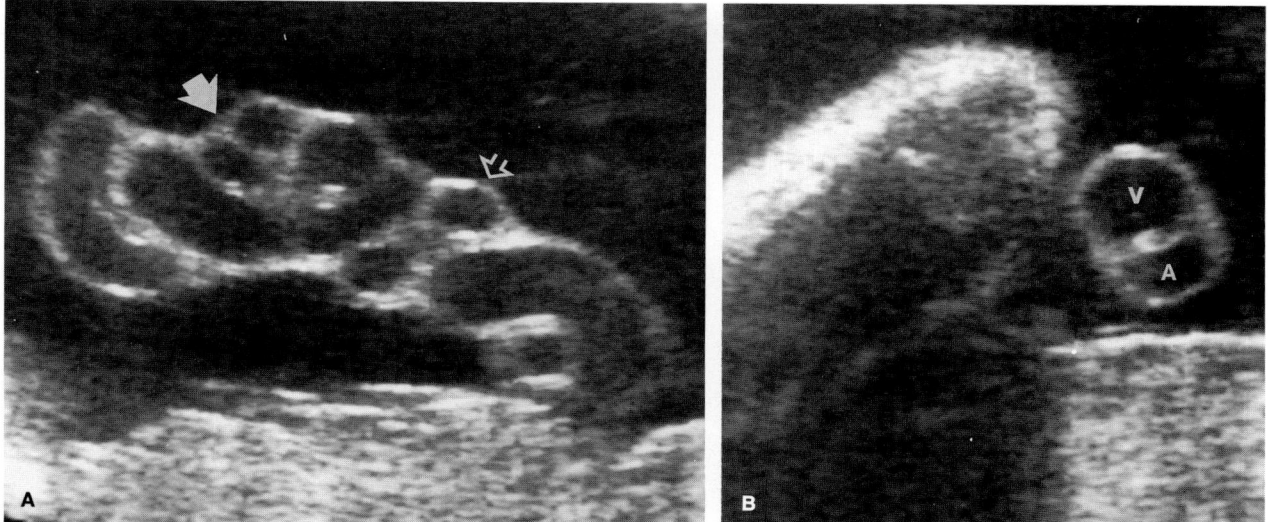

FIGURE 7-4. **(A)** Transition zone in umbilical cord from normal two-artery configuration toward fetal end (*closed arrow*) into single-artery segment toward placenta (*open arrow*). **(B)** Umbilical cord cross section at level of open arrow in **A** confirms single artery (A). (Two arteries were shown more proximally toward the fetus). V, vein.

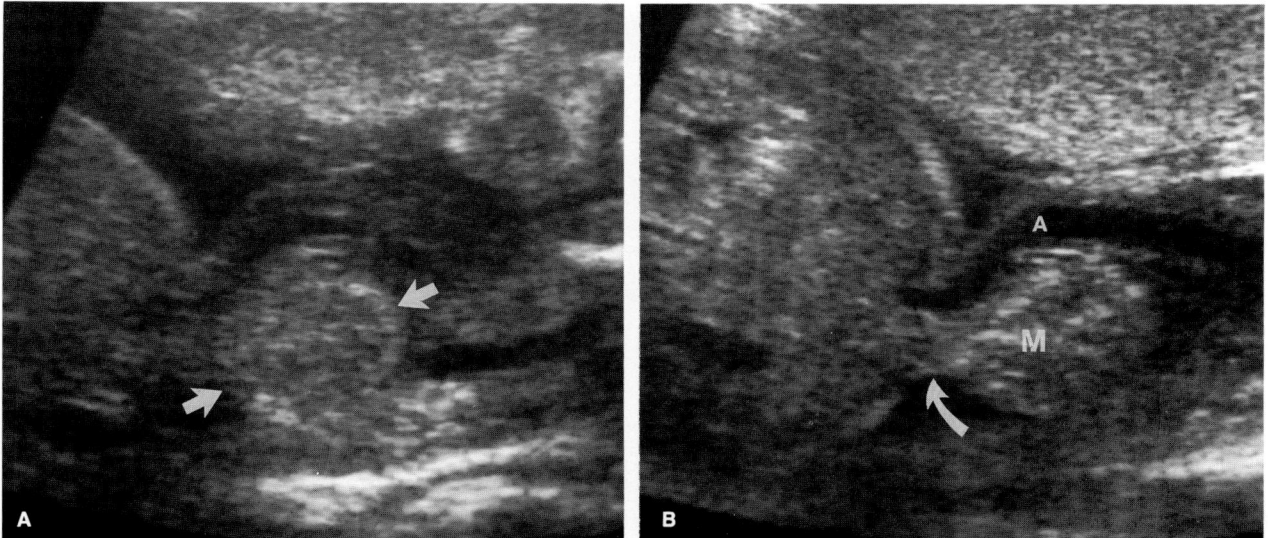

FIGURE 7-5. Pitfall: small omphalocele simulating a solid cord mass. **(A)** An echodense, 2-cm lesion (*arrows*) is seen within the umbilical cord at the fetal end. This could represent a tera-toma or hemangioma. **(B)** A view axial to the cord origin shows a stalk-like zone of similar echointensity (*curved arrow*), demonstrating continuity between cord mass (M) and the fetal intestine. An umbilical artery (A) deviating around the omphalocele is also shown.

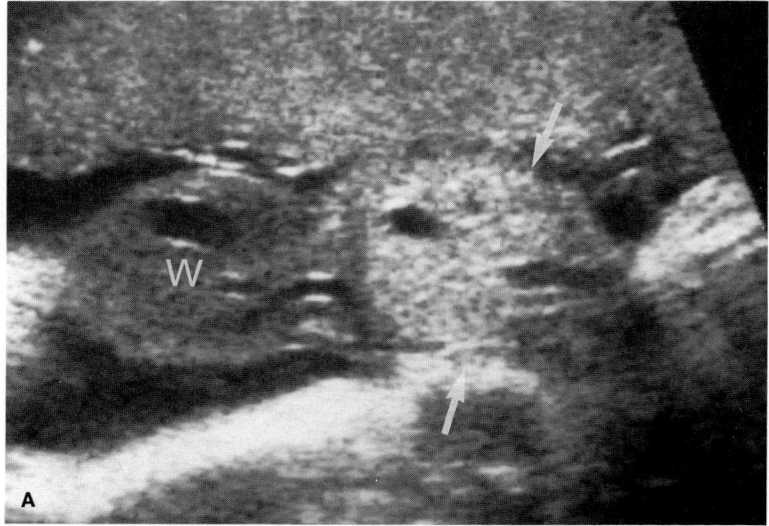

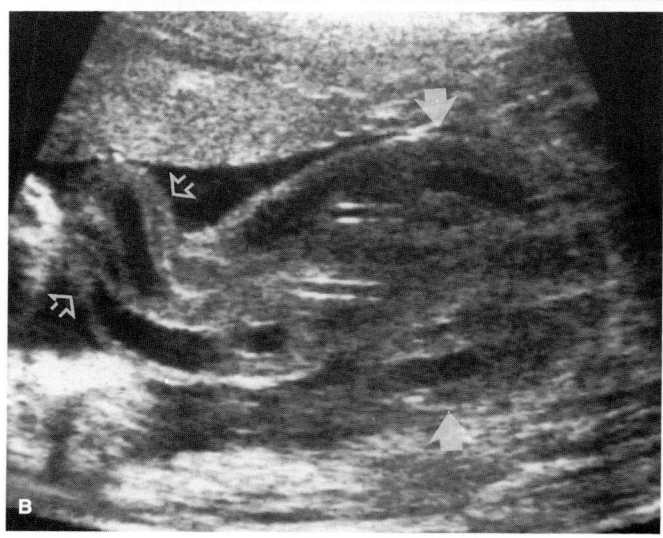

FIGURE 7-6. **(A)** Focal thickening of Wharton's jelly (W) is seen, enlarging the first several centimeters of the cord to 4-cm diameter at its origin along the anteroinferior surface of a large fetal omphalocele (*arrows*). **(B)** The three cord vessels are concentrically splayed in this segment (*arrows*), with the cord resuming a normal size and configuration more distally, to the left within the image (*open arrows*).

Differential Diagnosis of Umbilical Cord Abnormalities

Umbilical cord abnormalities may be grouped into five categories: Vascular development, cord formation, cord length and twist, cord masses, and trophotropism (Table 7-1).

Abnormalities of Vascular Development

An *SUA* is the most common intrinsic malformation of the umbilical cord, occurring in 0.6% to 1% of pregnancies, with higher frequencies in autopsy series and in first- and second-trimester delivery series[3] (Fig. 7-7). In a detailed review of this condition, Heifetz found a strong association between SUA and other fetal malformations, with additional anomalies occurring in about 20% of cases.[4] These abnormalities may affect any fetal organ sys-

tem without apparent predilection. Abnormalities were multiple in 15% or more of infants and in 50% of cases studied in autopsy series. When an SUA is detected along with an intrafetal anomaly, the risk that additional fetal anomalies is present and the risk that there will be aneuploidy increases. Nyberg and coworkers studied this phenomenon in 107 consecutive cases with a fetal central nervous system (CNS) malformation.[5] Among the 20 patients with SUA, all had additional extra-CNS malformations, as compared with only 35 of 87 (39%) who had other anomalies when a normal two-artery cord was present. Of 15 pregnancies with SUA tested, 8 (53%) had aneuploidy, while only 11 of 45 (24%) with a normal cord had an abnormal karyotype. It appears that chromosomal analysis is a reasonable part of the evaluation of all fetuses with CNS malformation regardless of SUA. A simi-

TABLE 7-1. Umbilical Cord Abnormalities and Associated Risks

Abnormality	Associated Risks
Vascular Development	
Single umbilical artery	50% risk of other anomalies
	With other anomalies, risk of aneuploidy
	Growth retardation even with single umbilical artery only
Gastroschisis	Intestinal obstruction and atresia
Persistent right umbilical vein	No definite risk itself
	Significant risk of other anomalies
Cord Formation	
Body stalk anomaly	Lethal exteriorization of thoracoabdominal organs
Omphalocele	Associated fetal anomalies, aneuploidy
Cord Length and Twist	
Short cord, nonspiraled vessels	Cord compression accidents
	Underlying fetal or maternal placental abnormalities
	Fetal distress
Long cord	
Nuchal Cord	Vascular compromise uncommon
True cord knot	Vascular compromise uncommon
Stricture or torsion	Rare but lethal
Trophotropism	
Marginal and velamentous cord insertion	Vasa previa if crosses internal cervical os
	Thrombosis or hemorrhage of cord vessels
	Obligate cord presentation and risk of cord compression or prolapse if near os.
Cord Masses	
Focal thickening of Wharton's jelly	No definite risk
	Normal variant
	Sequela of hydrops
Diffuse cord swelling	Sequela of hydrops
	Idiopathic
	Urine extravasation from patent urachus
Cysts	
Omphalomesenteric, allantoic, and degenerative	Vascular compromise rare
	? Risk of other anomalies or aneuploidy
Hemangioma, teratoma	Vascular compromise may occur
	? Risk of other anomalies or aneuploidy
Aneurysm or varix	Significant risk of vascular compromise
	? Risk of other anomalies or aneuploidy
False knot	No definite risk
Varix of intrafetal umbilical vein	Cases of stillbirth reported, but most cases normal
Thrombosis, hematoma	Severe risk of vascular compromise
	Embolic fetal or placental events

lar argument favoring karyotyping can be advanced for most congenital malformations detected prenatally.

What are the risks that other fetal anomalies or aneuploidy will be present when a detailed sonogram finds only an SUA, with no fetal malformations identified? Nyberg and colleagues evaluated 30 fetuses with prenatally diagnosed SUA.[6] Twelve fetuses had one or more major abnormality; 3 had minor abnormalities (pelvic kidney, uni-

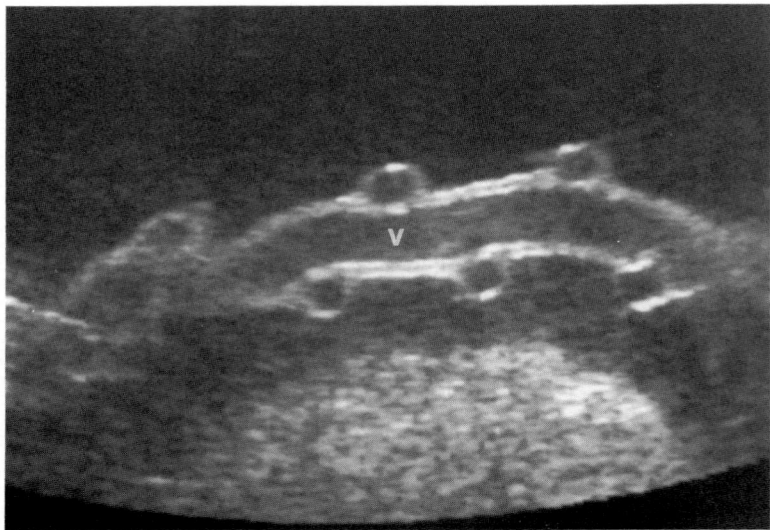

FIGURE 7-7. Single-artery umbilical cord. The single artery follows a helical course around the straighter umbilical vein (V).

lateral absent kidney, mild cerebral ventricular dilation); and 15 were sonographically normal. None of the 15 normal fetuses nor the 3 with minor anomalies had additional findings at birth, and none had aneuploidy. Of the 12 with SUA and major fetal malformations, 6 had abnormal karyotypes: 4 had trisomy 18, and 1 each had trisomy 13 and triploidy. Other aneuploidies may occur, but trisomy 21 is distinctly unusual.[7]

Based on Nyberg's studies and similar clinical experience at our center, identification of an SUA should prompt a detailed fetal anatomic survey, including the heart with outflow tracts, nuchal fold, face, hands, and feet. If no additional abnormalities are detected, the pregnancy and delivery are managed in routine fashion, and chromosome testing is not performed. Cases with anomalies undergo genetic testing and receive management appropriate to the specific abnormalities present.

According to Heifetz, the anatomically normal fetus with SUA may have an increased risk of intrauterine growth retardation associated with an abnormally small placenta.[4] Other groups studying SUA have not commented on this phenomenon, but it may be prudent to obtain a follow-up sonogram at 30 to 32 weeks of gestation to document satisfactory growth. A few additional observations about SUA are worth noting:

1. The risk of fetal anomalies is related to the cord architecture at the fetal end.[4] Two normal umbilical arteries may fuse into one toward the placental insertion of the cord without an increased incidence of anomalies. Cord vessel counting should be confirmed at or near the umbilicus or even within the fetal abdomen by identifying two hypogastric arteries (or absence of one of these in SUA) along the margins of the bladder. The iliac artery ipsilateral to an absent umbilical artery may be small at the aortic bifurcation, and the aorta may bow toward the contralateral iliac artery.[8]

2. SUA is considerably more frequent in multiple gestations, often discordant among the fetuses. The correlation with other fetal anomalies is less strong than SUA in singleton pregnancies, but it remains high enough to warrant a careful anatomic survey.

3. Remnants of a second umbilical artery are frequently detectable on microscopic examination of an SUA cord. Partially based on this observation, there is a widespread belief that most cases of SUA occur by atrophy of an existing artery rather than by the primary failure of its formation. Asymmetry in the size of the umbilical arteries, therefore, may be part of the spectrum of SUA. If one of the arteries is noticeably small, it is reasonable to check the fetal anatomy in detail.

4. There are no direct relations between SUA and maternal disease. An apparent relation with hydramnios actually is due to associated fetal anomalies.

Gastroschisis is also considered to be due to an abnormality in vascular development of the umbilical cord. The early embryologic cord has paired arteries and paired veins. Involution of the right

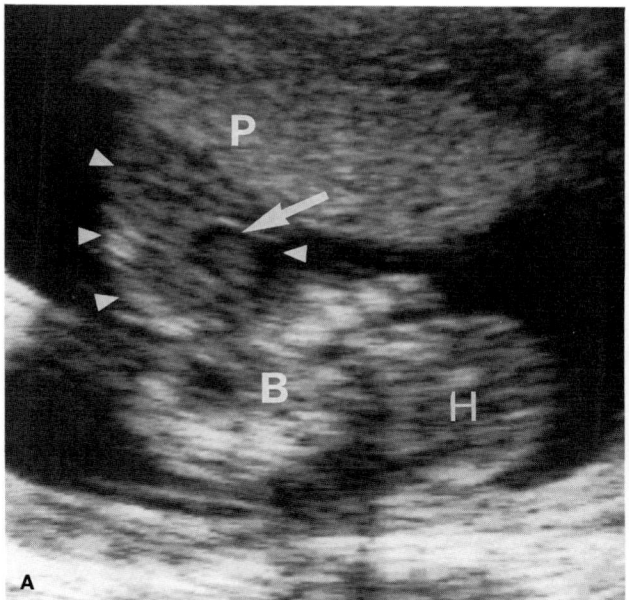 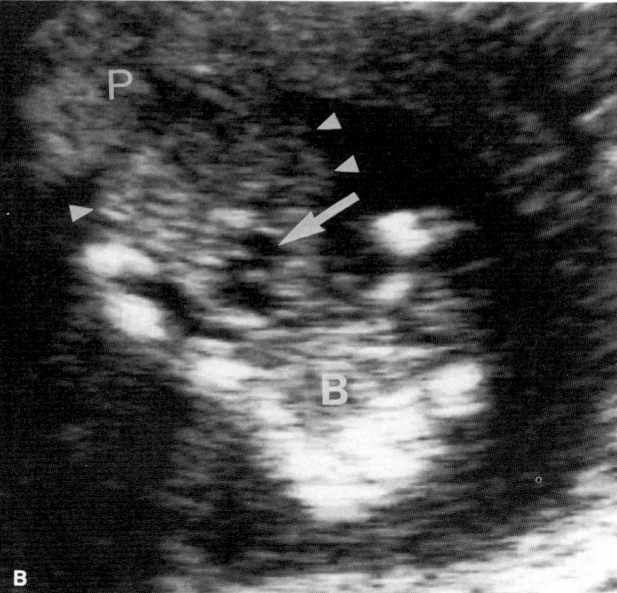

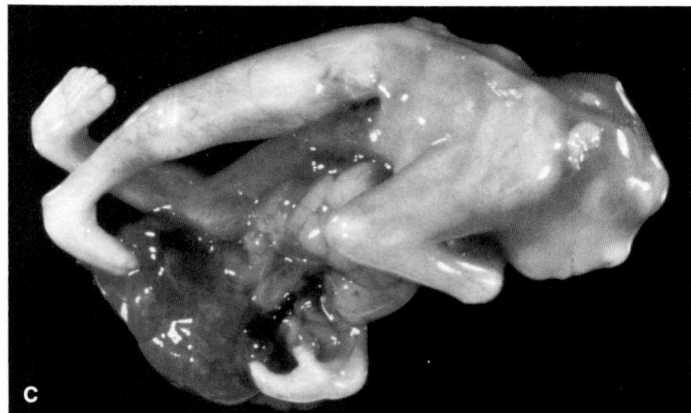

FIGURE 7-8. Body stalk anomaly in a 14-week fetus. **(A)** A longitudinal view of the fetus shows a thick connecting stalk (*arrowheads*) between the mid-body of the fetus (B) and the placenta. No separate umbilical cord was detected. The fluid-containing space in the stalk (*arrow*) is the beating heart. The fetal head (H) and dorsal contour are also abnormal in this fetus, representing inien-cephaly, a part of the overall malformation. **(B)** A view axial to the mid-body (B) of the fetus and body stalk, flanked by fetal limbs, again shows the heart (*arrow*) within the stalk (*arrowheads*) rather than in the thorax. P, placenta. **(C)** Fetal specimen demonstrates iniencephaly, exteriorized abdomi-nal and thoracic organs, and club feet as well.

umbilical vein leads to the normal, three-vessel configuration. Although the specific events are un-certain, exaggeration of this process may lead to the abdominal wall defect of gastroschisis, charac-teristically located immediately to the right of the umbilicus (see Chapter 16).

Persistent right umbilical vein occurs rarely and is due to involution of the left umbilical vein. The course of this vein, as described by Jeanty, sweeps in a cephalic direction to the right of the fetal gall-bladder.[9] This may enter and enlarge the right por-tal vein or enter directly into the right atrium. There is no definite clinical significance to this ana-tomic variant itself, but about half of the described cases have had other anomalies or anomaly com-plexes that may affect any organ system. Detection of this vascular abnormality should prompt a de-tailed fetal anatomic survey.

Abnormalities of Cord Formation

A defective embryonic folding process generates abnormalities of the fetal abdominal wall and um-bilical cord. Severe and generalized maldevelop-ment of all the folds leads to a failure of formation of the umbilical cord, with the fetus directly at-tached to the placental chorion by a persisting em-bryonic connecting stalk. The abdominal organs, including the intestine, liver, spleen, and pan-creas, lie within this stalk exterior to the fetal body. Incomplete formation of the diaphragm, sternum, and pericardium and exstrophy of the heart may also occur. This is referred to as the *body stalk anom-aly* or *congenital absence of the umbilical cord* and also as *limb–body wall complex*.[10,11] This anomaly is uni-formly lethal.

The sonographic findings (Fig. 7-8) include her-niation of the liver and viscera from the abdomen without an overlying membrane, as would be present in omphalocele. The organs extend from the fetal torso to the placenta and appear tethered to it. The heart may also be exteriorized. An umbilical cord is not identified. Amniotic band syndrome (discussed later) could simulate many or all of these findings in an individual case, even including poor umbilical cord development. With fetal tethering from amniotic bands, cord growth may be minimal.

More selective deficits in the embryonic body folding process may produce a variety of body wall anomalies, including pentalogy of Cantrell, large liver-containing and small bowel-containing types of omphalocele, and exstrophy of the bladder (see Chapter 16). An entity called the *short umbilical cord syndrome*, which combines a large omphalocele, exstrophy, imperforate anus, and spinal deformity with presence of a short umbilical cord, most likely is within the spectrum of body stalk anomaly.

Abnormalities of Cord Length and Twist

Abnormalities Related to Short Cords. Conditions that restrict or reduce fetal movements correlate with umbilical cords shorter than 40 cm. Oligohydramnios, tethering of the fetus as by amniotic bands, restricted space due to multiple gestation, and intrinsic fetal anomalies all may suppress fetal movement and lead to short cords. Presence of a short cord, regardless of cause, may predispose to inadequate fetal descent and fetal heart rate abnormalities related to cord compression.[12] Unfortunately, it is not practical to estimate cord length by ultrasound, but a related cord property can be evaluated by ultrasound.

The presence of spiral turns of the umbilical cord vessels is another characteristic that appears to be a consequence of fetal movement. Counterclockwise or left twists are consistently seven times as frequent as clockwise or right twists. Because the placental end of the cord is fixed and cannot rotate, this phenomenon implies that fetuses have a 7:1 predilection for rotating toward left rather than right within the uterus! Studies have demonstrated no relation to the eventually demonstrated child's or mother's handedness or to pregnancy location in the Northern versus Southern hemisphere. A number of theories for this phenomenon have been advanced, but none has been proved.[1]

The direction of cord twists can be determined by ultrasound, but perhaps of considerably greater clinical significance, the *absence of cord twist* can be identified[13] (Fig. 7-9). In live-born singleton pregnancies, only 5% of cords have absence of spiral-

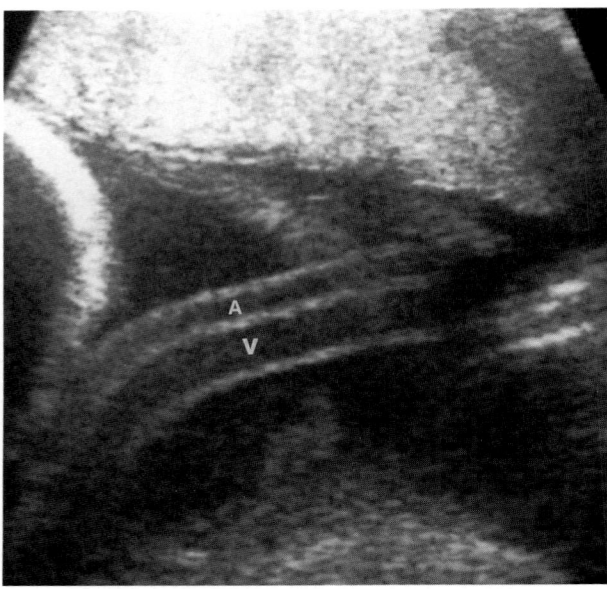

FIGURE 7-9.   Absence of coiling of the umbilical cord vessels. The arteries (A, one not shown) and vein (V) are all aligned with the long axis of the cord. This observation has been associated with increased perinatal morbidity and mortality.

ing. The frequency of noncoiled umbilical vessels in cases of intrauterine death is over three times higher at 18%.[2] Absent twists are also more common in SUA cords and in twins. Strong and coworkers recently confirmed the association of noncoiled cord vessels with increased perinatal morbidity and mortality.[14] Thirty-eight (4.3%) of 894 consecutively delivered infants had noncoiled cords and were compared with the normally coiled controls (determined by direct cord inspection at birth). The noncoiled cord cases had significantly increased incidence of fetal death (10.5% versus 2%; $P = .009$), preterm delivery, heart rate decelerations in labor, operative delivery for fetal distress, meconium staining, and anatomic and karyotypic abnormalities. It is not yet clear whether absent coiling is a cause or effect of factors leading to fetal morbidity. Strong's work on outcomes in cases with noncoiled cords detected prenatally by ultrasound is ongoing, but preliminary results appear to confirm this finding as a marker for increased perinatal morbidity and mortality (personal communication). Further prenatal studies are needed to validate the importance of this finding. If confirmed as a risk factor, presence of a noncoiled cord would trigger a management plan of heightened pregnancy surveillance as outlined in Table 7-2.

Abnormalities Related to Long Cords. Increased cord length may predispose the fetus to cord entanglements, including nuchal cord, to the development of true cord knots, to cord prolapse, and to cord compression events.[12]

Nuchal cord is remarkably common during pregnancy and at delivery. Miser found a nuchal cord in 167 (24%) of 706 consecutive deliveries in a community hospital.[15] There were no associated fetal deaths and no difference in operative delivery rates, 1- and 5-minute Apgar scores, or postnatal complications despite nearly twice the incidence in the nuchal cord group of fetal bradycardia and variable decelerations (18.6% versus 9.6%). Infants with nuchal cords had slightly lower birthweights than controls (3345 g versus 3468 g).

Any loop of cord by the fetal neck may be circumferential. When scans longitudinal to the neck show two adjacent cross sections, one can diagnose nuchal cord with confidence. The pitfall caused by a knuckle of cord simply passing by the neck and looping back on itself can be avoided with axial views showing portions of the cord conforming to the neck contour. If the nuchal cord appears loose, no alteration in pregnancy management need be undertaken, but if the loops of cord indent the soft tissues of the neck (Fig. 7-10), one should consider increased fetal surveillance. If there is flattening of the cross section of the umbilical vein, there should be strong concern for cord compromise and fetal strangulation. In this case,

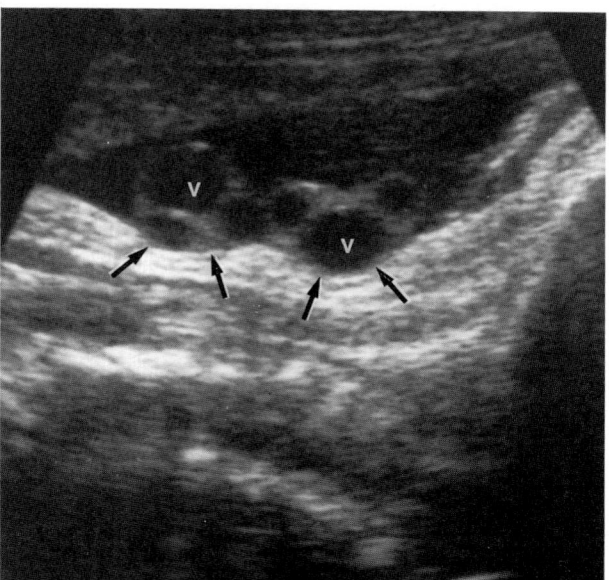

FIGURE 7-10.   Circumferential nuchal cord. Long axis view of the fetal neck demonstrates two adjacent cross sections of cord, sufficiently tight to indent the skin (*arrows*) but not enough to compress the umbilical vein (v). No fetal consequence was detected in this pregnancy.

immediate and intensive fetal monitoring is indicated. No nuchal cord with this degree of constriction has been detected in our practice.

True cord knots occur infrequently (0.5%) and are rarely detected by sonography.[16] A knot can be recognized by the characteristic looping of cord segments (Fig. 7-11). Simply seeing a cluster of cord segments is not sufficient for diagnosis (Fig. 7-12). *False cord knots* are focal redundancies of the cord vessels that alter the contour of the cord (Fig. 7-13). These are not of clinical significance. A true knot most often causes no problem but may occasionally be implicated in a fetal demise. Increased monitoring is recommended (see Table 7-2). Vaginal delivery is acceptable if there is no evidence of fetal compromise.

Umbilical cord compression may occur in a variety of circumstances. These include oligohydramnios and cord presentation. Particularly during uterine contractions, in these situations, there may be a reduction in flow of oxygenated blood from placenta to fetus through the umbilical vein, leading to hypoxia recognized by transient deceleration of the fetal heart rate. When there is compromise of the uteroplacental circulation, uterine contractions similarly may cause fetal heart rate decelerations, which is the basis for use of the contraction stress test as an early warning sign of fetal decompensa-

TABLE 7-2.   Management of Cord Abnormalities

1. Daily fetal movement counting

2. Twice-weekly fetal monitoring
   Biophysical profile, or
   Nonstress test with weekly amniotic fluid volume assessment

3. Umbilical artery Doppler: Are there reduced arterial diastolic velocities?

4. Vaginal delivery acceptable unless there is evidence of fetal compromise (cesarean section for vasa previa or obligate cord presentation)

5. Presence of a single-artery cord or of an intrinsic focal cord lesion should prompt a complete detailed fetal anatomic survey, searching for other anomalies

6. Consider karyotype determination for omphalocele, single-artery cord with additional fetal anomaly, and perhaps intrinsic focal cord lesions

7. Intensive monitoring and potential emergent delivery for cord thrombosis or hematoma and for stricture, if seen with live fetus

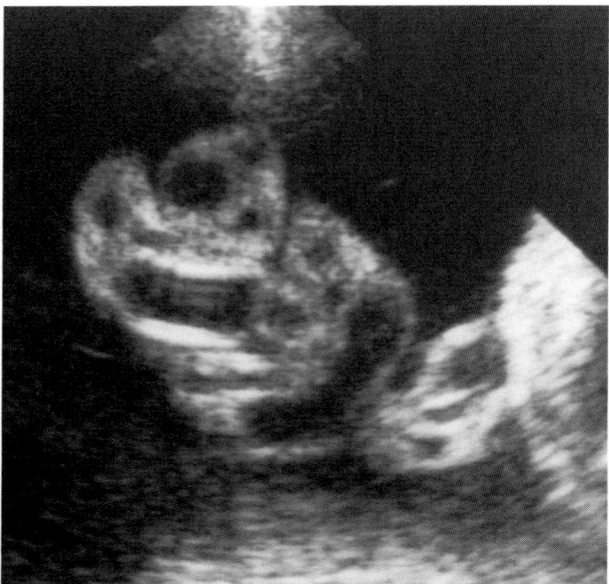

FIGURE 7-11. True cord knot, 32-week pregnancy. The visualized segments of cord are arranged in an orderly pattern produced by the crossings of a half-hitch knot. The patient was placed on twice-weekly fetal monitoring and daily fetal movement counts. No evidence of fetal compromise was detected, and the patient had a vaginal delivery of a healthy 9-lbs, 2-oz baby just past term.

thrombosis. Many references to individual cases of fetal demise attributable to a cord mass are found throughout umbilical cord literature, but, remarkably, most cases do not develop fetal distress and can be managed expectantly with eventual vaginal delivery.[3]

Nonetheless, the risk of morbidity and fetal demise must be borne in mind, and it is reasonable to place the patient on a program of frequent outpatient fetal monitoring, as outlined in Table 7-2. Umbilical artery Doppler analysis that shows abnormally low diastolic velocity ratios may justify the intensification of monitoring efforts, but the decision to perform an emergent preterm cesarean delivery generally is predicated on finding evidence of significant fetal distress by fetal heart rate monitoring and the biophysical profile.

As with other developmental fetal abnormalities, focal anomalies of the cord could be more prevalent in cases of aneuploidy. There are insufficient data to prove such a relation, but one could consider obtaining a fetal karyotype before committing the patient to long-term intensive monitoring.

Focal cord swelling due to a localized increased deposit of Wharton's jelly is generally of no clinical significance.[17] It may occur as an isolated finding but more frequently is seen in association with a

tion. Occasionally a transient cardiac deceleration is seen in an apparently healthy fetus without obvious explanation. One postulated cause is the fetus grabbing and squeezing the cord, becoming hypoxic, and releasing its grip, which returns normal circulation (Fig. 7-14).

Both cord length and the number of spiral turns of the cord vessels correlate with fetal activity. Longer cords tend to have an increased number of turns. Rare cases of extreme twisting have led to focal constriction and fetal demise. *Cord stricture* or *torsion* is usually at the fetal end, perhaps because there is less Wharton's jelly there to give the cord turgor. One can qualitatively recognize ranges of cord twisting from noncoiled through pronounced. I am unaware of any sonographic reports that recognize hypertwisting as a precursor to a fetal demise.

Cord Masses

Focal masses of many causes may enlarge the umbilical cord regionally. The chief concern with any cord swelling is the compromise of the fetal circulation, either by blood vessel compression or

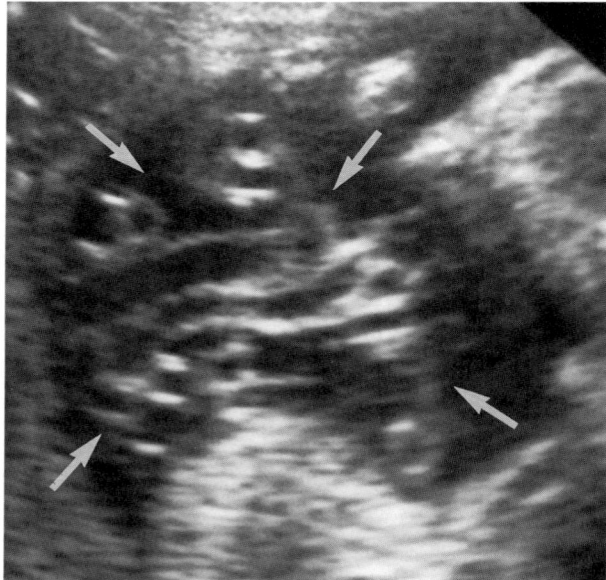

FIGURE 7-12. "Not a knot." Clustered segments of umbilical cord (*arrows*) are present but not in as orderly a fashion as in Figure 7-10. Possible knotting was questioned, but none was found at delivery.

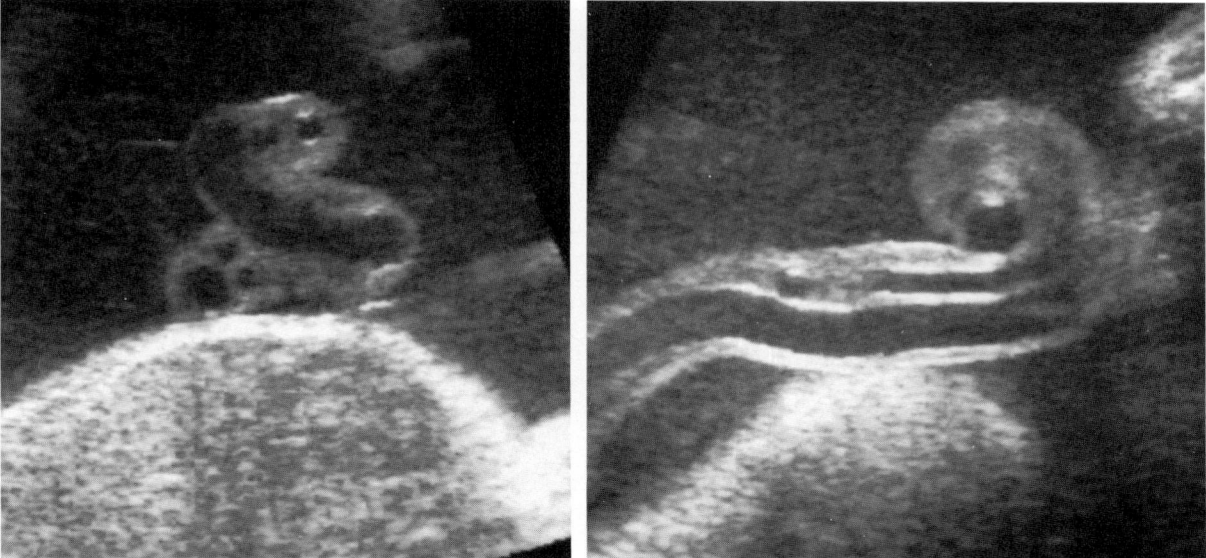

FIGURE 7-13.   False cord knot. A localized redundancy of the cord simulates a knot but is due to a simple loop or curlicue.

true focal cord lesion, such as a cyst (discussed later) or a fetal omphalocele (see Fig. 7-6). The umbilical vessels are usually splayed apart in a region of increased Wharton's jelly, indicating a diffuse, concentric enlargement of the cord rather than a focal mass, which would enlarge the cord eccentri-

cally with the vessels clustered together toward one surface. Small areas of watery accumulation or cystic degeneration may be seen within the thickened region of jelly (Fig. 7-15).

Diffuse cord swelling rarely may occur as an isolated finding (Fig. 7-16). Most often, it is seen as a

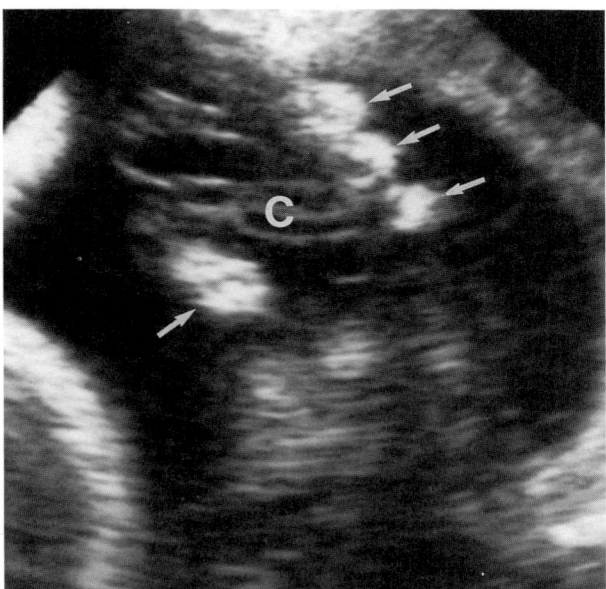

FIGURE 7-14.   Fetus grasping cord. The fetal digits (*arrows*) surrounded and partially compressed the cord (C), then gradually relaxed and released the cord. The heart rate, subsequently imaged, was normal.

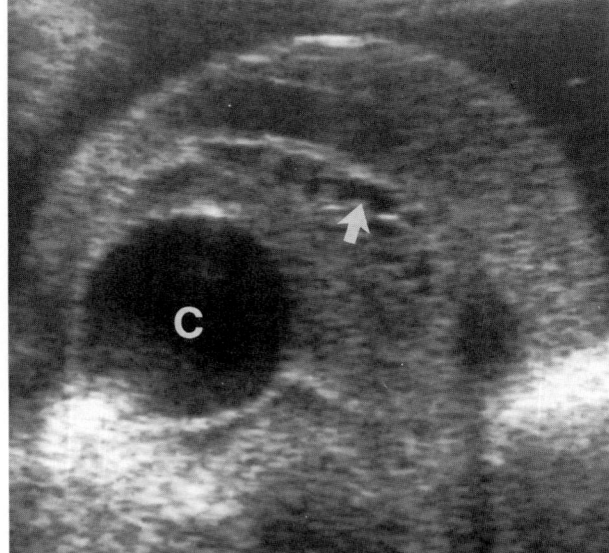

FIGURE 7-15.   A focal area of increased Wharton's jelly is seen adjacent to a 2-cm simple cyst (C) at the fetal end of the cord. Small beaded locules of fluid, cystic degeneration (*arrow*), are seen within the cord adjacent to the vein. Pregnancy outcome was normal.

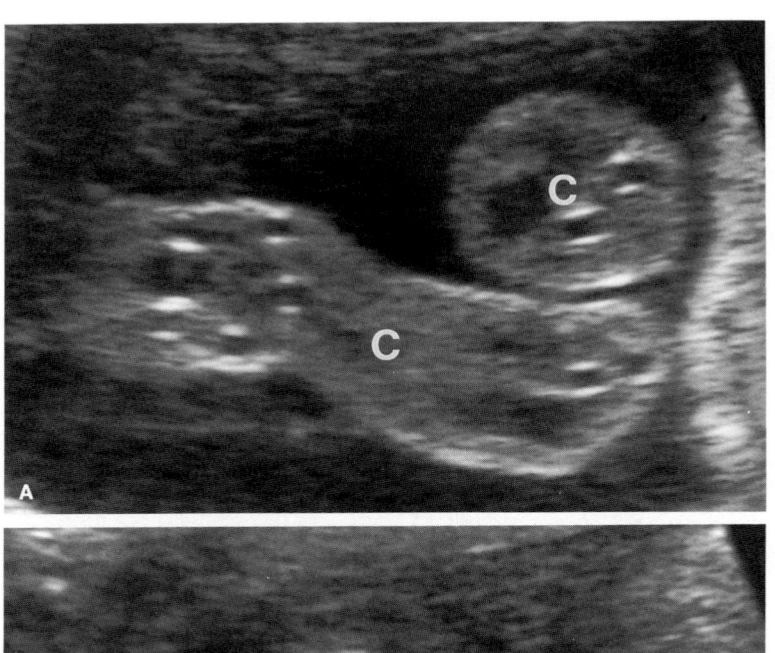

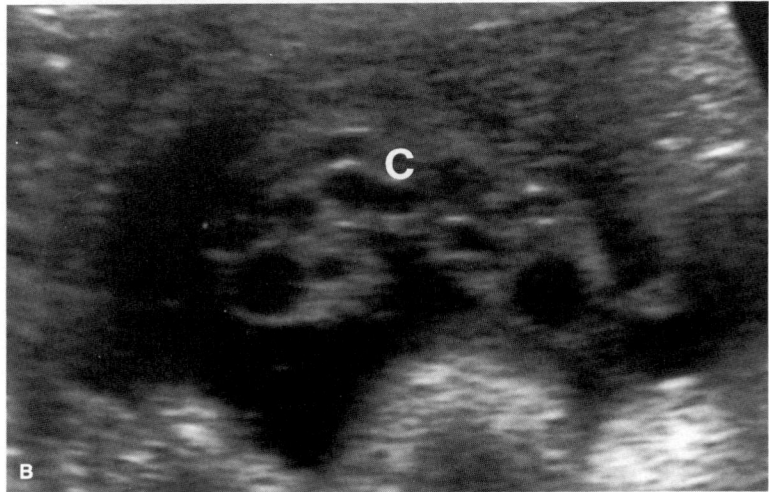

FIGURE 7-16. (A) Idiopathic diffuse swelling of the umbilical cord (C), measuring up to 2.5 cm in diameter at 25 weeks, was not associated with fetal hydrops or other anomaly. **(B)** Swelling gradually regressed, and the cord (C) appeared normal by sonography at 34 weeks and by inspection at delivery of a normal infant 2 weeks later.

consequence of fetal hydrops of any cause (Fig. 7-17). An unusual pathologic cause is a patent urachal duct, with extravasation of urine into the cord making it tense and distended. Live and stillborn outcomes have been recorded.[2]

Umbilical cord cysts may be of either omphalomesenteric or allantoic origin, distinguishable only by histology. These cysts tend to be closer to the fetal end of the cord. Most are small, 1 to 2 cm in diameter (Fig. 7-18), but they may attain large size. The cysts or associated thickening of Wharton's jelly may displace or splay the umbilical vessels, but the risk of vascular compromise appears low. Cords cysts may be considerably more prevalent in the first trimester and resolve by the second trimester in most cases[18] (Fig. 7-19).

Angiomas of the umbilical cord are unusual, and *teratomas,* the only other true neoplasm of the cord,

are much rarer. These both appear as well-circumscribed echogenic masses (Fig. 7-20). As with placental chorioangiomas, the cord angioma infrequently may be associated with fetal hydrops from high-output congestive failure. Fetal deaths from vascular obstruction have been reported, although the two cases in our practice had uneventful pregnancies. A full high-risk fetal monitoring program is warranted. Very high levels of α-fetoprotein have been reported in maternal serum and amniotic fluid in several cases.[19,20]

Aneurysm of the umbilical artery is a rare lesion. At least two reported cases, one diagnosed prenatally, ended in stillbirth, each near 36 weeks of gestation.[21] The thinned wall may dissect, causing umbilical vascular compression, or extensive intraaneurysmal clot may compromise circulation. Survival may also occur. A case seen in our prac-

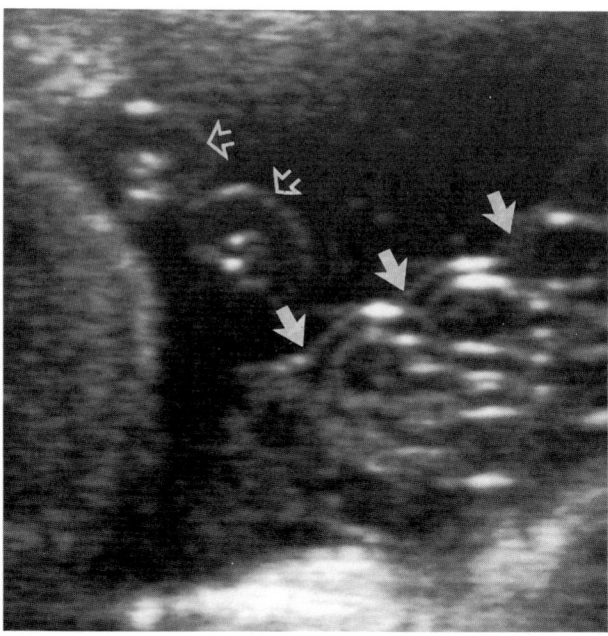

FIGURE 7-17.   Marked disparity in the size of the umbilical cords of a 25-week monochorionic, diamniotic twin pregnancy with twin-to-twin transfusion syndrome. The larger cord (*closed arrows*) is of the hydropic recipient twin, and the smaller cord (*open arrows*) is of the growth-retarded donor twin.

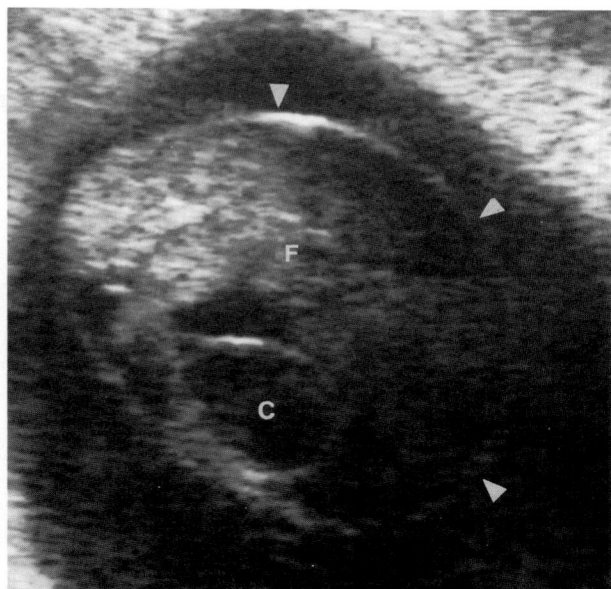

FIGURE 7-19.   Umbilical cord cyst (C), 6 mm in diameter, in a 9-week pregnancy imaged with a 7.5-MHz endovaginal transducer. The fetus (F), which appeared live and normal in other views, is enclosed within the amnion (*arrowheads*). The cyst resolved by the time of amniocentesis at 15 weeks, with normal karyotype and normal pregnancy outcome.

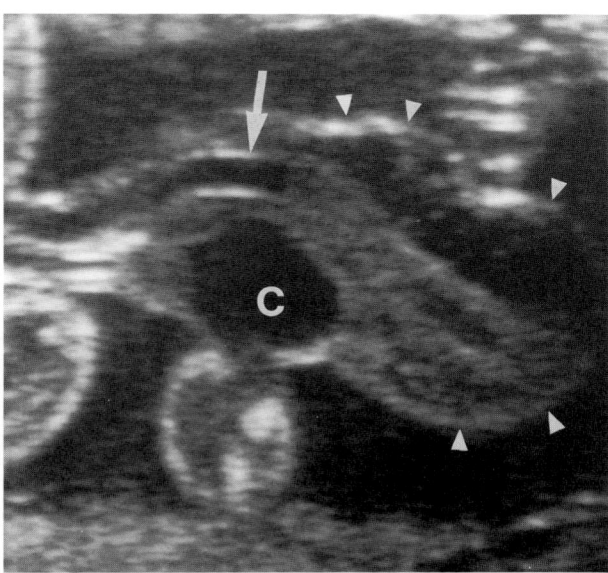

FIGURE 7-18.   A small omphalomesenteric cyst near the fetal origin of the cord at 22 weeks is associated with marked watery swelling of the cord and wide splaying of the vessels. The umbilical vein (*arrow*) is deviated by the cyst. *Arrowheads* show edge of cord.

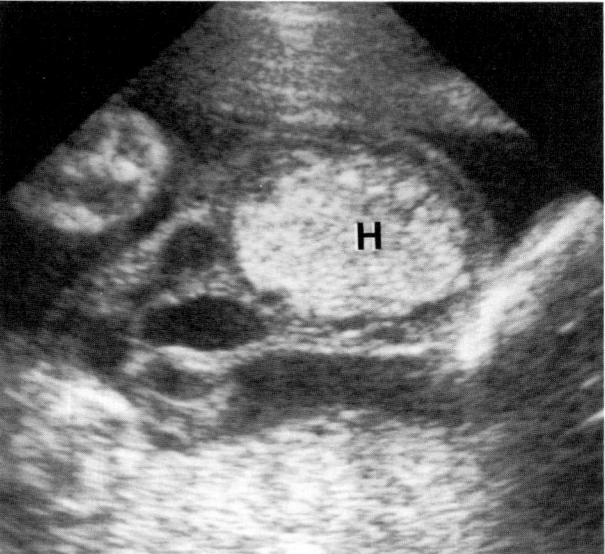

FIGURE 7-20.   Hemangioma of the umbilical cord. The echogenic lesion (H), at the fetal end of the cord, measured barely 2 cm diameter when first imaged at 18 weeks. It enlarged to 4 cm by the time of this study 1 month later and then stabilized. An omphalomesenteric cyst (not shown) distal to the hemangioma grew from barely detectable at 18 weeks to 10 cm in diameter at vaginal delivery of a normal infant. Intensive monitoring throughout the pregnancy showed no evidence of fetal compromise.

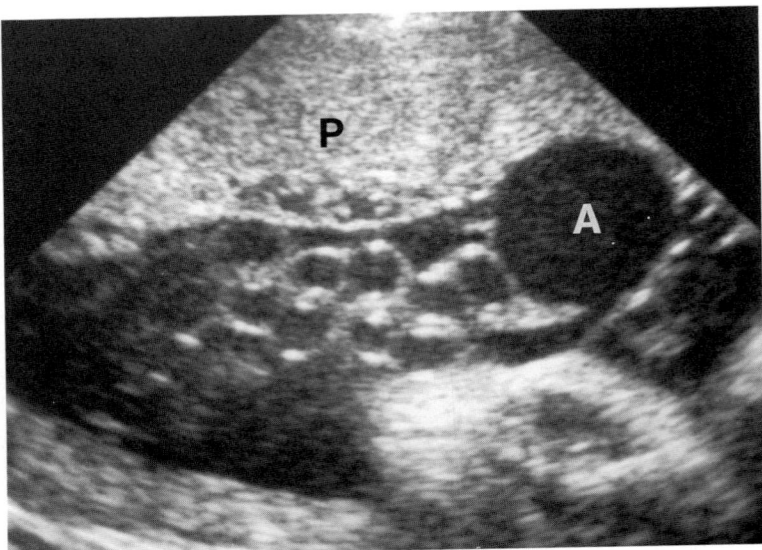

FIGURE 7-21. Umbilical artery aneurysm (A) adjacent to the placental (P) insertion of the cord in a 38-week pregnancy. The fetus was noted to have an endocardial cushion defect. Subsequent cordocentesis (avoiding the aneurysm) proved trisomy 18. Fetal size and amniotic fluid volume were in the normal range, suggesting no impairment of fetal perfusion. (Doppler was not available at the time of this pregnancy.)

tice was associated with a fetal endocardial cushion defect and was found to have trisomy 18 (Fig. 7-21). All the other focal cord lesions seen in our practice have not been associated with additional fetal anomalies, aneuploidy, or abnormal pregnancy outcomes.

A true *varix of the umbilical vein* is another rare anomaly that may be associated with fetal compromise. Fetal monitoring is advisable for both arterial and venous lesions.

Varix of the intrafetal umbilical vein, just deep to the umbilicus, is an infrequent finding, currently of controversial significance (Fig. 7-22). Mahoney and coworkers reported the finding in nine fetuses, with four dying in utero in the second trimester of unspecified causes. One had trisomy 21. Of the remaining five, one had transient nonimmune hydrops at 34 weeks of gestation, with all alive and well at 6 to 30 months after birth.[22] Estroff and Benacerraf reported five cases, with all

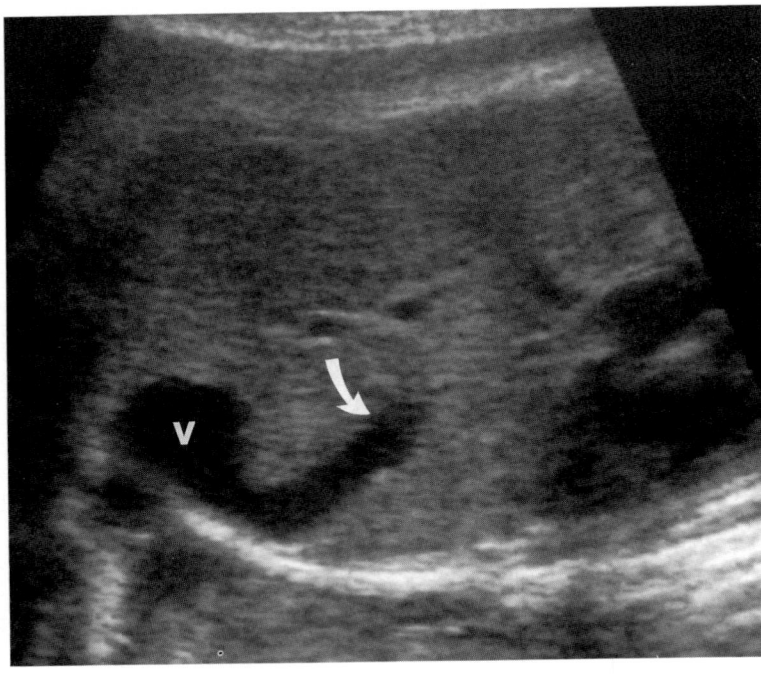

FIGURE 7-22. Varix of the intraabdominal portion of the umbilical vein (V), measuring 15 mm maximal cross-sectional diameter, is seen in a 31-week normally grown fetus with normal biophysical profile and subsequent normal outcome. The dilated segment tapers to normal caliber before the vein curves centrally into the liver.

infants delivered healthy at term.[23] Four cases seen in our practice had uncomplicated term deliveries as well. In view of the Mahoney report, fetal surveillance may still be prudent.

Thrombosis of umbilical vessels or *extravasated hematoma of the cord* may occur in several circumstances. Conditions that cause cord vessel compression or kinking may lead to thrombus formation. These include focal cord masses, cord knots or tight looping about the neck or extremities, velamentous cord insertions, and cord entanglement as in monoamniotic twinning or amniotic band syndrome. Thrombus or hematoma may result iatrogenically from cordocentesis[24] (Fig. 7-23) or even from amniocentesis. The risks are severe and include death or brain damage by asphyxia as well as embolic infarctions within the fetus or placenta. Sonographic detection of cord thrombus or hematoma should trigger immediate intensive fetal monitoring with consideration of possible emergent cesarean delivery. Bleeding into the amniotic space after cordocentesis is, on the other hand, a frequent occurrence that does not compromise the cord (Fig. 7-24). It does not jeop-

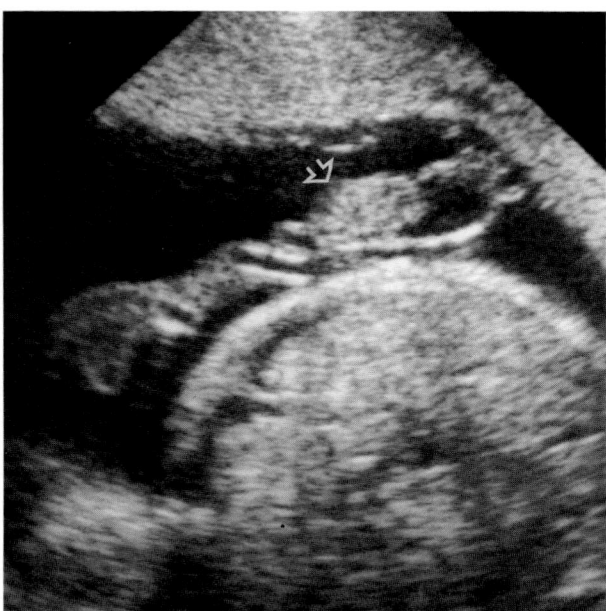

FIGURE 7-23. Thrombus of the umbilical vein: echogenic thrombus (*arrow*) occurring as an immediate complication of a cordocentesis. A fetal transfusion was performed for erythroblastosis fetalis due to Rh incompatibility at about 32 weeks. The thrombus developed during the transfusion, with constriction of the umbilical vein between the clotted segment and the fetus. The fetus developed profound bradycardia and could not be resuscitated despite emergency cesarean section.

ardize the fetus unless the blood loss is extreme. The bleeding usually stops spontaneously within 2 to 3 minutes.

Cord Abnormalities Resulting from Trophotropism

Trophotropism is defined as the preferential proliferation of trophoblastic villi of the placenta into regions of better endometrial blood supply along with atrophy of villi in areas of poorer blood supply. This phenomenon allows a placenta to change its position and remodel its shape within the uterus as the pregnancy progresses. It is generally accepted that at initial implantation and in early development, the placenta is a rounded disk with the cord insertion at the center. Differential proliferation of placental villi due to trophotropism may produce a placenta with an eccentrically located cord, even though the cord insertion remains in its original site relative to the underlying endometrium. With associated areas of villous atrophy, the cord insertion may end up at the margin of the placenta (Fig. 7-25) or even at some distance beyond the placental edge, the cord forming from fetal blood vessels extending from the placenta, running beneath the membranes. This latter case is called a velamentous or membranous cord insertion (Fig. 7-26). (Trophotropism is, incidentally, a useful unifying concept that also helps explain several placental phenomena, including resolution of placenta previa and the development of bilobed, succenturiate lobe, and other oddly shaped placentas.)

The vessels of the velamentous cord insertion are not protected by Wharton's jelly and are at risk of rupture or thrombosis. A significant risk is vasa previa (discussed later).

Competition for available endometrial surface explains the higher frequency of marginal and velamentous cords in multiple gestation. Low-lying initial implantations and uterine scarring or other uterine anomalies also predispose to these cord insertion variations. Marginal cords occur in 7% and velamentous cords in 1% of singleton pregnancies, with frequencies of 20% (marginal) and 12% (velamentous) in twins.[2]

Strong associations also exist between SUA cord and marginal (18%) and velamentous (9%) placental cord insertions. Evidence suggests that most SUA cords develop by atresia of a vessel rather than failure of formation. Heifetz theorized that in the absence of an anastomosis between the two umbilical arteries found toward the placental end of the cord in most pregnancies, atrophy of the

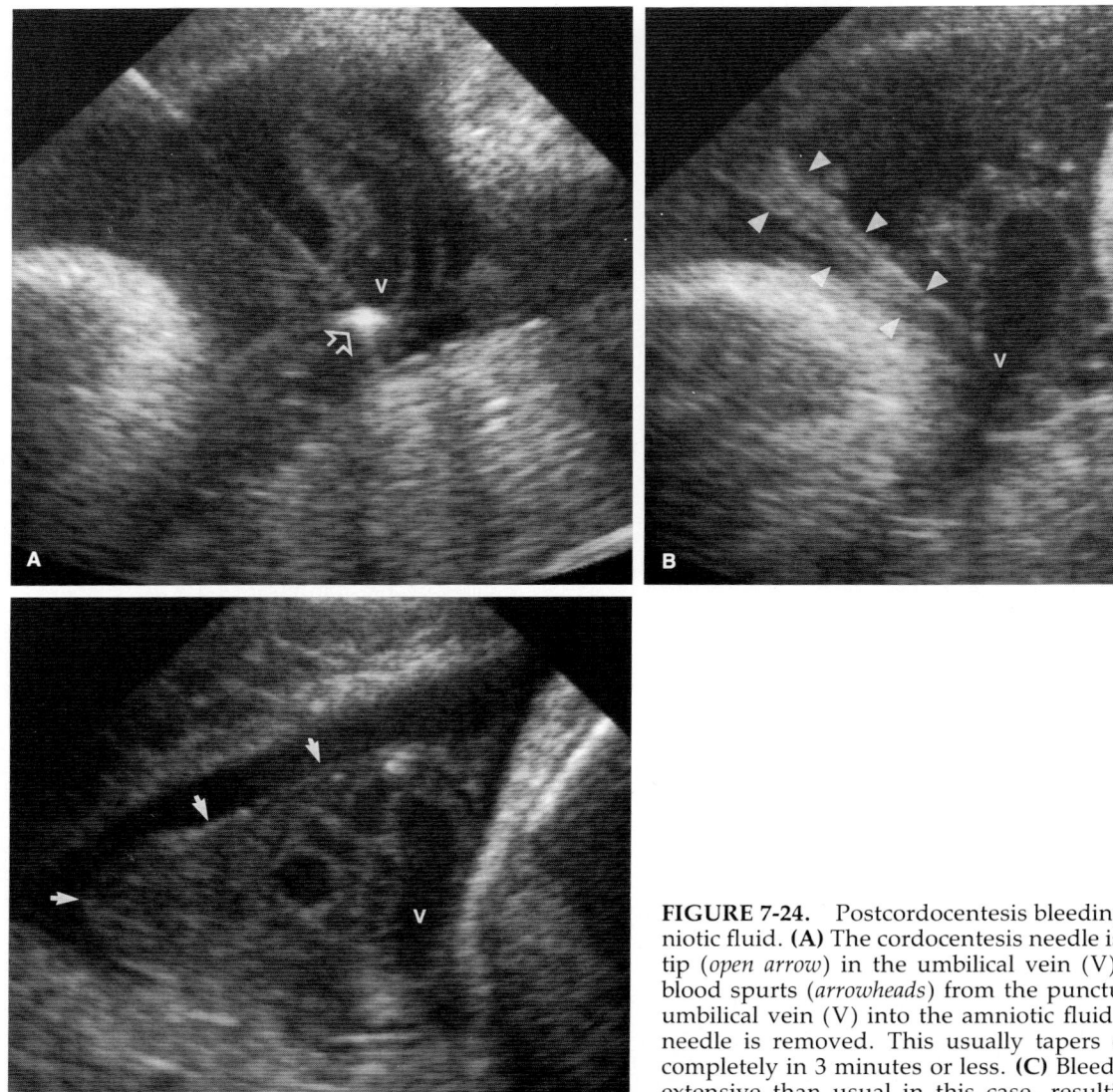

FIGURE 7-24. Postcordocentesis bleeding into the amniotic fluid. **(A)** The cordocentesis needle is seen with its tip (*open arrow*) in the umbilical vein (V). **(B)** A jet of blood spurts (*arrowheads*) from the puncture site in the umbilical vein (V) into the amniotic fluid just after the needle is removed. This usually tapers off and stops completely in 3 minutes or less. **(C)** Bleeding was more extensive than usual in this case, resulting in clotted blood (*arrows*) surrounding the cord. The fetus remained uncompromised, and on repeat scan 3 days later, the clot had lysed. V, umbilical vein.

portion of the placenta supplying one umbilical artery leads to atrophy of that artery and a peripheral cord insertion.[4]

Eddleman and coworkers reviewed all 82 cases of velamentous cord insertion found at delivery over 4 years, including 3 cases of vasa previa. None of the cases was detected by routine nontargeted obstetrical sonography. These authors believe that failure to diagnose this condition does not fall below the sonographic standard of care.[25]

Vasa Previa. The presence of fetal vessels from the placenta crossing the internal os of the cervix is referred to as *vasa previa*. This may be due either to a succenturiate placental lobe or to a velamentous cord insertion. Even with a marginal cord insertion, aberrant chorionic surface vessels may extend beyond the placental edge, raising concern for vasa previa in a low-lying placenta with a marginal cord near the cervix.[2] The fetal risk from rupture of vasa previa is extreme. Bleeding can be brisk, and there is no overlying placental tissue to help tamponade the flow, so the fetus can exsanguinate in minutes.

The diagnosis of vasa previa can be challenging. It should be suspected in any case of marginal or

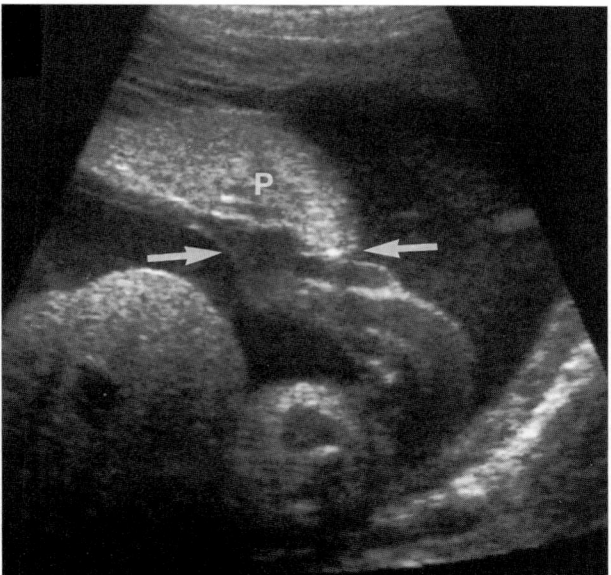

FIGURE 7-25.   Marginal cord insertion (*arrows*) into a narrow left lateral lobular extension of an anterior placenta (P) that is not a fully separated succenturiate lobe. Both the peripheral cord insertion and the oddly shaped placenta can be attributed to placental remodeling and repositioning due to trophotropism. There was normal attachment of this segment of the placenta to the underlying uterus, which is not shown in this oblique scan plane parallel to its endometrial surface.

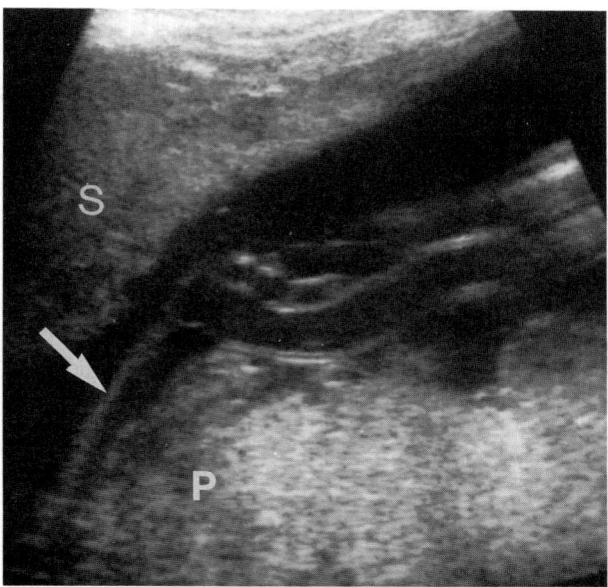

FIGURE 7-26.   Velamentous placental cord insertion arises along a membrane (*arrow*) between a posterior placenta (P) and a separate fundal succenturiate lobe (S). One cord artery could be traced to each placental lobe.

velamentous cord insertion in the lower uterine segment and whenever a succenturiate lobe is found that might connect to the main portion of the placenta by vessels passing near the cervix. Color flow Doppler offers the best chance for diagnosing vasa previa definitively.[26] If this is not available, duplex Doppler can be used to interrogate the area near the internal cervical os. When vasa previa is considered possible and cannot be definitely excluded by imaging and Doppler studies, it is most prudent to deliver the pregnancy by cesarean section in view of the grave risk of fetal loss from this condition.

Obligate Cord Presentation. Even in the absence of vasa previa, a marginal or velamentous cord insertion in the lower uterine segment near the cervix may fix the cord so that it presents in front of the fetus (Fig. 7-27). With cervical dilation, this can prolapse. With a closed os, uterine contractions may cause cord compression by the adjacent fetal presenting part, resulting in fetal distress. These risks provide justification for elective cesarean de-

livery when there is a lower uterine segment marginal or velamentous cord insertion, even if vasa previa is proved not to be present.

Other Causes of Cord Presentation. Any condition in which the presenting fetal pole does not completely fill the pelvic inlet may be complicated by umbilical cord presentation (also called *funic presentation*) with its associated risk of cord prolapse. Predisposing factors include fetal malpresentation, nonengagement of the fetus due to prematurity, multiple gestation, long cord, contracted or otherwise distorted bony pelvic inlet, and uterine fibroids.[27] Lange and coworkers found cord presentation in 9 of 1471 consecutively scanned, singleton high-risk pregnancies at more than 37 gestational weeks, persistent in the 5 patients not delivered in the first 48 hours.[28] Cord presentations were confirmed at cesarean section in 7 patients. One patient underwent spontaneous breech to cephalic version with resolution, and the final patient had an acute fetal death from cord prolapse within 1 day of sonographic diagnosis. The sonographic

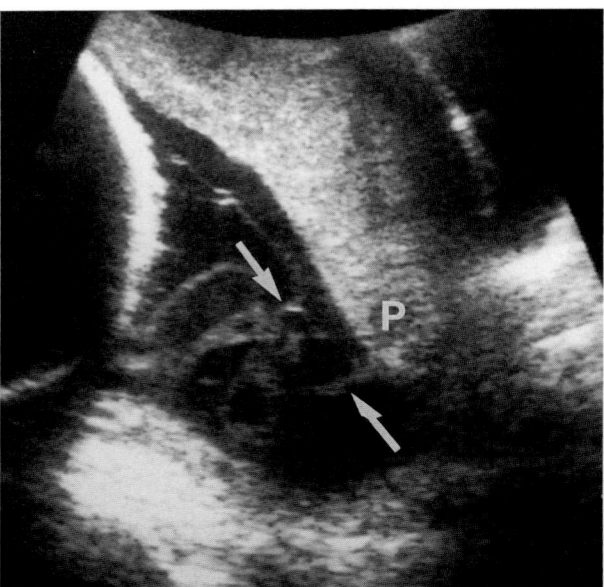

FIGURE 7-27. Cord insertion (*arrows*) along the caudal margin of a low-lying anterior placenta (P), which extended to within 2 cm of the internal os as seen on transvaginal sonograms (not shown). The anatomy indicates an obligate cord presentation. There is also the risk of aberrant chorionic surface fetal vessels, which could cross the os, although none were seen in this case.

identification of cord presentation should prompt close observation of the pregnancy, possibly with hospitalization, and with consideration of cesarean delivery.

AMNIOTIC MEMBRANES: SHEETS, STRANDS, AND SHELVES

Sheetlike membranes, filamentous strands, and ridges or shelves extending inward from the endometrium or placenta may all be encountered within the amniotic space. Analysis of their sonographic details permits differentiation among those that may directly injure the fetus, those related to intercurrent obstetrical events, and those likely to be of little clinical significance.

Membrane Development

The outer cell layer of the blastocyst stage of the dividing fertilized ovum is the trophoblast, which is capable of attachment to the endometrium. At the site of attachment, the trophoblastic villi proliferate and are called the *chorion frondosum*, eventually becoming the fetal tissue of the placenta with a

chorionic plate at the fetal surface. Away from the implantation site, the trophoblast becomes smooth and flat, called the *chorion laeve*.

Connective tissue cells of the secretory endometrium, in response to progesterone from the corpus luteum, differentiate into decidua. At the implantation site of the ovum, the *decidua basalis* thickens, becoming the maternal component of the placenta. A thin layer of *decidua capsularis* overlies the remainder of the developing ovum and, with the chorion laeve, becomes the chorionic membrane of the gestational sac. The *decidua vera* lines the endometrial cavity away from the placenta. The decidua capsularis atrophies with advancing gestation, and the chorion of the growing pregnancy lies against the decidua vera but does not firmly adhere to it.

The chorion surrounds the extraembryonic coelom within which the embryo, with its primary yolk sac and amniotic sac, is developing. The amniotic sac enlarges, eventually enveloping the fetus. The amniotic membrane pushes out, obliterating the extraembryonic coelom, and lies in apposition to the chorion (see Fig. 7-1). The membranes normally adhere to each other, but the amnion can be stripped from the chorion.

Two potential spaces thus exist. Between decidua vera and chorion, the *subchorionic space* is in continuity with the endocervical canal and can provide a pathway for vaginal egress of pregnancy-related bleeding. This space does not extend under the placenta unless there is subplacental abruption. Between amnion and chorion, there is a contained *subamniotic space*. Fluids do not escape from this space unless the membranes rupture. The subamniotic space may extend over the placenta because the amnion is firmly adherent only at the umbilical cord insertion and along the cord.

Membranes imaged in the amniotic space may be characterized as strands, sheets, or shelves (Fig. 7-28).

> *Strands* generally are linear structures that lie within the amniotic fluid space and can entangle or trap the fetus (Table 7-3).
> *Sheets* are portions of the amnion or combined amnion and chorion that divide off a fluid loculus or compartment, completely separating it from the perifetal amniotic space (see Table 7-3).
> *Shelves* are produced by an anatomic feature, often ridgelike, lying external to the amnion and indenting it (Table 7-4).

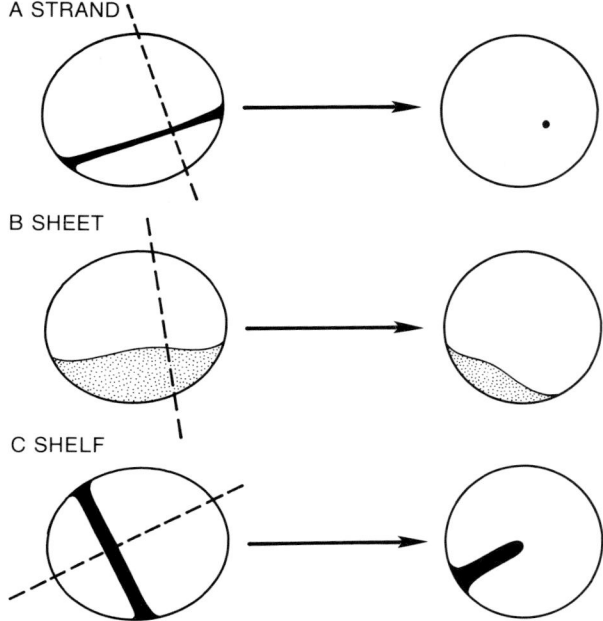

FIGURE 7-28. Membranes that may be seen within the amniotic space. (Dotted line in the left-hand image indicates the plane of the right-hand image.) **(A)** *Strands:* A linear strand lies within the amniotic fluid. Scans axial to the strand show a small round or linear mass completely surrounded by fluid. Entities include amniotic band and disrupted amnion. **(B)** *Sheets:* A linear or curvilinear membrane completely separates a volume of fluid from the amniotic space. Scans in all planes show that the sheet is continuous, extending to the margins of the amniotic cavity. Entities include inter-twin membrane, chorionic–amniotic elevation (subchorionic collection), and chorionic–amniotic separation (subamniotic collection). **(C)** *Shelves:* An extraamniotic ridge-like feature indents the amniotic cavity, so that the amnion or combined amnion and chorion drape over it. Scans axial to a shelf show a structure with a free edge projecting into the amniotic fluid and with a thin or thick membrane or tissue band extending from the free edge to the margin of the amniotic cavity (see Table 7-4). At the margin, the draped amniotic membranes curve away from each other to lie against the endometrial wall. Entities include uterine synechia, circumvallate placenta, and uterine septum.

Pitfalls in the Evaluation of Amniotic Membranes

Evaluation of the various membranes and other structures that may be found in the amniotic space is generally straightforward if one analyzes the details of their appearance with care. The main pitfall comes from noticing an abnormal amniotic strand or sheet and jumping to a conclusion, such as

equating it with the presence or risk of amniotic band syndrome.

Many of the membranes encountered are thin and may be relatively weakly echogenic specular reflectors. If the incident sound beam is off from orthogonal, the membrane returns no echo to the transducer. This is a frequent problem with the delicate membrane of a monochorionic diamniotic twin pregnancy and may lead to an erroneous diagnosis of the considerably higher-risk monoamniotic form of twin pregnancy.

Differential Diagnosis of Amniotic Sheets and Strands

Membranes in Multiple Gestations

The subject of multiple gestations is discussed in detail in Chapter 20. In the context of membranes that may be found in the amniotic space, suffice it to say that identification of an intertwin membrane is important in excluding the occurrence of monoamniotic twins, a form of twin pregnancy with a mortality rate approaching 50%. When a membrane is seen, its thickness provides reasonably accurate, although imperfect, differentiation between monochorionic diamniotic twins, which have a wispy, hard-to-image membrane less than 2 mm thick, and dichorionic diamniotic twins, which have a more echogenic membrane 2 mm or greater in thickness. Recognition of two separate placentas or of a *chorionic peak* of placental tissue extending into the intertwin membrane at its junction with a single, fused placental zone also confirms a dichorionic twin pregnancy.[29]

A twin membrane also may be encountered with one live fetus and the other dead and macerated, or even so small as to go undetected (*blighted twin*). In such a case, an empty amniotic fluid compartment separate from that surrounding the live fetus may be seen. Close inspection of the membrane at its intersection with the endometrial wall may identify Y-shaped splitting of the membrane, showing it to be composed of two layers and supporting twin pregnancy as its cause (Fig. 7-29).

Posthemorrhagic Membrane Elevation

Bleeding that occurs in an intrauterine pregnancy may collect in the amniotic cavity, in the potential space between amnion and chorion (subamniotic), or in the endometrial cavity extrinsic to the chorionic membrane (subchorionic). Many bleeds are due to abruptions developing along the margin of the placenta, likely in relation to the marginal sinus. These are usually low-pressure venous bleeds

TABLE 7-3.   Sheets and Strands Within Amniotic Space

Diagnosis	Findings
Intertwin Membrane	
Dichorionic, diamniotic	Two separate placentas or both placentas fused
	Thicker membrane ≥2 mm
	Chorionic peak
Monochorionic, diamniotic	One placenta
	Thinner, wispy membrane <2 mm
	Delicate T intersection of membrane and placenta
Failed twin gestation	Membrane completely separates a loculus of fluid
	Membrane may have Y-shaped division at endometrial margin, indicating two layers
	Detectable fetal remnant?
Posthemorrhagic Membrane Elevation (Subchorionic Collection)	Usually with vaginal bleeding
	Often at placental margin, but may be remote from placenta
	Solid material, strands, or echogenic fluid in contained space
	Lens-shaped
	Membrane ≥ 1 mm, strong reflector
	Subchorionic collection stops at placental edge.
Chorionic–Amniotic Separation	
Primary	Before 15 weeks of gestation
	Thin, weakly reflective membrane seen only where membrane is orthogonal to sound beam
	Seen near uterine contraction or other structure that indents smoothly rounded contour of gestational sac
Secondary	Second or third trimester
	Thin membrane, weakly reflective
	Parallels contour of endometrial margin
	May continue over placenta to cord insertion
	Predisposing event or condition:
	Amniocentesis
	Bleeding
	Polyhydramnios, especially after amniodrainage
Extraamniotic Pregnancy	Multiple, flaccid, sheet-like membranes freely mobile, randomly positioned in amniotic fluid
	Membrane attached at placental cord insertion
	No fetal deformity or tethering
Early Amnion Rupture Sequence (Amniotic Band Syndrome)	Fetal deformities: constrictions, amputations, abdominal or cranial defects
	Strands may extend from fetus to amniotic space margin
	Fetus may be tethered or restricted

and track away from the placenta under or between the membranes rather than dissecting under the placenta, further interrupting its endometrial attachment. The extravasated blood may form collections that elevate the membranes locally, creating a lens-shaped bulging inward on the amniotic space. Blood clot, fibrin strands, and echogenic fluid may be seen in this space (Fig. 7-30). The collection may be at the placental margin or in a remote location, not infrequently overlying the internal cervical os.

It usually is not possible to differentiate sonographically between fluid in the subamniotic space and fluid in the subchorionic space. When there is vaginal bleeding, at least some of the blood must lie in the endometrial cavity beyond the chorion. The chorion becomes adherent to the placenta at its margin, while the amnion may strip from the

TABLE 7-4. Shelf-like Membranes That May Indent the Amniotic Space

Diagnosis	Findings
Uterine synechia 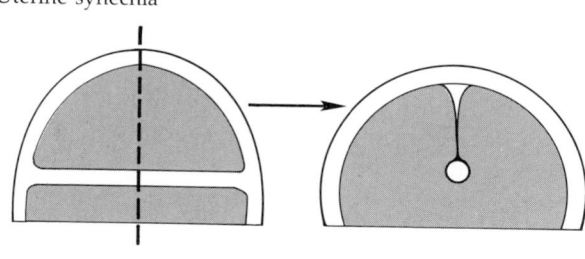	Thick, linear, hypoechoic band with more echodense edge traverses amniotic space from wall to wall. Scan axial to band shows a shelf with bulbous free edge, hypoechoic in center. Remainder of shelf is thin, extending to endometrial margin. Y-shaped splitting at membrane at endometrium Placenta may extend to, around, or along strand. Curettage or cesarean section may predispose
Circumvallate placenta 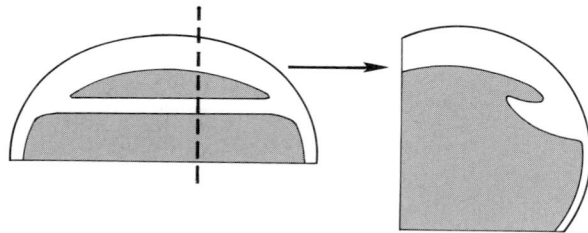	Edge of placenta lifted away from uterine wall and folded back in on itself within the amniotic space along entire circumference (complete) or segment (partial) of the placenta Tangential scan shows linear band traversing amniotic space, paralleling placenta. Axial scan, aligned radially, shows shelf to have triangular cross section, apex inward toward amniotic fluid, with free edge arcuate, conforming to curvature of the placental shape.
Uterine septum 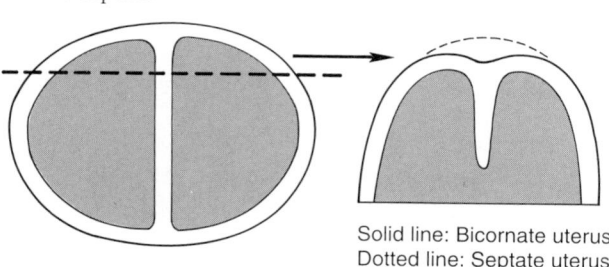 Solid line: Bicornate uterus Dotted line: Septate uterus	Transverse scans near fundus show septum oriented anterior to posterior. Coronal scan from fundus, indenting maternal abdomen cephalad to fundus, shows shelf extending from fundus, tapering to a point. Outer margin of uterus smoothly domed indicates subseptate uterus. Outer margin of uterus indented indicates bicornuate uterus.

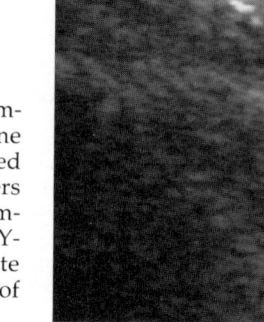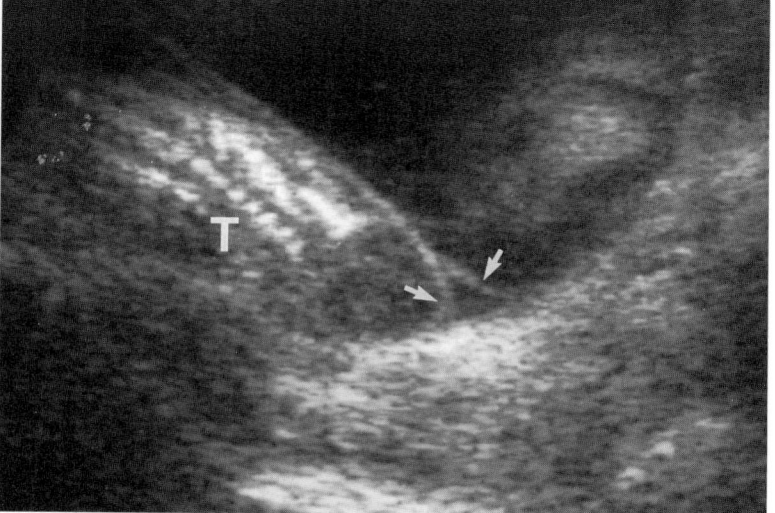

FIGURE 7-29. Sheet-like inter-twin membrane of a dichorionic pregnancy with one live twin (not shown) and a macerated remnant of the other twin. The two layers of the membrane, each composed of combined chorion and amnion, show Y-shaped splitting (*arrows*) as they separate from each other to lie against the margin of the endometrial cavity.

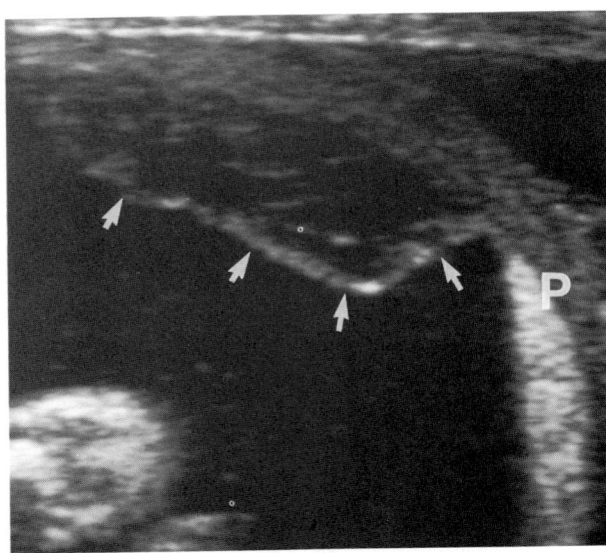

FIGURE 7-30. Submembrane blood collection (*arrows*) 1 week after a bleeding episode. The collection stops at the edge of the placenta (P), consistent with a subchorionic location. The fibrin strands within the contained fluid are consistent with a nonacute bleed in which there has been time for clot lysis.

chorion all the way to the cord insertion. Those submembrane collections that stop at the edge of the placenta are likely subchorionic, while collections extending along the placental surface are more probably subamniotic. Preplacental, subchorionic abruptions may occur infrequently.

All bleeding episodes in pregnancy are of concern for possible progression, leading to fetal (and occasionally maternal) compromise and necessitating emergent delivery or, earlier on, therapeutic abortion. Those bleeds that do not produce a detectable subplacental abruption tend to be less severe and resolve more frequently without need for urgent intervention.

Chorionic–Amniotic Separation

The amnion forms as an embryonic structure within and separate from the chorion. The amniotic cavity grows progressively throughout the first trimester, so that the amniotic membrane become contiguous with the chorion by the 15th or 16th week of gestation and then adheres to it. The primary separation before this time is a normal phenomenon (Fig. 7-31). One clinical implication is that amniocentesis before 16 weeks of gestation may be technically more difficult. The amnion may indent in front of the advancing needle rather than being pierced. Near 16 weeks of gestation, the membranes may lie against each other but have

not yet joined. A uterine contraction or other structure that indents the smoothly rounded contour of the gestational sac may elevate the amnion away from the chorion locally.

Chorionic–amniotic separation may recur later in pregnancy, usually in response to a predisposing event such as hemorrhage or amniocentesis, especially amniodrainage for polyhydramnios (Fig. 7-32). The separation generally is not of clinical consequence itself. Even if it leads to frank amniotic disruption, the risk of fetal entrapment and amniotic disruption sequence appears to be extremely small beyond 10 to 12 weeks of gestation. With separation, there may be some predisposition to premature rupture of the chorion also, but this is not certain.

In chorionic–amniotic separation, the thin, poorly reflective amnion is seen parallel to the chorion, best visualized where the membrane is orthogonal to the transducer. If the separation is secondary to hemorrhage, the intermembrane fluid may be more echogenic than the amniotic fluid. In third-trimester postamniocentesis separation, the subamniotic fluid may be less echogenic. Care should be taken in any subsequent amniocentesis for lung maturity studies to obtain amniotic rather than subamniotic fluid to avoid falsely immature results.

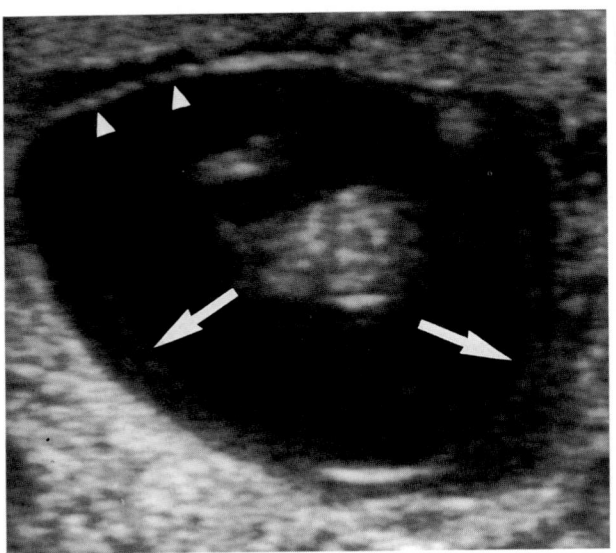

FIGURE 7-31. Primary chorionic–amniotic separation in a normal 13-week pregnancy. The thin, faintly echogenic amnion (*arrows*) has not yet fused with the thicker, more echogenic chorion. A small amount of subchorionic (endometrial cavity) fluid demarcates the chorion clearly (*arrowheads*). The subchorionic fluid may be a normal observation in the first trimester and does not necessarily imply a bleeding episode.

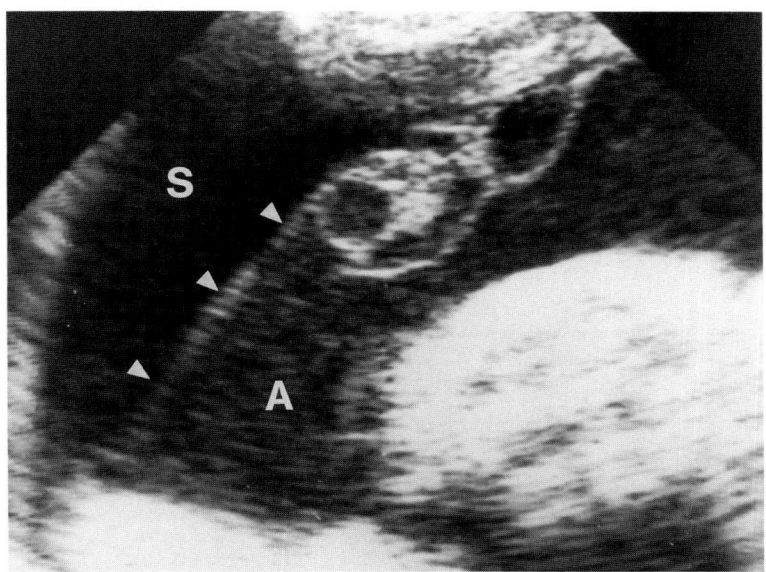

FIGURE 7-32. Acquired chorionic–amniotic separation occurring after an amniocentesis in a 37-week pregnancy. The amniotic fluid (A) contains particulate matter consistent with vernix, while the subamniotic fluid (S) is clear. This, along with the smooth amniotic contour (*arrowheads*), suggests a small amniotic membrane perforation rather than a large disruption. Umbilical cord is seen adjacent to the amnion.

Extraamniotic Pregnancy

Rupture of the amniotic membrane may progress, so that the amnion collapses away from the chorion entirely, retracting around the insertion of the umbilical cord as flaccid sheets (Fig. 7-33). The fetus escapes from the amniotic space, continuing to develop within the preserved intrachorionic cavity (or extraembryonic coelom; Fig. 7-34). The amniotic rupture sequence of fetal damage has not been reported in this condition despite fetal contact with the chorionic, nonfetal surface of the amnion. This is attributed to extraamniotic pregnancy occurring in the second trimester, beyond the stage when fetal deformities of amniotic band syndrome are believed to occur.[30]

Amniotic Band Syndrome or Early Amnion Rupture Sequence

Amniotic band syndrome is distinguished from other types of membranes that may be seen in pregnancy in that the presence of fetal deformities is integral to the diagnosis, whether or not actual amniotic bands are identified. There is some controversy over the pathogenesis of the condition, but the primary theory is that disruption of the amnion, perhaps accompanied by transient oligohydramnios, allows the fetus to contact the chorionic side of the amnion. This surface can be thought of as sticky such that the portions of the fetus that touch this membrane surface become enmeshed by adherent fibrous bands. These bands may deform, constrict, or slice through the entrapped fetal structures. The highly variable resultant anomalies include ring constriction, lymphedema, amputations of limbs, facial clefts, open defects of the chest or abdomen wall, and cranial deformities.

The common feature of these abnormalities is that they do not occur in the locations or symmetric distributions anticipated in congenital deviations from embryologic development. An encephalocele occurring off midline, for example, is strongly indicative of amniotic band syndrome. The severity of the defects may vary from a single, subtle constriction ring of a finger detected only postnatally to absolutely devastating, lethal body clefts and amputations (Fig. 7-35).

Visualization of bands extending from the deformed fetal regions to the endometrial wall, or recognition that the fetus is tethered to the margin of the gestational sac, is confirmatory.

Fetal defects from amniotic band syndrome do not appear to occur when there is amniotic disruption (as from an amniocentesis or a spontaneous extraamniotic pregnancy) after the first trimester. Significant fetal malformations probably require early amniotic rupture, likely before 10 weeks of gestation, hence the alternative designation, *early amnion rupture sequence.*

Shelves

Shelves projecting into the amniotic cavity can be distinguished from strands, which lie within the amniotic space, as in amniotic band syndrome, and from sheetlike membranes, which completely isolate a fluid-containing compartment, as in an

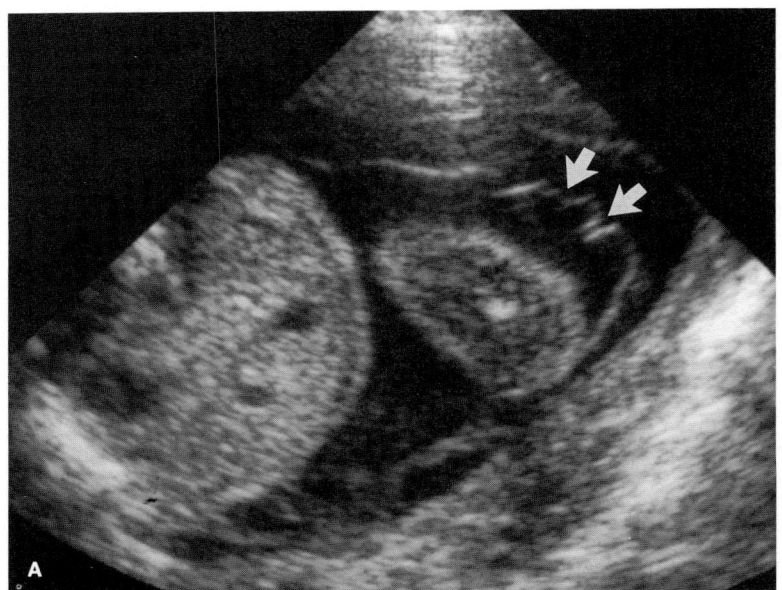

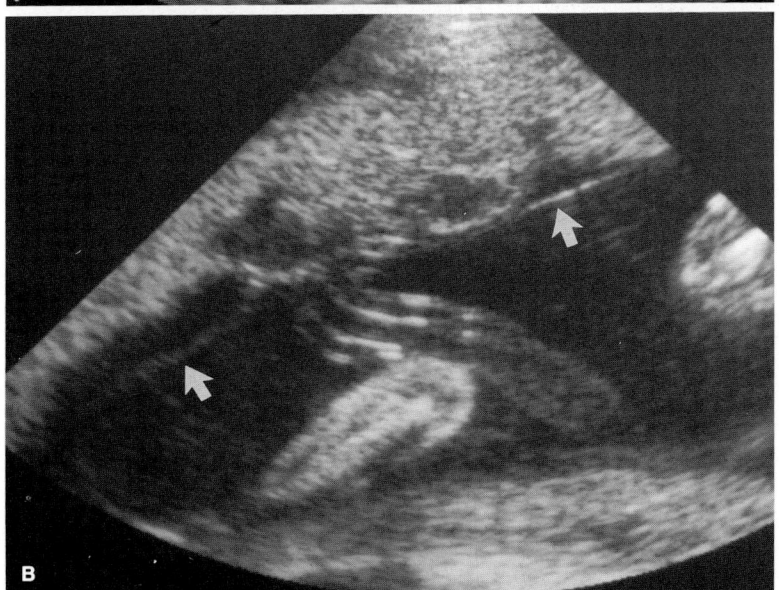

FIGURE 7-33. Chorionic–amniotic separation occurring spontaneously in a 23-week pregnancy. **(A)** The flaccid nature of the amnion (*arrows*) suggests significant membrane distortion. **(B)** The amniotic membrane (*arrows*) is separate from the chorion except at the umbilical cord insertion into the placenta. There was clinical rupture of the membranes at 27 weeks, with delivery of a normal but premature infant at 30 weeks. (Nyberg DA, Mahoney BS, Pretorius DH [eds]: Diagnostic Ultrasound of Fetal Anomalies: Text and Atlas. Chicago: Mosby–Year Book, 1990.)

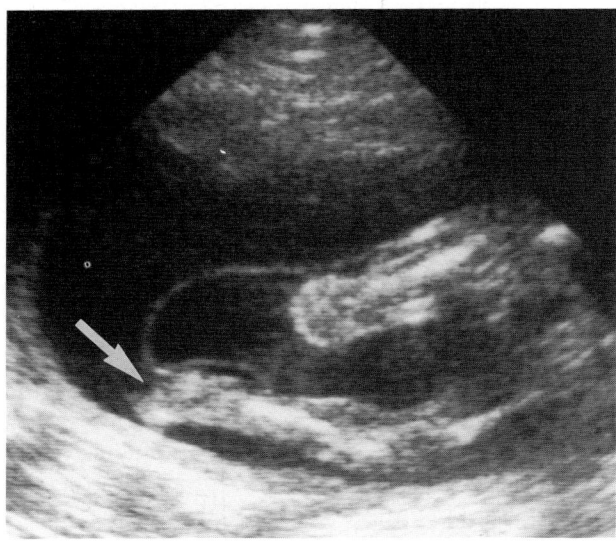

FIGURE 7-34. Extraamniotic pregnancy. Complete chorionic–amniotic separation occurred in this 19-week, clinically uncomplicated pregnancy. Amniotic disruption is present, with one fetal leg seen outside the amnion (*arrow*). On subsequent scans, the fetus was fully extraamniotic. A normal infant was delivered near term.

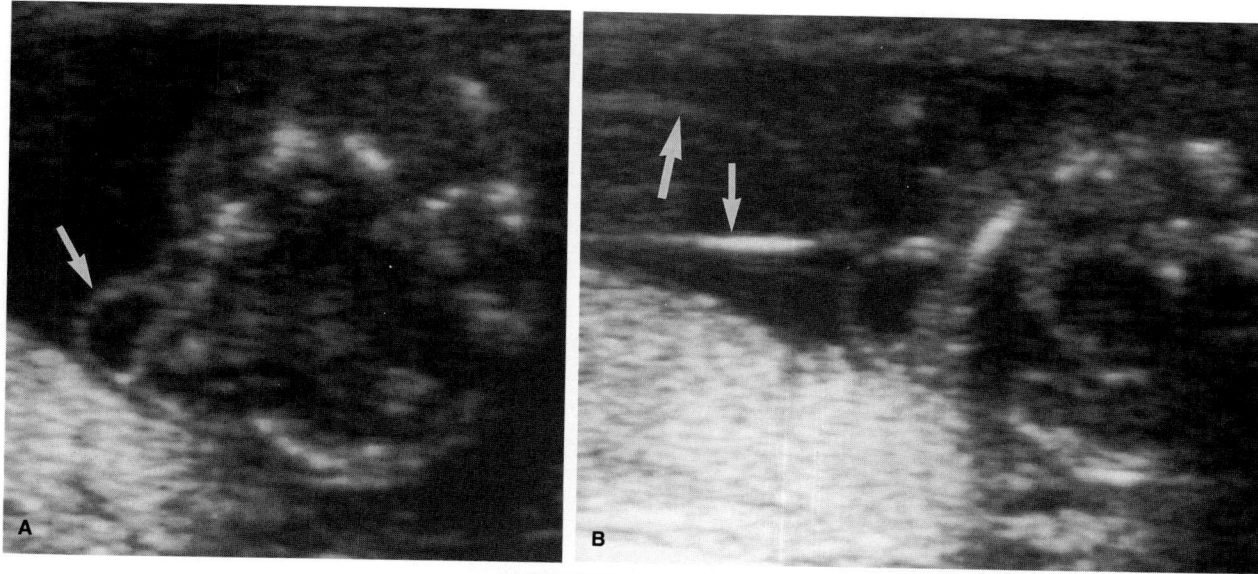

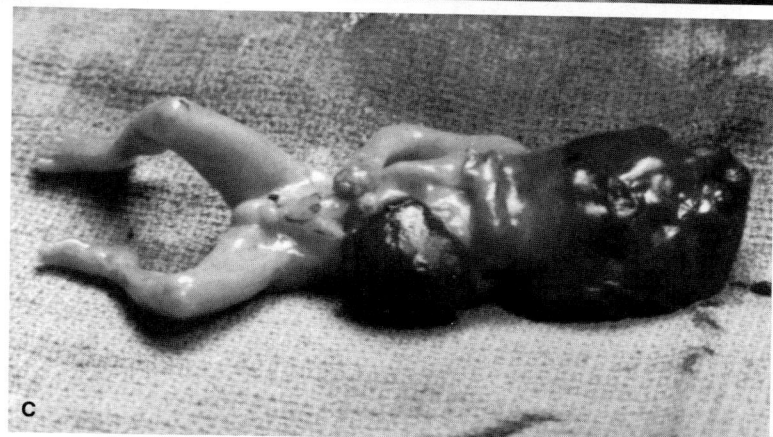

FIGURE 7-35. Amniotic band syndrome, producing eccentric encephalocele, obliterated facial features, abdominal wall defect with herniated liver, intestine, and heart, and tethered left arm in a 17-week pregnancy. **(A)** A left temporal–parietal encephalocele is seen (*arrow*). Intracranial and facial landmarks are not identified. **(B)** Amniotic bands (*arrows*) are seen between the encephalocele and the gestation wall. (Additional bands extended to the midtorso at the area of the herniated organs.) **(C)** The aborted fetal specimen confirms the devastating fetal malformations.

intertwin membrane or submembrane hemorrhage. Conditions that produce a shelf have in common a ridgelike configuration or a strut that is extraamniotic and provides a contour indenting the amniotic space, with the amnion draped over it. Thus, the shelf always extends to the margin of the gestational cavity and has a free edge projecting inward on the amniotic space. No portion of the amniotic fluid is loculated or isolated by the shelf. Because these processes are all extraamniotic, they can neither entrap nor deform the fetus. They include uterine synechia, circumvallate placenta, and uterine septum (see Table 7-4).

Uterine Synechia. A uterine synechia or endometrial adhesion develops most commonly as a consequence of dilation and curettage, less often after other uterine surgeries such as cesarean section,

and occasionally in the absence of any recognizable antecedent event. As the endometrial cavity of a uterus with a synechia enlarges during pregnancy, the adhesion stretches across the cavity, forming a taut, column-like strand. The chorionic–amniotic membrane encounters this band, folds over it, and extends to the endometrial margin, where the folded membrane layers separate. The resultant ultrasound appearance has the following characteristics (Fig. 7-36):[31]

- An echo-poor zone, representing the fibrous synechia, within the linear free edge of a shelflike membrane extending to the endometrium
- A free edge that is bulbous and thicker than the remainder of the shelf, as seen in axial views, because this contains the synechia,

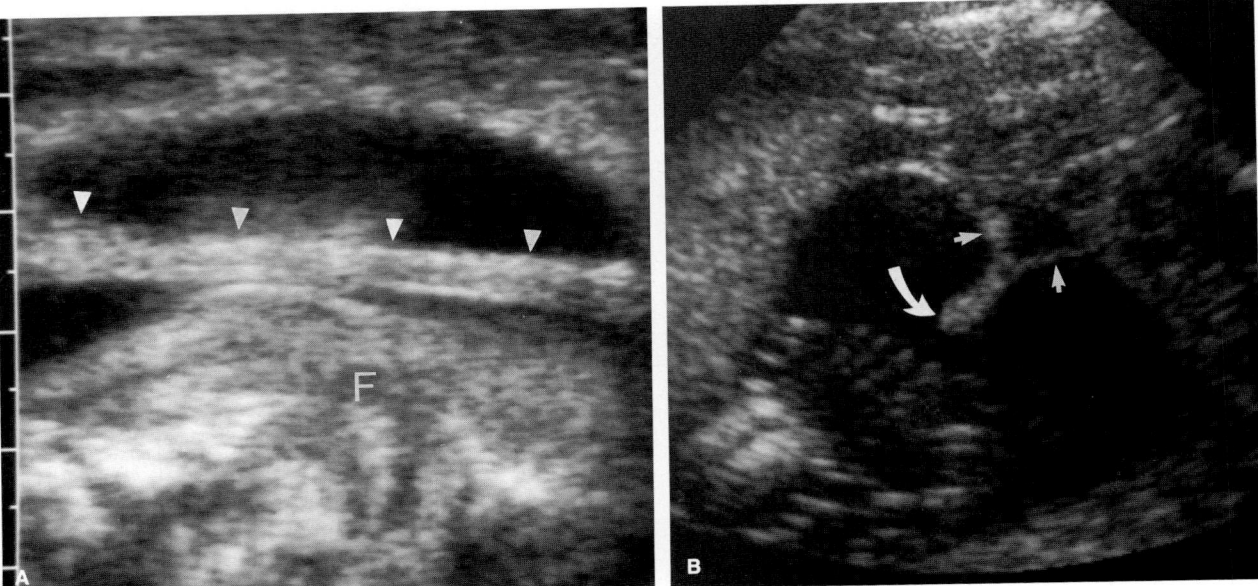

FIGURE 7-36. Uterine synechiae. **(A)** Scan along the axis of the adhesion shows a linear structure (*arrowheads*) centrally hypoechoic, extending to the endometrial margin at both ends. The fetus (F) is neither tethered nor deformed by the synechia. **(B)** Scan axial to the synechia, in a different patient, shows the free edge to be bulbous (*curved arrow*), with the overlying membranes separating from each other at the endometrial margin, producing a Y-shaped split (*arrows*).

while the remainder of the shelf is thin, made up only of two adjacent layers of combined chorion-amnion

- Y-shaped splitting of the membrane layers as they separate from each other to lie against the endometrium

In about half of cases, the placenta extends to, is indented by, or actually grows out along the synechia, and the placental tissue may obscure some of the anticipated sonographic features (Fig. 7-37).

Most synechiae are not of clinical importance, but in some cases, particularly when the adhesion is in the lower portion of the uterus, fetal malpresentation may result. There may also be a tendency toward low placental implantations and bleeding, but the data supporting this as a consequence of synechiae are limited.

Circumvallate Placenta. The shape of a circumvallate placenta and the resultant sonographic appearance can be difficult to conceptualize. In this condition, the membranes, decidua, and villi at the periphery of the placenta lift away from the endometrium, becoming raised and folded back toward the center of placenta along the fetal surface. The shape is closely analogous to a mushroom cap (with the top of the cap against the endometrium and the stem side representing the chorionic surface). The circumvallate configuration may affect the entire circumference of the placenta or only a portion of it.

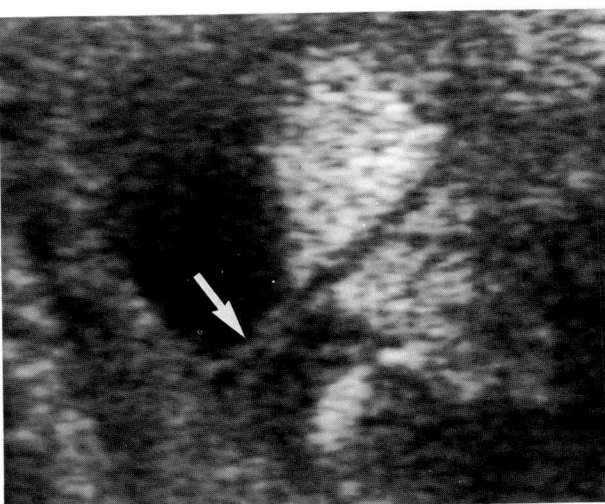

FIGURE 7-37. Much of the length of this synechia indents the placenta. The enveloped adhesion is seen only as a hypoechoic linear structure, except where it traverses the amniotic space (*arrow*).

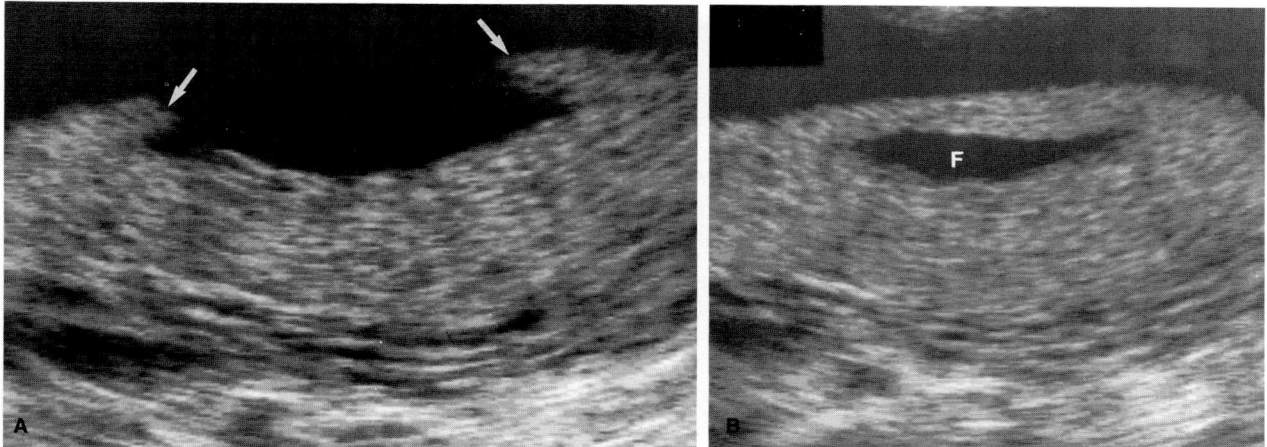

FIGURE 7-38. Circumvallate placenta in an 18-week, asymptomatic pregnancy. **(A)** Scan along a diameter of the placenta shows the infolded margins (*arrows*). **(B)** Scan along a more peripheral arc of the placenta shows the infolded margin as a continuous linear band parallel to the chorionic surface with fluid (F) trapped in the fold.

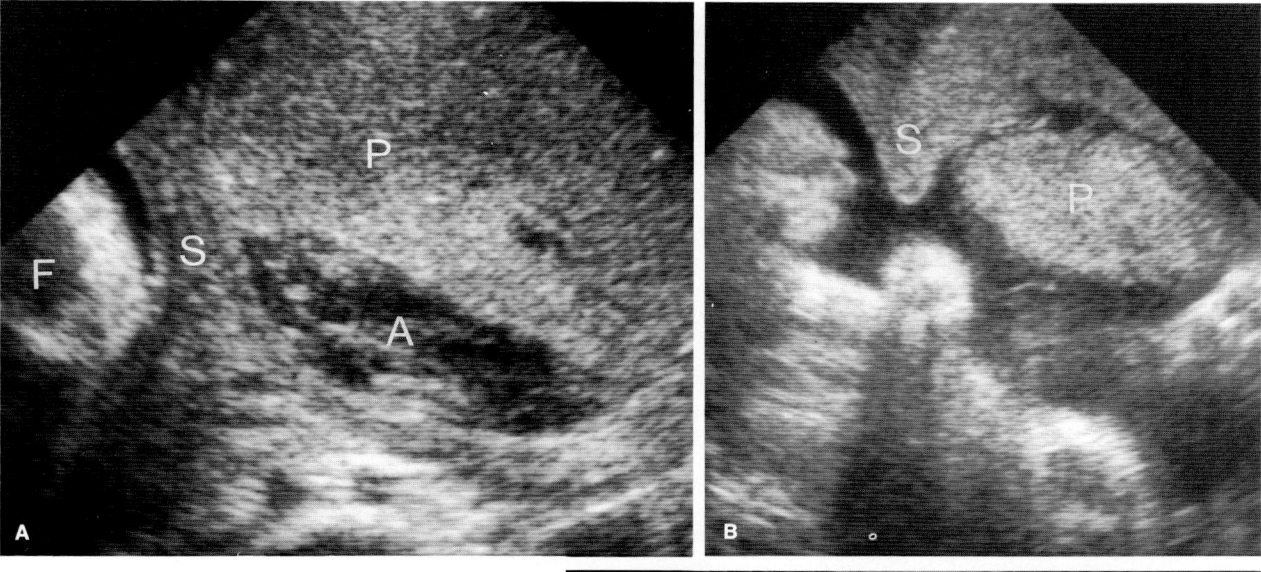

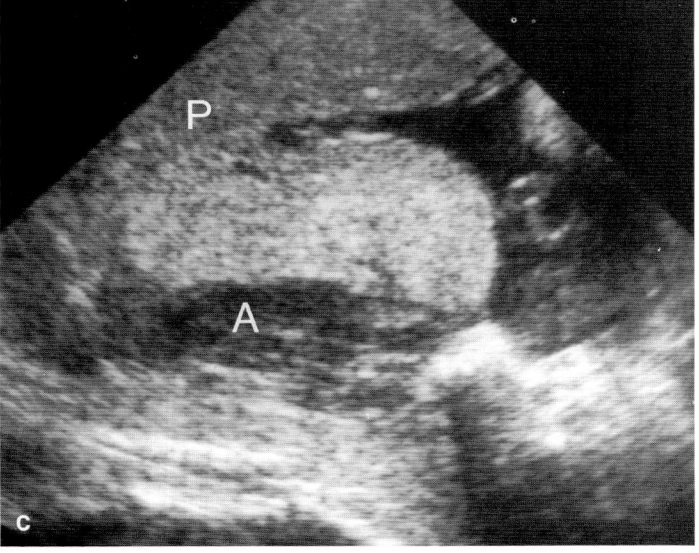

FIGURE 7-39. Septate uterus with left fundal placenta partially implanted on the septum and with a retroplacental abruption posteriorly. The patient presented with painless vaginal bleeding at 29 weeks. A live infant in breech presentation was delivered by cesarean section with confirmation of a large abruption. **(A)** Transverse scan at uterine fundus shows a septum (S), with the placenta (P) to the left and a posterior abruption (A). The fetal head (F) is to the right of the septum. **(B)** Coronal scan obtained by indenting the maternal abdomen just above the uterine fundus and angling caudally shows the septum (S) as a short, ridge-like peak. P, placenta. **(C)** Sagittal scan through the left fundus shows the large posterior abruption (A), estimated at 25% of the placental attachment.

Scans oriented radially to the placenta show a triangular tissue fold, thickest at the placental edge, tapering to an apex that points into the amniotic space and back toward the center of the placenta. Scans that intersect a peripheral arc of the placenta may show a continuous linear band just deep to the placenta, with both its surfaces outlined by amniotic fluid (Fig. 7-38). Although this superficially may simulate a synechia, the fact that the free edge is curvilinear, following the contour of the placenta, as well as the triangular cross section of the circumvallate placental fold, allow easy differentiation of these two conditions.

Little clinical significance is related to the presence of a circumvallate placenta. Its occurrence may be due to low uteroplacental blood flow, and conditions associated with reduced blood flow, such as preeclampsia and smoking, may predispose to this placental variant. The risks to fetal growth and well-being are predominantly those of the underlying cause of lessened uteroplacental blood flow, but a circumvallate placenta is associated with an independent, additional slight increase in risk of fetal growth retardation. A subtle relation to antepartum hemorrhage from marginal abruptions has also been suggested.

Uterine Septum. A congenital septum of the uterus extends from the fundus, oriented in a mid-sagittal plane. In transverse scans, it is seen as a band of tissue, running anterior to posterior and usually several millimeters to more than 1 cm thick. It is thickest at the fundus, tapering and eventually disappearing at a variable distance toward the cervical end of the uterus. A useful view to show the length of the septum is obtained in a plane coronal to the uterine fundus. The transducer is held almost parallel to the maternal abdominal surface, pointing toward the pelvis and indenting the skin over the fundus (Fig. 7-39). With a septate uterus, the outer contour of the fundus is convex upward. With a bicornuate uterus, the fundal contour is indented or heart-shaped.

A uterine septum may predispose to malpresentation by preventing the fetus from rotating within the uterus; it similarly may prevent successful external version for breech presentation. The blood supply to the septum is less adequate than to the rest of the uterine corpus. Placental implantations on the septum may be associated with increased risk for fetal growth retardation and placental abruption.

REFERENCES

1. Lacro RV, Jones KL, Benirschke K: The umbilical cord twist: Origin, direction, and relevance. Am J Obstet Gynecol 1987; 157:833.
2. Benirschke K, Kaufman P: Umbilical cord and major fetal vessels. In Pathology of the Human Placenta, 2nd ed. New York: Springer-Verlag 1990: 180.
3. Clausen I: Umbilical cord abnormalities and antenatal fetal deaths. Obstet Gynecol Surv 1989; 44:841.
4. Heifetz SA: Single umbilical artery: A statistical analysis of 237 autopsy cases and review of the literature. Perspect Pediatr Pathol 1984; 8:345.
5. Nyberg DA, Shepard T, Mack LA, et al: Significance of a single umbilical artery in fetuses with central nervous system malformations. J Ultrasound Med 1988; 7:265.
6. Nyberg DA, Mahoney BS, Luthy D, Kapur R: Single umbilical artery: Prenatal detection of concurrent anomalies. J Ultrasound Med 1991; 10:247.
7. Saller DN, Keene CL, Sun CCJ, Schwartz S: The association of single umbilical artery with cytogenetically abnormal pregnancies. Am J Obstet Gynecol 1990; 163:922.
8. Jeanty P: Fetal and funicular vascular anomalies: Identification with prenatal US. Radiology 1989; 173:367.
9. Jeanty P: Persistent right umbilical vein: An ominous prenatal finding? Radiology 1990; 177:735.
10. Giacoia GP: Body stalk anomaly: Congenital absence of the umbilical cord. Obstet Gynecol 1992; 80:527.
11. Lockwood CJ, Scioscia AL, Hobbins JC: Congenital absence of the umbilical cord resulting from maldevelopment of embryonic body folding. Am J Obstet Gynecol 1986; 155:1049.
12. Rayburn WF, Beynen A, Brinkman DL: Umbilical cord length and intrapartum complications. Obstet Gynecol 1981; 57:450.
13. Finberg HJ: Avoiding ambiguity in the sonographic determination of the direction of umbilical cord twists. J Ultrasound Med 1992; 11:185.
14. Strong TH, Elliott JP, Radin TG: Non-coiled umbilical blood vessels: A new marker for the fetus at risk. Obstet Gynecol 1993; 81:409–411.
14a. Strong TH, Finberg HJ, Mattox JH: Antepartum diagnosis of non-coiled umbilical cords. Am J Obstet Gynecol [forthcoming].
15. Miser WF: Outcome of infants born with nuchal cords. J Fam Pract 1992; 34:441.
16. Collins JH: First report: Prenatal diagnosis of a true cord knot. Am J Obstet Gynecol 1991; 165:1898.
17. Ramanathan K, Epstein S, Yaghoobian J: Localized deposition of Wharton's jelly: Sonographic findings. J Ultrasound Med 1986; 5:339.
18. Skibo LK, Lyons EA, Levi CS: First-trimester umbilical cord cysts. Radiology 1992; 182:719.
19. Pollack MS, Bound LM: Hemangioma of the umbili-

cal cord: Sonographic appearance. J Ultrasound Med 1989; 8:163.

20. Resta RG, Luthy DA, Mahoney BS: Umbilical cord hemangioma associated with extremely high alpha-fetoprotein levels. Obstet Gynecol 1988; 72:488.
21. Siddiqi TA, Bendon R, Schultz DM, Miodovnik M: Umbilical artery aneurysm: Prenatal diagnosis and management. Obstet Gynecol 1992; 80:530.
22. Mahoney BS, McGahan JP, Nyberg DA, Reisner DP: Varix of the fetal intra-abdominal umbilical vein: Comparison with normal. J Ultrasound Med 1992; 11:73.
23. Estroff JA, Benacerraf BR: Fetal umbilical vein varix: Sonographic appearance and postnatal outcome. J Ultrasound Med 1992; 11:69.
24. Keckstein G, Tschurtz S, Schneider V, et al: Umbilical cord hematoma as a complication of intrauterine intravascular blood transfusion. Prenat Diagn 1990; 10:59.
25. Eddleman KA, Lockwood CJ, Berkowitz GS, et al: Clinical significance and sonographic diagnosis of velamentous umbilical cord insertion. Am J Perinatal 1992; 9:123.
26. Nelson LH, Melone PJ, King M: Diagnosis of vasa previa with transvaginal and color flow Doppler ultrasound. Obstet Gynecol 1990; 76:506.
27. Strong TH, Phelan JP: Umbilical cord prolapse. The Female Patient 1991; 16:19.
28. Lange IR, Manning FA, Morrison MB, et al: Cord prolapse: Is antenatal diagnosis possible? Am J Obstet Gynecol 1985; 151:1083.
29. Finberg HJ: The "twin peak" sign: Reliable evidence of dichorionic twinning. J Ultrasound Med 1992: 11:571.
30. Jeanty P, Laucirica R, Luna SK: Extra-amniotic pregnancy: A trip to the extraembryonic coelom. J Ultrasound Med 1990; 9:733.
31. Finberg HJ: Uterine synechiae in pregnancy: Expanded criteria for recognition and clinical significance in 28 cases. J Ultrasound Med 1991; 10:547.

John P. McGahan and Manuel Porto:
DIAGNOSTIC OBSTETRICAL ULTRASOUND.
© 1994 J.B. Lippincott Company.

John P. McGahan   Amy S. Thurmond

Chapter 8

The Fetal Head

NORMAL ANATOMY

Evaluation of the fetal central nervous system (CNS), including the brain and the cerebral ventricles, has been recommended as a standard of care.[1] In the second and third trimesters, visualization of (1) the ventricular atrium, (2) the cisterna magna, and (3) the cavum septi pellucidi allows exclusion of most intracranial abnormalities.[2]

Ventricular Atrium

The downside ventricular atrium can be visualized in 99% of normal fetuses.[2] The ventricular atrium is best visualized on a standardized transaxial plane taken through the fetal cranium. The ventricular atrium, at this level, remains fairly stable in size throughout the second and third trimesters of pregnancy. The normal ventricular atrium has a mean diameter of between 6 and 7 mm. A measurement of 10 mm is 4 standard deviations above the mean and is considered the cut-off point between normal and abnormal size of the ventricular atrium[2,3] (Figs. 8-1 and 8-2).

Recent data have shown the feasibility of demonstrating the proximal, or upside, cerebral ventri-

cle throughout pregnancy using an angled technique.[4,5] Normal measurements of the body of the upside cerebral ventricle remain fairly stable throughout pregnancy, with the upper limits of normal for mean plus 3 standard deviations being 9 mm (see Figs. 8-1 and 8-2).

Cisterna Magna

An image of the posterior fossa in the transaxial plane is obtained by angling caudally from the plane used to visualize the ventricular atrium. This shows the brain stem and the vermis of the cerebellum outlined by the cisterna magna.[6,7] The anteroposterior measurement of the cisterna magna obtained in the midline from the posterior margin of the cerebellar vermis to the inner wall of the occipital bone is about 5 mm. The cisterna magna measurement should be no more than 10 mm in depth and no less than 2 mm.[6] The diameter of the two cerebellar hemisphere increases by about 1 mm/week of pregnancy between 14 and 21 menstrual weeks (Fig. 8-3).

In the fetus, arachnoid septations typically are visualized within the cisterna magna. These septations are normal and should not be confused with

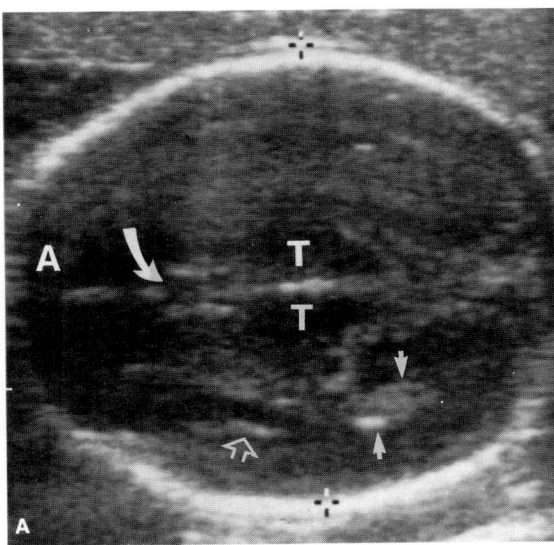

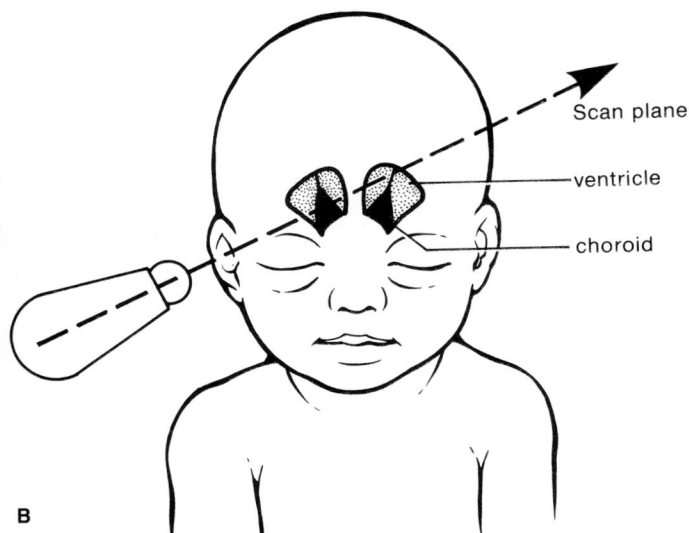

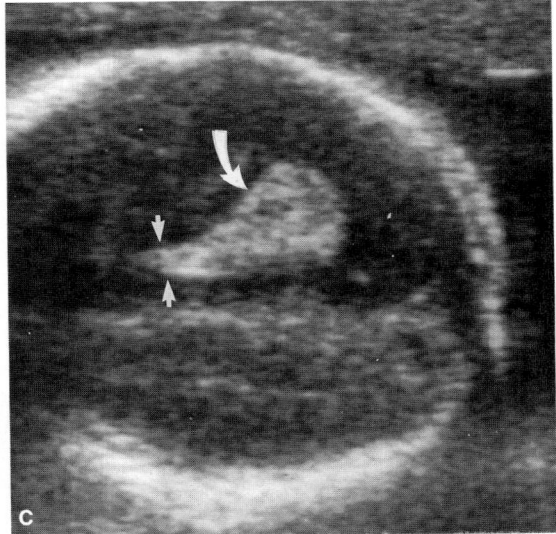

FIGURE 8-1. Normal cerebral ventricles at 21 menstrual weeks. **(A)** Real-time image demonstrating choroid plexus filling the trigone of the cerebral ventricle (*arrows*) farthest from the transducer, with no visualization of the cerebral ventricle closer to the transducer. A, anterior; T, thalami; *open arrow*, sylvian cistern; *curved arrow*, cavum septum pellucidum. **(B)** The plane of the transducer is positioned so that the calvarium is scanned through the region of the temporal bone, with the plane angled tangentially through the cerebral ventricle lying closer to the transducer, as illustrated. **(C)** Real-time image demonstrating the upside choroid plexus (*curved arrow*) filling the lateral ventricle. The medial and lateral walls of the upside lateral ventricle are seen (*arrows*). (Cronan MS, McGahan JP: A new ultrasound technique to visualize the proximal fetal cerebral ventricle. J Diagn Med Sonography 1990; 6:333–335.)

vascular structures[7] (Fig. 8-4). If a ventricular atrial view and posterior fossa view are satisfactorily obtained and are normal, the risk for a CNS anomaly is about 0.005%.[2,8]

Cavum Septi Pellucidi

Identification of a third anatomic structure, the cavum septi pellucidi, may be helpful to detect subtle midline abnormalities such as agenesis of the corpus callosum or lobar holoprosencephaly.[2] The cavum septum pellucidi typically is identified on a transaxial plane with the anteriorly placed cavum septi pellucidi as a structure that contains cerebrospinal fluid (CSF) and that is positioned between the frontal horns of the lateral ventricles (see Figs. 8-1 and 8-2). When scanning through this region, the shape of the cranium can also be assessed.[9]

ARTIFACTS

Pseudohydrocephalus

Within the early second trimester of pregnancy, the brain parenchyma on the side farthest from the transducer is hypoechoic and may be confused with hydrocephalus.[10] Additionally, adjacent to the dependent portion of the bony calvarium is an echogenic interface thought to represent the fetal

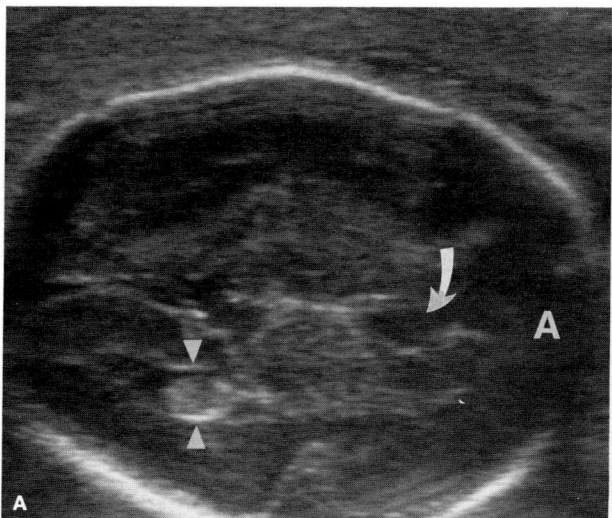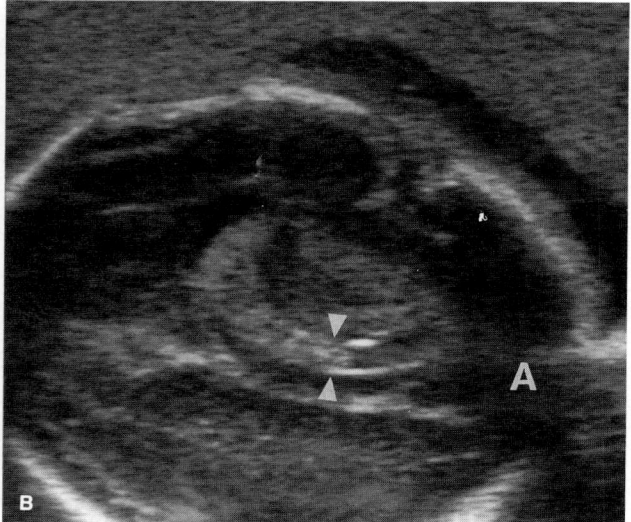

FIGURE 8-2. Normal cerebral ventricles: downside and upside. **(A)** Real-time ultrasound of the fetal brain demonstrates a scan through the cavum septi pellucidi (*curved arrow*) and the choroid plexus filling the trigone of the lateral ventricle (*arrowheads*). The upside lateral ventricle is not seen. Measurement from the medial to lateral wall of the trigone of the lateral ventricle should be less than 10 mm throughout pregnancy. A, anterior. **(B)** Using the angle technique, the choroid plexus is noted filling the lateral ventricle (*arrowhead*). Medial to lateral wall diameter of the body of the upside lateral ventricle should be less than 9 mm throughout pregnancy.

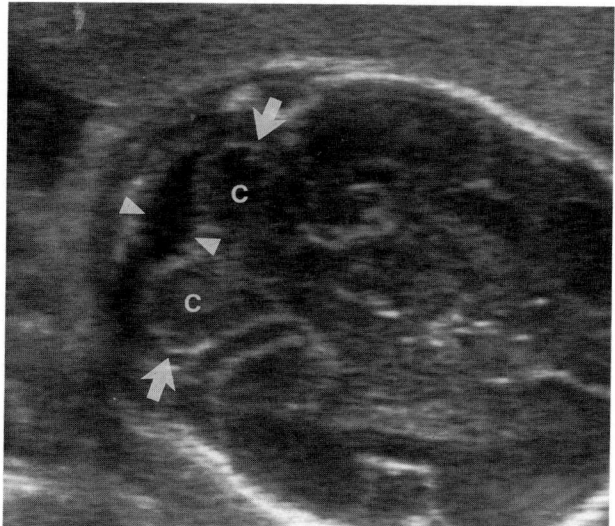

FIGURE 8-3. Normal posterior fossa. Scan through the posterior fossa demonstrates the cisterna magna with the normal anteroposterior diameter (*arrowheads*) to be no greater than 10 mm throughout pregnancy. The side-to-side measurement (*arrows*) of the cerebellar hemispheres (C) should increase by about 1 mm per week of menstrual age from 14 to 21 weeks.

subarachnoid space, which may be misinterpreted as the lateral ventricular wall, causing further confusion.[11] Misdiagnosis of hydrocephalus may be overcome by noting the points outlined in Table 8-1 and depicted in Figure 8-5.[12]

Unilateral Versus Bilateral Hydrocephalus

Unilateral hydrocephalus is incorrectly diagnosed when the upside fetal cerebral ventricle is not visualized to the artifact created by the bony calvarium in the near field.[10] This misdiagnosis may be overcome by angling the transducer through the anterolateral fontanel or the thinner squamosal portion of the temporal bone to visualize the obscured fetal cerebral ventricle[4,5] (see Figs. 8-1 and 8-2).

Reverberation Artifact

Reverberation artifact from the anterior cranial vault may be identified within the fetal cranium. This source of confusion may be remedied by noting that there is no distortion of the intracranial anatomy or by using a technique such as the an-

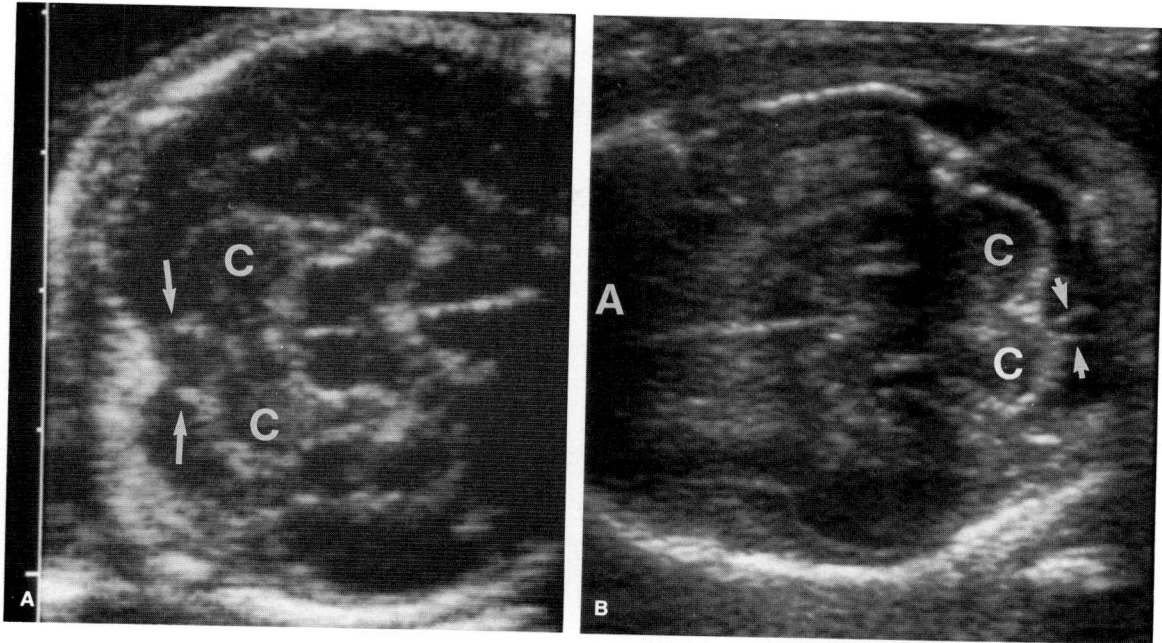

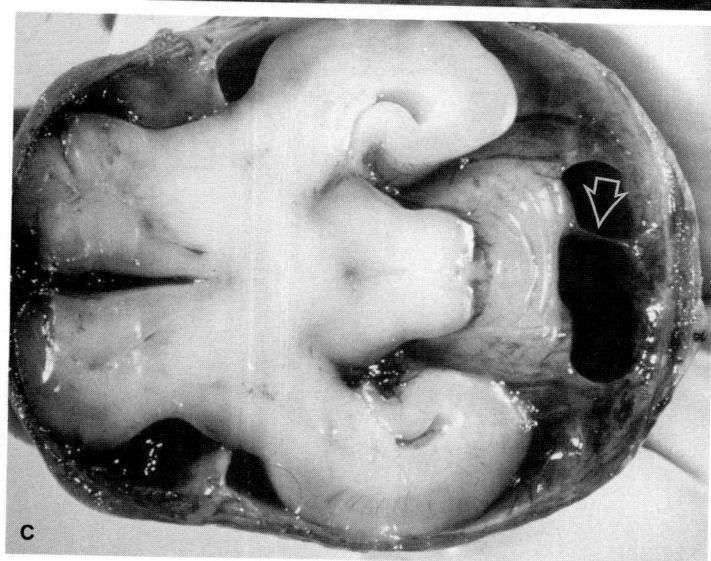

FIGURE 8-4. Posterior fossa septations. **(A)** Cyst-like structure in the cisterna magna corresponding to normal bridging septations (*arrows*). C, cerebellar hemispheres. **(B)** These normal septations may have a variable appearance, with from one to four septations normally being identified with careful scanning (*arrows*). C, cerebellar hemispheres; A, anterior. **(C)** Gross dissected specimen demonstrating a septum bridging the subarachnoid space (*arrows*) posterior to the cerebellar hemispheres. This is a normal finding. (Knutzen R, McGahan JP, Salamat MS, Brant WB: Fetal cisternal magna septa: A normal anatomical finding. Radiology 1991; 180:799–801.)

TABLE 8-1. Hydrocephalus Versus Pseudohydrocephalus

The misdiagnosis of hydrocephalus may be avoided by:
- Noting that there is a specular reflection anteriorly that represents the normal sylvian cistern with the accompanying middle cerebral artery
- Scanning more cephalad in the fetus, so that the true walls of the frontal horn of the lateral ventricle can be seen
- Noting that both the medial and lateral walls of the ventricular atrium can be recognized with meticulous scanning
- Noting that the ventricular choroid plexus remains relatively parallel to the long axis of the lateral ventricle (absence of dangling choroid)

gled approach to visualize the proximal intracranial structures (see Figs. 8-1 and 8-2).

Choroid Plexus Pseudocyst

An oval hypoechoic structure can be visualized in the inferior and lateral aspect of the atrium of the lateral ventricle. This should not be mistaken for a true choroid plexus cyst. This artifact may be recognized based on its oval shape, small size, and constant location and by noting that the structure is without a strong acoustic interface (wall), which occurs with a true cyst[13] (Fig. 8-6).

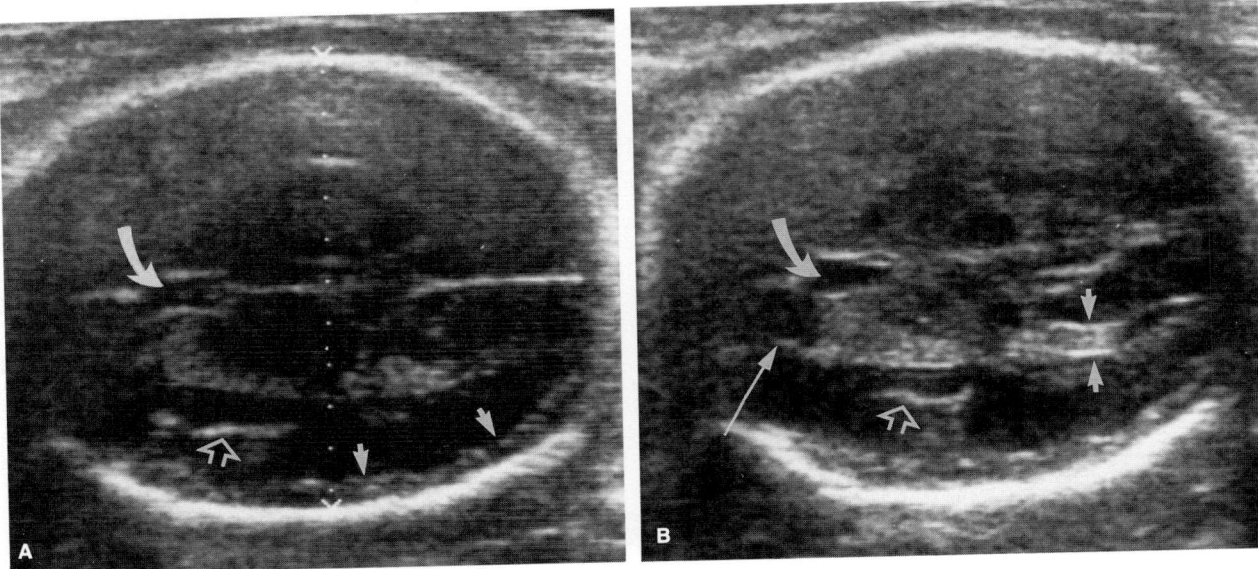

FIGURE 8-5.   Pseudohydrocephalus. **(A)** Twenty-six weeks of menstrual age fetal head demonstrating hypoechoic area adjacent to the dependent portion of the calvarium, which may be misinterpreted as hydrocephalus. Note echogenic interface of the subarachnoid space (*arrows*), which may be misinterpreted as the lateral wall of the lateral ventricle. Curved arrow, cavum septum pellucidi; open arrow, sylvian cistern. **(B)** To avoid this pitfall, note: (1) the normal appearance of the cavum septi pellucidi (*curved arrow*), (2) the frontal horns of the lateral ventricle (*long arrow*), (3) the sylvian cistern (*open arrow*), and most important, (4) the two walls of the trigone of the lateral ventricle (*small arrows*); also (5), note that the choroid plexus does not dangle to a more dependent portion within the cerebral hemisphere.

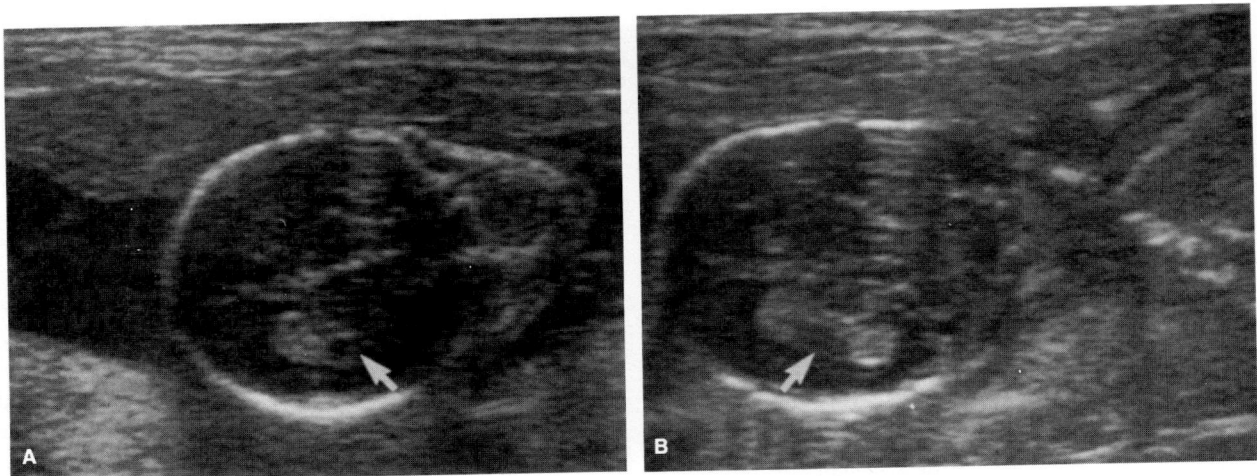

FIGURE 8-6.   Pseudo choroid plexus cyst. **(A)** Off-axis coronal image through the lateral ventricle of a 17.4-week fetus showing a hypoechoic region in the inferior lateral aspect of the atrium. **(B)** With change in the angle of the transducer, this appears as an oval hypoechoic structure that is thought to represent the corpus striatum projecting into the choroid plexus. (Nelson NL, Callen PW, Filly RA: The choroid plexus pseudocyst: Sonographic identification and characterization. J Ultrasound Med 1992; 11:597–601.)

TABLE 8-2.   Ultrasound Features of Ventriculomegaly

- Enlargement of the downside fetal cerebral ventricle atrium greater than 10 mm
- Enlargement of the upside fetal cerebral ventricle greater than 9 mm
- Minimal separation of the choroid plexus in either proximal or distal cerebral ventricle
- Dangling choroid plexus with an abnormal choroid angle

THE ABNORMAL FETAL HEAD

Ventriculomegaly

The term *ventriculomegaly* strictly defines enlargement of the cerebral ventricles without defining the cause. Sonographic features of ventriculomegaly are listed in Table 8-2, with examples shown in Figures 8-7 through 8-10.

The *choroid angle* is the measurement of the long axis of the dependent choroid in relation to the midline. The normal choroid angle is between 16 and 22 degrees, with choroid angles greater than 29 degrees indicative of ventriculomegaly. In most

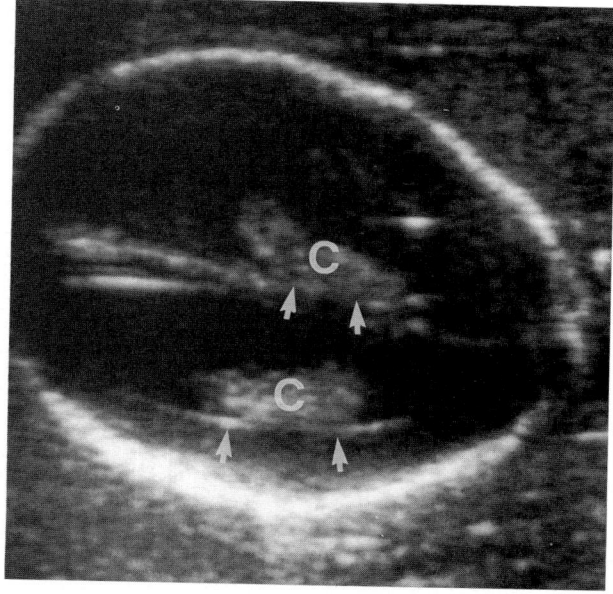

FIGURE 8-8.   Moderate hydrocephalus. Compare this scan with a pseudohydrocephalus appearance in which the choroid plexus (C) of both the downside and upside lateral ventricles dangle on the dependent ventricular wall (*arrows*). Identification of the choroid plexus, which is dangling or dependent within the lateral ventricle, may be a helpful sign in distinguishing true hydrocephalus from pseudohydrocephalus.

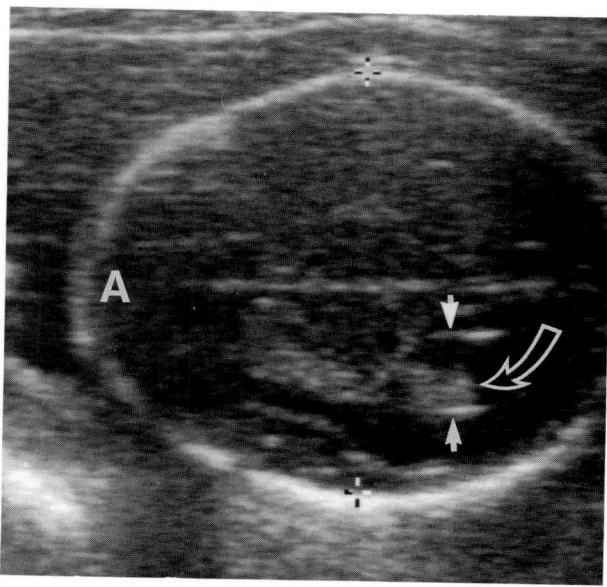

FIGURE 8-7.   Mild ventriculomegaly. The trigone of the lateral ventricle is mildly dilated to 11 mm (*arrows*). Also note the separation of the echogenic choroid plexus (*open curved arrow*) from the medial wall of the ventricle, which may be another feature of mild ventriculomegaly. A, anterior.

instances, however, it is easy to recognize dangling choroid without measuring it.[12]

Ventriculomegaly indicates enlargement of the cerebral ventricles and is not synonymous with hydrocephalus, which implies the ventriculomegaly based on obstruction of flow of the CSF. Causes of ventriculomegaly can be classified into three major categories: hydrocephalus, brain atrophy, or abnormal development of the brain.

Hydrocephalus usually implies blockage of the flow of CSF and rarely results from overproduction of CSF by tumor. CSF is produced within the choroid plexus and flows within the ventricles and over the subarachnoid space to be absorbed in the arachnoid granulations. Obstructive hydrocephalus within the fetus is most commonly noncommunicating (blockage within ventricles) rather than communicating (extraventricular blockage) (Table 8-3).

Another cause of ventriculomegaly is underdevelopment of the brain in or around the trigone region of the lateral ventricle; this is called *colpocephaly*. Colpocephaly is seen commonly with agenesis of the corpus callosum and does not re-

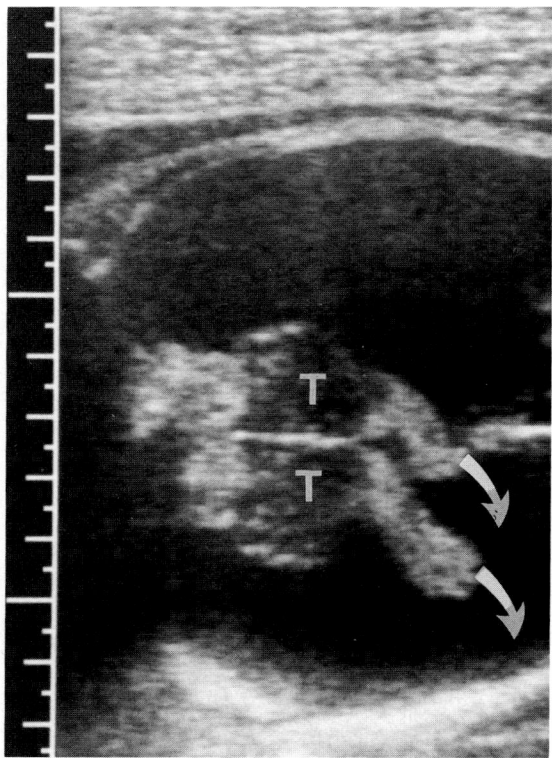

FIGURE 8-9. Massive hydrocephalus. Scan through midline structures and thalami (T), brain stem, and bilateral dangling choroid plexus (*curved arrows*). Note that the choroid plexus from the upside lateral ventricle dangles through midline into the dependent ventricle. This observation of dangling choroid may be an important feature in distinguishing true hydrocephalus from pseudohydrocephalus or other causes of massive cerebrospinal fluid collections.

spond to ventricular shunting. Also, in *lissencephaly* (smooth brain), there may be an absence of gyri and sulci and occasionally ventriculomegaly.

Brain destruction is another cause of ventriculomegaly and may include in utero damage due to a CNS infection. CNS infections may be associated with brain atrophy, with resultant microcephaly and ventriculomegaly. These infections are discussed in more detail later in this chapter.

Often, a single cause may produce ventriculomegaly by more than one mechanism. For instance, a fetus with intracranial infection may develop ventriculomegaly secondary to cerebral atrophy as well as meningitis, with resultant blockage in the sylvian aqueduct and hydrocephalus.

No definitive cut-off point has been determined to distinguish normal from abnormal ventricular size. For instance, in slight ventriculomegaly, pa-

tients with slightly enlarged ventricular size and normal postnatal outcome overlap those with similar ventriculomegaly but with a poorer or a poor postnatal outcome. In fetuses with mild ventriculomegaly, with a trigone measurement between 10 and 14 mm, the outcome is normal in about 40% of newborns.[14] Conversely, patients with certain intracranial malformations, such as Arnold-Chiari type II malformation or Dandy-Walker malformation (DWM), may have only minimal ventriculomegaly.[9,15]

When ventriculomegaly is detected, a careful anatomic survey of the fetus is necessary to determine any associated anomalies. Furthermore, hydrocephalus is associated with a significant risk of chromosomal abnormalities.[8] Distinguishing features and more common causes of ventriculomegaly are listed in Table 8-4.[16]

Open Neural Tube Defect
Ventriculomegaly related to open neural tube defect (ONTD) and Arnold-Chiari type II malformation may be manifest as so-called lemon and banana signs.[9] The lemon sign in the fetal head is caused by overlapping of the frontal bones, which

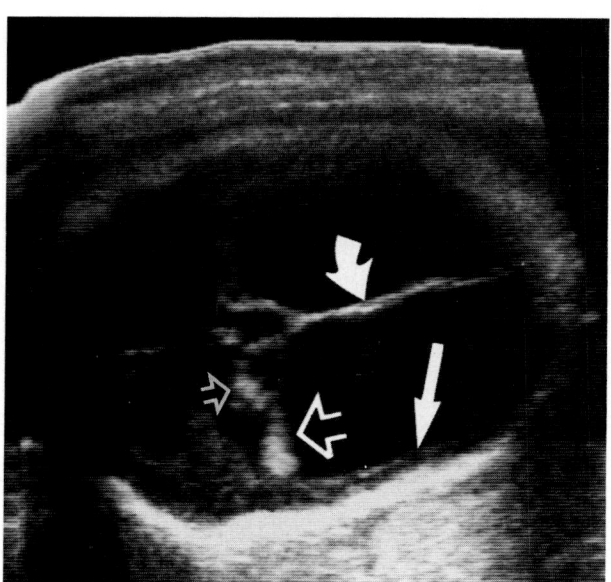

FIGURE 8-10. Massive hydrocephalus. Transaxial scan through the fetal head demonstrates massive cerebrospinal fluid collection with intact dura and midline structures (*curved arrow*) and compressed cerebral tissue (*long arrow*). Note the prominent dangling choroid plexus (*large open arrow*) in the downside ventricle and the choroid plexus from the upside lateral ventricle, which dangles into the contralateral ventricle (*small open arrow*).

TABLE 8-3. Causes and Associations of Ventriculomegaly

Cause	Associations
Neural tube defects	Spina bifida (Arnold-Chiari type II malformation)
	Cephaloceles
Other central nervous system malformations	Dandy-Walker malformation
	Agenesis of the corpus callosum
	Lissencephaly
Aqueductal stenosis	Sporadic
	Postinflammatory
	X-linked recessive
	Autosomal
Masses	Neoplasms
	Arachnoid cysts
Obstruction of cerebral spinal fluid flow in subarachnoid space	Postinflammatory
	Posthemorrhage
	Thanatophoric dysplasia
	Achondroplasia
	Osteogenesis imperfecta
Vascular anomalies	Aneurysm of Galen's vein
Multiple anomaly syndromes	Meckel-Gruber syndrome
	Walker-Warburg syndrome
	Apert's syndrome
	Smith-Lemli-Opitz syndrome
	Nasal–facial–digital syndrome
	Albers-Schönberg disease
	Robert's syndrome
	Fragile X syndrome
	Trisomy 18
	Trisomy 13

(Nyberg DA, et al: Cerebral malformations. In Nyberg DA, Mahony BS, Pretorius DH [eds]: Diagnostic Ultrasound of Fetal Anomalies: Text and Atlas. Chicago: Year Book Medical Publishers, 1990: 93.)

gives the head a lemon shape rather than an oval shape. This appearance can also occur with cephalocele[17] (discussed later). The banana sign is caused by downward displacement of the cerebellum, which gives a banana shape and also results in effacement of the cisterna magna (Fig. 8-11). An associated spinal defect occurs with this abnormality and is discussed in Chapter 9.

Dandy-Walker Malformation

Dandy-Walker malformation consists of a large posterior fossa cyst of variable size, vermian agenesis, hypoplasia of the cerebellar hemispheres, and variable amounts of hydrocephalus (Figs. 8-12 and 8-13). DWM is discussed in more detail in the section on massive intracranial fluid collections.[15,18]

Agenesis of the Corpus Callosum

The corpus callosum is a midline structure above the third ventricle that connects the cross fibers between the cerebral hemispheres. Agenesis of the corpus callosum may be complete or partial and may be accompanied by hydrocephalus. Only cases of complete agenesis of the corpus callosum have been diagnosed in utero. In many cases, isolated enlargement of the occipital horns (culpocephaly) is seen without hydrocephalus but with a high-riding third ventricle. These cases may be more difficult to diagnosis. Scanning anteriorly through the ventricles, however, shows an absence of the cavum septum pellucidum in agenesis of the corpus callosum.[19] In situations associated with hydrocephalus, the diagnosis can be made with certainty by noting the lateral displacement of both lateral ventricles by an enlarged third ventri-

(text continues on p. 145)

TABLE 8-4. Causes and Distinguishing Features of Ventriculomegaly

Malformation	Features
Arnold-Chiari type II malformation	Deformed cranium (lemon sign), usually disappears in third trimester
	Obliteration of cisterna magna (banana sign)
	Associated open spinal defect
	Minimal hydrocephalus
	Large massa intermedia
	Pointed frontal horns
Dandy-Walker malformation	Midline posterior fossa cyst
	Cyst communicates with fourth ventricle
	Vermian agenesis
	Hypoplastic cerebellar hemispheres
	Elevated tentorium
	Mild to moderate hydrocephalus
Agenesis of the corpus callosum	Third ventricle elevated
	Separation of frontal horns
	Associated colpocephaly
	Mild hydrocephalus
Aqueductal stenosis	Moderate to massive hydrocephalus
	Normal fourth ventricle
	Normal posterior fossa
	Normal cranial configuration
Cephalocele	Open defect, usually occipital skull base
	Obliteration of the cisterna magna
	Occasional lemon sign
	Mild to moderate hydrocephalus
	Polyhydramnios

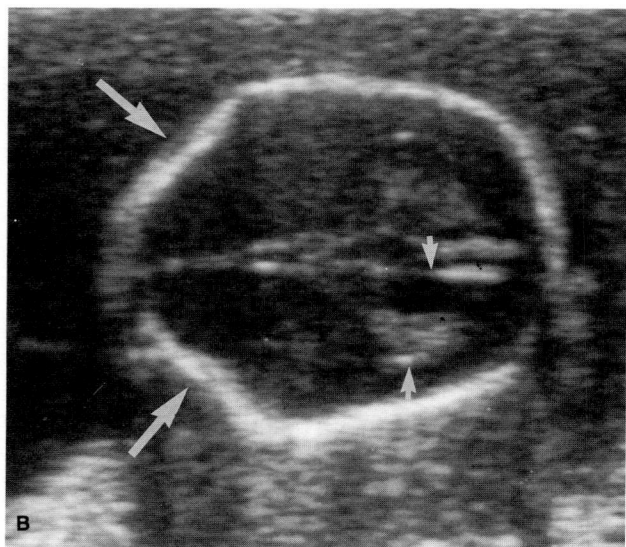

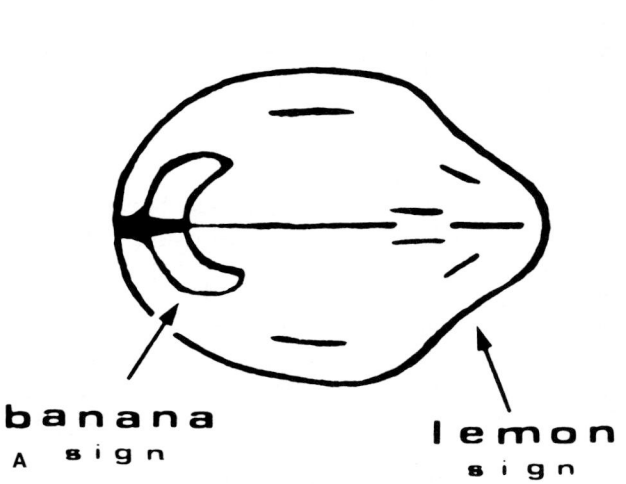

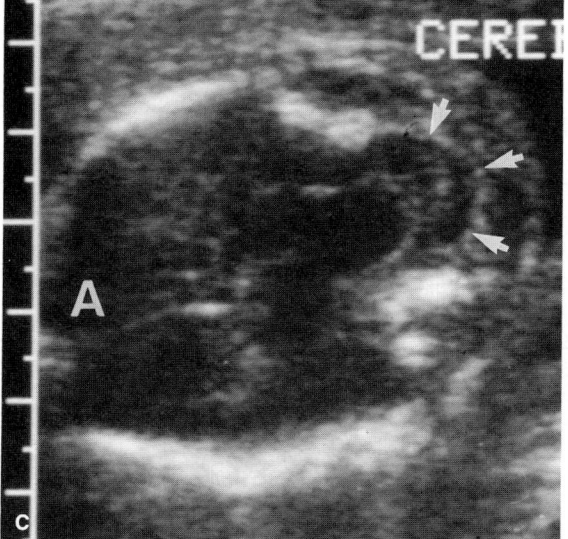

FIGURE 8-11. "Lemon" and "banana" signs. **(A)** Diagram demonstrating the overlapping coronal sutures of the fetal head, which has been termed the *lemon sign*. Also, the cerebellar hemispheres within the posterior fossa are compressed, which has been termed the *banana sign*. These are important features for ultrasound screening for open neural tube defects. (Nicolaides KH, Campbell S, Gabbe SG, Guidetta R: Ultrasound screening for spina bifida: Cranial and cerebellar signs. Lancet 1986; 2:72.) **(B)** Axial ultrasound of the fetal head demonstrates overlapping of the coronal sutures, so-called lemon head (*large arrows*), occurring with an open neural tube defect. Also note mild enlargement of the trigone of the lateral ventricle to 12 mm, which often occurs with open neural tube defect (*small arrows*). **(C)** Scans of the posterior fossa do not demonstrate the normal appearance of the cisterna magna but rather associated compression of the cerebellar hemispheres, or so-called banana sign (*arrows*). There is complete obliteration of the cisterna magna.

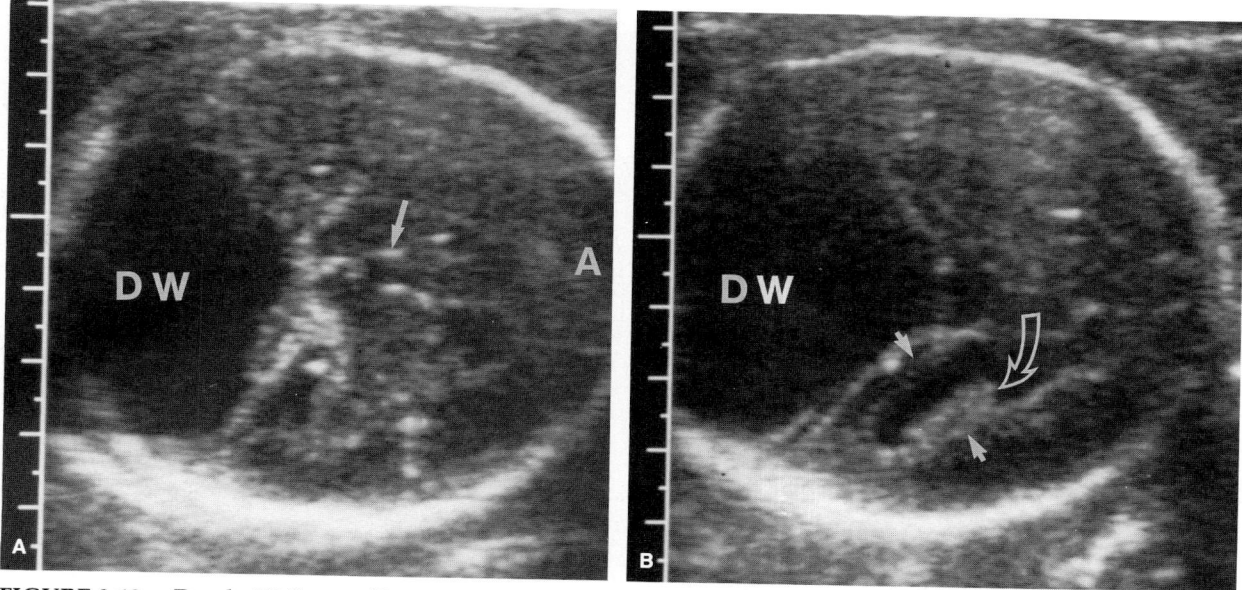

FIGURE 8-12.   Dandy-Walker malformation. **(A)** Axial scan of the fetal cranium demonstrates a large, symmetric, posterior fossa cyst (DW) with minimal enlargement of the third ventricle (*arrow*). The posterior fossa cyst communicates with the fourth ventricle. In this case, there is not only agenesis of the cerebellar vermis but also near complete absence of the cerebellar hemispheres. A, anterior. **(B)** A scan slightly more cephalad demonstrates the Dandy-Walker cyst (DW) and enlargement of the lateral ventricle (*arrows*). The choroid plexus (*open curved arrow*) is separated from the medial wall of the lateral ventricle.

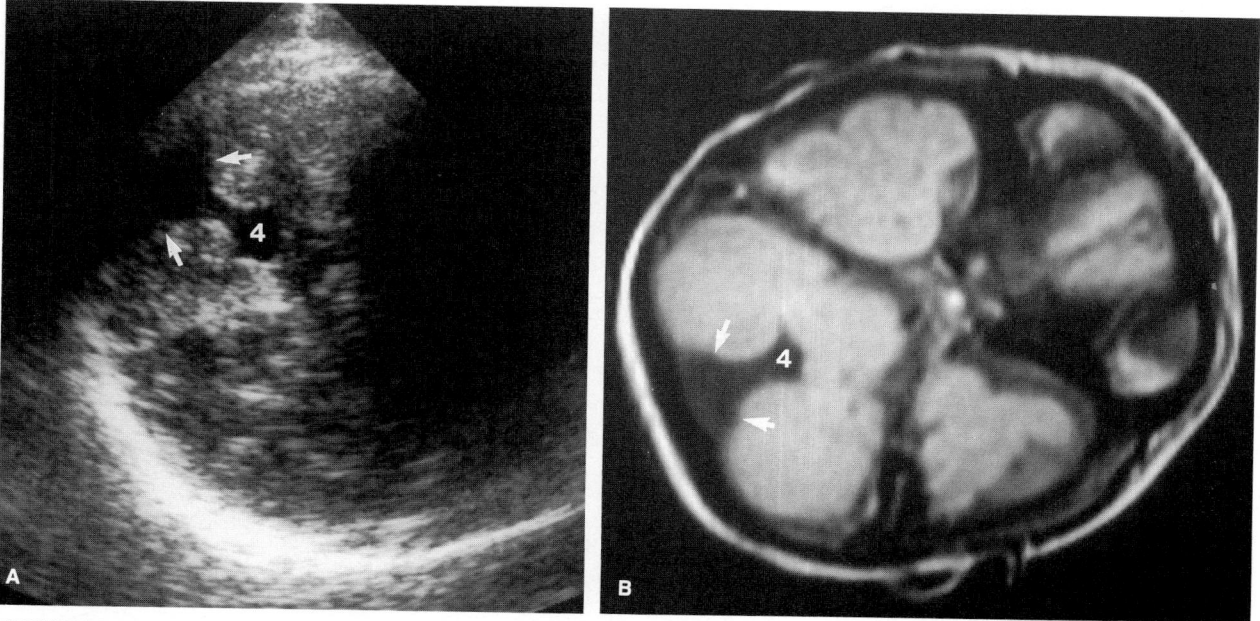

FIGURE 8-13.   Dandy-Walker variant. **(A)** In utero axial ultrasound showing cystic posterior fossa defect (*arrows*), which communicates with the fourth ventricle (4). **(B)** Corresponding magnetic resonance image that shows the defect (*arrows*) communicating with the fourth ventricle (4) secondary to partial vermian agenesis. (Estroff JA, Scott MR, Benacerraf BR: Dandy-Walker variant: Prenatal sonographic features and clinical outcome. Radiology 1992; 185:755–758.)

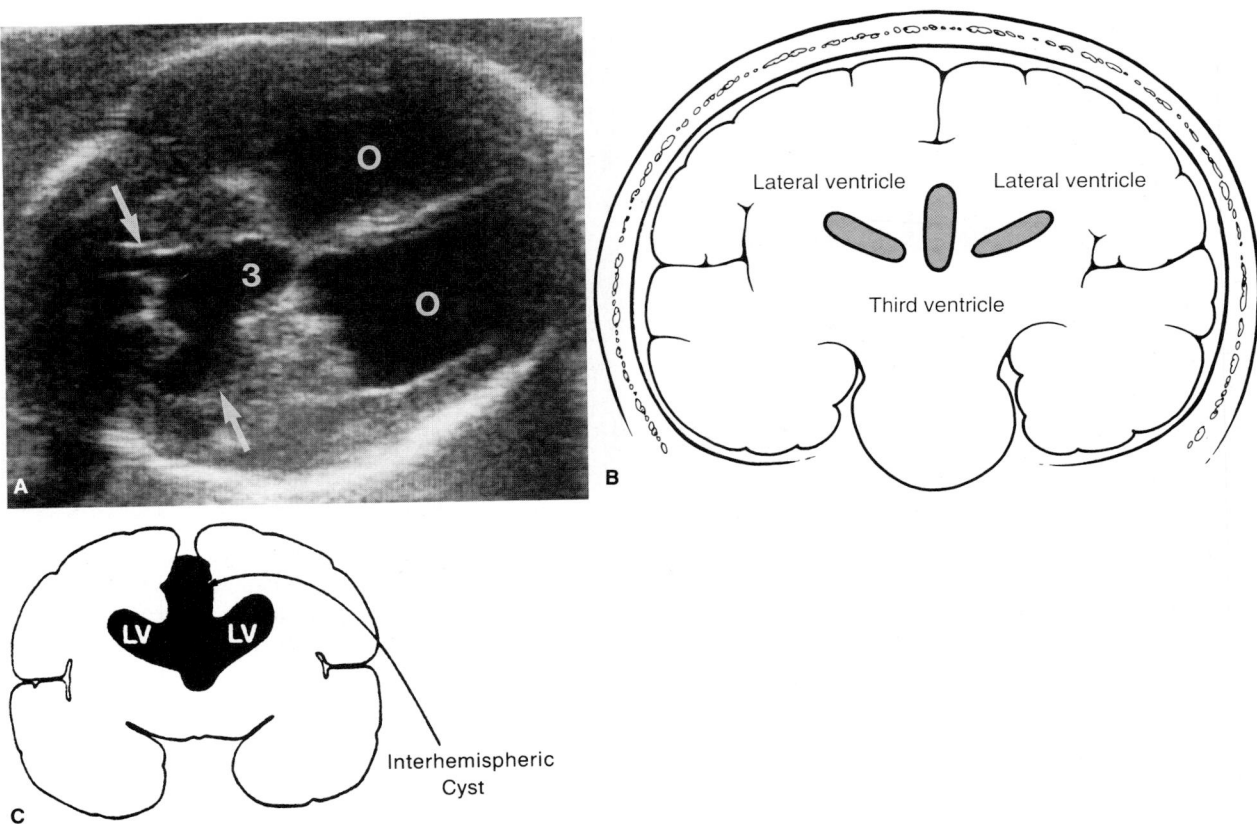

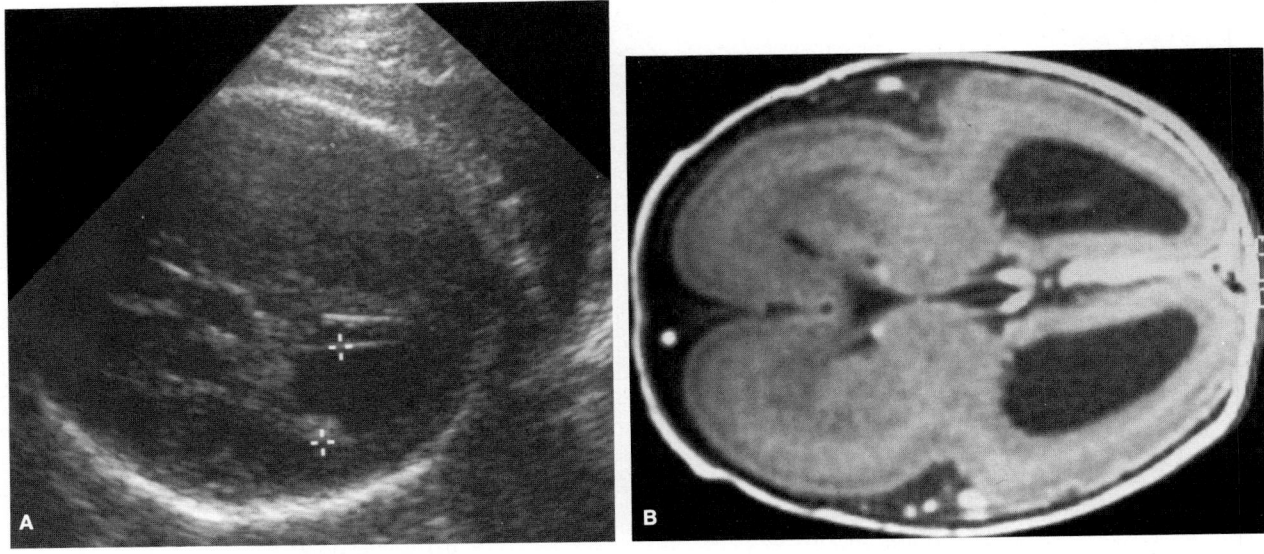

FIGURE 8-15.   Lissencephaly. **(A)** In utero ultrasound demonstrates mild dilation of the trigone and occipital horn of the lateral ventricle. The frontal horn was not dilated. **(B)** Postnatal magnetic resonance image demonstrates smooth appearance of the brain surface with dilation of the trigone in the occipital horn in this infant with lissencephaly.

FIGURE 8-14. Agenesis of the corpus callosum. **(A)** In utero axial ultrasound scan demonstrates a dilated third ventricle (3), which lies between the frontal horns (*arrows*), and an accompanying disproportionate dilation of the occipital horns (O), that is, culpocephaly. (McGahan JP, Ellis W, Lindfors KK, Lee BCP, Arnold JP: Congenital cerebrospinal fluid-containing intracranial abnormalities: A sonographic classification. J Clin Ultrasound 1988; 16:531–544.) **(B)** Coronal diagram of the third ventricle displaced between the lateral ventricles. **(C)** Schematic diagram of agenesis of the corpus callosum with interhemispheric cyst representing portions of the mildly dilated and elevated third ventricle. (Nyberg DA, Mahony BS, Pretorius DH: Cerebral malformation. In Diagnostic Ultrasound of Fetal Abnormalities. Chicago: Year Book Medical Publisher, 1990: 113.)

TABLE 8-5. Causes of Massive Intracranial Fluid Collections

Common

Hydrocephalus

Uncommon

Holoprosencephaly
Hydranencephaly

---

cle (Fig. 8-14). Often, other associated CNS anomalies or non-CNS anomalies of the limb or urinary tract are seen and are associated with agenesis of the corpus callosum.

Lissencephaly

Lissencephaly is a term used to described a brain with absent or poor sulci formation. Lissencephaly is also called *smooth brain* and may be associated with dilated trigone, occipital horns, and temporal horns of the lateral ventricles. This ventriculomegaly is probably secondary to incomplete development of the calcarine sulci and the hippocampus.[20] Lissencephaly is probably not recognized prenatally until the dilated lateral ventricles are identified[21] (Fig. 8-15).

Aqueductal Stenosis

Aqueductal stenosis is one of the more common causes of in utero hydrocephalus. The cause of aqueductal stenosis often is never found, but specific causes may exist. For instance, in utero infections, such as viral infections due to cytomegalovirus, may cause adhesive arachnoiditis and lead to obstruction of flow of the CSF at a number of different sites, including the sylvian aqueduct. A defective recessive gene on the X chromosome has also been associated with aqueductal stenosis. Male infants with this defect have hydrocephalus and often severe mental retardation.[22] Moderate to massive dilation of the lateral ventricles is easily identified. There may be mild dilation of the third ventricle with a normal fourth ventricle. Usually, the diagnosis of aqueductal stenosis is by exclusion, noting no other specific cause for the hydrocephalus. The ventriculomegaly in aqueductal stenosis is often progressive throughout pregnancy. Infrequently, CNS anomalies or chromosomal abnormalities are associated with aqueductal stenosis (see Fig. 8-10).

Massive Intracranial Fluid Collections

The three common causes of massive intracranial fluid collections with intact cranial vault are hydrocephalus, holoprosencephaly, and hydranencephaly[23] (Table 8-5). Distinguishing features are listed in Table 8-6, and a flow chart for abnormal CSF fluid collections is listed in Flow Diagram 1. CSF collections may be divided into generalized and focal. In generalized, symmetric CSF collections, considerations include hydrocephalus, holoprosencephaly, and hydranencephaly. If no corti-

TABLE 8-6. Distinguishing Features of Hydrocephalus, Hydranencephaly, and Alobar Holoprosencephaly

	Cerebral Tissue	Falx	Fused Thalami	Midline Cavity	Dangling Choroid	Midface Abnormalities
Hydrocephalus	Yes	Yes	No	No	Yes	No
Holoprosencephaly	Yes	No	Yes	Yes	Minimal	Yes
Hydranencephaly	No	Yes	No	No	Minimal	No

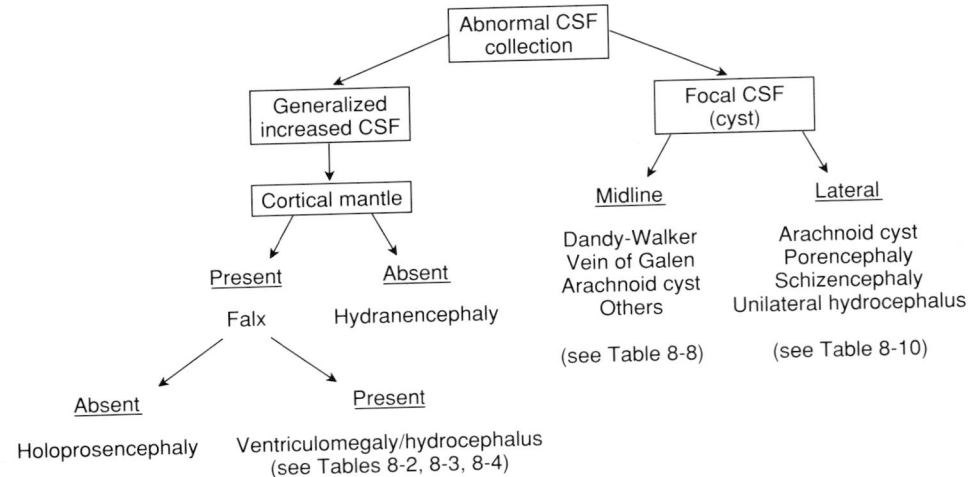

Flow Diagram 1. Flow chart for intracranial abnormalities.

cal mantle is present, but there is a falx, the anomaly is most probably hydranencephaly. If there is a cortical mantle, absent falx, and midline intracranial and facial abnormalities, holoprosencephaly is the diagnosis. Otherwise, the abnormality is probably hydrocephalus (see Table 8-6).

Massive Hydrocephalus

Massive hydrocephalus is usually secondary to an obstructive phenomenon, such as aqueductal stenosis (see Figs. 8-9 and 8-10), rather than cerebral malformations, such as Arnold-Chiari type II malformation. The ultrasound features are listed in Table 8-6.

Alobar Holoprosencephaly

Holoprosencephaly may exhibit a sonographic spectrum of abnormalities classified as alobar, semilobar, and lobar (Table 8-7). The lobar form of holoprosencephaly has only fused frontal horns, with the rest of the brain tissue appearing grossly normal. The most common form of holoprosencephaly is the alobar form. This results in a monoventricular cavity with fused thalami (Figs. 8-16 and 8-17). Alobar holoprosencephaly is secondary to failure of the development of the cleavage of the prosencephalon.[23] Separation of the prosencephalon is induced by the prenotochordal mesoderm, which is needed for normal development of the midline facial structures. Thus, alobar holoprosencephaly is often associated with significant facial abnormalities, including cyclopia, ethmoidocephaly, cebocephaly, and cleft lip (see Chapter 10). Alobar holoprosencephaly also is often associated with trisomy 13.[24]

Alobar holoprosencephaly may have three separate configurations: pancake, cup, or ball forms[16,23] (see Fig. 8-17). The pancake type, which is the rarest, occurs when the residual brain is minimal and compressed over the skull base. The ball variation occurs when the cerebral cortex covers the monoventricular cavity. The cup form is intermediate between the two, with the residual brain having a cup-like configuration on sagittal view (see Figs. 8-16 and 8-17).

Other authors divide cases of alobar holoprosencephaly into those with and without a dorsal sac. Thus, alobar holoprosencephaly without a dorsal sac is similar to the ball form, while the cup and pancake forms have a dorsal sac.[23]

TABLE 8-7. Classifications and Features of Holoprosencephaly

Classification	Features
Alobar (most common in utero)	Fused thalami
	Facial abnormalities
	Monoventricular cavity
	Absent falx cerebra
Semilobar (rarest form)	Fused thalami
	Facial abnormalities
	Monoventricular cavity with increased cerebral tissue, especially in the occipital lobes
Lobar (usually identified in infants)	Squared frontal horns
	Absent cavum septi pellucidi
	Possible ventriculomegaly
	Otherwise fairly normal intracranial anatomy

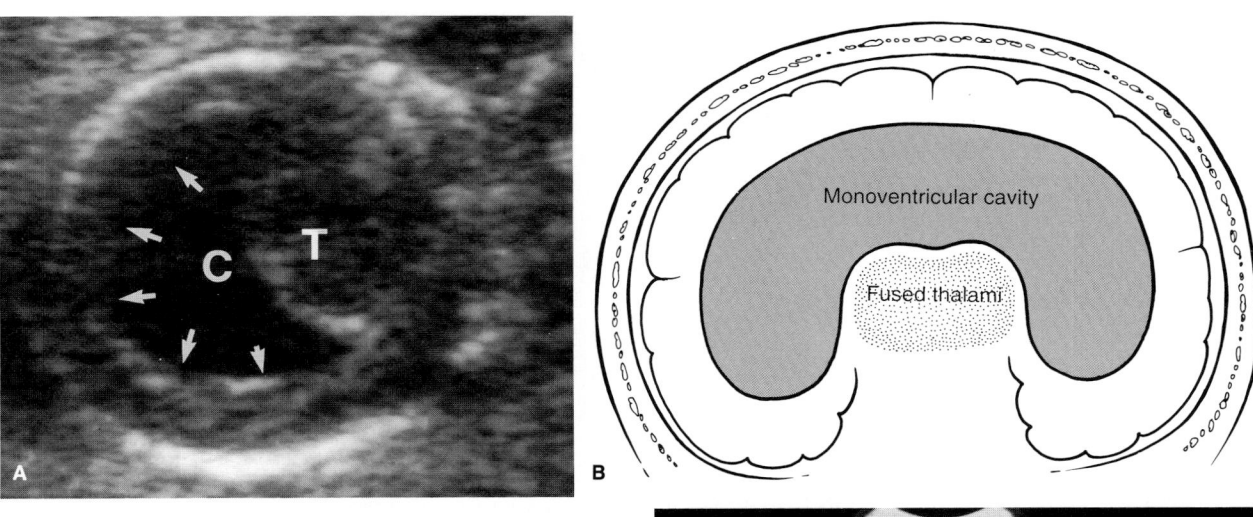

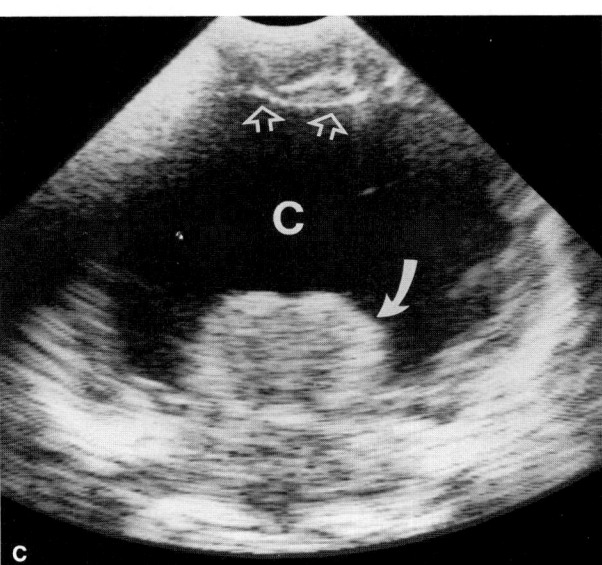

FIGURE 8-16.   Alobar holoprosencephaly. **(A)** In utero coronal ultrasound of the fetal head demonstrates a monoventricular cavity (C) surrounded by cerebral tissue (*arrows*) with fused thalami (T), which is diagnostic of alobar holoprosencephaly. **(B)** Drawing of coronal ultrasound demonstrates that in alobar holoprosencephaly, there is absence of midline structures, a large monoventricular cavity, and fused thalami. **(C)** Coronal ultrasound of the newborn head demonstrates monoventricular cavity (C) surrounded by cerebral tissue (*open arrows*) with fused thalami (*curved arrow*), compressed choroid, and absence of dural coverings. (Modified from McGahan JP, Ellis W, Lindfors KK, et al: Congenital cerebrospinal fluid-containing intracranial abnormalities: A sonographic classification. J Clin Ultrasound 1988; 16:531–544.)

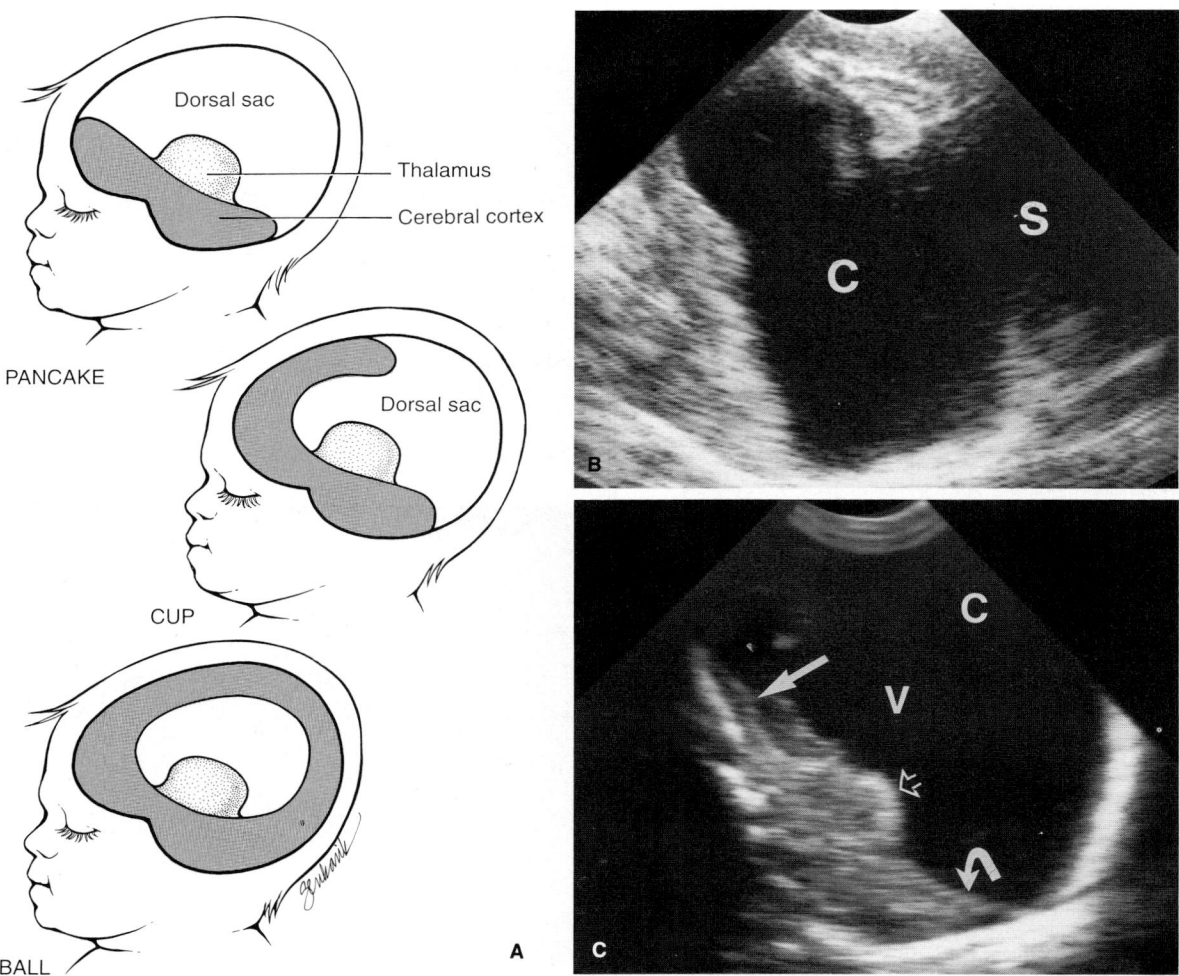

FIGURE 8-17. **(A)** Sagittal conception of the (A) "pancake," (B) "cup," or (C) "ball" type of configuration that occurs with alobar holoprosencephaly. This concept is based on the amount of cerebral tissue that covers the monoventricular cavity; the residual tissue is similar in appearance to either a pancake, cup, or ball. In both the pancake and cup forms, a dorsal sac protrudes from the monoventricular cavity. **(B)** Sagittal sonogram of the neonatal head with a cup form of alobar holoprosencephaly shows monoventricular cavity (C) that extends posteriorly as a dorsal sac (S). **(C)** Sagittal ultrasound scan demonstrating the pancake form of alobar holoprosencephaly monoventricular cavity (V), which continues as a dorsal sac (C). Cerebral tissue was present in the occipital (*curved arrow*) and frontal (*straight arrows*) regions, and there was compressed choroid plexus (*open arrow*). See Fig. 8-16 for the ball form of alobar holoprosencephaly. (Modified from McGahan JP, Ellis W, Lindfors KK, et al: Congenital cerebrospinal fluid-containing intracranial abnormalities: A sonographic classification. J Clin Ultrasound 1988; 16:531–544.)

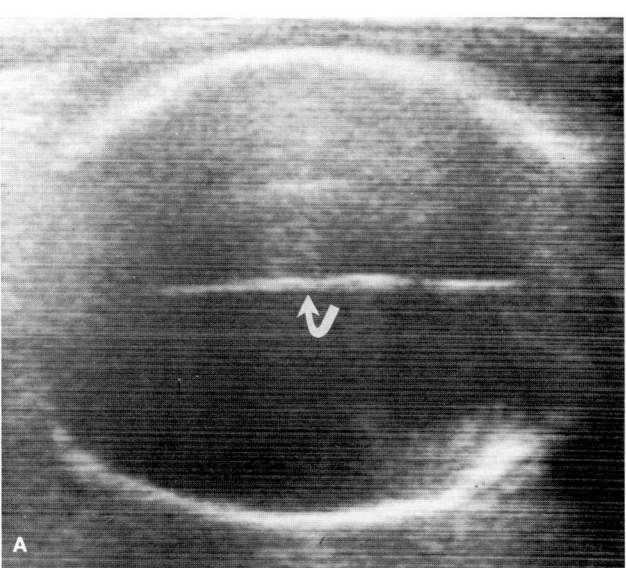 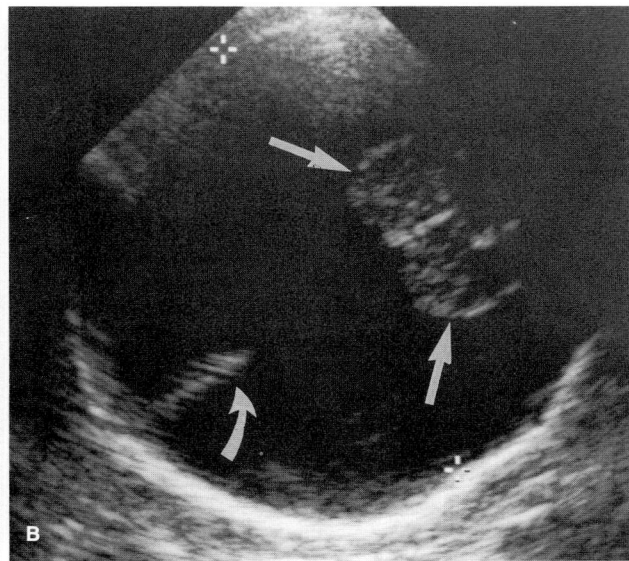

FIGURE 8-18. Hydranencephaly in utero. **(A)** In utero axial scan performed in a cephalad location within the fetal head demonstrates a midline falx (*curved arrow*) with no brain tissue adjacent to the bony calvarium. **(B)** Coronal in utero ultrasound shows midline falx (*curved arrow*) and no cerebral tissue with nonfused thalami (*straight arrows*), diagnostic features of hydranencephaly.

Distinguishing ultrasound features are listed in Table 8-6.

Hydranencephaly

The term *hydranencephaly* is derived from the combination of the words *hydrocephalus* and *anencephaly*. Hydranencephaly is different from both these entities. In contrast to hydrocephalus, hydranencephaly is characterized by a complete lack of cerebral tissue; and in contrast to anencephaly, there is covering by bone, skin, dura, and leptomeninges[25] (Fig. 8-18). Hydranencephaly is thought to result from bilateral in utero internal carotid artery infarction. Ultrasound features are listed in Table 8-6 (Fig. 8-19).

Cystic Abnormalities of the Brain

A number of focal cystic abnormalities of the brain have been identified. Some may be associated with other intracranial abnormalities, such as hydrocephalus, while others are isolated findings. Some cystic intracranial abnormalities are typically midline. These include DWM and vein of Galen aneurysm. Other cystic intracranial abnormalities are usually lateral but can occur within the midline, such as arachnoid cyst or brain tumors. Complex intracranial abnormalities, such as agenesis of the corpus callosum or alobar holoprosencephaly, may have midline cystic components as well (Table 8-8).

Dandy-Walker Malformation

One of the more common midline cystic abnormalities is DWM. DWM is characterized by a midline cyst located within the posterior fossa that communicates with the fourth ventricle (see Fig. 8-12). This cyst is posterior to the ventricle and is associated with near or complete absence of the cerebellar vermis and enlarged posterior fossa. There is associated hydrocephalus in 80% of cases, concurrent CNS malformations in greater than 50% cases, and often systemic or chromosomal abnormalities.[15]

On occasion, there may be a variant of DWM in which there is only partial absence of the cerebellar vermis with a small posterior fossa cyst (see Fig. 8-13). In these fetuses, ventriculomegaly occurs less frequently (in about 25% of cases), but there is a high incidence of concurrent non-CNS abnormalities and often an abnormal karyotype. A significant number of these fetuses with no concurrent abnormalities develop normally after birth.[18]

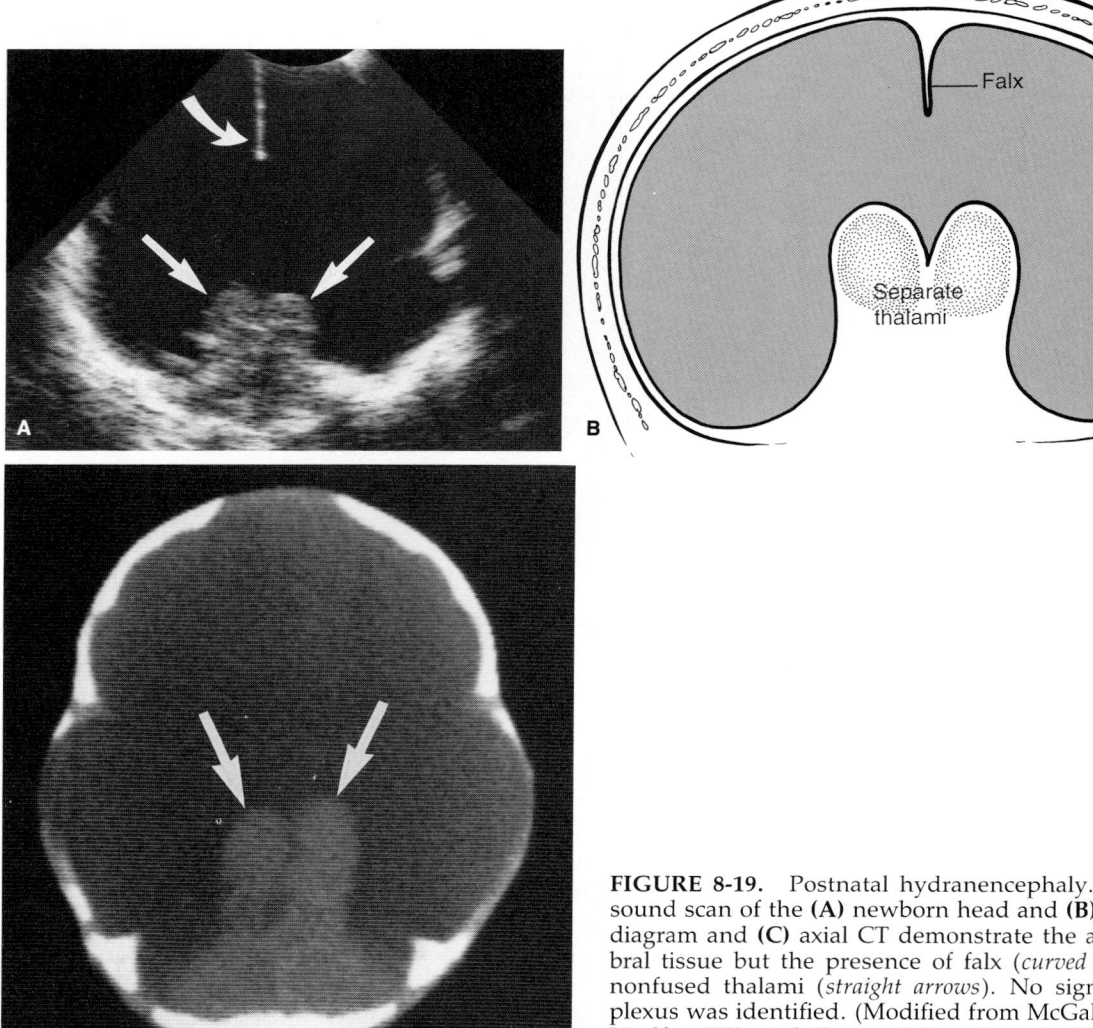

FIGURE 8-19. Postnatal hydranencephaly. Coronal ultrasound scan of the **(A)** newborn head and **(B)** corresponding diagram and **(C)** axial CT demonstrate the absence of cerebral tissue but the presence of falx (*curved arrow*) and the nonfused thalami (*straight arrows*). No significant choroid plexus was identified. (Modified from McGahan JP, Ellis W, Lindfors KK, et al: Congenital cerebrospinal fluid-containing intracranial abnormalities: A sonographic classification. J Clin Ultrasound 1988; 16:531–544.)

TABLE 8-8.   Distinguishing Features of Midline Intracranial Cysts

	Location	Features
Dandy-Walker	Posterior fossa	Communication with fourth ventricle Concomitant hydrocephalus
Vein of Galen aneurysm	Supratentorial, posterior to corpus callosum	Doppler signal within cyst Arteriovenous shunting
Arachnoid cyst	Any location	Smooth wall Asymmetric location Mass effect Possibly hydrocephalus (dependent on location)
Cystic neoplasm	Any location	Solid mass Cystic components Irregular outline Mass effect
Agenesis of the corpus callosum with interhemispheric cyst	Interhemispheric between frontal horns of the lateral ventricles	Communication with cephalad displaced third ventricle
Alobar holoprosencephaly	Posterior–supratentorial	Typical features of alobar holoprosencephaly (see previous tables)

Vein of Galen Aneurysm

An uncommon but pathognomonic midline intracranial cyst is the vein of Galen aneurysm. The vein of Galen is a major draining vein that lies posterior and slightly superior to the thalami within the subarachnoid space. Within the aneurysm, there is abnormal rapid flow between the artery and the vein and resultant aneurysmal dilation of the vein of Galen. Thus, a moderate-size midline cyst with Doppler flow is diagnostic of an arteriovenous malformation[26] (Fig. 8-20).

Other Midline Cystic Abnormalities

Other midline cystic abnormalities may be associated with more complex malformations. In *agenesis of the corpus callosum,* the cavum septum pellucidi is absent, and the third ventricle is elevated between the laterally displaced frontal horns. A *midline interhemispheric cyst* may communicate with the third ventricle[19] (see Fig. 8-14). *Posterior midline fluid collection* may be related to holoprosencephaly as previously described (see Figs. 8-16 and 8-17). This is a dorsal sac that originates from a monoventricular cavity and extends posteriorly.[23] Other cystic abnormalities are typically located laterally but may be in the midline. These include *arachnoid cyst* (Fig. 8-21) and the rare *cystic neoplasm*[27] (Fig. 8-22).

Lateral or Asymmetric Cysts

The most common lateral cystic abnormality is the choroid plexus cyst, but a number of other lateralizing cystic brain abnormalities may occur (Tables 8-9 and 8-10).

Choroid Plexus Cysts. Choroid plexus cysts frequently are identified prenatally. Most of these cysts are benign and regress spontaneously (Fig. 8-23); however, reports have been made of these cysts being associated with abnormal karyotypes, including Down's syndrome (trisomy 21), Klinefelter's syndrome, and Turner's syndrome (XO). The most frequent chromosomal abnormality associated with choroid plexus cyst is trisomy 18.[28,29] It is therefore important to be familiar with the features of trisomy 18[30] (see Chapter 21). These include a high incidence of certain abnormalities that may be recognized sonographically, such as rocker-bottom feet or overlapping fingers. Nyberg and colleagues presented some major sonographic findings in fetuses with trisomy 18, including choroid plexus cyst, cystic hygroma, intrauterine growth retardation, and club or rocker-bottom feet.[31] (This is better detailed in Chapter 21.)

Much debate has surrounded the adequacy of ultrasound in detecting features of chromosomal

(text continues on p. 154)

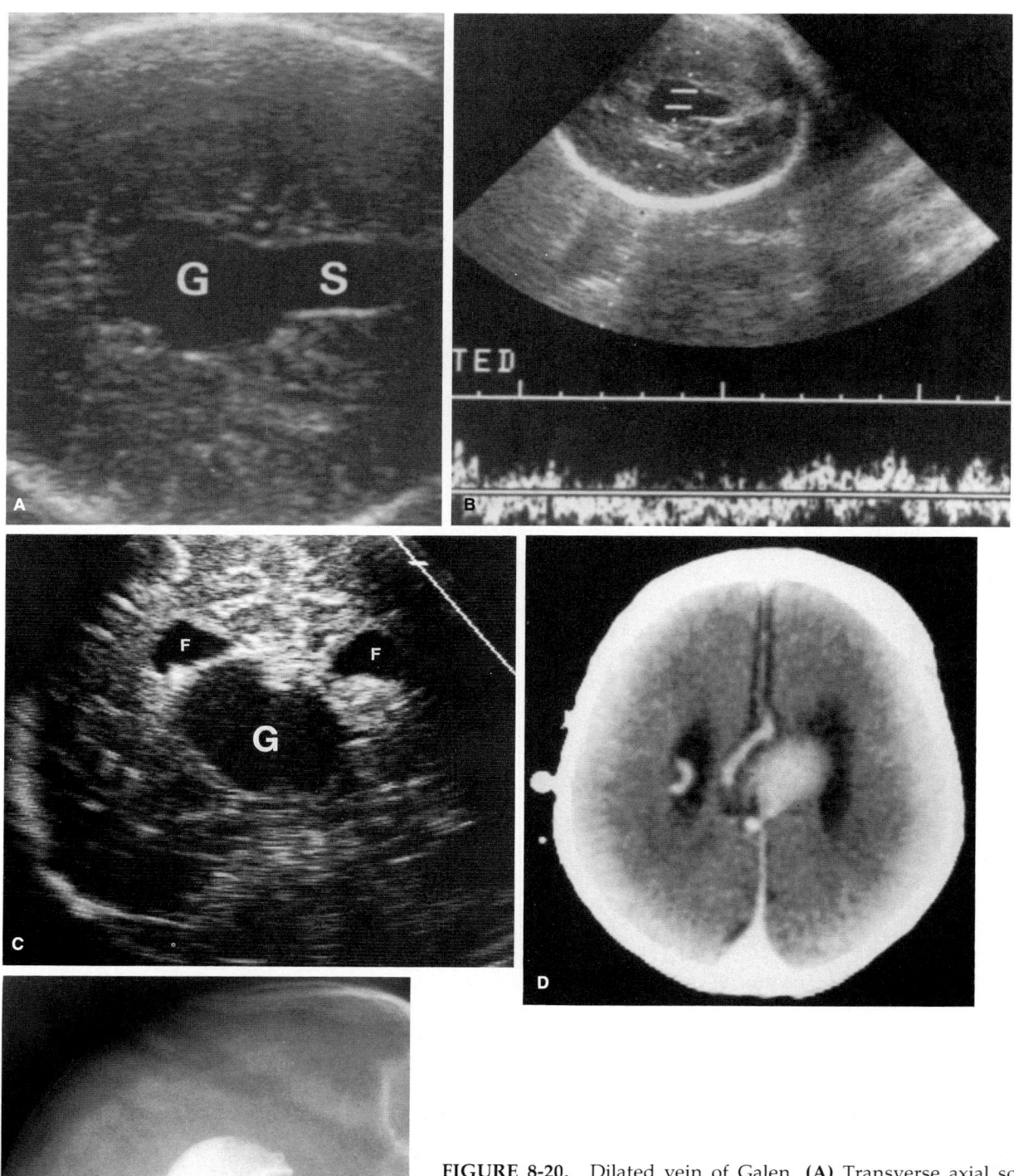

FIGURE 8-20. Dilated vein of Galen. **(A)** Transverse axial sonogram of the fetal brain showing a central and posterior midline fluid collection. The larger, central component in the dilated vein of Galen (G) (the so-called aneurysm). The smaller, posterior component is the dilated straight sinus (S). **(B)** That the pathologic structure is a dilated vein is easily shown with pulse-gated Doppler ultrasound, which demonstrates the turbulent flow in the venous side of the arteriovenous malformation. (Filly RA: Fetus with a CNS malformation—ultrasound evaluation. In Harrison MR, Golbus MS, Filly RA [eds]: The Unborn Patient. Philadelphia: WB Saunders, 1991: 424.) **(C)** Postnatal coronal ultrasound in another case showing frontal horns (F) displaced by midline mass representing dilated vein of Galen (G). **(D)** Corresponding enhanced CT. **(E)** Direct-stick angiograms showing dilated vein of Galen (G).

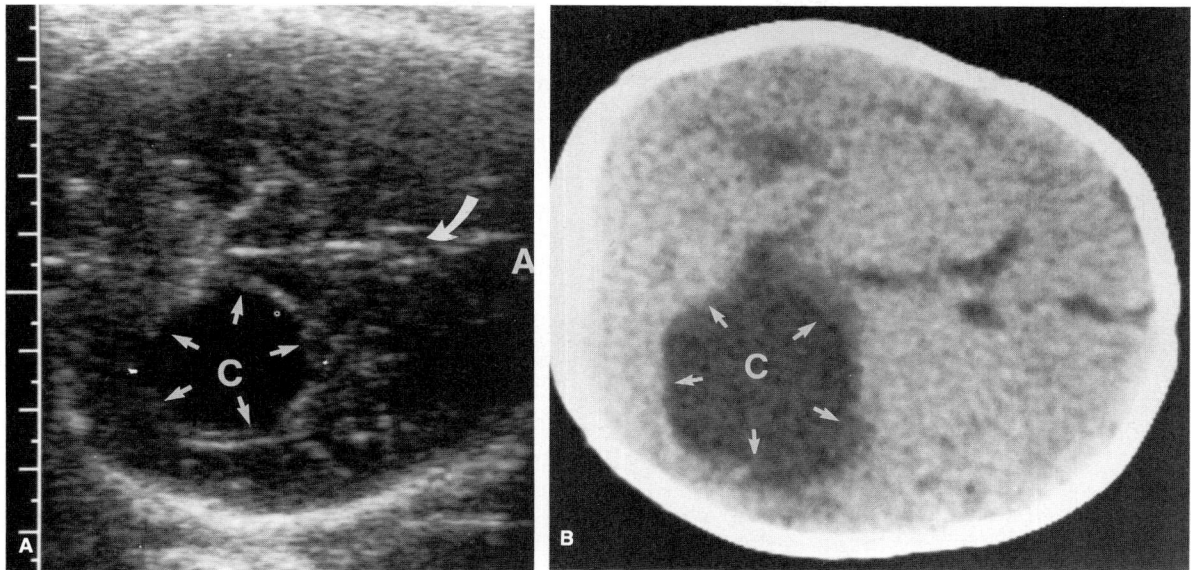

FIGURE 8-21. Arachnoid cyst. **(A)** In utero axial ultrasound demonstrating a cystic area in the temporal occipital area (C). A, anterior; curved arrow, cavum septi pellucidi. **(B)** Corresponding CT scan demonstrates a cystic area in the temporal occipital region (C) that corresponds to an arachnoid cyst. (McGahan JP, Ellis W, Lindfors KK, et al: Congenital cerebrospinal fluid-containing intracranial abnormalities: A sonographic classification. J Clin Ultrasound 1988; 16:531–544.)

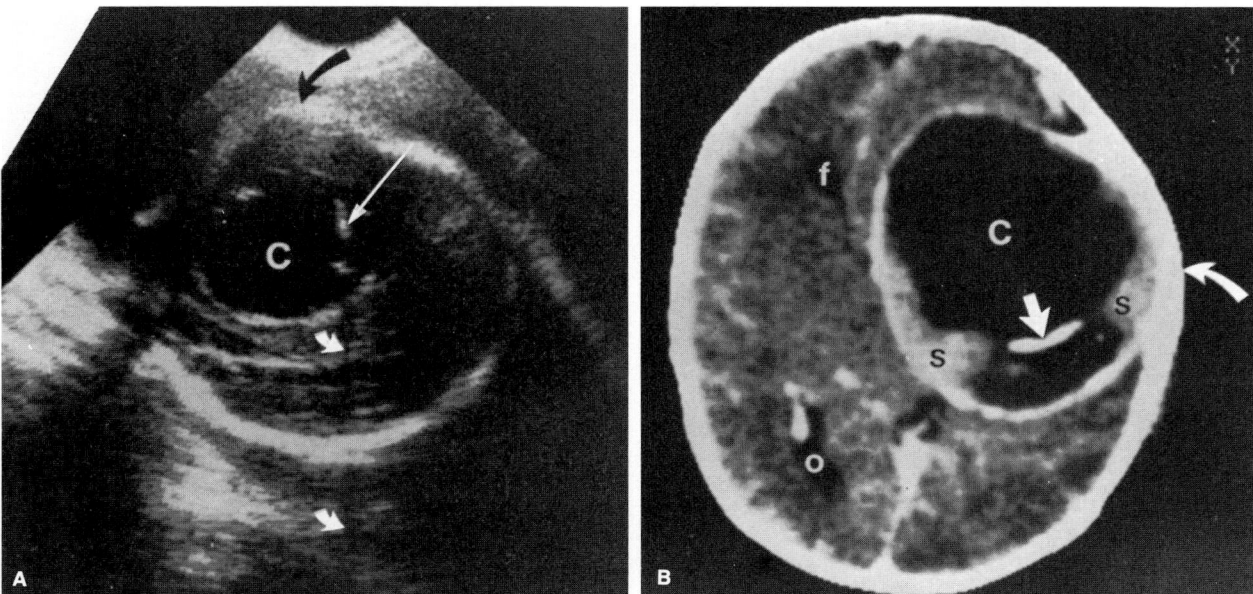

FIGURE 8-22. Cystic neoplasm. **(A)** Axial scan at 31 weeks demonstrates a large cystic mass (C) in the left cerebral hemisphere, with internal septation (*long straight arrow*). Acoustic shadow (*short curved arrows*) suggests calcification. Note asymmetric bulge of left cranial vault (*curved arrow*). **(B)** CT scan shows cystic mass (C) displacing midline structures to right. Note peripheral solid components (S) and calcified septation (*arrow*) of mass and asymmetric bulge of cranial vault (*curved arrow*). f, frontal horn; o, occipital horn. (Sauerbrei EE, Cooperberg PL: Cystic tumors of the fetal and neonatal cerebrum: Ultrasound and computed tomographic evaluation. Radiology 1983; 147:689–692.)

TABLE 8-9.   Causes of Lateral Intracranial Cysts

Common

Choroid plexus cysts

Uncommon

Arachnoid cyst
Porencephaly
Schizencephaly
Unilateral hydrocephalus
Cystic neoplasm
Intracranial hemorrhage

abnormalities such as trisomy 18 when choroid plexus cysts are detected. Many authors believe that amniocentesis should be offered based on certain criteria, such as size of the cysts (>5 mm or <10 mm); bilateralness of the cysts; and lack of regression of the cysts. Appropriate genetic counseling must be given to the patient that is based on the most recently published data, prior personal experience, and familiarity with possible abnormalities associated with trisomy 18[30,31] (see Chapter 21).

Porencephaly. Two abnormalities, porencephaly and schizencephaly, are often considered together because of their similar appearance. Some authors, however, believe that these two entities have separate origins. Porencephaly (Fig. 8-24) results from localized brain destruction during early gestation. This destructive process results in a smooth-walled, fluid-filled cavity that communicates directly with the cerebral ventricle and extends to the cranial vault. Porencephaly is usually unilateral, with the defect increasing in size the farther it is from the ventricle. The destructive process involves the entire thickness of the cerebral cortex.[23,32] Therefore, the lining of the cavity contains white matter, which may be imaged by postnatal magnetic resonance imaging[32] (Fig. 8-25).

Schizencephaly. Schizencephaly (Fig. 8-26) may appear similar on ultrasound to porencephaly. This defect may be either unilateral or bilateral. Schizencephaly is considered to be a migrational abnormality rather than a destructive process.[33] The walls of the schizencephalic defect are usually separate, but on occasion, they may be fused.[33] Because schizencephaly is a migrational abnormality, the cavity is completely lined by gray matter,

which distinguishes it from porencephaly when postnatal magnetic resonance imaging is performed[32] (see Fig. 8-25).

Arachnoid Cysts. Arachnoid cysts may be midline or lateral. These cysts are thought to arise from either the arachnoid separating into two layers that secrete CSF and form a cyst or from a cyst that arises between the arachnoid and pia mater. The cells lining the cyst wall produce CSF, which is trapped and produces a well-demarcated cystic cavity. Sonographically, these cysts are well circumscribed, are often circular, and may occur anywhere within the subarachnoid space. They may produce hydrocephalus owing to their mass effect[23] (see Fig. 8-21).

(*text continues on p. 158*)

TABLE 8-10.   Distinguishing Features of Lateral Intracranial Cysts

Abnormality	Features
Choroid plexus cyst	Cyst present within the choroid plexus of the lateral ventricle
	Bilateral or unilateral
Arachnoid cyst	Smooth wall
	Asymmetric
	Mass effect
	Possibly hydrocephalus (dependent on location)
Porencephaly	Usually unilateral
	Communicates with ventricle
	Cavity size increases with distance from ventricle
	Decreased size of ipsilateral bony calvarium
	Cavity lined by white matter (postnatal MRI)
Schizencephaly	Unilateral or bilateral
	May or may not communicate with ventricle
	Cavity size increases with distance from ventricle
	Defect lined by gray matter (postnatal MRI)
Unilateral hydrocephalus	Unusual: Check opposite ventricle after changing fetal position or perform angled scanning (see text)
Cystic neoplasm	Mass effect
	Solid or irregular with cystic components
Intracranial hemorrhage	Initial echogenic clot in ventricle
	Later echogenic clot plus ventriculomegaly on side of hemorrhage

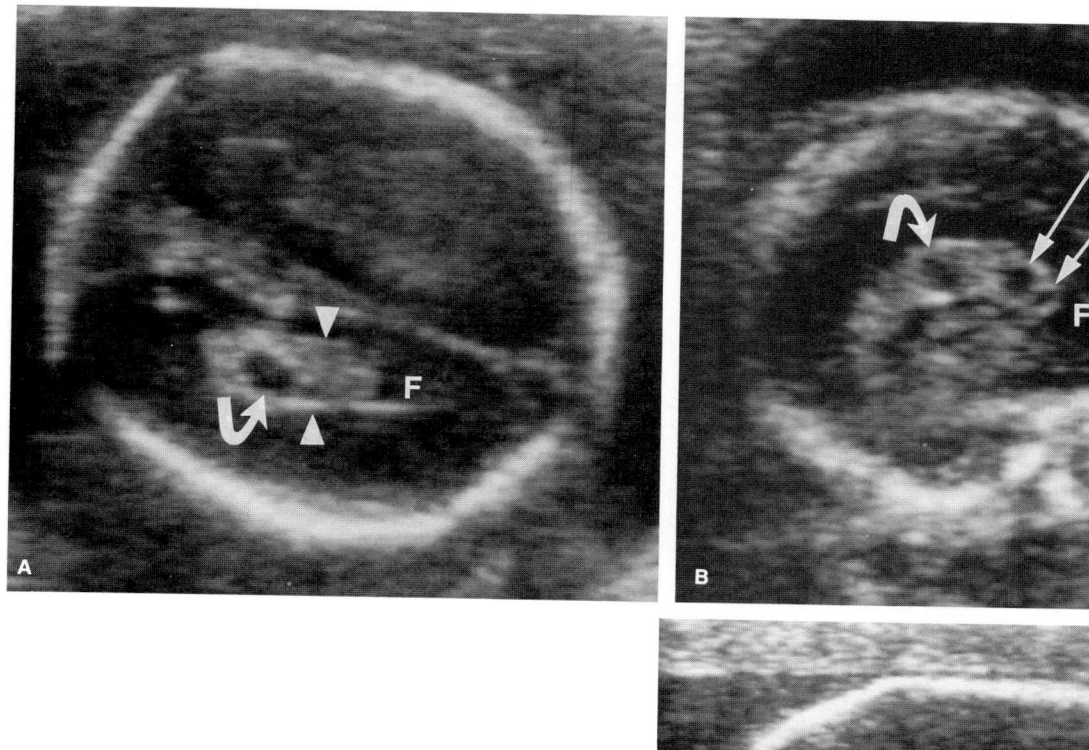

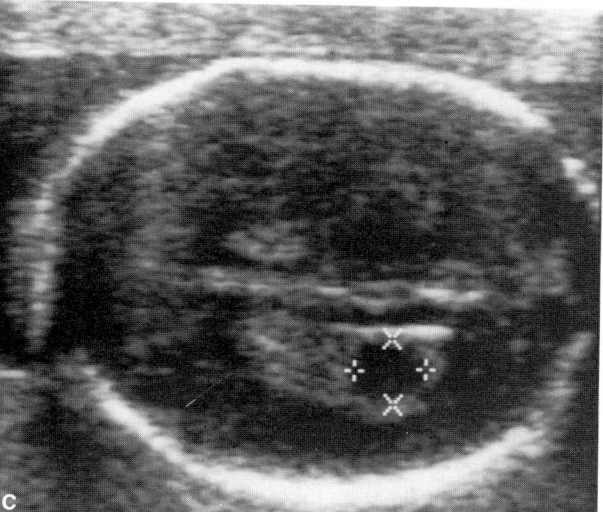

FIGURE 8-23.   Choroid plexus cyst. **(A)** Axial ultrasound demonstrating a single well-demarcated choroid plexus cyst (*curved arrow*). Note the choroid occupying the full diameter of the medial to lateral wall (*arrowheads*) of the lateral ventricle and its absence in the frontal horn (F), which is normal. **(B)** Sagittal ultrasound confirms a larger choroid plexus cyst (*curved arrow*) but also two smaller choroid plexus cysts (*long arrows*). F, frontal horn of the lateral ventricle. **(C)** Another case with a single cyst (*calipers*).

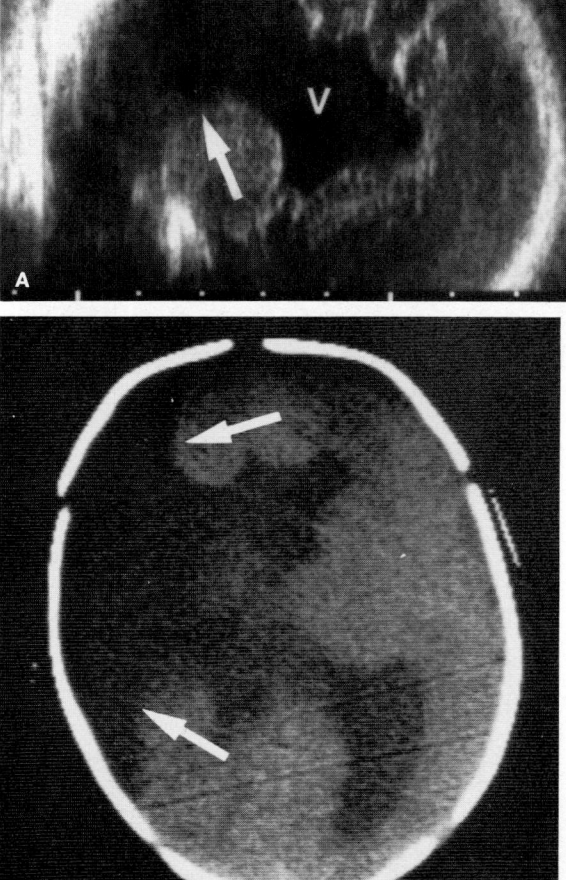

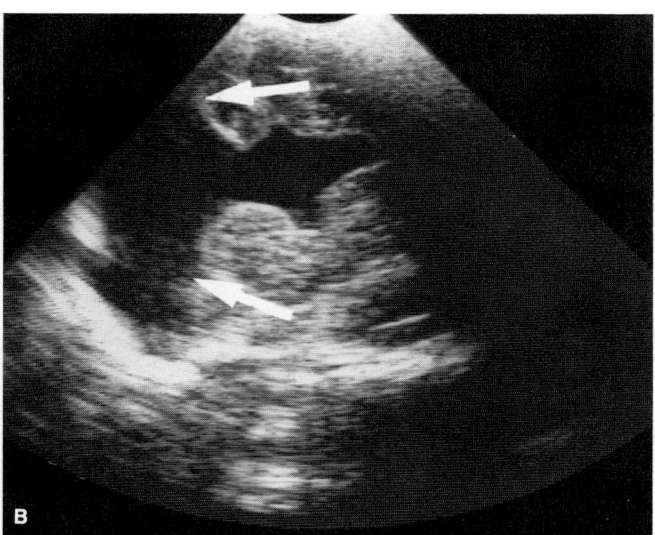

FIGURE 8-24. Porencephaly. **(A)** In utero coronal ultrasound scan demonstrating absence of the septum pellucidum with dilated ventricles (V) and a large wedge-shaped cystic area originating from one ventricle (*arrows*), which extends to bony calvarium. **(B)** Coronal ultrasound and **(C)** corresponding axial CT of the newborn demonstrating similar findings as described in **A**. (McGahan JP, Ellis W, Lindfors KK, et al: Congenital cerebrospinal fluid-containing intracranial abnormalities: A sonographic classification. J Clin Ultrasound 1988; 16:531–544.)

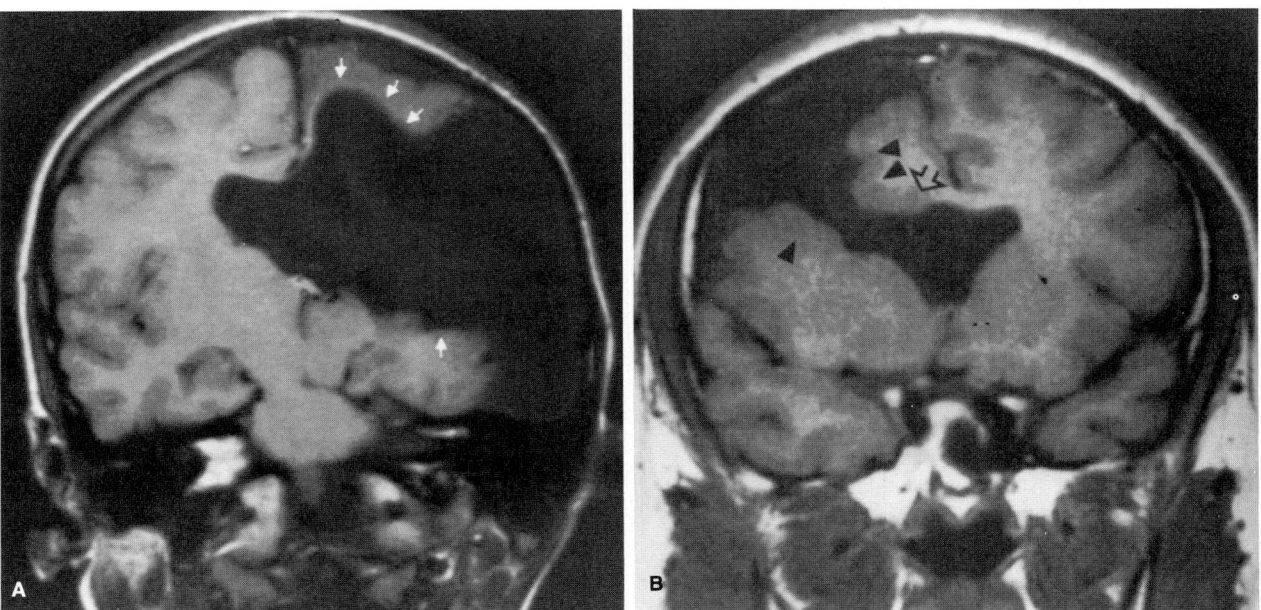

FIGURE 8-25.   MRI: porencephaly versus schizencephaly. **(A)** Coronal spin-echo 600/20 image shows a large cavity extending from the left lateral ventricle through the entire cerebral hemisphere. Note that the cavity is covered by white matter. Thus, MRI defines this to represent porencephaly. **(B)** Unilateral schizencephaly with a coronal spin-echo 600/200 MRI showing a similar defect as with porencephaly, except the gray matter rather than white matter covers the entire cleft. Thus, MRI defines this to represent schizencephaly, which is a form of polymicrogyria, a developmental abnormality, as opposed to porencephaly, which is thought to represent an in utero cerebral infarction. (Barkovich AJ: Metabolic and destructive brain disorders. In Barkovich AJ [ed]: Contemporary Neuroimaging, Vol. 1: Pediatric Neuroimaging. New York: Raven Press, 1990: 60, 99.)

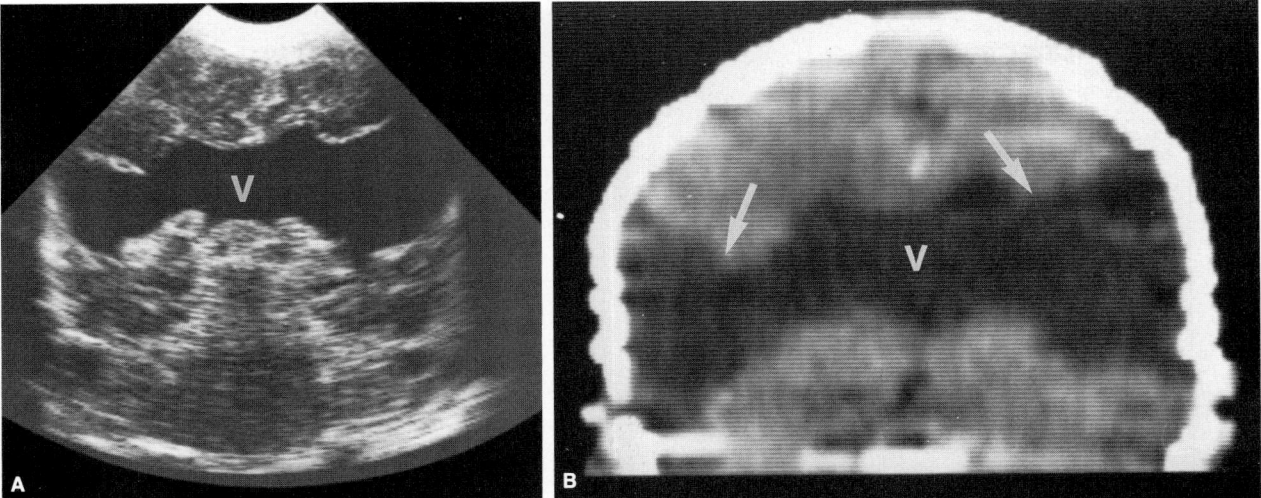

FIGURE 8-26.   Schizencephaly. **(A)** Coronal ultrasound and **(B)** corresponding reconstructed CT scan of the newborn head demonstrating absent pellucidum with bilateral cerebrospinal fluid–containing defects (*arrow*) originating from the ventricles (V) and extending to the bony calvarium. Note that there is a normal amount of choroid plexus within the cerebral ventricles. (McGahan JP, Ellis W, Lindfors KK, et al: Congenital cerebrospinal fluid-containing intracranial abnormalities: A sonographic classification. J Clin Ultrasound 1988; 16:531–544.)

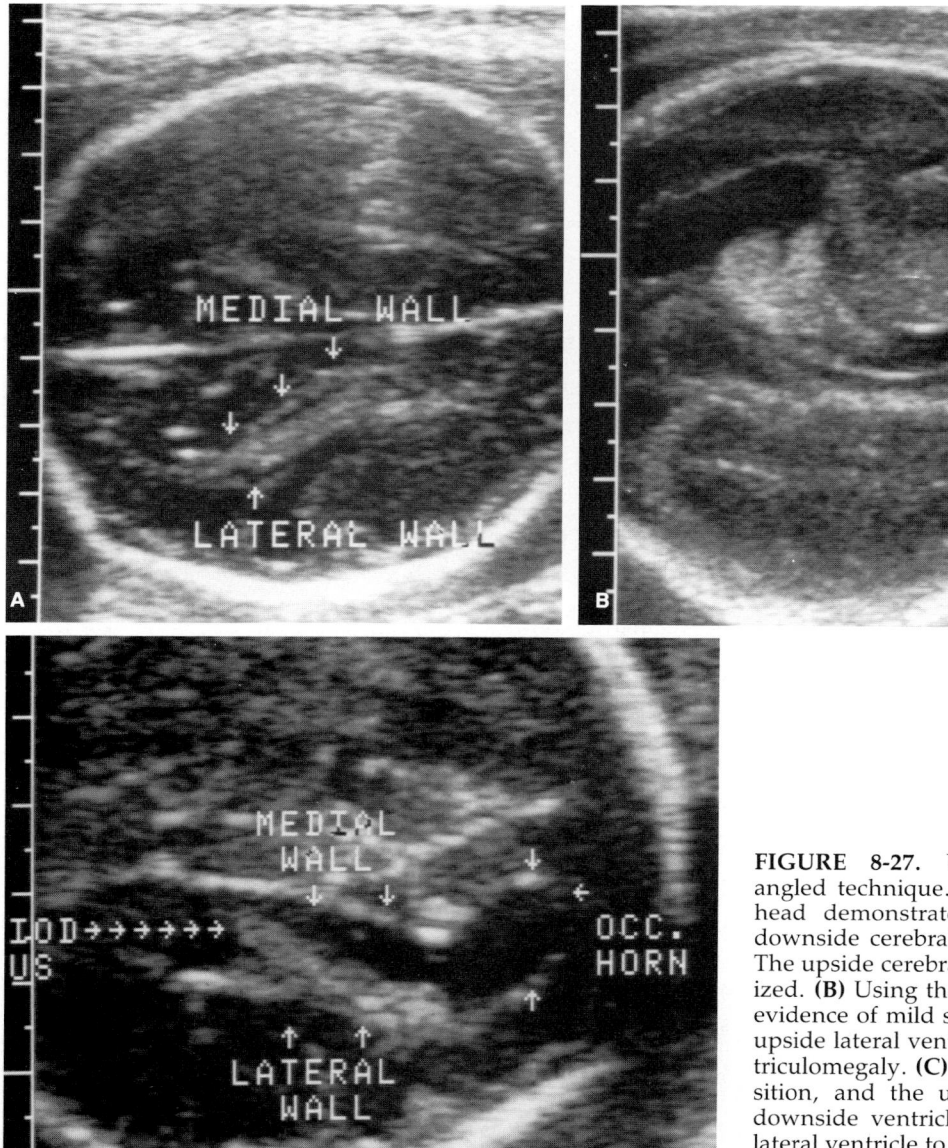

FIGURE 8-27. Unilateral ventriculomegaly angled technique. **(A)** Ultrasound of the fetal head demonstrates that the trigone of the downside cerebral ventricle is normal in size. The upside cerebral ventricle is not well visualized. **(B)** Using the angled techniques, there is evidence of mild separation of the walls of the upside lateral ventricle, indicative of mild ventriculomegaly. **(C)** Later, the fetus changed position, and the upside ventricle became the downside ventricle. Mild enlargement of the lateral ventricle to 12 mm is identified. (Browning BP, Laorr A, McGahan JP, et al: Ultrasound assessment of the "upside" cerebral ventricle. Radiology [forthcoming].)

Intracranial Neoplasms. Intracranial neoplasms are rare in the newborn or the fetus. Intracranial tumors occurring in the perinatal period are most commonly teratomas.[34] Gliomas are the second most common intracranial newborn tumors.[35] Intracranial neoplasms with cystic components are usually teratomas[34] (see Fig. 8-21). These tumors may appear anywhere within the brain, are usually irregular in appearance, and are mostly echogenic, with occasional cystic portions.

Unilateral Hydrocephalus. Unilateral hydrocephalus is a rare abnormality caused by focal obstruction of the CSF pathway at the level of Monro's foramen. Examination of the fetal cerebral ventricle using the angled technique helps to distinguish between unilateral and bilateral hydrocephalus (Fig. 8-27).

In Utero Intracranial Hemorrhage. Fetal intracranial hemorrhage has been reported in the early

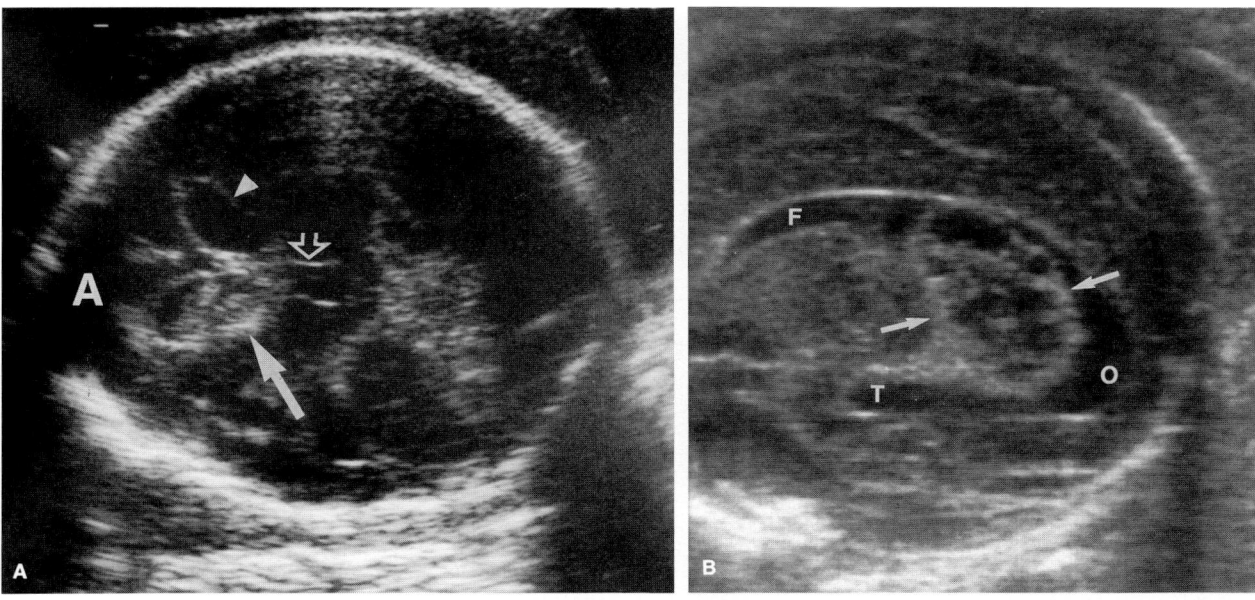

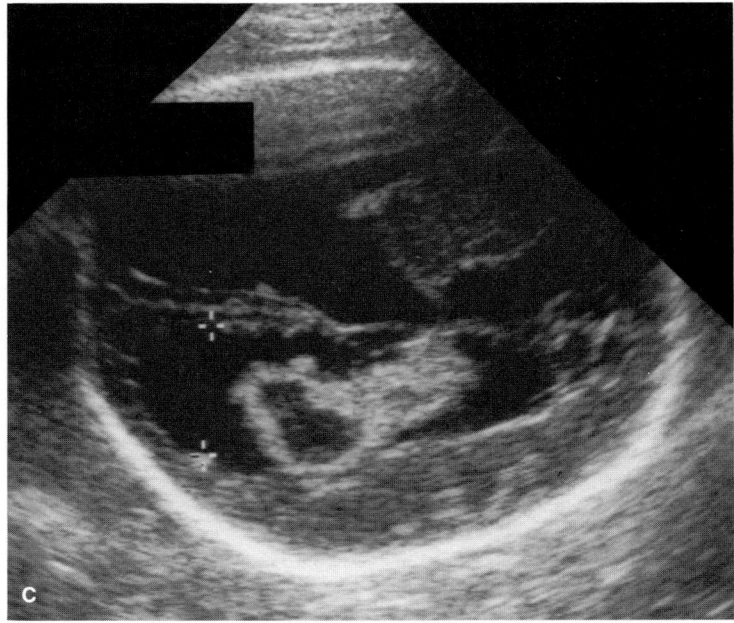

FIGURE 8-28. Sonographic spectrum of intracranial hemorrhage. **(A)** Ultrasound of fetal head at 32 weeks, with acute hemorrhage showing echogenic clot well identified in the dilated frontal horn of one of the lateral ventricles (*closed arrow*). Contralateral dilated frontal horn is without clot (*arrowhead*), and there is dilatation of the third ventricle (*open arrow*). A, anterior. **(B)** Sagittal ultrasound of dilated ventricle in another fetus with probable 10-day-old hemorrhage, showing mixed echogenic clot (*arrows*) adhered to the trigone region of the lateral ventricle. F, frontal horn; O, occipital horn; T, temporal horn. **(C)** Axial scan of the fetus with hemorrhage greater than 2 weeks old, showing regular ventricular walls, ventriculomegaly, and mixed echogenic clot adherent to choroid plexus.

third trimester of pregnancy. Intracranial hemorrhage is thought to occur in the germinal matrix of newborns. The cause of germinal matrix hemorrhage is explained by the extreme capillary permeability of the vascular germinal matrix, which makes it susceptible to hemorrhage. Elevation in blood pressure caused by fetal hypoxia may lead to hemorrhage in the germinal matrix. The mechanism for in utero intraventricular hemorrhage is less clear and often is secondary to maternal factors, such as pancreatitis, hepatitis, preeclampsia, or bleeding disorders. Often, the cause of in utero

intraventricular hemorrhage is never found.[34] Unlike neonatal hemorrhage, fetal intracranial hemorrhage is most often intraventricular. Sonographically, there is first an echogenic clot filling the ventricles; later, this may result in hydrocephalus[36] (Fig. 8-28). In utero hemorrhage usually occurs in the beginning of the third trimester of pregnancy. Later, there may be hydrocephalus with mixed echogenic debris layering within the ventricles. Occasionally, mixed echogenic, enlarged choroid plexus results from hemorrhage into the choroid plexus (see Fig. 8-28).

TABLE 8-11.   Causes of Cranial Defects and Deformed Cranium

Abnormality	Possible Causes
Cranial defects	Anencephaly
	Acrania
	Limb–body–wall complex
	Amniotic band syndrome
	Cephalocele
Undermineralized	Hypophosphatasia
	Osteogenesis imperfecta
	Achondrogenesis type I
Deformed cranium	Fetal demise
	Open neural tube defect (lemon sign)
	Microcephaly
	Craniosynostosis
	Amniotic band syndrome
	Limb–body–wall complex
	Cloverleaf skull (thanatophoric dwarf)

Cranial Defects

Cranial defects may be partial or complete. Partial defects are usually secondary to cephalocele, amniotic band syndrome (ABS), or limb–body–wall complex (LBWC; Table 8-11). Complete defects are secondary to exencephaly with acrania or due to anencephaly. Severe bone demineralization, which occur with such abnormalities as osteogenesis imperfecta, may give the appearance of a complete cranial defect.

The differential diagnosis for deformed cranium is comprehensive, including anything from physiologic head compression to ONTD or fetal demise (see Table 8-11). The distinguishing features of the more common abnormalities are cited in Table 8-12, and a general flow chart for calvarial abnormalities is provided in Flow Diagram 2. In addition, considerable overlap may be found in these features among abnormalities. For instance, the lemon sign was originally described with ONTD;

TABLE 8-12.   Distinguishing Features of Cranial Defects and Deformed Cranium

Abnormality	Features	Abnormality	Features
Anencephaly	Absent bony calvarium above orbits	Open neural tube defects	Lemon sign
	Orbits well visualized		Banana sign
	Absence of supratentorial brain		Mild hydrocephalus
	Residual brain (angiomatous stroma)		Spinal defect
	Possibly spina bifida	Fetal demise	Overlapping sutures (Spalding's sign)
	Polyhydramnios		Poor visualization of intracranial structures
Exencephaly secondary to acranium	Calvarium absent		Associated findings of fetal demise
	Disorganized supratentorial brain tissue	Microcephaly	Calvarium present
Amniotic band syndrome (ABS)	Asymmetric cephalocele		Decreased brain tissue
	Fixed fetal parts		Head circumference 2–3 standard deviations below expected for menstrual age
	Other deformities, including limb amputation		
Limb–body–wall complex	Asymmetric encephaloceles	Craniosynostosis	Complete or partial
	Similar to ABS except fetal body adherent to placenta		Deformed skull
	Usually more severe than ABS, associated bizarre defects of fetal body		Possibly microcephaly (see above)
Cephalocele	Midline defect		Abnormal cephalic index
	Extracranial cyst or brain tissue		
	Possibly ventriculomegaly		
	Lemon sign may be present		

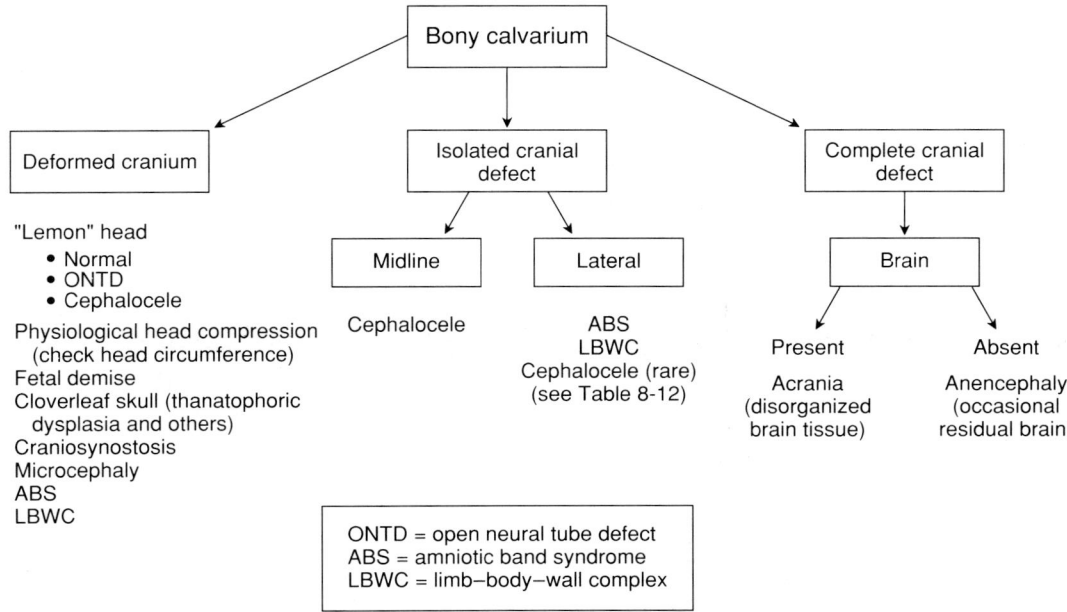

Flow Diagram 2. Flow chart for cranial defects and deformed cranium.

however, it may not be present in an ONTD identified in the third trimester of pregnancy, and a mild lemon sign may be identified in normal fetuses (Table 8-13).

Anencephaly

Anencephaly is the single most common ONTD. Anencephaly is characterized by absence of the cerebral hemispheres and lack of bony calvarium above the orbits (Fig. 8-29). There are normal midbrain and posterior fossa structures but a lack of normal development of the cerebral hemisphere. In about one third of cases, there is a variable amount of angiomatous stroma, which may mimic

TABLE 8-13. Differential Diagnosis of Lemon Sign of Fetal Head

Common

Normal fetus

Less Common

Open neural tube defect (Arnold-Chiari type II)

Uncommon

Cephalocele

Rare

Oligohydramnios
Thanatophoric dwarf (cloverleaf deformity)

rudimentary brain.[37] Anencephaly may be accompanied by polyhydramnios, which is thought to be secondary to severe brain dysfunction resulting in ineffective fetal swallowing.

Exencephaly (Acrania)

Acrania is a developmental abnormality characterized by partial or complete absence of the cranial vault. Exencephaly is acrania with protrusion of brain tissue into the amniotic cavity. Exencephaly is different but similar to anencephaly.[38] Like anencephaly, there is absence of the fetal crania; however, unlike anencephaly, brain tissue is always present. With exencephaly, the brain tissue appears heterogeneous and disorganized. The hypothesis of a continuum of findings between exencephaly and anencephaly is supported by the observation of residual brain tissue (angiomata stroma) in about one third of cases of anencephaly[37] (Fig. 8-30).

Cephalocele

The sonographic appearance of cephalocele is variable. Most cephaloceles are midline and occipital extracranial masses.[22] If the cephalocele is large, the residual brain size is small. Cephalocele may be associated with the lemon-shaped appearance of the bony calvarium that occurs with ONTD and with the Arnold-Chiari type II malformation (Fig. 8-31). Cephalocele may also occur in other intracranial locations (see Chapter 9).

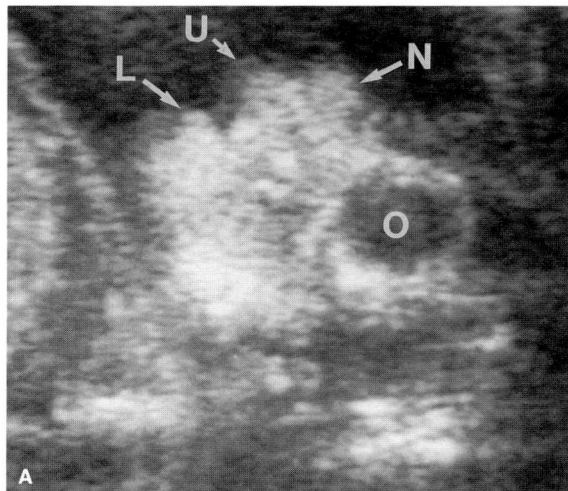

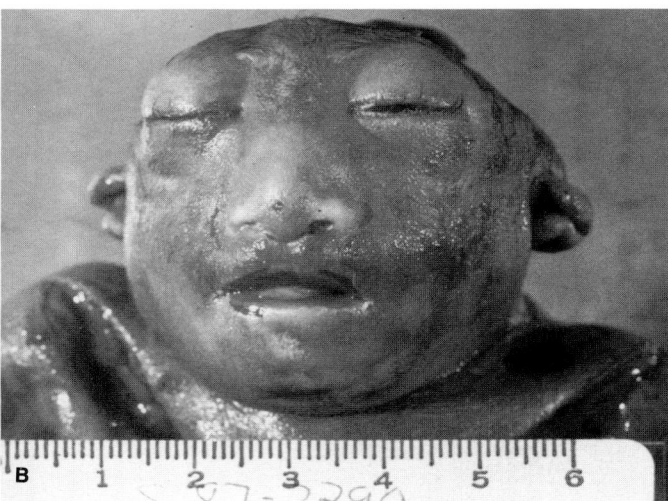

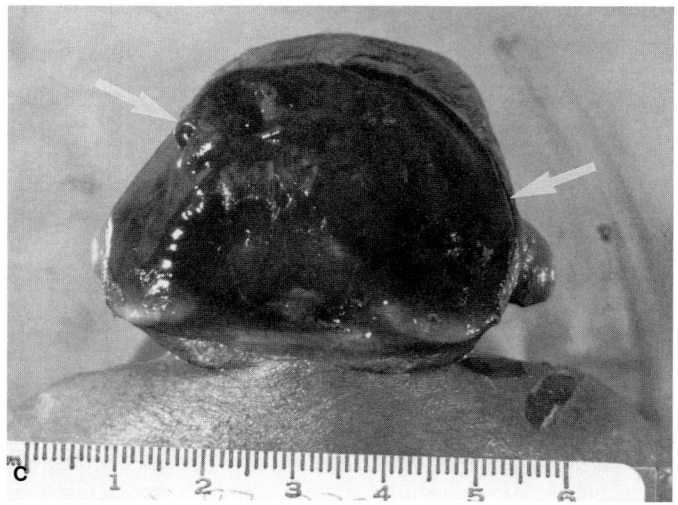

FIGURE 8-29. Anencephaly. **(A)** In utero ultrasound of the fetal face and head demonstrating normal fetal facial structures, including lower lip (L), upper lip (U), nose (N), prominent orbit (O), and no cerebral tissue above the orbits. **(B** and **C)** Corresponding anatomic specimen of the fetal head demonstrates essentially no brain tissue above the orbits. Image of the posterior head, however, demonstrates residual brain tissue, so-called angiomatous stroma.

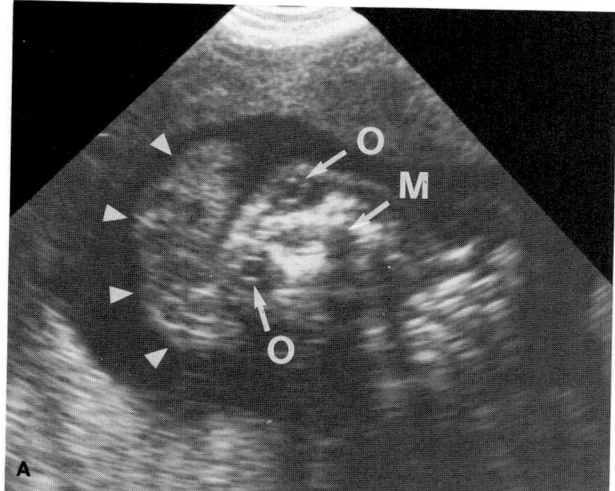

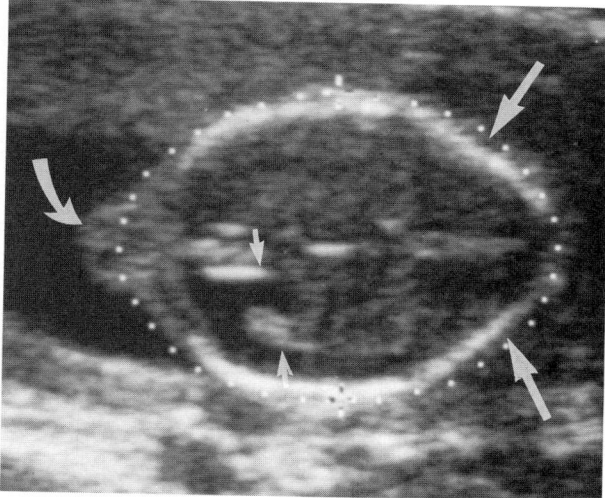

FIGURE 8-31. Ultrasound of fetal head demonstrates small encephalocele (*curved arrow*), lateral ventricle dilated to 12 mm (*small arrows*), and mild overlapping of the cranial sutures (*large arrows*), the so-called lemon sign.

Amniotic Band Syndrome and Limb–Body–Wall Complex

Amniotic band syndrome[39] or LBWC[40] should be considered when there is an extremely bizarre and asymmetric cranial defect (Fig. 8-32). Both ABS and LBWC may be associated with a number of abnormalities thought to result from disruption of the amnion in utero. LBWC is the more severe defect, with the fetal body usually adhered to the placenta and with absent umbilical cord. Many consider LBWC and ABS as separate entities, while some consider them to be a variation of the same syndrome. They may be similar entities based on a common cause, such as disruption of the amnion, but with different features. LBWC is also called the body-stalk anomaly, usually with a defect of the amnion extending from the placenta to the fetal body wall and incorporating the umbilical cord. This is a severe anomaly associated with bizarre intracranial defects, abdominal wall defects, and amputations (see Fig. 8-32).

ABS is characterized by a disruption of the amnion, with the fetal body part sticking to the chorion. The resultant amputational defects may be minor to severe, depending on the timing of the amnion disruption. In ABS, the fetus is fixed in the amniotic defect at a site separate from the placenta. The amnion is thought to protect the fetus from the chorion. Thus, with disruption of the fetal amnion, the fetal part becomes stuck to the chorion.

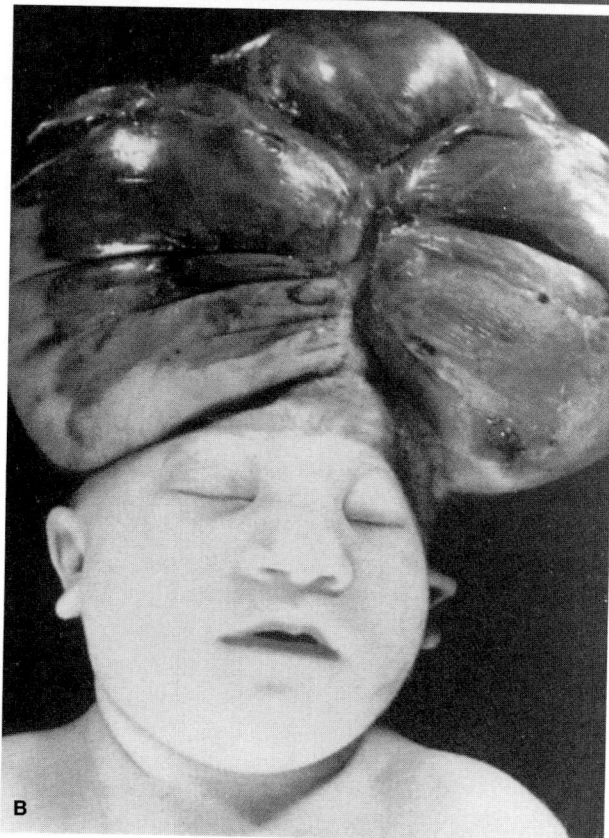

FIGURE 8-30. Exencephaly (acrania). **(A)** In utero coronal ultrasound demonstrates bony orbits (O), fetal mouth (M), and large amount of brain tissue above the bony orbits (*arrowheads*). This case is different from anencephaly in that a large amount of residual brain tissue is present. **(B)** Postmortem specimen of a 38-week-gestation stillborn shows a large, multilobed cerebral tissue covered by a highly vascular layer of skin. The flat bones of the cranium were absent, and the brain remained disorganized but symmetric and intact. (Naidich TP, Altman NR, Braffman BH, et al: Cephaloceles and related malformations. AJNR 1992; 13:655–690.)

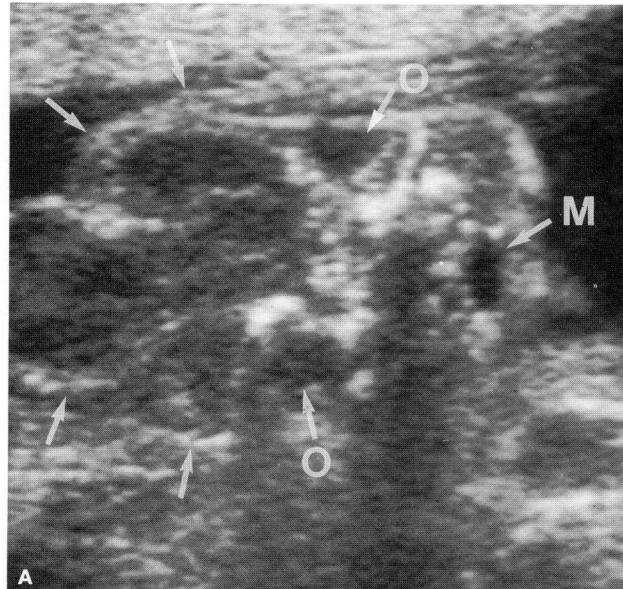
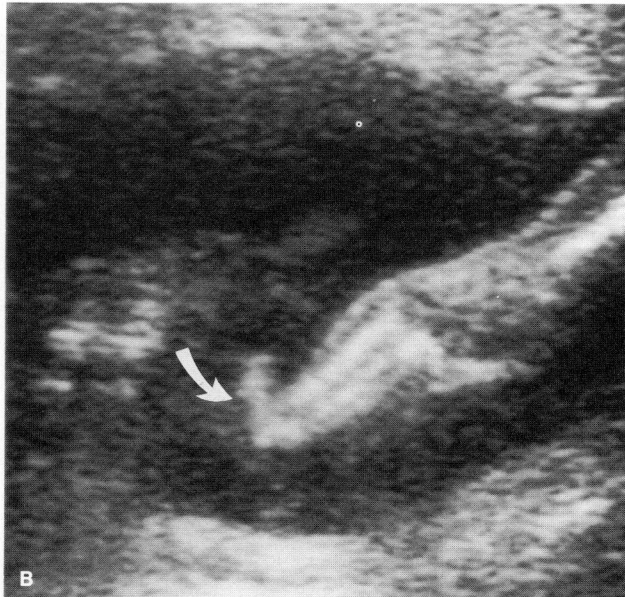
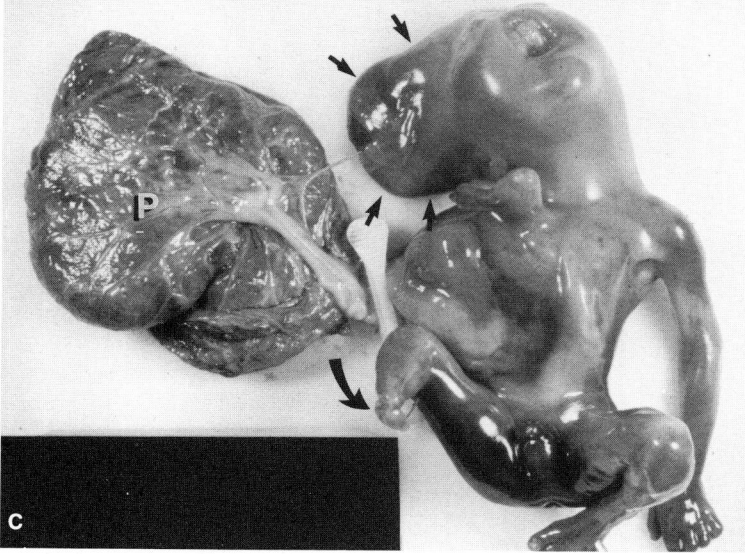

FIGURE 8-32. Severe amniotic bands. **(A)** Coronal ultrasound demonstrates orbits (O), open fetal mouth (M), and disorganized brain tissue (*arrows*). **(B)** Amputational defect of the foot of the lower extremity (*curved arrow*). **(C)** Corresponding anatomic specimen demonstrates asymmetric cranial defect (*arrows*), amputation of the upper and lower limbs (*curved arrow*), and abdominal defect contiguous with placenta and umbilical cord, as with limb–body–wall complex.

With continual growth, constriction of the fetal part results in asymmetric amputational defects.

Bony Demineralization

Diffuse demineralization may occur with osteogenesis imperfecta, hypophosphatasia, or achondrogenesis type I. This is presented in more detail in Chapter 19. In cases of severe demineralization of the bony calvarium, there may be supervisualization of the intercranial structures. This increased visualization of the intracranial structures may be confused with such abnormalities as exencephaly due to acrania. Unlike exencephaly, how-

ever, there is intact but poorly mineralized cranial vault. Careful scanning reveals concomitant limb abnormalities. For instance, osteogenesis imperfecta is associated with bowed limbs combined with supervisualization of the intracranial structures[41] (Fig. 8-33).

Small or Deformed Cranium

Microcephaly

Severe microcephaly may be difficult to distinguish from anencephaly. Microcephaly is reduction of brain mass and head size with an intact

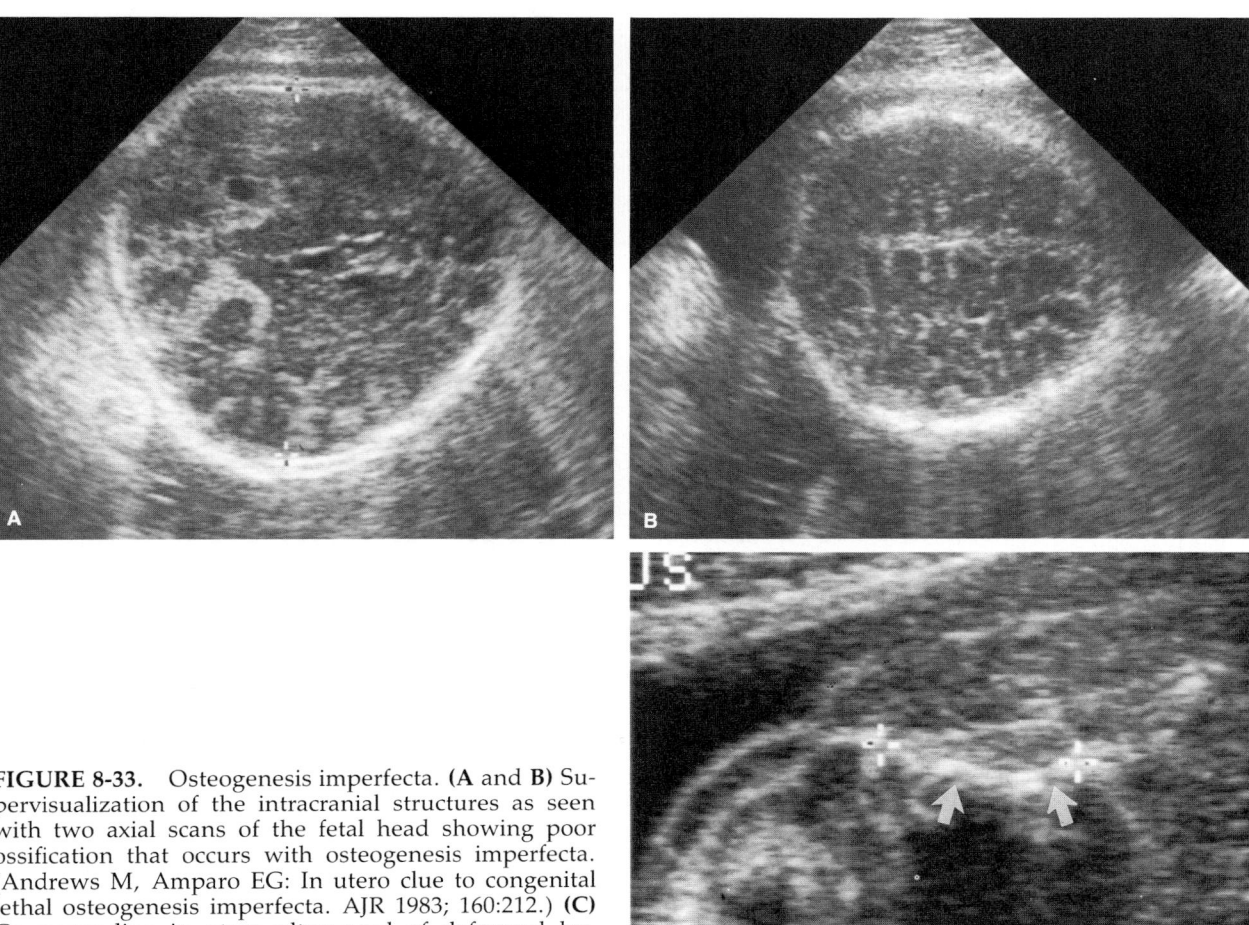

FIGURE 8-33.   Osteogenesis imperfecta. **(A and B)** Supervisualization of the intracranial structures as seen with two axial scans of the fetal head showing poor ossification that occurs with osteogenesis imperfecta. (Andrews M, Amparo EG: In utero clue to congenital lethal osteogenesis imperfecta. AJR 1983; 160:212.) **(C)** Corresponding in utero ultrasound of deformed humerus *(arrows)*.

bony calvarium. Microcephaly is defined as a fetal head circumference either 2[42] or 3[43] standard deviations below the mean of that expected for menstrual age. Most would define microcephaly as being less than 3 standard deviations below the mean of expected head circumference. The head circumference is used to define microcephaly rather than the biparietal diameter because the biparietal diameter is affected by normal head compression (Table 8-14). Chervenak and colleagues found that ratios of head circumference (perimeter) to abdominal circumference at 4 standard deviations had no false-positive diagnoses, while femur length/head circumference ratios at 3 standard deviations were a sensitive threshold without false-positive diagnosis of microcephaly[43] (Tables 8-15 and 8-16). Causes of microcephaly are numerous and include in utero infections, anoxia, and chromosomal abnormalities (Fig. 8-34).

Fetal Demise

When fetal demise has occurred, there may be poor visualization of the intracranial structures and overlapping of the cranial sutures, or so-called Spalding's sign[44] (Fig. 8-35). Other, more definitive signs of fetal demise, including absence of fetal movement and lack of cardiac motion, confirm the diagnosis.

Lemon Sign of the Fetal Head

Mild overlapping of the cranial sutures occurs most commonly as a variant of normal pregnancy. It also may occur with ONTD, as previously described. Careful scanning of the posterior fossa and the spine is indicated in these cases. Even with ONTD in the third trimester of pregnancy, the cranial shape reverts to a more normal oval shape rather than to a lemon shape. As previously de-

(text continues on p. 168)

TABLE 8-14. Mean and Standard Deviation of Head Perimeter as a Function of Gestational Age

Week No.	SD Above Mean		Mean	SD Below Mean				
	+2	+1		−1	−2	−3	−4	−5
20	204	189	175	160	145	131	116	101
21	216	201	187	172	157	143	128	113
22	228	213	198	184	169	154	140	125
23	239	224	210	195	180	166	151	136
24	250	235	221	206	191	177	162	147
25	261	246	232	217	202	188	173	158
26	271	257	242	227	213	198	183	169
27	282	267	252	238	223	208	194	179
28	291	277	262	247	233	218	203	189
29	301	286	271	257	242	227	213	198
30	310	295	281	266	251	236	222	207
31	318	304	289	274	260	245	230	216
32	327	312	297	283	268	253	239	224
33	334	320	305	290	276	261	246	232
34	341	327	312	297	283	268	253	239
35	348	333	319	304	289	275	260	245
36	354	339	325	310	295	281	266	251
37	360	345	330	316	301	286	272	257
38	364	350	335	320	306	291	276	262
39	369	354	339	325	310	295	281	266
40	372	358	343	328	314	299	284	270
41	375	360	346	331	316	302	287	272
42	377	363	348	333	319	304	289	275

(Chervenak FA, Jeanty P, Cantraine F, et al: The diagnosis of fetal microcephaly. Am J Obstet Gynecol 1984; 149:512–517.)

TABLE 8-16. Mean and Standard Deviation of Femur Length to Head Perimeter Ratio as a Function of Gestational Age

Week No.	SD Below Mean					Mean	SD Above Mean				
	−5	−4	−3	−2	−1		+1	+2	+3	+4	+5
20	0.107	0.122	0.137	0.152	0.167	0.180	0.197	0.212	0.227	0.242	0.257
21	0.111	0.126	0.141	0.156	0.171	0.190	0.201	0.216	0.231	0.246	0.261
22	0.115	0.130	0.145	0.160	0.175	0.190	0.205	0.220	0.235	0.250	0.265
23	0.118	0.133	0.148	0.163	0.178	0.190	0.208	0.223	0.238	0.253	0.268
24	0.121	0.136	0.151	0.166	0.181	0.200	0.211	0.226	0.241	0.256	0.271
25	0.123	0.138	0.153	0.168	0.183	0.200	0.213	0.228	0.243	0.258	0.273
26	0.125	0.140	0.155	0.170	0.185	0.200	0.215	0.230	0.245	0.260	0.275
27	0.127	0.142	0.157	0.172	0.187	0.200	0.217	0.232	0.247	0.262	0.277
28	0.129	0.144	0.159	0.174	0.189	0.200	0.219	0.234	0.249	0.264	0.279
29	0.130	0.145	0.160	0.175	0.190	0.200	0.220	0.235	0.250	0.265	0.280
30	0.131	0.146	0.161	0.176	0.191	0.210	0.221	0.236	0.251	0.266	0.281
31	0.132	0.147	0.162	0.177	0.192	0.210	0.222	0.237	0.252	0.267	0.282

(Chervenak FA, Jeanty P, Cantraine F, et al: The diagnosis of fetal microcephaly. Am J Obstet Gynecol 1984; 149:512–517.)

TABLE 8-15.   Mean and Standard Deviation of Head Perimeter to Abdominal Perimeter Ratio as a Function of Gestational Age

Week No.	SD Above Mean		Mean	SD Below Mean				
	+2	+1		−1	−2	−3	−4	−5
20	1.43	1.34	1.25	1.16	1.07	0.98	0.89	0.8
21	1.42	1.33	1.24	1.15	1.06	0.97	0.88	0.79
22	1.41	1.32	1.23	1.14	1.05	0.96	0.87	0.78
23	1.4	1.31	1.22	1.13	1.04	0.95	0.86	0.78
24	1.39	1.3	1.21	1.12	1.03	0.94	0.86	0.77
25	1.38	1.29	1.2	1.11	1.02	0.94	0.85	0.76
26	1.37	1.28	1.19	1.1	1.02	0.93	0.84	0.75
27	1.36	1.27	1.18	1.1	1.01	0.92	0.83	0.74
28	1.35	1.26	1.17	1.09	1	0.91	0.82	0.73
29	1.34	1.25	1.17	1.08	0.99	0.9	0.81	0.72
30	1.33	1.25	1.16	1.07	0.98	0.89	0.8	0.71
31	1.33	1.24	1.15	1.06	0.97	0.88	0.79	0.7
32	1.32	1.23	1.14	1.05	0.96	0.87	0.78	0.69
33	1.31	1.22	1.13	1.04	0.95	0.86	0.77	0.68
34	1.3	1.21	1.12	1.03	0.94	0.85	0.76	0.68
35	1.29	1.2	1.11	1.02	0.93	0.84	0.76	0.67
36	1.28	1.19	1.1	1.01	0.92	0.84	0.75	0.66
37	1.27	1.18	1.09	1.00	0.92	0.83	0.74	0.65
38	1.26	1.17	1.08	1.00	0.91	0.82	0.73	0.64
39	1.25	1.16	1.08	0.99	0.90	0.81	0.72	0.63
40	1.24	1.16	1.07	0.98	0.89	0.80	0.71	0.62
41	1.24	1.15	1.06	0.97	0.88	0.79	0.70	0.61
42	1.23	1.14	1.05	0.96	0.87	0.78	0.69	0.60

(Chervenak FA, Jeanty P, Cantraine F, et al: The diagnosis of fetal microcephaly. Am J Obstet Gynecol 1984; 149:512–517.)

Week No.	SD Below Mean					Mean	SD Above Mean				
	−5	−4	−3	−2	−1		+1	+2	+3	+4	+5
32	0.134	0.149	0.164	0.179	0.194	0.210	0.224	0.239	0.254	0.269	0.284
33	0.135	0.150	0.165	0.180	0.195	0.210	0.225	0.240	0.255	0.270	0.285
34	0.136	0.151	0.166	0.181	0.196	0.210	0.226	0.241	0.256	0.271	0.286
35	0.138	0.153	0.168	0.183	0.198	0.210	0.228	0.243	0.258	0.273	0.288
36	0.140	0.155	0.170	0.185	0.200	0.210	0.230	0.245	0.260	0.275	0.290
37	0.142	0.157	0.172	0.187	0.202	0.220	0.232	0.247	0.262	0.277	0.292
38	0.144	0.159	0.174	0.189	0.204	0.220	0.234	0.249	0.264	0.279	0.294
39	0.147	0.162	0.177	0.192	0.207	0.220	0.237	0.252	0.267	0.282	0.297
40	0.151	0.166	0.181	0.196	0.211	0.230	0.241	0.256	0.271	0.286	0.301
41	0.155	0.170	0.185	0.200	0.215	0.230	0.245	0.260	0.275	0.290	0.305
42	0.160	0.175	0.190	0.205	0.220	0.230	0.250	0.265	0.280	0.295	0.310

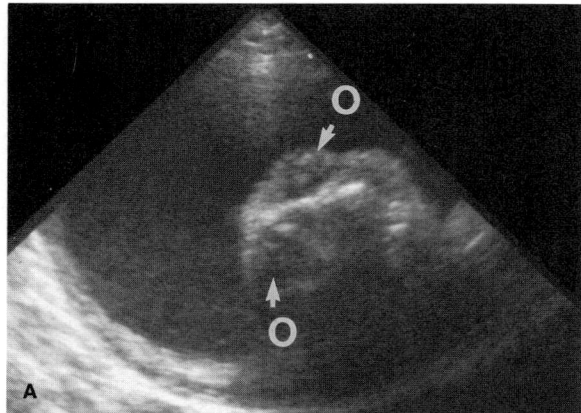

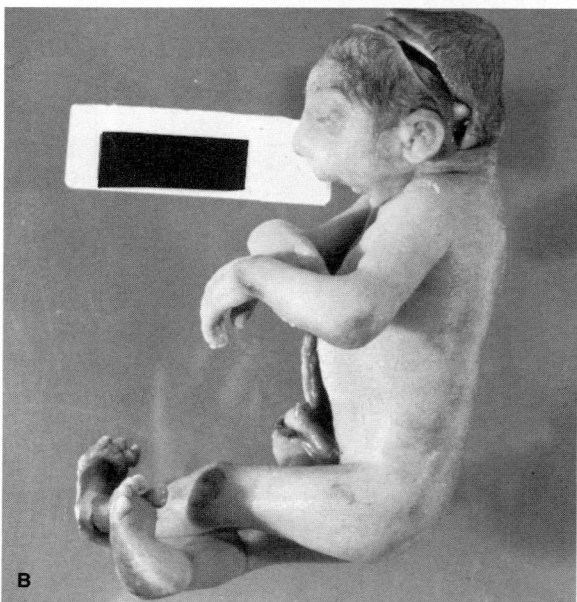

FIGURE 8-34. Microcephaly. **(A)** In utero cranial ultrasound of the fetal head demonstrates prominent orbits (O) and essentially no brain above the bony orbits, which may be confused with anencephaly. **(B)** In this case, there was severe microcephaly with an intact bony calvarium and decreased cerebral tissue. (The skull was dissected after delivery.)

scribed, the lemon sign also may occur with fetal cephalocele (see Figs. 8-11 and 8-30 and Table 8-13).

Cloverleaf Deformity of the Skull

The cloverleaf deformity is characterized by a skull in which there is frontal and bitemporal bulging of the calvarium. This pronounced deformity of the fetal cranium may occur with thanatophoric dwarfism (Fig. 8-36) or homozygous achondroplasia. Cloverleaf appearance is not pathogno-

monic of dwarfism, however, and may occur with Apert's, Carpenter's, Crouzon's, and Pfeiffer's syndromes.[45] If the cloverleaf skull is identified with a limb shortening and abnormally small thoracic circumference, this is nearly pathognomonic of thanatophoric dwarfism. This is discussed in more detail in Chapter 19.

Intracranial Calcifications

In utero cerebral calcifications are rare, subtle, and difficult to recognize on prenatal ultrasound. Most commonly, these calcifications are a result of in utero infection,[46,47] but they may be secondary to fetal brain tumors.[34] In utero infections are most commonly viral in origin and secondary to cytomegalic inclusion disease. This may manifest as a faint, subependymal calcification with accompanying ventriculomegaly and possible microcephaly (Fig. 8-37). Herpes simplex virus type II can be acquired in utero and may have a similar appearance.[46] Alternatively, calcifications from toxoplasmosis in the neonate are scattered, and calcifications from rubella are rare.[47] Intracranial calcifications as a result of intracranial tumor are associated with a mass effect and calcifications localized to one portion of the brain[47] (see Fig. 8-22).

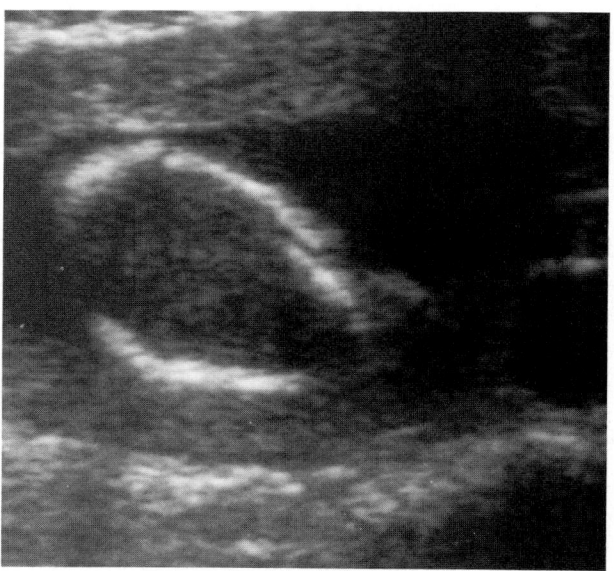

FIGURE 8-35. Fetal demise. Ultrasound image of the fetal cranium demonstrates poor visualization of the fetal cranial structures and overlapping of the cranial sutures (Spalding's sign), as occurs with in utero fetal demise.

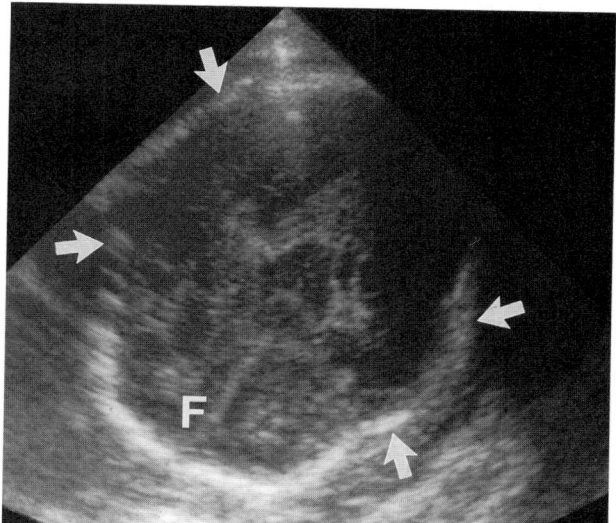

FIGURE 8-36. Thanatophoric dwarf. Mild cloverleaf deformity of the fetal cranium with prominent bitemporal region (*arrows*) and frontal region (F). This defect may be seen in a number of other malformations (see text). If cloverleaf deformity of the skull is identified with limb shortening and small thorax, this is diagnostic of thanatophoric dwarf.

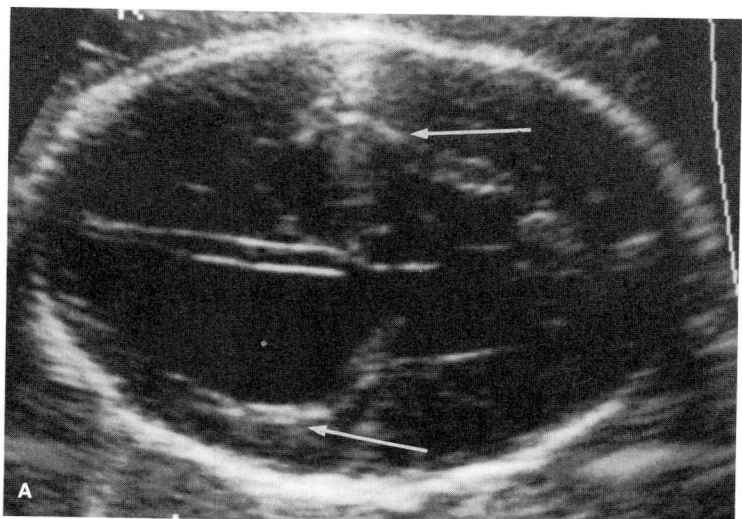

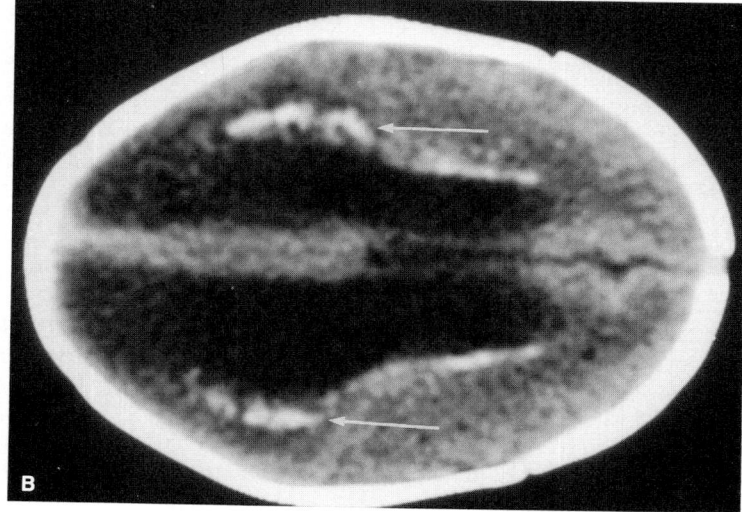

FIGURE 8-37. Intracranial infection. **(A)** Ultrasound of the fetal head showing dilated lateral ventricles with bilateral periventricular echogenicity (*arrows*), which corresponds to calcifications. **(B)** Postnatal, nonenhanced CT demonstrates periventricular calcifications (*arrows*).

REFERENCES

1. AIUM guidelines. J Ultrasound Med 1991; 10(10):576–578.
2. Filly RA, Cardoza JD, Goldstein RB, Barkovich AJ: Detection of fetal central nervous system anomalies: A practical level of effort for a routine sonogram. Radiology 1989; 172:403–408.
3. Cardoza JD, Goldstein RB, Filly RA: Exclusion of fetal ventriculomegaly with a single measurement: The width of the lateral ventricular atrium. Radiology 1988; 169:711–714.
4. Cronan MS, McGahan JP: A new ultrasound technique to visualize the proximal fetal cerebral ventricle. J Diagn Med Sonography 1991; 6:333–335.
5. Browning BP, Laorr A, McGahan JP, et al: Ultrasound assessment of the "upside" cerebral ventricle. Radiology (in press).
6. Mahony BS, Callen PW, Filly RA, Hoodick WK: The fetal cisterna magna. Radiology 1984; 153:773–776.
7. Knutzon R, McGahan JP, Salamat MS, Brant WB: Fetal cisterna magna septa: A normal anatomic finding. Radiology 1991; 180:799–801.
8. Filly RA: Fetal neural axis: Practical approach to identify anomalous development. In Rifkin MD, Charboneau JW, Laing FC (eds): Syllabus: Special Course, Ultrasound 1991. Presented at 77th Scientific Assembly and Annual Meeting of the Radiological Society of North America, 1991: 103–110.
9. Nicolaides KH, Campbell S, Gabbe SG, Guidetti R: Ultrasound screening for spina bifida: Cranial and cerebellar signs. Lancet 1986; 2:72–74.
10. Schoenecker S, Pretorius D, Manco-Johnson M: Artifacts seen commonly on ultrasonography of the fetal cranium. J Reprod Med 1985; 30:541–544.
11. Laing F, Stamler C, Jeffrey B: Ultrasonography of the fetal subarachnoid space. J Ultrasound Med 1983; 2:29–32.
12. Cardoza JD, Filly RA, Podrasky AE: The dangling choroid plexus: A sonographic observation of value in excluding ventriculomegaly. AJR 1988; 151:767.
13. Nelson NL, Callen PW, Filly RA: The choroid plexus pseudocyst: Sonographic identification and characterization. J Ultrasound Med 1992; 11:597–601.
14. Mahony BS, Nyberg DA, Hirsch J, et al: Mild idiopathic lateral cerebral ventricular dilatation in utero: Sonographic evaluation. Radiology 1988; 169:715–721.
15. Russ P, Pretorius D, Johnson M: Dandy-Walker syndrome: A review of 15 cases evaluated by prenatal sonography. Am J Obstet Gynecol 1989; 161:401–406.
16. Nyberg DA, Pretorius DH: Cerebral malformation. In Diagnostic Ultrasound of Fetal Abnormalities. Chicago: Year Book Medical Publishers, 1990: 83–145.
17. Goldstein RB, LaPidus AS, Filly RA: Fetal cephaloceles: Diagnosis with ultrasound. Radiology 1991; 180:803–808.
18. Estroff JA, Scott MR, Benacerraf BR: Dandy-Walker variant: Prenatal sonographic features and clinical outcome. Radiology 1992; 185:755–758.
19. Bertino RE, Nyberg DA, Cyr DR, et al: Prenatal diagnosis of agenesis of the corpus callosum. J Ultrasound Med 1988; 7:251–260.
20. Barkovich AJ, Gressen P, Evrard P: Formation, maturation and disorders of brain neocortex. Am J Neuroradiol 1992; 13:423–426.
21. McGahan JP: Prenatal diagnosis of lissencephaly. J Clin Ultrasound (in press).
22. Friedman JM, Santos-Ramos R: Natural history of X-linked aqueductal stenosis in the second and third trimesters of pregnancy. Am J Obstet Gynecol 1984; 150:104–106.
23. McGahan JP, Ellis W, Lindfors KK, et al: Congenital cerebrospinal fluid-containing intracranial abnormalities: A sonographic classification. J Clin Ultrasound 1988; 16:531–544.
24. Jones KL: Trisomy 13 syndrome. In Smith's Recognizable Patterns of Human Malformation, 4th ed. Philadelphia: WB Saunders, 1988: 20–25.
25. Dublin AB, French BN: Diagnostic image evaluation of hydranencephaly and pictorially similar entities, with emphasis on computed tomography. Radiology 1980; 137:81.
26. Dan U, Shalev E, Greif M, et al: Prenatal diagnosis of fetal brain arteriovenous malformation: The use of color Doppler imaging. JCU 1992; 20:149–151.
27. Sauerbrei EE, Cooperberg PL: Cystic tumors of the fetal and neonatal cerebrum: Ultrasound and computed tomographic evaluation. Radiology 1983; 147:689–692.
28. Benacerraf BR, Harlow B, Figoletto FD: Are choroid plexus cysts an indication for second trimester amniocentesis? Am J Obstet Gynecol 1990; 162:1001–1006.
29. Porto M, Murata Y, Warneke L, Keegan KA: Fetal choroid plexus cysts: An independent risk factor for chromosomal anomalies. J Clin Ultrasound 1993; 21:103–108.
30. Jones KL: Trisomy 18 syndrome. In Smith's Recognizable Patterns of Human Malformation, 4th ed. Philadelphia: WB Saunders, 1988: 16–19.
31. Nyberg DA, Kramer D, Resta RG, et al: Prenatal sonographic findings of trisomy 18: Review of 47 cases. J Ultrasound Med 1993: 12:103–113.
32. Barkovich AJ: Metabolic and destructive brain disorders. In Barkovich AJ (ed): Contemporary Neuroimaging, Vol 1: Pediatric Neuroimaging. New York: Raven Press, 1990: 35–76.
33. Yakovlev PI, Wadsworth RC: Schizencephalies. II. Clefts with hydrocephalus and lips separated. J Neuropathol Exp Neurol 1946; 5:169–206.
34. Crade M: Ultrasonic demonstration in utero of an intracranial teratoma. JAMA 1982; 247:1173.
35. Osborn RA, McGahan JP, Dublin AB: Sonographic appearance of congenital malignant astrocytoma. AJNR 1984; 5:814–815.

36. McGahan JP, Hasslein HC, Meyers M, Ford KB: Sonographic recognition of in utero intraventricular hemorrhage. AJR 1984; 142:171–173.

37. Goldstein RB, Filly RA: Prenatal diagnosis of anencephaly: Spectrum of sonographic appearances and distinction from the amniotic band syndrome. AJR 1988; 151:547–550.

38. Cox GG, Rosenthal SJ, Holsapple JW: Exencephaly: Sonographic findings and radiologic-pathologic correlation. Radiology 1985; 155:755–756.

39. Mahony BS, Filly RA, Callen PW, et al: The amniotic band syndrome: Antenatal diagnosis and potential pitfalls. Am J Obstet Gynecol 1985; 152: 63–68.

40. Gorczyca DP, Lindfors KK, McGahan JP, Hanson FW: Limb-body-wall complex: Another cause for elevated maternal serum alpha fetoprotein. J Clin Ultrasound 1990; 18:198–201.

41. Andrews M, Amparo EG: In utero clue to congenital lethal osteogenesis imperfecta. AJR 1983; 160:212.

42. Kurtz A, Wapner R, Rubin C, et al: Ultrasound criteria for in utero diagnosis of microcephaly. J Clin Ultrasound 1980; 8:11–16.

43. Chervenak FA, Jeanty P, Cantraine F, et al: The diagnosis of fetal microcephaly. Am J Obstet Gynecol 1984; 149:512–517.

44. Platt LD, Manning FA, Murata Y, et al: Diagnosis of fetal death in utero by real-time ultrasound. Obstet Gynecol 1980; 55(2):191–193.

45. Isaacson G, Blakemore KJ, Chervenak FA: Thanatophoric dysplasia with cloverleaf skull. Am J Dis Child 1983; 137:896.

46. Dublin AB, Merten DF: Computed tomography in the evaluation of herpes simplex encephalitis. Radiology 1977; 125:133–134.

47. Hayden CK, Swischuk LE: The head and spine. In Grayson T (ed): Pediatric Ultrasonography. Baltimore: Williams & Wilkins, 1987: 1–80.

John P. McGahan and Manuel Porto:
DIAGNOSTIC OBSTETRICAL ULTRASOUND.
© 1994 J.B. Lippincott Company.

Keith B. Lescale   Keith A. Eddleman   Frank A. Chervenak

Chapter 9

The Fetal Neck and Spine

NECK

Although it is a small region of the body, the neck contains vital conduits of respiration, deglutition, and blood to and from the brain as well as important endocrine and neural structures. Anomalies of the neck are fairly infrequent but often are associated with poor fetal outcome. Examination of the posterior neck and the base of the skull is important to detect abnormalities such as cystic hygroma, occipital cephalocele, and cervical meningomyelocele. This may be done with both transverse and longitudinal scanning (Fig. 9-1). A specific transverse view through the posterior fossa and the base of the occiput has been used to assess the thickness of the skin and soft tissues over the neck (Fig. 9-2). Finally, assessment of the anterior and anterolateral neck is important to detect such abnormalities as goiter, hemangioma, and teratoma.

Pitfalls

Certain normal anatomic variations, or pitfalls, may be encountered when examining the fetal neck.

Nuchal Cord

The fetal umbilical cord may overlie or wrap around the fetal neck; this is called *nuchal cord*. The nuchal cord is especially common in the third trimester of pregnancy. The exact significance of nuchal cord and its in utero frequency are unknown. When examining the fetal neck for nuchal thickening, the overlying cord may be mistaken for increased skin thickness of the neck (Fig. 9-3). This pitfall may be overcome by performing either pulse Doppler or color Doppler over the presumed skin thickening to ascertain whether this in fact represents the umbilical cord.

Nonfused Amnion Versus Cystic Neck Mass

When examining the fetal occiput or spine in the first trimester of pregnancy, nonfused amnion may overlap the fetal neck and give the artificial appearance of a cystic mass in or around the occiput (see Fig. 9-3). This may be remedied by checking elsewhere within the uterus for incomplete fusion of the amnion and the chorion or by checking the fetus when it has moved into a different anatomic position in which the neck is separate from the amnion.

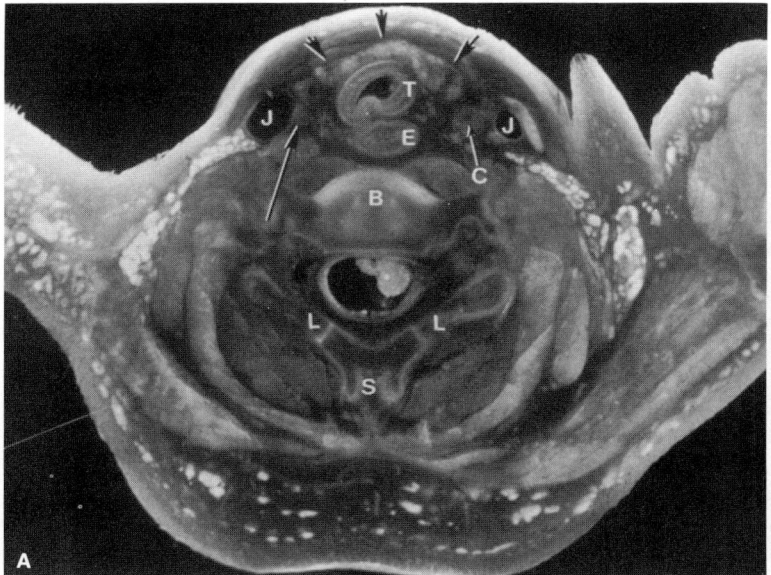
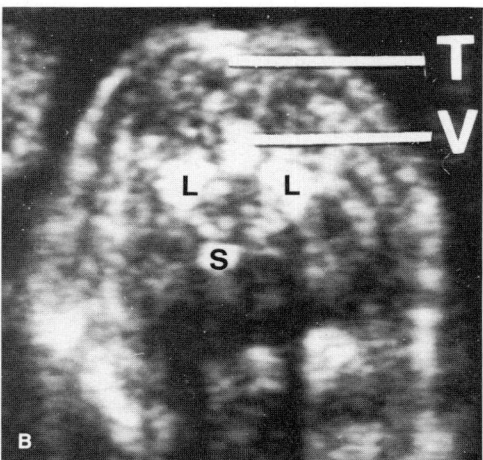

FIGURE 9-1. Normal neck. **(A)** Transverse section of lower neck in a fetal specimen of 20 weeks. J, jugular vein; C, carotid artery; T, trachea; E, esophagus; B, body of cervical vertebra; L, ossification centers of laminae; S, spinous process; arrows point at vagus nerve; arrowheads outline thyroid isthmus. (Chervenak FA, Isaacson G, Campbell S: Ultrasound in Obstetrics and Gynecology. Boston: Little, Brown, 1992.) **(B)** Corresponding transverse sonogram of the neck with smooth anterior contours, trachea (T), and cervical vertebra (V). L, ossification of the laminae; S, spinous process. (Chervenak FA, Isaacson G, Lorber J: Anomalies of the Fetal Head, Neck, and Spine: Ultrasound Diagnosis and Management. Philadelphia: WB Saunders, 1988.)

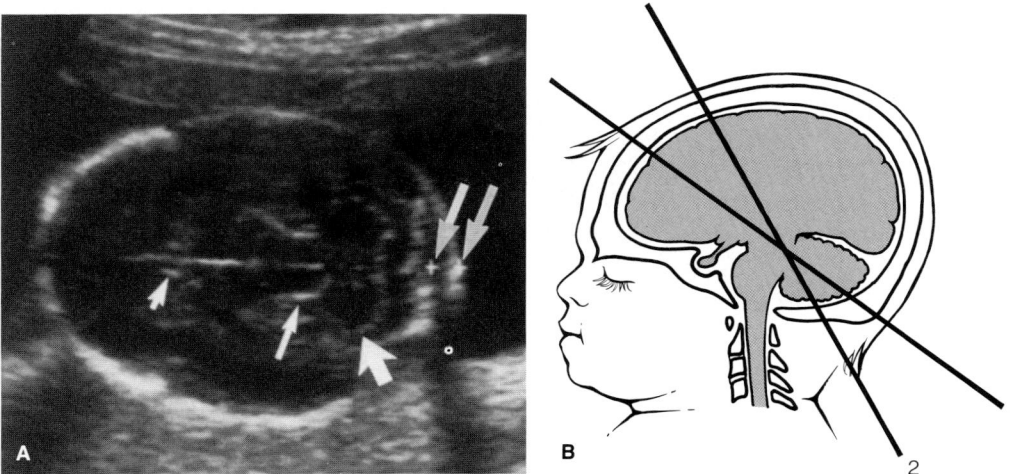

FIGURE 9-2. Nuchal skin thickness. **(A)** Correct plane and technique for measuring nuchal skinfold thickness. Critical landmarks include the cavum septi pellucidi (*short arrow*), cerebral peduncles (*long arrow*), and cerebellar hemispheres (*broad arrow*). Calipers (+) (*arrows*) are placed from the outer skull table to the outer skin surface. (Crane JP, Gray DL: Sonographically measured nuchal skinfold thickness as a screening tool for Down syndrome: Results of a prospective clinical trial. Obstet Gynecol 1991; 77:533.) **(B)** If the transducer is not angled in the correct plane (1) but is too steep (2), this will produce incorrect measurement for nuchal skin thickness.

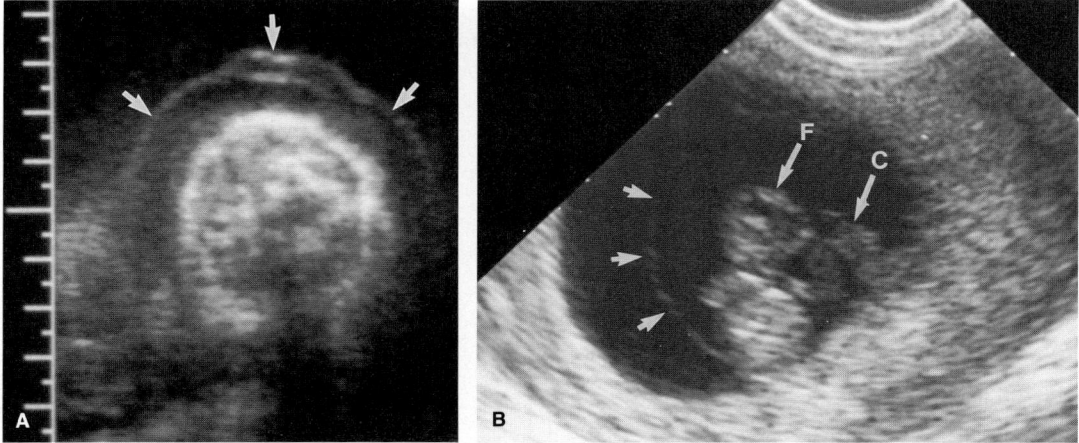

FIGURE 9-3. Pseudo neck masses. **(A)** Nuchal cord—hypoechoic cord (*arrows*) posterior to the neck should not be mistaken for increased skin thickness. Color Doppler sonography may help to demonstrate that this represents the umbilical cord. **(B)** Normal amnion—when scanning in the first trimester of pregnancy, the amnion (*arrows*) may potentially be confused for a cystic fetal neck mass. This may be especially confusing in the late first trimester of pregnancy, when only a portion of the amnion is not fused to the chorion. F, fetus; C, umbilical cord. (Courtesy of John P. McGahan, MD, Sacramento, CA.)

Pseudonuchal Thickening

When examining the fetal neck for nuchal thickening, a specific anatomic plane must be obtained. If angulation is too steep and a more coronal plane is obtained, this will artificially have the appearance of increased thickness of the skin over the posterior occiput (see Fig. 9-3).

TABLE 9-1. Possible Causes of Fetal Neck Masses

Type	Possible Cause
Common	Cystic hygroma
Uncommon	Cervical meningomyelocele
	Occipital cephalocele
	Amniotic band syndrome*
	Goiter
	Cervical teratoma
	Hemangioma
Rare	Neuroblastoma
	Hemangioendothelioma
	Lipoma, fibroma
	Branchial cleft cyst
	Thyroglossal duct cyst
	Metastases

* See Chapters 8 and 10.

Fetal Neck Abnormalities

A list of some possible causes of fetal neck abnormalities is given in Table 9-1. Cystic hygroma is the most common neck mass visualized in the fetus. A less common neck mass of major concern is occipital cephalocele. Other uncommon and rare neck masses are listed in Table 9-1.

Classification of neck masses can be made by a number of criteria, including location, ultrasound characteristics, and associated findings (Tables 9-2 through 9-4). For instance, fetal cystic hygroma and occipital cephalocele typically have a posterior cervicooccipital location. Other typical locations are listed in Table 9-2. There are a number of exceptions to locations, however, with cephaloceles occasionally occurring in the frontal-ethmoid, parietal, or other regions of the skull. Although cystic hygromas typically are multiseptated cystic structures, cephaloceles may be cystic, complex, or solid, depending on the contents of the herniated sac (see Table 9-3.) Differential features of cystic hygroma, occipital cephalocele, and cervical meningomyelocele, are listed in Table 9-5.

Cystic Hygroma

The most common neck mass identified in the fetus is cystic hygroma, which is a congenital malformation of the lymphatic system. Cystic hygroma most likely develops from a defect in the formation

TABLE 9-2.   Characteristic Location of Fetal Neck Masses

Neck Mass	Characteristic Location
Cystic hygroma	Posterolateral, bilateral
Cervical meningomyelocele	Posterior, midline
Occipital cephalocele	Posterior, midline
Goiter	Anterior, bilateral
Cervical teratoma	Anterolateral, unilateral
Hemangioma	Variable

of lymphatic vessels. The fetal lymphatic vessels drain into two large sacs lateral to the jugular veins (Fig. 9-4). If the lymphatic and venous structures fail to connect, the jugular lymph sacs enlarge, resulting in cystic hygromas of the posterior triangles of the neck.[1] There is often concomitant fetal hydrops (Figs. 9-5 through 9-7). These cysts are characteristically found in the posterolateral region of the neck (Fig. 9-8) and are frequently divided by random, incomplete septa.[2] A dense midline septum extending from the fetal neck across the full width of the hygroma is found. This septum represents the nuchal ligament[2] (see Fig. 9-5; Table 9-6). Once a cystic hygroma is detected, a careful search is made for associated skin edema, ascites, and pleural or pericardial effusions (see Figs. 9-6 through 9-8). The outcome of fetuses with cystic hygromas is variable but can result in in utero demise or partial regression, leaving a webbed neck. Rarely, they may be localized with a fairly normal outcome (Figs. 9-6 and 9-9).

A recent series by Bernstein and colleagues found that 65% (29 of 45) of fetuses diagnosed with

cystic hygroma had abnormal karyotypes.[3] In fetuses diagnosed during the first trimester (see Fig. 9-8), the incidence of abnormal karyotype is about 50%[4] (Table 9-7). A more recent study by Shulman and colleagues corroborated these findings: 15 of 33 fetuses (46.9%) diagnosed with cystic hygroma in the first trimester had an abnormal karyotype.[5] Turner's syndrome is the most frequently reported karyotypic abnormality associated with fetal cystic hygroma, but trisomy also is often encountered with cystic hygromas (see Table 9-7).

When first-trimester cystic hygroma occurs in the presence of a normal karyotype, an entirely normal outcome is possible.[4-6] When hydrops is present, however, the outlook is grave. In reports of cases in which the hydropic fetuses were alive at initial ultrasound examination and the pregnancies were not electively terminated, all fetuses died within the next few weeks.[2,7,8] It is possible that some cystic hygromas regress in utero, leaving only a webbed neck (see Fig. 9-9). Such a process is postulated to account for neck webbing seen in patients with Turner's syndrome (see Fig. 9-8) or possibly the nuchal thickening of Down's syndrome. Isolated cystic hygromas (ie, those not occurring as part of a jugular lymphatic obstruction sequence) may be surgically corrected and have a good prognosis.

Emphasis of obstetrical management should be on ultrasound detection of the extent of the hygroma, associated findings, and determination of karyotype for genetic counseling. Furthermore, cytogenic studies of several tissues may be required after abortion or birth to confirm that the fetus may have chromosomal mosaicism. In cases detected later in pregnancy, if the cystic hygroma is so large

(text continues on page 179)

TABLE 9-3.   Ultrasound Features of Fetal Neck Masses

Neck Mass	Ultrasound Features
Cystic hygroma	Multicystic, midline septation
Cervical meningomyelocele	Cystic → complex → solid (depending on contents of sac)
Occipital cephalocele	Cystic → complex → solid (depending on contents of sac)
Goiter	Generalized hypoechoic (solid)
Cervical teratoma	Solid with cystic components
Hemangioma	Echogenic (occasional cystic form depending on histology)

TABLE 9-4.   Ultrasound Findings Associated With Fetal Neck Masses

Neck Mass	Associated Findings
Cystic hygroma	Hydrops
Cervical meningomyelocele	Spinal dysplasia
Occipital cephalocele	Bony defect of the skull
	Polyhydramnios
Goiter	Polyhydramnios
	Maternal thyroid disease
Cervical teratoma	Polyhydramnios
Hemangioma	Positive Doppler signals

TABLE 9-5. Differential Ultrasound Features Among Cystic Hygroma, Occipital Cephalocele, and Cervical Meningomyelocele

Ultrasound Feature	Fetal Cystic Hygroma (Common)	Occipital Cephalocele (Uncommon)	Cervical Meningomyelocele (Rare)
Body defect	No	Yes (skull)	Yes (spine)
Intracranial abnormalities	No	Common	Common
Symmetric abnormalities	No	Yes	Yes
Septations	Yes	No	No
Acute angle with skin	No	Yes	Yes
Hydrops	Common	No	No

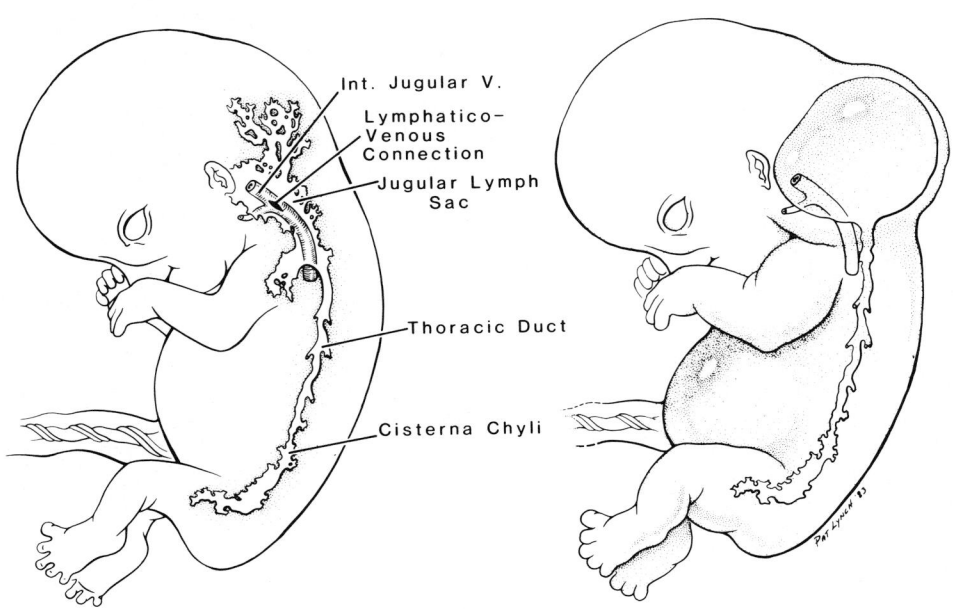

FIGURE 9-4. **(Left)** Lymphatic system in a normal fetus with a patent connection between the jugular lymph sac and the internal jugular vein. **(Right)** Cystic hygroma and hydrops from a failed lymphatovenous connection. (Chervenak FA, Isaacson G, Blakemore KJ, et al: Fetal cystic hygroma: Cause and natural history. N Engl J Med 1983; 309:822.)

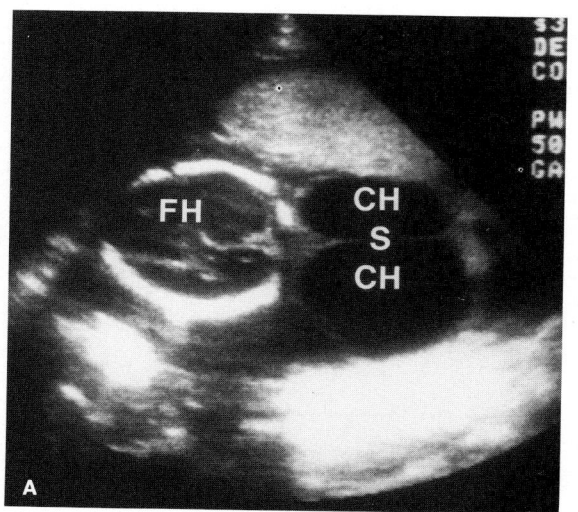

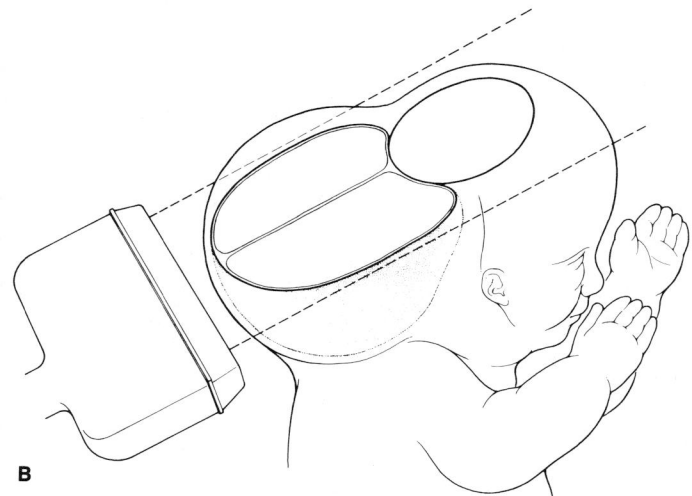

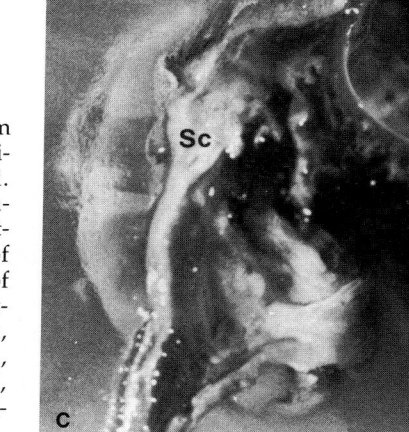

FIGURE 9-5. Cystic hygroma. **(A)** Sonogram demonstrating a nuchal cystic hygroma (CH) divided by a midline septum (S). FH, fetal head. (Chervenak FA, Isaacson G, Campbell S: Ultrasound in Obstetrics and Gynecology. Boston: Little, Brown, 1992.) **(B)** Corresponding depiction of scan plane through cystic hygroma. **(C)** Section of hygroma embedded in gelatin with arrow pointing to midline septum. H, hygroma; Sc, scalp; Sk, skin covering hygroma. **(B, C,** Chervenak FA, Isaacson G, Lorber J: Anomalies of the Fetal Head, Neck, and Spine: Ultrasound Diagnosis and Management. Philadelphia: WB Saunders, 1988.)

FIGURE 9-6. Natural history of cystic hygroma. Generalized hydrops results from jugular lymphatic obstruction sequence (JLOS), which may result in either isolated hygroma, generalized edema and death, or partial regression of hygroma. (Chervenak FA, Isaacson G, Lorber J: Anomalies of the Fetal Head, Neck, and Spine: Ultrasound Diagnosis and Management. Philadelphia: WB Saunders, 1988.)

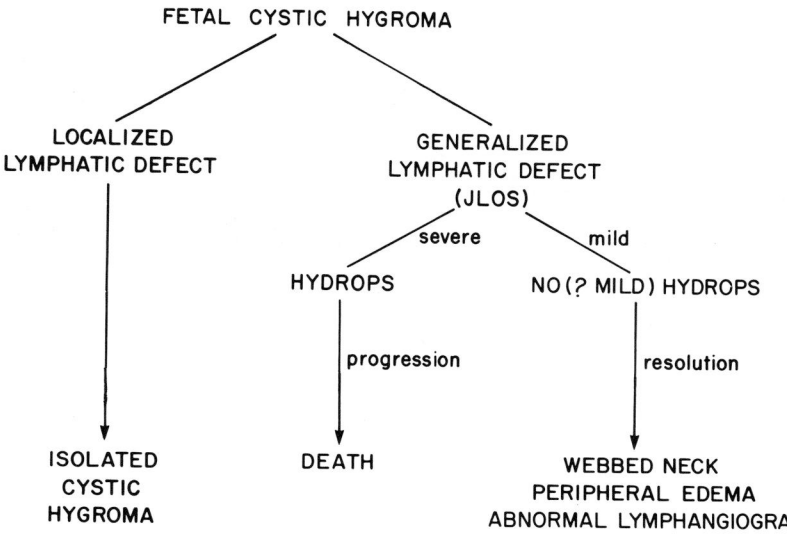

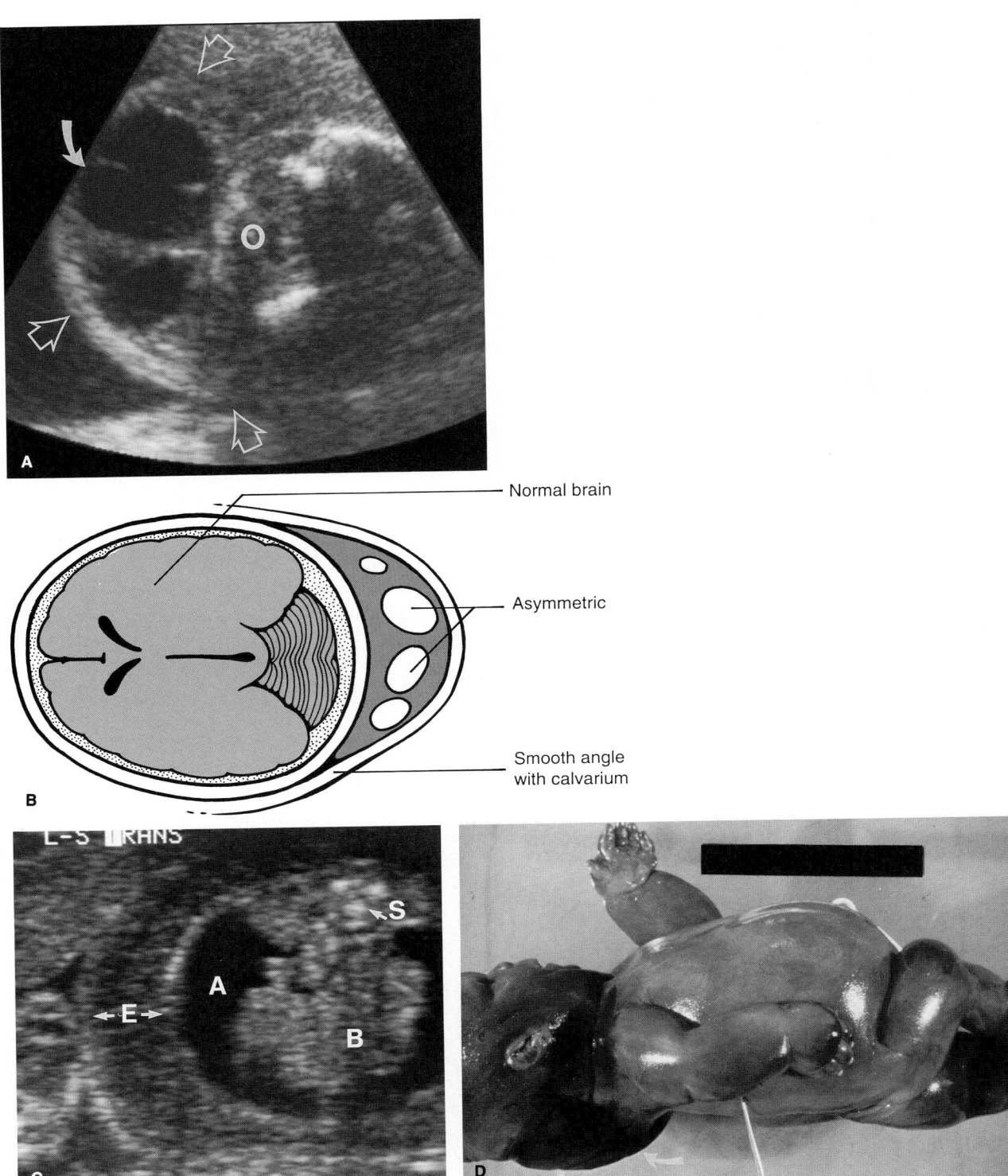

FIGURE 9-7.   Cystic hygroma plus hydrops. **(A)** Septated cystic hygroma (*curved arrow*) posterior to the occiput (O) with associated skin thickening (*open arrows*). **(B)** Diagram demonstrating typical features of cystic hygroma. **(C)** Scan through the fetal abdomen demonstrates evidence of abdominal ascites (A), with floating bowel (B), as well as cutaneous edema (E). S, fetal spine. **(D)** Gross specimen shows large cystic hygroma (*curved arrow*) with marked associated fetal hydrops. (Courtesy of John P. McGahan, MD, Sacramento, CA.)

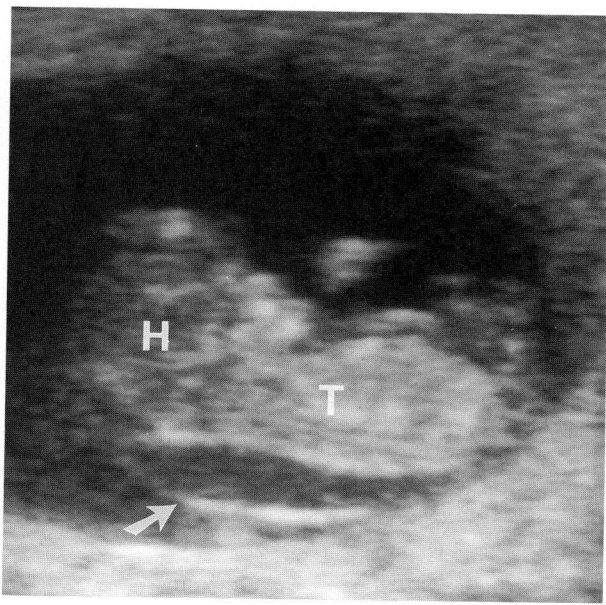

FIGURE 9-8. Early nuchal thickening (Turner's syndrome). Typical nuchal membrane (*arrow*) as observed in the first-trimester fetus with a cystic hygroma and associated Turner's syndrome. Transverse scanning and scanning of the fetus after movement are helpful in these cases to confirm true nuchal thickening. H, head; T, thorax. (Courtesy of John P. McGahan, MD, Sacramento, CA.)

that it interferes with delivery, a transabdominal needle aspiration of cyst fluid may be indicated to allow vaginal delivery or to facilitate cesarean section.

Occipital Cephalocele

A cephalocele is a protrusion of the meninges, and frequently brain substance, through a defect in the cranium. There may be a number of different types, including *cranial gliocele,* which is protrusion of a glial-lined cyst; *atretic cephalocele,* which is residual of a cephalocele; *cranial meningocele,* which is

TABLE 9-6. Sonographic Features That Differentiate Cystic Hygroma From Other Craniocervical Masses

- Intact skull and spinal column
- Lack of a solid component in the mass
- Typical posterior lateral position of the mass relative to the fetal head
- Cysts separated by septa
- Dense midline septation (nuchal ligament)
- Normal intracranial contents

protrusion of cerebrospinal fluid (CSF) and meninges; *cranial meningoencephaloceles,* which is protrusion of CSF, leptomeninges, and brain; and *meningoencephalocystocele,* which is protrusion of CSF, leptomeninges, brain, and ventricles. Most commonly, cephaloceles are either meningoceles or meningoencephaloceles. The incidence is about 1 in 2000 live births, with more than two thirds occurring in the occiput.[9] Cephaloceles also may occur in the parietal, frontal, ethmoid (sincipital), or nasopharyngeal regions, to name a few.

Ultrasound Findings. Sonographically, a cephalocele appears as a saclike protrusion around the head that is not covered by bone (Fig. 9-10). The diagnosis can be made with certainty only if a bony defect in the skull is detected. The position of the defect may be determined using the bony structures of the face, the spine, and if possible, the midline echo of the brain for orientation (Fig. 9-11). If brain has herniated, the contents of the sac have a heterogeneous appearance. A diligent search for skull defects, using serial examinations if necessary, may help to improve diagnostic accuracy. If a defect in the skull is still not found, differential possibilities include cystic hygroma, teratoma, hemangioma, and branchial cleft cyst. Fetal hair, the ear, a scalp tumor, and cephalhematoma can each mimic the sonographic appearance of cephalocele.[10–12] Differential points between cystic hygroma and cephalocele are listed in Table 9-5.

A bony defect in the occipital vault is a distinguishing feature between cystic hygroma and cephalocele[13] (see Figs. 9-7 and 9-11). Septation is a second important sign to distinguish hygroma from cephalocele. A third differential diagnostic feature between hygroma and cephalocele is the echogenic appearance of the malformation. A cystic hygroma has a translucent appearance, whereas meningoencephalocele with protruding brain appears more echogenic[13] (see Table 9-5). Also, the margin between the cephalocele and the cranium is often an acute angle, whereas there is a fairly smooth angle between the skin covering the cystic hygroma and the cranium.

Prognosis. In cases of cephalocele or cervical meningomyelocele, the prognosis depends on the location, size, and content of the herniated sac and concomitant CNS malformations. In the presence of other defects, such as microcephaly or hydrocephalus, or as part of a genetic syndrome, the outlook is uniformly poor. A number of other syndromes are associated with cephalocele (Table 9-8

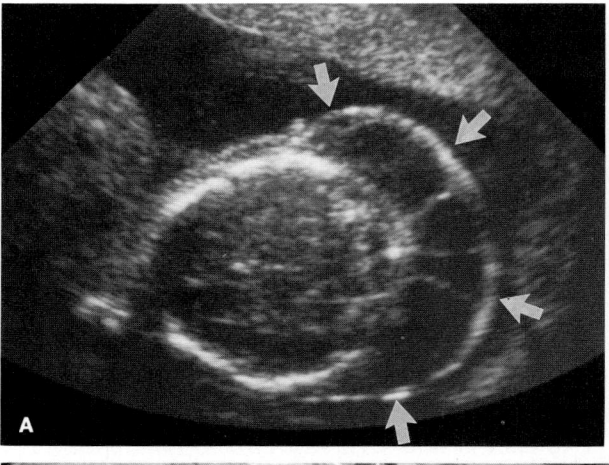

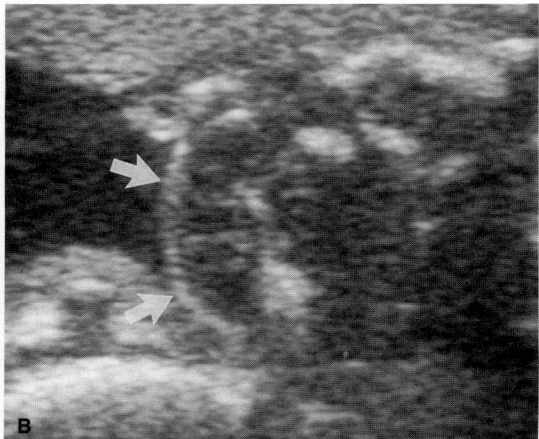

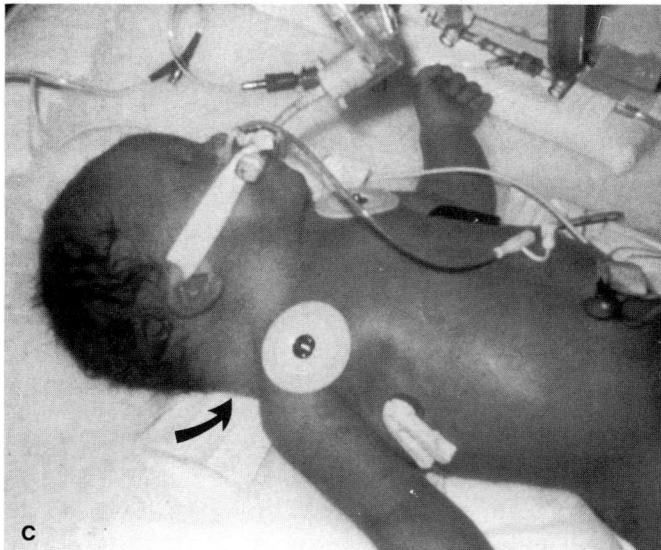

FIGURE 9-9. Regression of fetal cystic hygroma. **(A)** Ultrasound of the head demonstrating septated fetal cystic hygroma (*arrows*). **(B)** Follow-up ultrasound obtained 4 weeks later demonstrated partial regression of the cystic hygroma (*arrows*). (Courtesy of John P. McGahan, MD, Sacramento, CA.) **(C)** Neonatal photograph of another newborn demonstrating neck webbing. (Chervenak FA, Isaacson G, Lorber J: Anomalies of the Fetal Head, Neck, and Spine: Ultrasound Diagnosis and Management. Philadelphia: WB Saunders, 1988.)

TABLE 9-7. Karyotypes in Embryos With the Prenatal Diagnosis of Cystic Hygroma in the First Trimester

Karyotype	n	%
Total patients	30	100
Chromosomes available	29	97
Aneuploid	15	52
47,XY, +21	4	14
47,XX, +21	2	7
45,X	4	14
47,XY, +18	2	7
47,XY, +15/46,XY	1	3
49,XXXXY	1	3
47,XX, −21, +der(21)t(18q;21p)	1	3
Euploid	14	48

(Cullen MT, Gabrielli S, Green JJ, et al: Diagnosis and significance of cystic hygroma in the first trimester. Prenatal Diagn 1990; 10:643.)

and Fig. 9-12). If a large amount of brain tissue is observed in the sac, and especially if there are associated CNS anomalies, the parents should be counseled that the chance for a good outcome is remote and cesarean section is probably not advisable. Decompression of a large sac or associated hydrocephalus may be necessary to allow vaginal delivery.[14] There are, however, certain situations when cesarean section should be considered. These include: (1) a cephalocele sufficiently large and solid enough to indicate possible dystocia, (2) other obstetrical considerations (eg, previous low vertical cesarean section), (3) a viable coincident twin with an indication for cesarean section, and (4) an isolated cephalocele sonographically identified in which the parents accept the risks of significant developmental defects. In such cases, cesarean section might minimize birth trauma and improve neonatal outcome.[15]

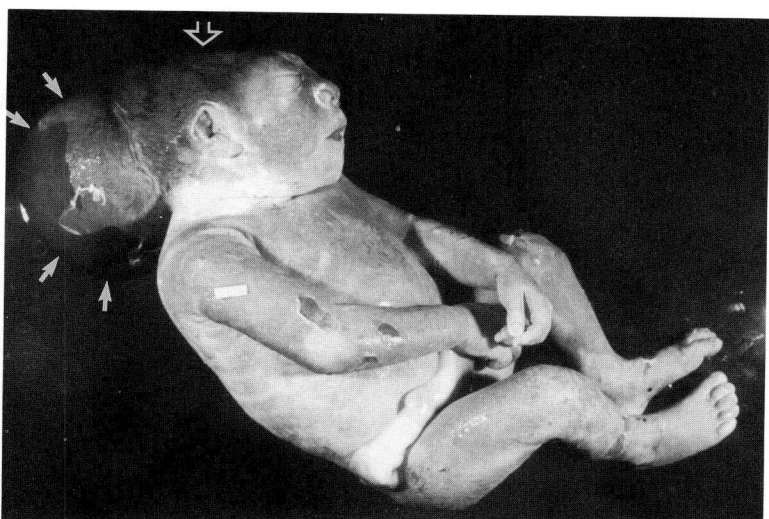

FIGURE 9-10. Postmortem cephalocele (*arrows*) with resultant microcephaly (*open arrow*). (Chervenak FA, Isaacson G, Mahoney MJ, et al: Diagnosis and management of fetal cephalocele. Obstet Gynecol 1984; 64:86.)

Cervical Meningomyelocele

Although far less common than cystic hygroma and cephalocele, cervical meningomyelocele may present as posterior neck masses. Cervical meningomyeloceles are usually located in the midline of the dorsum of the neck and most often are cystic in nature, but because of prolapsing ossification centers of the spine, they often appear complex. Splaying of the posterior ossification centers of the spine distinguishes this lesion from other neck masses (Fig. 9-13).

Goiter

Goiter, a massively enlarged thyroid gland, can be associated with variable maternal thyroid states but most often occurs in pregnancies in which maternal ingestion of iodides or other thyroid-blocking agents have been used.[16] Goiter has also occurred secondary to maternal Graves' disease as a result of transplacental passage of a thyroid-stimulating substance, such as long-acting thyroid stimulant. Congenital hypothyroidism occurs in about 1 in 3700 births.[16]

Ultrasound Findings. Fetal goiter is typically characterized sonographically as a solid, bilobed, anterior neck mass (Figs. 9-14 and 9-15). The mass is usually homogeneous and, although solid, may appear hypoechoic. Displacement of the common carotids posteriorly or hyperextension of the fetal head also may be noted. Associated findings include hydramnios, presumably due to impaired fetal swallowing.

Prognosis. Evidence of hypothyroidism, based on elevated levels of thyroid-stimulating hormone in the amniotic fluid, may help to confirm the diagnosis of fetal goiter during the second trimester. Wenstrom and colleagues used fetal blood sampling for the measurement of fetal thyroid function.[17] This appears to be an accurate method of diagnosing fetal hypothyroidism as well as a guide for therapeutic management.

The possibility of airway obstruction at birth from tracheal compression by a large goiter, as well as the risk of cretinism and mental retardation secondary to hypothyroidism, underscores the importance of early prenatal diagnosis, serial ultrasound surveillance, and delivery in a tertiary center.

Cervical Teratoma

Teratomas are neoplasms derived from pluripotent cells and composed of a diversity of tissues foreign to the anatomic site in which they arise.[18] These tissues are derived from precursors in two or three different embryonic germ layers. With an incidence 1 in 20,000 to 1 in 40,000 live births, the neck accounts for about 5% of teratomas.[19] Since 1983, only 137 cases have been reported in the literature.[20]

Ultrasound Findings. Sonographically, these tumors are typically unilateral with an anterolateral location. They are generally cystic masses early in gestation, becoming larger and more complex as

(text continues on page 184)

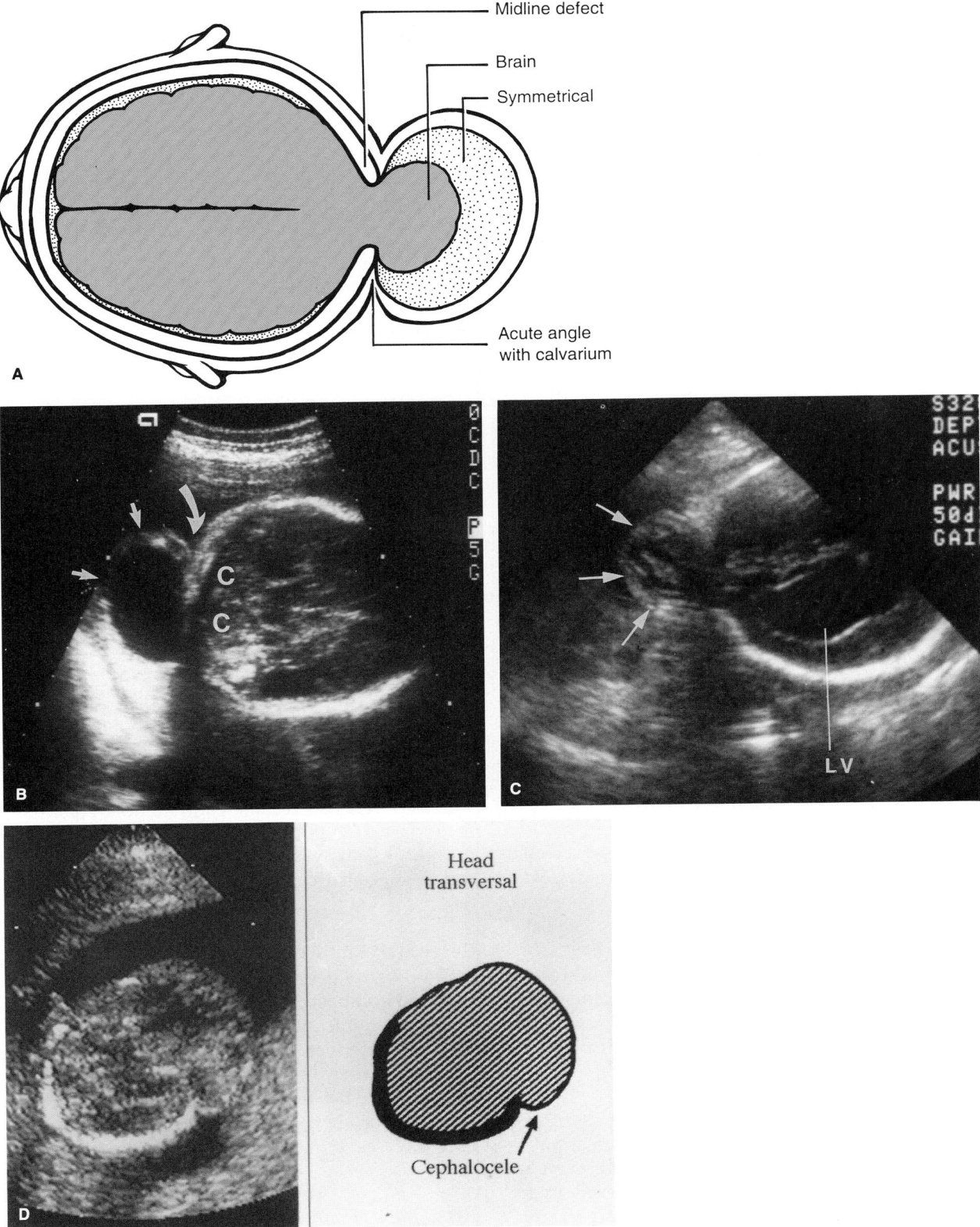

FIGURE 9-11.

TABLE 9-8.   Partial List of Conditions Associated With Cephaloceles

Condition	Striking Features	Cause
Meckel's syndrome	Polydactyly, multicystic kidneys	Autosomal recessive
Knobloch's syndrome	Myopia, vitreoretinal degeneration	Autosomal recessive
Chemke's syndrome	Hydrocephaly, agyria	Autosomal recessive
Dyssegmental dwarfism	Lethal dwarfism	Autosomal recessive
Pseudo-Meckel's syndrome	Arhinencephaly, absent corpus callosum	Autosomal recessive t(p+)
Frontonasal dysplasia	Ocular hypertelorism	? Sporadic
Amniotic band syndrome	Amputational defects	? Sporadic

(Naidich TP, Altman NR, Braffman BH, McLone DG, Zimmerman RA: Cephaloceles and related malformations. Am J Neuroradiol 1992; 64:666–667.)

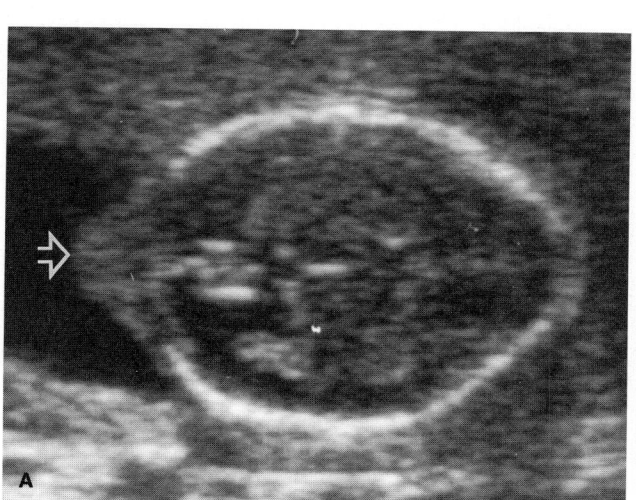
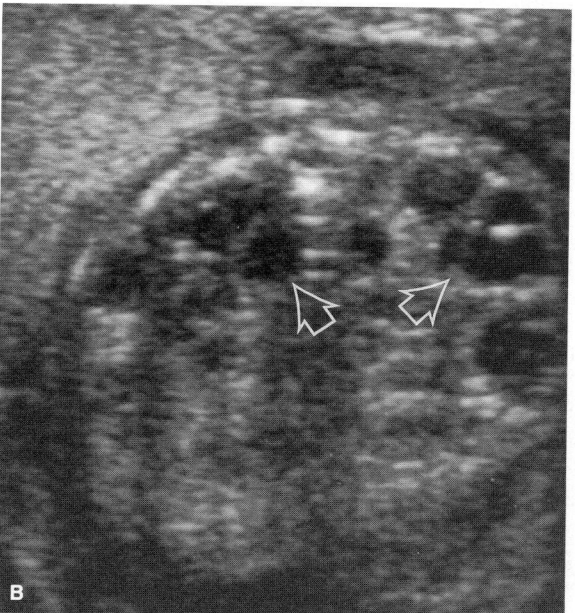

FIGURE 9-12.   Meckel-Gruber syndrome. **(A)** Small echogenic encephalocele noted in the midline occipital region (*open arrow*). **(B)** Scans of the kidneys demonstrate multiple cysts of varying sizes identified within both kidneys, consistent with multicystic dysplastic kidneys. There was also associated polydactyly in this case of Meckel-Gruber syndrome. (Courtesy of John P. McGahan, MD, Sacramento, CA.)

FIGURE 9-11.   Various appearances of cephaloceles. **(A)** Diagram of a cephalocele demonstrating several common features, including occipital location, bony defect, and variable herniation of brain into cephalocele sac. Note acute angulation of the margin of the cephalocele and the bony calvarium. **(B)** Cystic cephalocele (*arrows*) with herniation of meninges but little or no brain. Note acute angulation of cephalocele with bony calvarium (*curved arrow*). Cerebellar hemispheres are identified (C), but with obliteration of cisterna magna. **(C)** Occipital cephalocele (outlined by *arrows*) is a complex mass due to both herniated meninges and brain tissue. LV, dilated lateral ventricles. **(B, C,** courtesy of John P. McGahan, MD, Sacramento, CA.) **(D)** Ultrasound of a fetus at 13 weeks' gestation showing solid cephalocele as identified on transvaginal sonography. (Van Zalen-Sprock MM, van Vugt JM, van der Harten HJ, van Geijn HP: Cephalocele and cystic hygroma: Diagnosis and differentiation in the first trimester of pregnancy with transvaginal sonography. Report of two cases. Ultrasound Obstet Gynecol 1992; 2:289.)

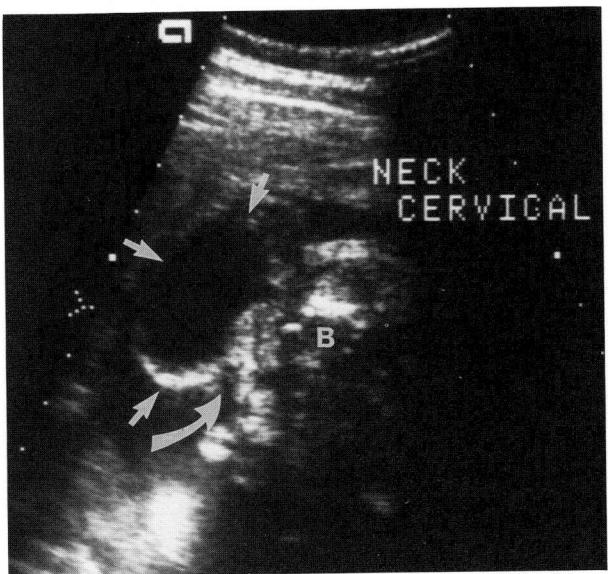

FIGURE 9-13. Cervical meningocele at level of C1 (*arrows*) demonstrating cystic component of herniated meninges and cerebrospinal fluid. Also note acute angulation of the meningocele (*curved arrow*) and the posterior neck. B, vertebral body of spine.

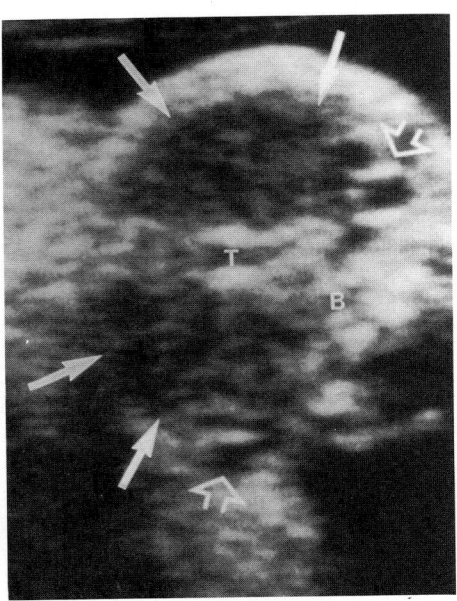

FIGURE 9-15. Fetal goiter. Axial scan of the neck (*arrows*) demonstrating a goiter. The neck vessels are indicated by open arrows. The trachea (T) can be seen between the lobes of the thyroid. B, vertebral body of spine. (Bromley B, et al: The fetal thyroid: Normal and abnormal sonographic measurements. J Ultrasound Med 1992; 11:25.)

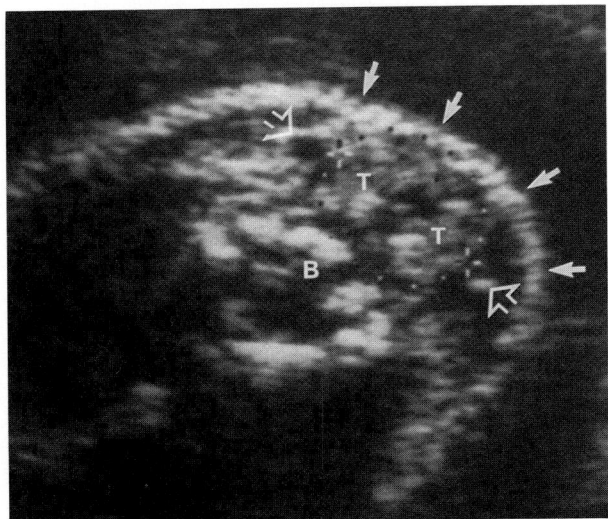

FIGURE 9-14. Fetal thyroid. Axial scan of the thyroid in a fetus without thyroid disease. The transverse limits of the thyroid are shown with calipers, and the diameter and circumference measurements are displayed. B, vertebral body; T, thyroid; open arrows point to jugular vein and carotid artery; and skin surface is outlined by small arrows. (Bromley B, et al: The fetal thyroid: Normal and abnormal sonographic measurements. J Ultrasound Med 1992; 11:25.)

the gestation progresses. They can undergo calcification or exhibit bone formation. Calcification is present in about 45% of cases (Fig. 9-16). Tumor sizes of 8 to 10 cm in diameter are not uncommon. Hydramnios is noted in 30% of cases.[21]

Prognosis. More than 90% of these lesions are benign, and a surgical cure is possible; however, operative mortality is 9% to 15%.[21,22] Mortality rates as high as 80% to 100% are reported in untreated neonates, most often due to respiratory obstruction.[21] With prenatal diagnosis, however, a good outcome is possible. Cesarean section with prompt airway management at the time of birth is necessary. Debulking procedures and definitive surgery may be performed with a good outcome.[23]

Hemangioma

Hemangiomas are localized proliferations of vascular endothelium that may occur anywhere in the body; they rarely present as a neck mass prenatally. Because hemangiomas may be a number of different types (eg, capillary, arteriovenous, venous angiomas), the sonographic appearance is variable. Most hemangiomas appear solid owing

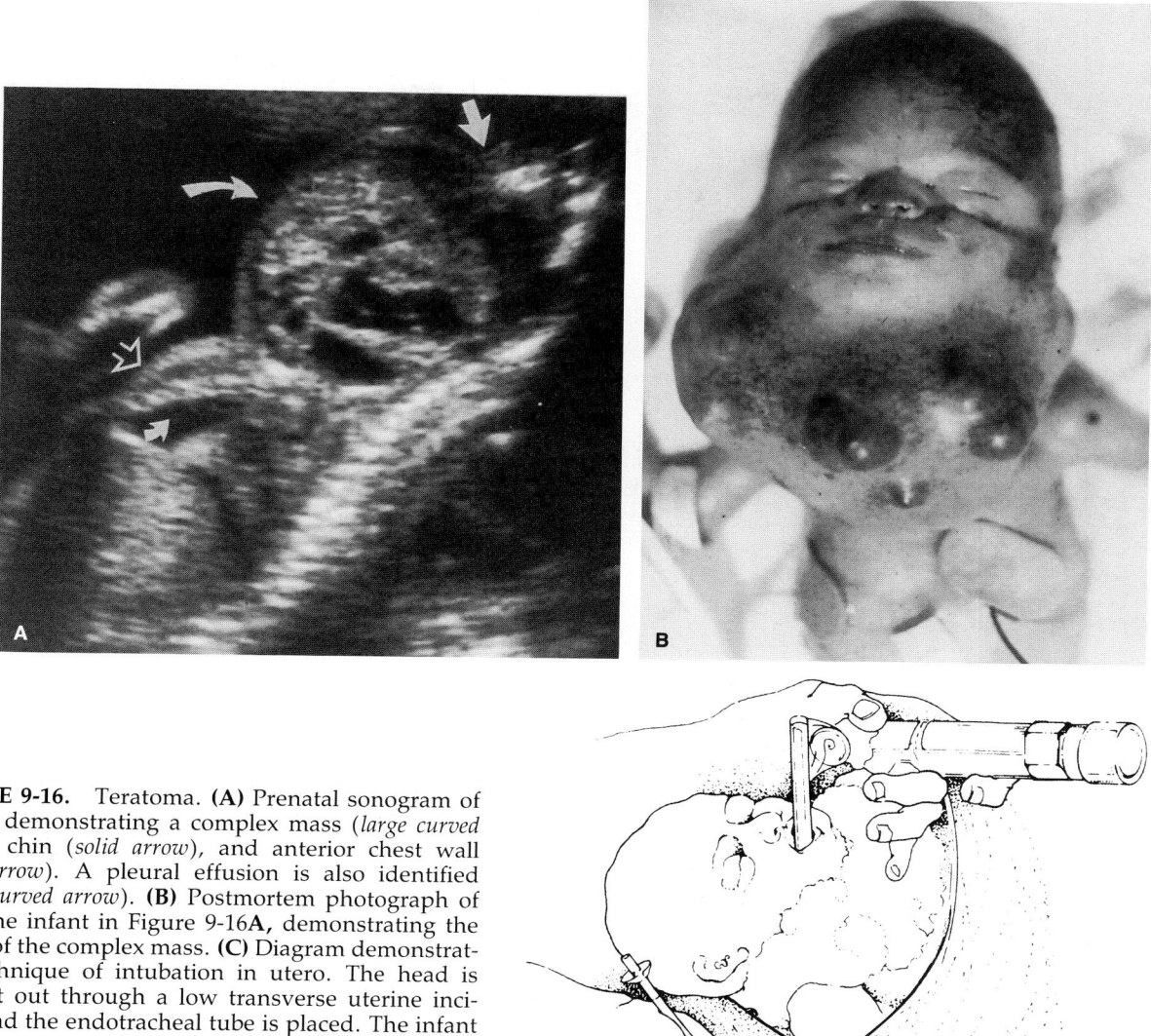

FIGURE 9-16.   Teratoma. **(A)** Prenatal sonogram of a fetus demonstrating a complex mass (*large curved arrow*), chin (*solid arrow*), and anterior chest wall (*open arrow*). A pleural effusion is also identified (*small curved arrow*). **(B)** Postmortem photograph of the same infant in Figure 9-16**A,** demonstrating the extent of the complex mass. **(C)** Diagram demonstrating technique of intubation in utero. The head is brought out through a low transverse uterine incision, and the endotracheal tube is placed. The infant is then delivered and the cord clamped. (Langer JC, Tabb, T, Thompson P, et al: Management of prenatally diagnosed tracheal obstruction: Access to the airway in utero prior to delivery. Fetal Diagn Ther 1992; 7:12.)

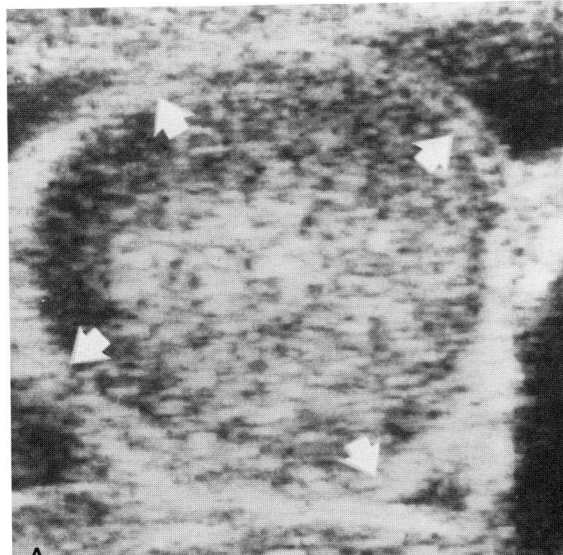

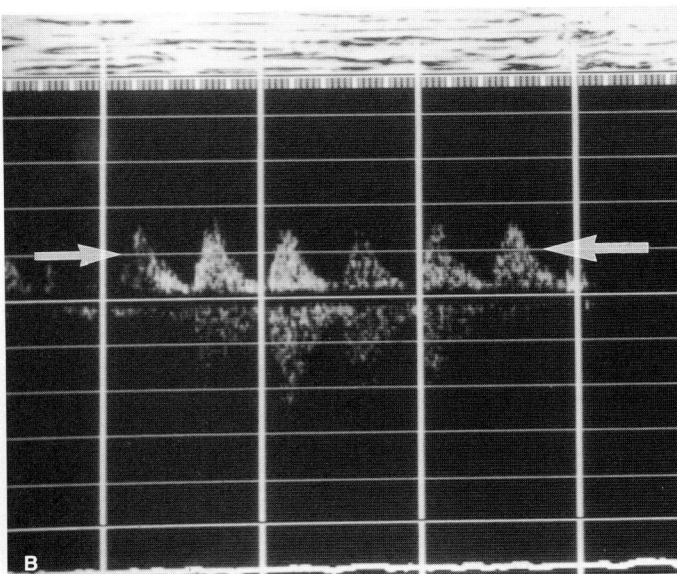

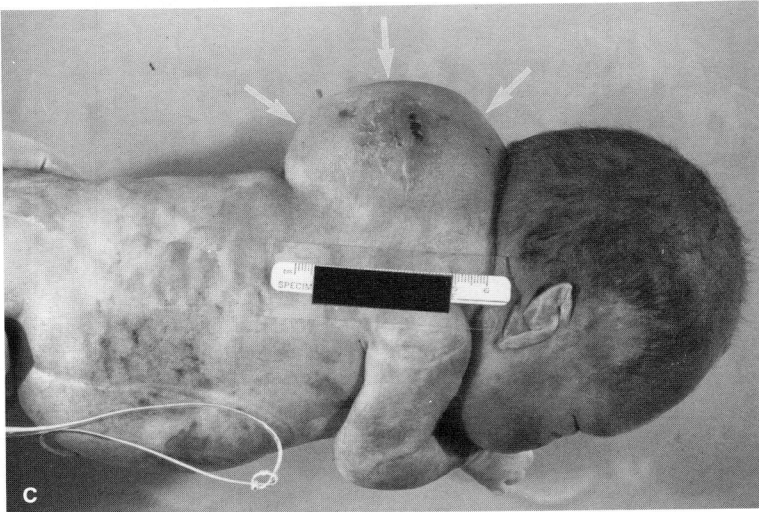

FIGURE 9-17. Hemangioendothelioma. **(A)** Prenatal ultrasound demonstrates well-circumscribed echogenic mass (*arrows*) located posterior to the neck. **(B)** Doppler tracing from the base of the mass demonstrates multiple areas with arterial waveform (*arrows*). **(C)** Postmortem specimen demonstrates mass in the posterior neck (*arrow*), which was a hemangioma at the base of the neck. (McGahan JP, Schneider JM: Fetal neck hemangioendothelioma with secondary hydrops fetalis: Sonographic diagnosis. J Clin Ultrasound 1986; 14:384–388.)

to innumerable small vascular channels that act as multiple interfaces.[24] Occasionally, small internal hypoechoic spaces may be observed. Many times, the spaces are so small that the mass appears uniformly echogenic (Fig. 9-17). Pulse Doppler, placed at the base of the mass, often reveals significant blood flow and helps to distinguish hemangioma from other neck masses. Occasionally, the hemangioma contains large vascular spaces. In these cases, the mass appears hypoechoic owing to the dilated vascular channels (Fig. 9-18). Color flow mapping is also useful in the diagnosis. Most often, there are no associated findings; however, in the case of a massive hemangioma, high-output congestive heart failure may lead to subsequent

fetal hydrops and death in utero. Therefore, close ultrasound follow-up of these pregnancies is suggested. Mode of delivery depends on the size of the hemangioma; if it is large, prompt airway management and debulking surgery are necessary.

Nuchal Thickening

Originally described by Benacerraf and colleagues in 1985, the sonographic sign of a thickened posterior nuchal fold has been used as a marker for detecting second-trimester fetuses with Down's syndrome.[25] The reason for nuchal thickening is not known, but it may be secondary to resolution of cystic hygroma. Recent studies by Nicolaides and colleagues[26] and Ville and colleagues[27] have dem-

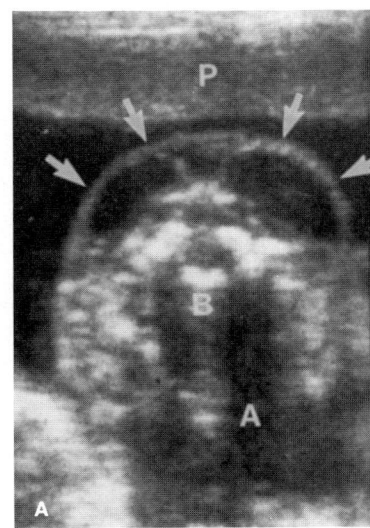
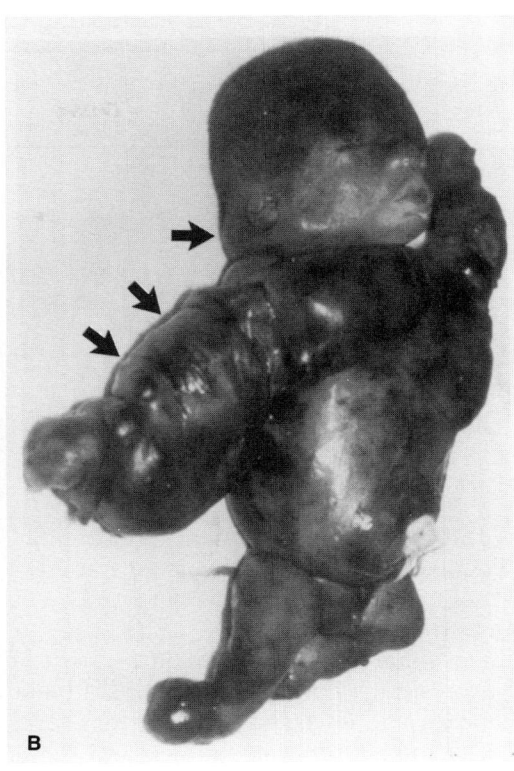

FIGURE 9-18. Hemangioma. **(A)** Transverse section of a fetal neck illustrating a hypoechoic lesion (*arrow*) in the posterior neck. B, vertebral body of spine; A, anterior neck; P, placenta. **(B)** Fetus with multiple massive hemangiomas (*arrows*) and other multiple defects. (Grundy H, et al: Hemangioma presenting as a cystic mass in the fetal neck. J Ultrasound Med 1985; 4:147.)

onstrated that this association exists in the first trimester. Nuchal skinfold thickness can be measured on axial view of the skull in which the following internal landmarks are identified: cavum septi pellucidi, cerebral peduncles, cerebellar hemispheres, and cisterna magna[28] (see Fig. 9-2). A soft tissue thickening of 6 mm or greater between 16 and 20 weeks of gestation is considered abnormal (Fig. 9-19). A recent study by Crane and Gray[28] supported the earlier findings by Benacerraf and colleagues (Table 9-9).

In the first trimester, nuchal skin thickening (as defined by Nicolaides and colleagues) is present if, in the mid-sagittal plane of the neck, there is subcutaneous edema that produces a characteristic tremor on ballottement of the fetal head.[26] In this series, an abnormal karyotype was noted in 53 of 145 fetuses (35.5%); the most common abnormality was trisomy 21 (32 of 53 abnormal karyotypes; see Fig. 9-19). Ville and colleagues consider nuchal thickening in the first trimester to be the presence of a unilocular collection of nuchal fluid 3 mm.[27] Eight of 28 fetuses (28.6%) by this definition had abnormal karyotypes. Appropriate genetic counseling should be offered to women with fetuses

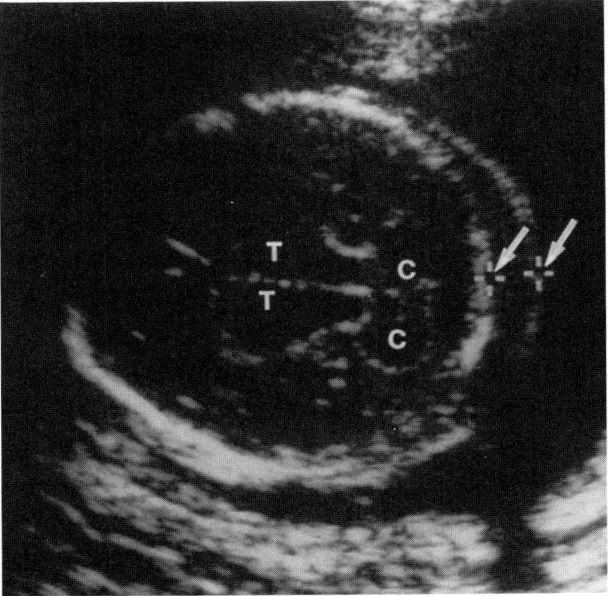

FIGURE 9-19. Nuchal thickening (Down's syndrome). Transverse view of the head in a second-trimester fetus with Down's syndrome. Note the thickened nuchal fold of 6.2 mm (*arrows*). (Benacerraf BR, et al: Prenatal sonographic diagnosis of congenital hemivertebra. J Ultrasound Med 1986; 5:257.)

TABLE 9-9.   Screening Criteria for Down Syndrome Detection

Method	Sensitivity (%)	False-Positive (%)	PPV
Maternal age ≥ 35[62]	20	5	1/110
Low MSAFP (general population)[63]	33	5	1/161
Nuchal skinfold:			
Crane and Gray (current study)	75	1	1/13
Benacerraf, et al.[60]	39	0.1	1/5.5
Perrella, et al.[61]	21	11	

PPV, positive predictive value; MSAFP, maternal serum α-fetoprotein.

(Crane JP, Gray DL: Sonographically measured nuchal skinfold thickness as a tool for Down syndrome: Results of a prospective clinical trial. Obstet Gynecol 1991; 77:533.)

with this abnormal soft tissue thickening whether diagnosed in the first or second trimester.

Iniencephaly

Iniencephaly is a malformation consisting of four features: (1) a defect of the occipital bone with accompanying enlarged foramen magnum, (2) partial or total absence of thoracic and cervical vertebrae, (3) significant shortening of the spine as a result of an extreme lordosis and hyperextension (retroflexion) of the malformed spinal column at the neck and thorax, and (4) an upturned face.[29] It is usually combined with a cervical neural tube defect and sometimes with fusion to the cranium. The resultant extreme cervical retroflexion, which may be fixed, gives affected infants their character-istic appearance. Iniencephaly is both rare and heterogeneous in terms of associated intracranial and skeletal anomalies. Sonographically, a diagnosis is based on an inability to locate the entire fetal spine on longitudinal scan in conjunction with visualization of the head when scanning the thorax transversely[30,31] (Fig. 9-20). Death usually occurs within hours of birth.

SPINE

The spine is composed of a series of bones that provide skeletal support to the body, and it houses a major portion of the central nervous system and the spinal cord (Fig. 9-21). To begin to approach

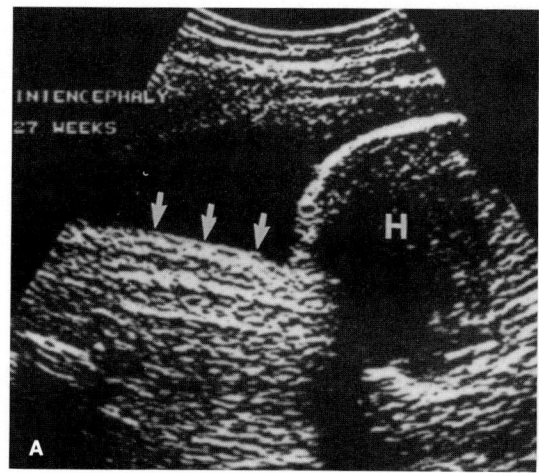
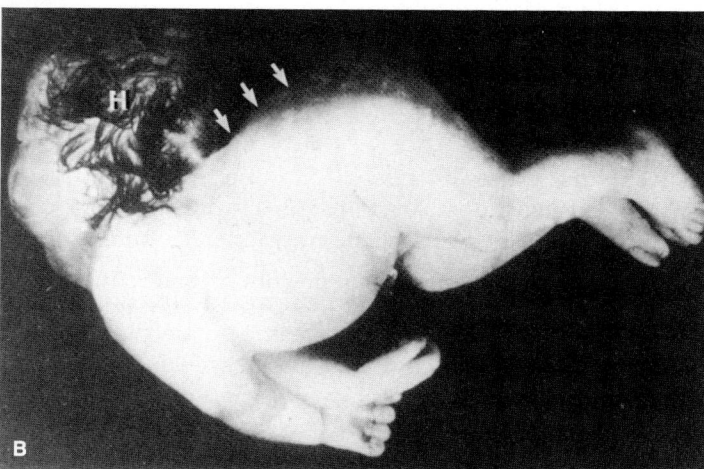

FIGURE 9-20.   Iniencephaly. **(A)** Ultrasound and **(B)** photograph of fetus with iniencephaly at 27 weeks' gestation. Retroflexion of the head (H) and the ingrown neck are clearly visible (arrows point to spine). (Hrgovic Z, Panitz A, Kurjak A, Jurkovic D: Contribution to the recognition of iniencephaly on the basis of a new case. J Perinat Med 1989; 17:375.)

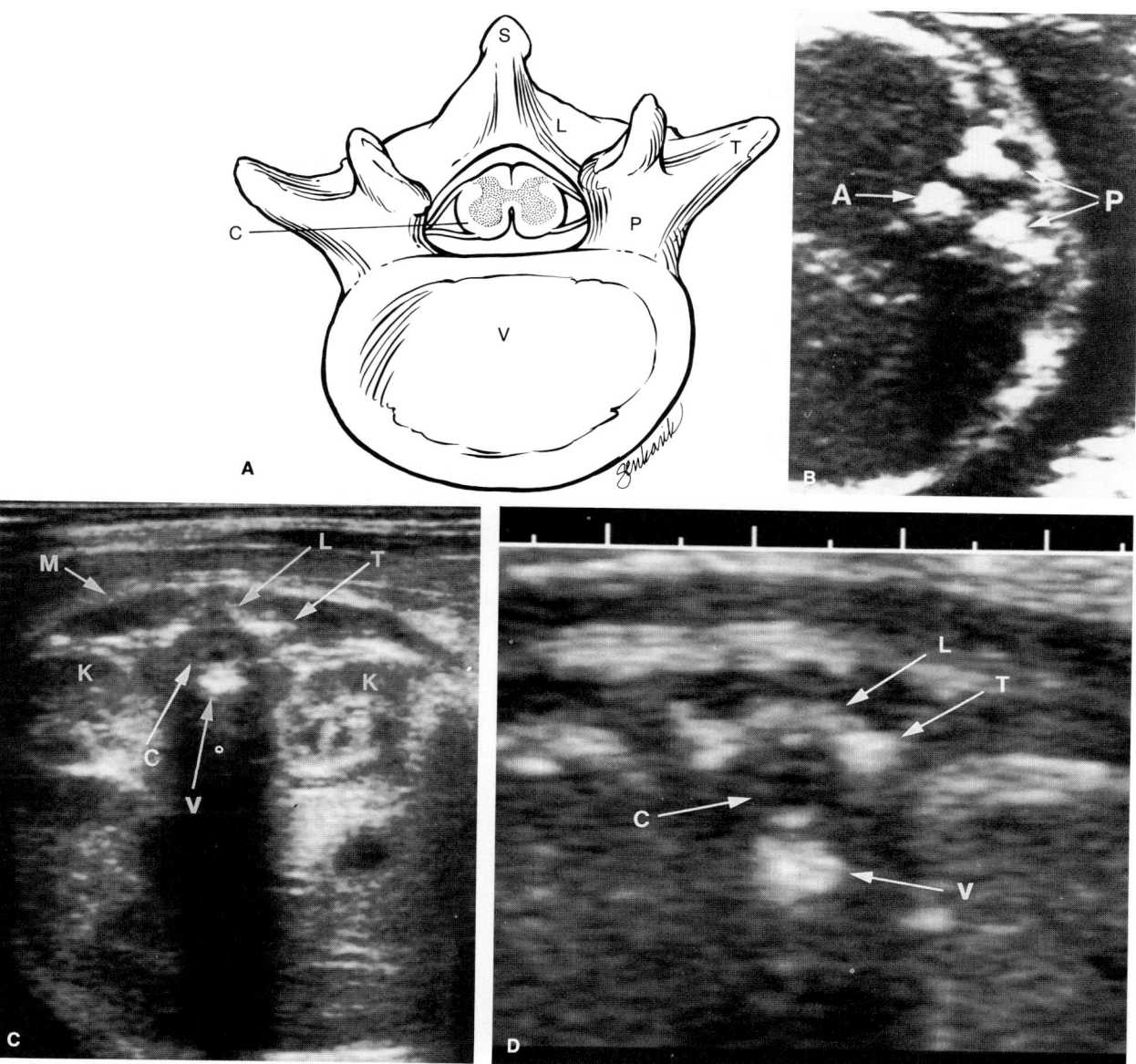

FIGURE 9-21. Normal transverse view of fetal spine. **(A)** Depiction of fetal vertebra. V, vertebral body; P, pedicle; L, lamina; T, transverse process; S, spinous processes; C, spinal cord. **(B)** Transverse sonogram of thoracic fetal spine at 18 weeks of gestation demonstrating two posterior (P) and one anterior (A) ossification centers. **(A, B,** Chervenak FA, Isaacson G, Lorber J: Anomalies of the Fetal Head, Neck, and Spine: Ultrasound Diagnosis and Management. Philadelphia: WB Saunders, 1988.) **(C)** Fetal abdominal ultrasound at 30 weeks demonstrating the anterior ossification center of vertebral body (V), the posterior ossification center in which the laminae (L) are converging posterior toward the midline. Also note the hypoechoic spinal cord (C). T, transverse process; M, paraspinal muscles; K, kidneys. **(D)** Magnified transverse ultrasound of the lumbar fetal spine at 30 weeks demonstrating posterior ossification centers from which the laminae (L) are converging toward the midline. Note the hypoechoic spinal cord (C). T, transverse process; V, vertebral body. **(C, D,** Courtesy of John P. McGahan, MD, Sacramento, CA.)

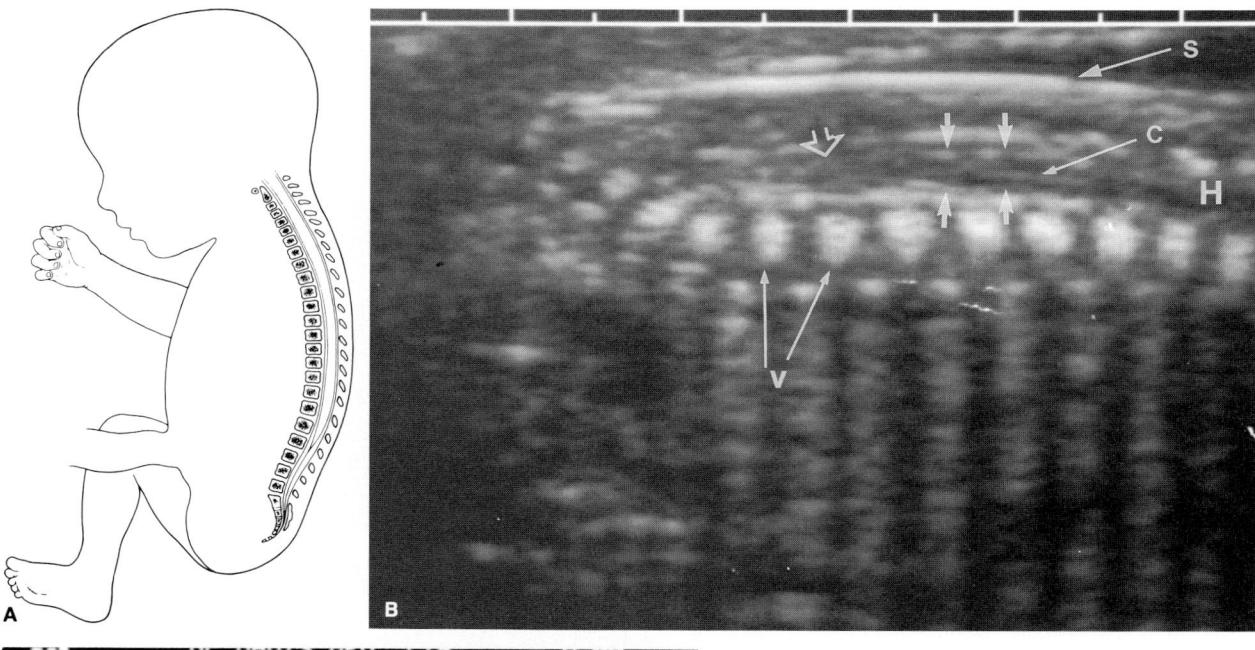

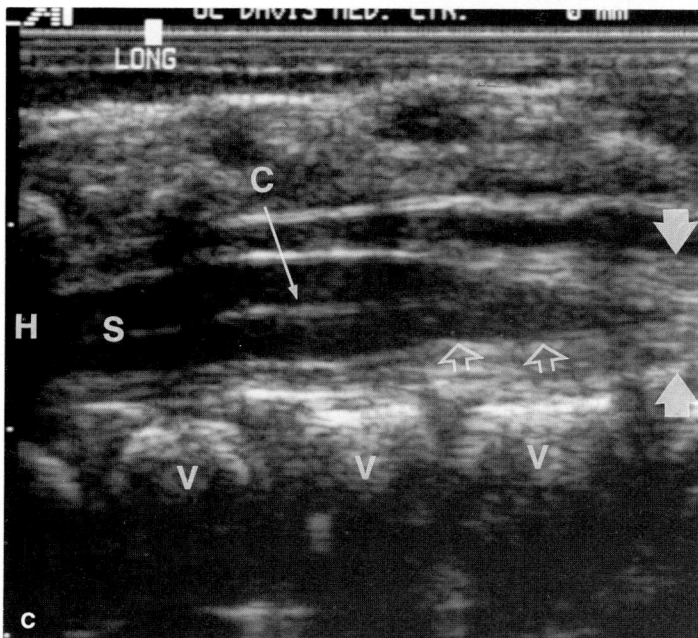

FIGURE 9-22. Normal sagittal spine. **(A)** Sagittal view of fetal spine demonstrating vertebral bodies and varying angles of spinous processes. (Chervenak FA, Isaacson G, Lorber J: Anomalies of the Fetal Head, Neck, and Spine: Ultrasound Diagnosis and Management. Philadelphia: WB Saunders, 1988.) **(B)** Longitudinal view of the spine of the 20-week fetus demonstrating echogenic vertebral bodies (V) and hypoechoic spinal cord (*arrows*), with echogenic central canal of the cord (C). Note the cord tapering to the region of the conus medullaris (*open arrows*). Note at this time the spinous process is not ossified in this true sagittal view, permitting visualization of the spinal cord. Also note echogenic lines forming the skin surface (S). H, toward the head of the fetus. **(C)** Longitudinal view of the spine of the newborn demonstrating hypoechoic spinal cord (S), which tapers in the region of the conus medullaris (*open arrows*), and the more echogenic spinal nerve roots noted distally (*closed arrows*). Also note vertebral bodies (V) and central canal of the cord (C). H, toward the head of the fetus. (**B, C,** Courtesy of John P. McGahan, MD, Sacramento, CA.)

anomalies of the spine in a systematic way requires an appreciation of the embryologic events leading to the formation of these structures.

Embryology

The neural tube is the basic embryologic structure that gives rise to the central nervous system. It arises from an infolding of the neural plate, a midline thickening of ectoderm, during the third week of intrauterine life. This infolding, or *neurulation,* starts from the region of the fourth somite (the center of the plate) and proceeds both rostrally and caudally. The rostral end of the tube (anterior neuropore) closes on or about day 23 of embryonic life. The caudal end of the tube (posterior neuropore) closes on or about day 28. If this process is interrupted, defects may occur in both the lumbosacral

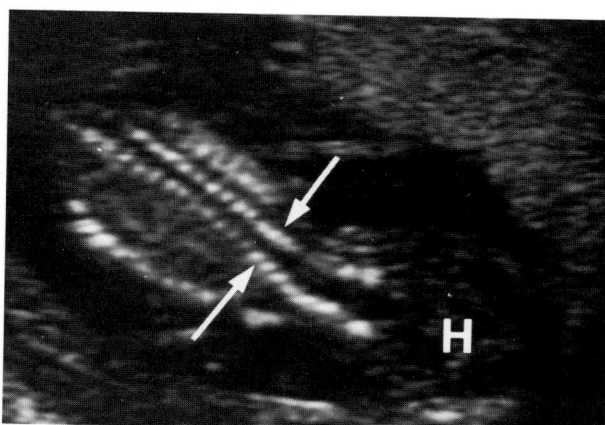

FIGURE 9-23. Normal cervical widening. Coronal sonogram of fetal spine at 13 weeks of gestation demonstrating normal cervical widening (*arrows*) of posterior ossification centers. H, head. (Chervenak FA, Isaacson G, Lorber J: Anomalies of the Fetal Head, Neck, and Spine: Ultrasound Diagnosis and Management. Philadelphia: WB Saunders, 1988.)

and cranial ends of the neural tube, thus explaining the association of cephalocele and anencephaly with spina bifida.

Normal Anatomy

To differentiate small defects in the spine from normal anatomic features, it is important to appreciate the variability in the shapes of the vertebral bodies and the changing sonographic appearance of the spine during gestation. By 16 weeks of gestation, individual vertebrae may be identified sonographically by the observation of their echogenic ossification centers in the transverse plane (see Fig. 9-21). Two of these are posterior to the spinal canal in the laminae, and one is anterior, representing the vertebral body (see Fig. 9-21).

During the third trimester, the vertebral body, pedicles, transverse processes, laminae, and spinous processes may all be identified as echogenic structures in transverse scans (see Fig. 9-21). The spinal canal and intervertebral foramina may be seen as nonechogenic areas. In the sagittal plane, the posterior aspects of the vertebral bodies become more complex. The cord is hypoechoic, and the central canal of the spinal canal can be identified with careful scanning (Fig. 9-22).

A systemic approach to sonographic examination of the spinal region is necessary to reveal the numerous possible abnormalities in this complex region. To avoid distortions in the spinal anatomy,

a continuous scanning of the entire spine in both transverse and sagittal planes is essential.

Pitfalls

Pseudosplaying of the Cervical Spine
In the coronal plane, the two rows of echogenic posterior ossification centers are seen to diverge progressively in both the cervical and lumbar regions. This is especially pronounced close to the base of the skull and should not be misinterpreted as a spinal dysraphism (Fig. 9-23).

Off-Axis Sagittal Scans
Scanned sagittally (longitudinally), a parallel line of vertebral bodies may be identified anterior to the nonechogenic spinal canal. In the second trimester of pregnancy, the posterior elements are not identified if scanned in a true sagittal plane because the spinous process is incompletely ossified. The posterior elements are identified only if there is angulation of the sagittal image through the two posterior ossification centers (Figs. 9-22 and 9-24). A small spinal defect may be missed when scanning in an off-axis rather than a true sagittal plane.

Pseudodysraphism of the Lumbosacral Spine
Possible pitfalls encountered when scanning the fetal spine include incorrect assessment of fetal position and errors in maintaining the proper scanning angle. Oblique transverse angulation of the ultrasound transducer creates a plane in which the anterior vertebral elements are included but posterior elements are missed, thus simulating spina bifida.[32] This reemphasizes the import of maintaining a true transverse orientation along the normal curvature of the spine.

Incomplete Ossification
Early in the pregnancy, especially the early second trimester, the ossification of the lateral masses occurs first in the region of the laminae. Later ossification progresses both anteriorly toward the pedicle and posteriorly toward the spinous process. Early scanning reveals incomplete ossification of the lateral masses, which may appear parallel rather than converging posteriorly; this may be erroneously misinterpreted as spinal dysraphism.

Open Neural Tube Defects
Small, flat, or cystic open neural tube defects may be easily missed when scanning in the early sec-

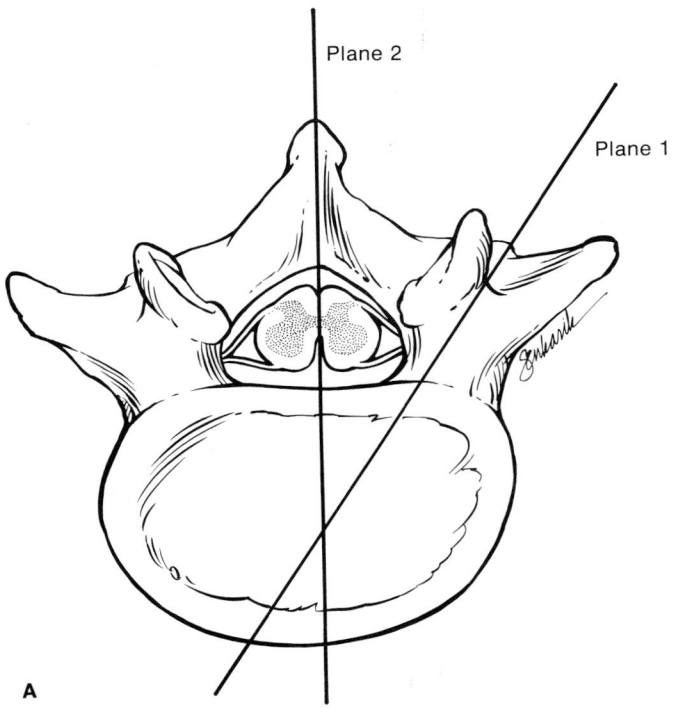

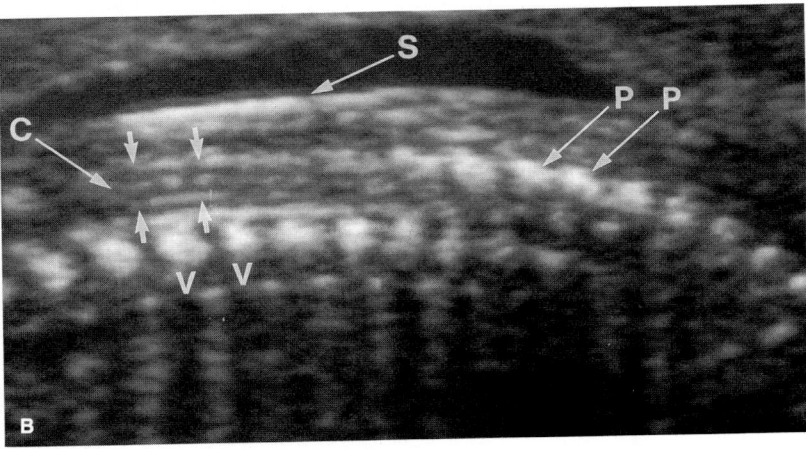

FIGURE 9-24. Oblique versus true sagittal scan plane. **(A)** Diagram demonstrating true sagittal plane (2) versus oblique sagittal plane (1) in which scanning through both the vertebral body and the lateral echogenic masses is obtained. **(B)** Ultrasound of the thoracic and lumbar spine demonstrating using oblique sagittal plane in the thoracic spine. The posterior ossification centers (P) obscure visualization of the spinal cord. Scanning at a true sagittal plane in the lumbar spine allows better visualization of the spinal cord (*arrows*) and central canal of cord (C). V, vertebral body; S, skin surface. (Courtesy of John P. McGahan, MD, Sacramento, CA.)

ond trimester (Figs. 9-25 and 9-26). Sagittal and meticulous transverse imaging is needed with optimally focused transducers to evaluate if the posterior ossification centers are diverging rather than converging toward the midline. Rescanning of the spine may be necessary in certain cases if ultrasound examination is obtained early in the first trimester of pregnancy. More important, recognition of such signs of Arnold-Chiari type II malformation, including the lemon sign or banana sign, is helpful.[33]

Spinal Abnormalities

The differential diagnosis for spinal curvature is presented in Table 9-10. This is a partial list of causes of abnormal spinal curvature but should include spinal dysraphism, amniotic band syndrome, and limb–body–wall complex, to name a few. It is also plausible that such anomalies as isolated hemivertebra may be missed in utero; therefore, their true incidence may be higher than is reflected in this table.

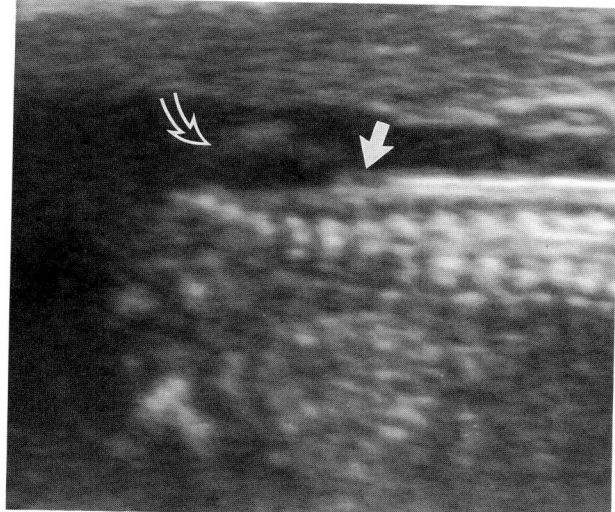

FIGURE 9-25. Cystic open neural tube defect. A potential limitation of scanning in the longitudinal plane is the cystic appearance of an open neural tube defect (*open arrow*). It may be difficult on longitudinal images to visualize a cystic open neural tube defect; however, disruption of the skin line (*closed arrow*) and transverse images would show separation of the lateral masses of the lumbosacral spine. (Courtesy of John P. McGahan, MD, Sacramento, CA.)

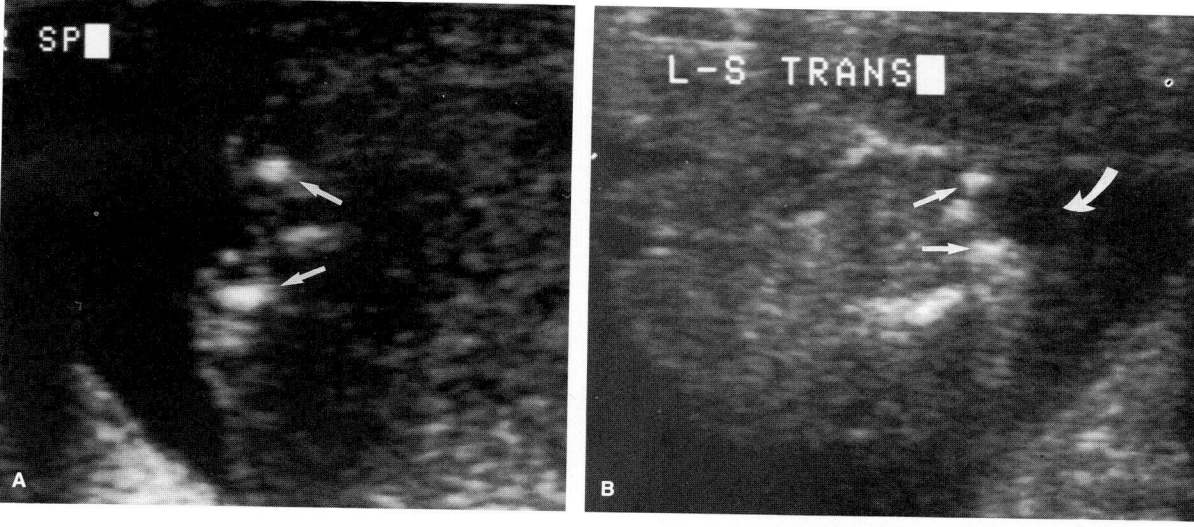

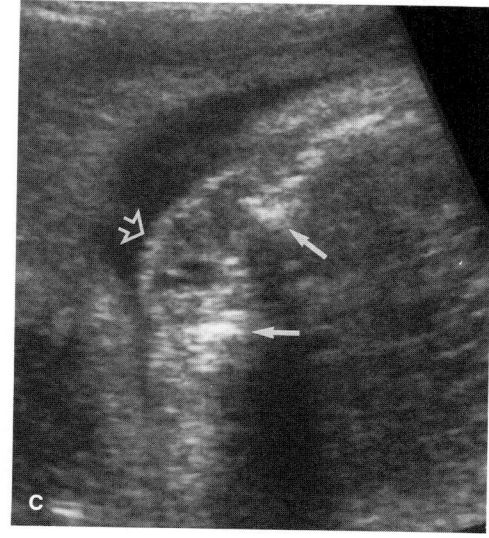

FIGURE 9-26. Variable appearance of open neural tube defects. Open neural tube defects may have a variety of appearances on ultrasound. These transverse views of the lumbar sacral spine show they may be **(A)** flat, contain a sac that may be **(B)** cystic (*curved arrow*), or **(C)** complex (*open arrow*), depending on the amount of neural elements herniated into the sac. *Straight arrows* point to the splayed posterior ossification centers. (Courtesy John P. McGahan, MD, Sacramento, CA.)

TABLE 9-10. Diagnoses in Fetuses With Abnormal Spinal Curvature

Diagnosis	Number (n = 20)
Neural tube defect	12
Myelomeningocele	6
Frontal encephalocele with ectrodactyly	1
Exencephaly	1
Anencephaly	1
Anencephaly with trisomy 18	1
Iniencephaly	1
Craniorachischisis	1
Limb–body–wall complex (LBWC)	2
Amniotic band syndrome (ABS)	1
Multiple congenital anomalies, likely LBWC or ABS	2
Caudal regression syndrome	1
Thoracic dysplasia with multiple anomalies	1
Hemivertebrae, no other anomalies	1

(Harrison LA, Pretorius DH, Budorick NE: Abnormal spinal curvature in the fetus. J Ultrasound Med 1992; 11:473.)

The differential diagnosis for lumbosacral mass is given in Table 9-11. Most commonly, these masses are open neural tube defects, but they may include a symmetric defect such as amniotic band syndrome or limb–body–wall complex. Early tumors, such as sacrococcygeal teratomas or other tumors, may occur in this region.

Spina Bifida Aperta

Spina bifida is a general term used to describe the open forms of spinal dysraphism that result from failure of closure of the posterior neuropore. *Aperta* is derived from the Latin, meaning *open*. Spina bifida is the most common malformation of cranial and spinal dysraphism (Table 9-12). The incidence of spina bifida varies greatly, and it has long been recognized as one of the most common congenital malformation in the Western world. With an incidence ranging from 0.3 per 1000 births in Japan to more than 4 to 8 per 1000 births in parts of Great Britain, the average incidence of spina bifida in the United States is about 0.5 to 2 per 1000 births.[34,35] Incidence also varies depending on specific risk factors, as shown in Table 9-13.

Meningoceles are cystic lesions that result from protrusion of the dura and arachnoid through the spinal defect (see Fig. 9-25). They usually occur at the upper and lower ends of the neural axis (ie, occipital, cervical, upper thoracic, and low sacral positions). In contrast, meningomyeloceles (or myelomeningoceles) contain abnormal central nervous system tissue (ie, a malformed, maldeveloped spinal cord) in the defect. These lesions are usually large and covered by a *neural plaque* composed of a membrane of meningeal origin and mal-

TABLE 9-11. Typical Lumbosacral Masses and Associated Ultrasound Features

Type	Abnormality	Ultrasound Features
Common	Open neural tube defects	Symmetric cystic complex or solid mass in the lumbosacral region
		Associated with cranial defect and lemon or banana sign
Uncommon	Amniotic band syndrome	Asymmetric defect with scoliosis
		Cystic to complex mass
		Associated amputational defects
	Limb–body–wall complex	Limb–body–wall complex
		Similar to amniotic band syndrome
		Plus fetus in continuity with placental surface
	Sacrococcygeal teratoma	Usually solid mass from buttocks
		Often intrapelvic components
		Rarely a cystic mass
Rare	Tumors	Rare tumors, such as lipomas, which are echogenic, or other neural or cutaneous tumors
		Ultrasound appearance depending on tumor type

TABLE 9-12. Classification of Cranial and Spinal Dysraphism

Spina bifida aperta
  Myeloschisis
  Myelomeningocele
  Hemimyelomeningocele
  Syringomyelomeningocele
  Spinal meningocele
Arnold-Chiari malformation
Dandy-Walker malformation
Cranium bifidum
  Cranial meningocele
  Encephalomeningocele
Occult cranial dysraphism
  Cranial dermal sinus
Occult spinal dysraphism
  Spinal dermal sinus
  Tethered cord syndrome
  Lumbosacral lipoma
  Diastematomyelia
  Neurenteric cyst
  Combined anterior and posterior spina bifida
  Anterior sacral meningocele
  Occult intrasacral meningocele
Nondysraphic malformations
  Perineurial (Tarlov's) cyst
  Spinal extradural cyst
  Nondysraphic spinal meningocele
  Caudal regression syndrome
  Sacrococcygeal teratoma

(Youmans JR: Neurological Surgery. Philadelphia: WB Saunders, 1982: 1082.)

formed spinal cord substance. Meningomyeloceles typically occupy the lower thoracolumbar, lumbar, and lumbosacral areas. They typically are single and only rarely are multiple.

Ultrasound Findings. Sonographically, spina bifida is seen as a splaying of the posterior ossification centers of the spine, giving the vertebra a U-shaped appearance instead of the normal triangular appearance (Fig. 9-27). The posterior ossification centers in a defective vertebra should be more widely spaced than those in vertebrae above and below the defect. Although spina bifida may be visualized on longitudinal scanning, meticulous transverse examination of the entire vertebral ossification centers is necessary to detect smaller defects.

Associated anomalies include the Arnold-Chiari malformation. Chiari originally described three types of this malformation. The most common type detected in utero is the type II malformation. This includes hindbrain anomalies with displacement of the inferior cerebellar vermis into the upper cervical canal and caudal dislocation of the medulla and the fourth ventricle. This is probably caused by tension due to the spinal dysraphism and resulting in the spinal cord pulling the cerebellum and the medulla caudally. Most of these cases have accompanying hydrocephalus.[33] Nicolaides and colleagues have described two characteristic sonographic signs due to the Arnold-Chiari malformation (see Fig. 9-27). A scalloping of the frontal bones gives a lemon-like configuration to the skull of an affected fetus in axial section during the second trimester (the lemon sign). The caudal displacement of the cranial contents within a pliable skull is thought to produce this scalloping effect. Similarly, as the cerebellar hemispheres are displaced into the cervical canal, they are flattened rostrocaudally, and the cisternal magna is obliterated. This produces a flattened, centrally curved,

TABLE 9-13. Estimated Incidence of Neural Tube Defects Based on Specific Risk Factors in the United States

Population	Incidence per 1000 Live Births
Mother as Reference	
General incidence	1.4–1.6
Women undergoing amniocentesis for advanced maternal age	1.5–3
Women with diabetes mellitus	20
Women on valproic acid in first trimester	10–20
Fetus as Reference	
One sibling with NTD	15–30
Two siblings with NTD*	57
Parent with NTD	11
Half sibling with NTD	8
First cousin (mother's sister's child)	10
Other first cousins	3
Sibling with severe scoliosis secondary to multiple vertebral defects	15–30
Sibling with occult spinal dysraphism	15–30
Sibling with sacrococcygeal teratoma or hamartoma	≤ 15–30

* Risk is higher in British studies. Risk increases further for three or more siblings or combinations of other close relatives.

NTD, neural tube defect.

(Main DM, Mennuti MT: Neural tube defects: Issues in prenatal diagnosis and counseling. Obstet Gynecol 1986; 67:1.)

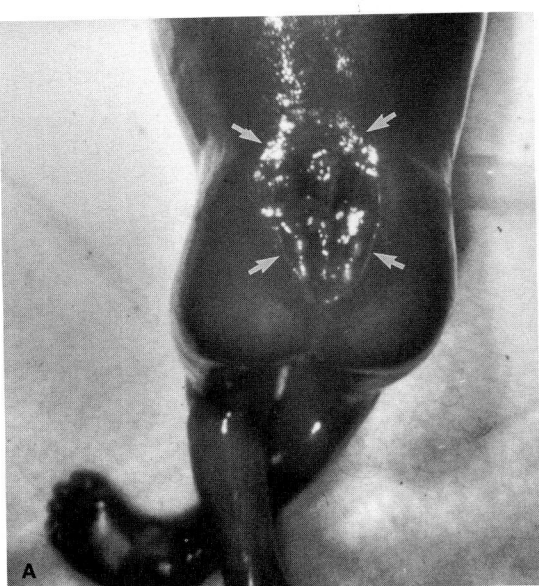
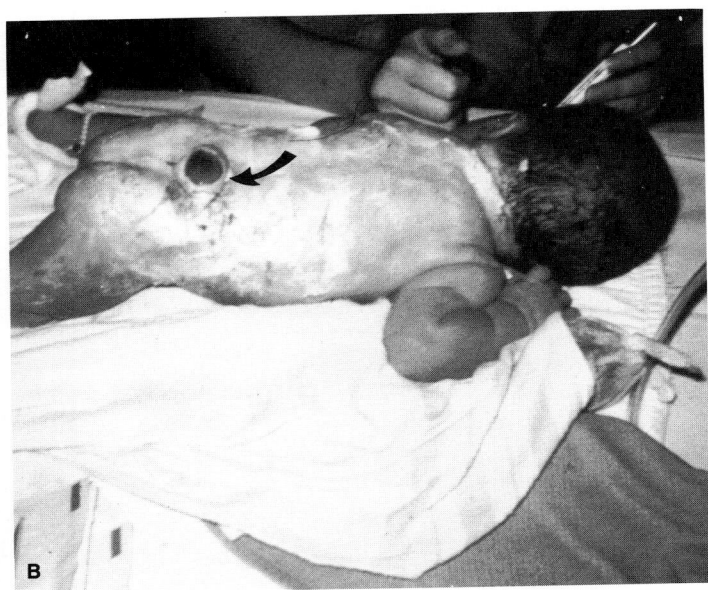

FIGURE 9-27. Variable appearance of open neural tube defects. **(A)** Large, flat, open spina bifida (*arrows*) found as a result of α-fetoprotein screening. **(B)** Meningomyelocele sac bulges from the lumbosacral region (*curved arrow*) in this neonate. (Chervenak FA, Isaacson G, Lorber J: Anomalies of the Fetal Head, Neck, and Spine: Ultrasound Diagnosis and Management. Philadelphia: WB Saunders, 1988.)

banana-like sonographic appearance (the banana sign; Table 9-14). These signs are also discussed in Chapter 8.

Prognosis. The prognosis in any case of spina bifida depends on a number of factors. Most important are the presence or absence of neural tissue in the meningeal sac and the spinal level and extent of the lesion (ie, number of neural arches involved). Lower-extremity paralysis and incontinence of bowel and bladder are common, and intelligence may be affected.[38,39] The survivors of this disorder have significant multiple and permanent handicaps relating to almost every system in the body. Early closure of defects, ventriculoperitoneal or ventriculoatrial shunting of hydrocephalus, and management and biofeedback techniques are partly responsible for recent improvement in these patients.[40] In contrast, a simple meningocele (constituting only 5% of the total cases of spina bifida) carries a better prognosis.

If a meningomyelocele is diagnosed in the third trimester, fetal surveillance consists of heart rate monitoring and serial sonography to assess fetal growth, head size, and severity of hydrocephalus. Ventriculoamniotic shunting does not alter long-term outcome and is not recommended.[41] In view of the potential dangers and the lack of clinical data demonstrating that vaginal delivery of the infant with a meningomyelocele can be nontraumatic, elective cesarean section before the onset of labor should be offered to the parents as a potentially beneficial procedure[42] (Fig. 9-28).

Diastematomyelia

Diastematomyelia is a splitting of the spinal cord into halves, usually by a bony spicule or fibrous band in an area of spina bifida. This defect may be covered by intact skin.[43]

Ultrasound demonstrates broadening of the lateral masses of the spine (Fig. 9-29). The point of greatest diastasis may be identified in the images of the double vertebral column, and this confirms the diagnosis. When diastematomyelia presents as a closed neural tube defect, the prognosis for neurologic function may be enhanced by early surgical removal of the septum dividing the spinal cord.[43]

Lipomyelomeningocele

Lipomyelomeningocele (intraspinal lipoma) is a histologically benign fatty tumor associated with occult spina bifida. The fatty tissue often originates in the spinal cord or cauda equina and is covered with skin. It is nearly always asymmetric.[44]

In a report by Seeds and Jones, the lesion appeared sonographically as a discrete echogenic

TABLE 9-14.   Frequencies of Cranial Signs Compared With Those in Other Reports With Open Neural Tube Defects*

Investigation	Lemon Sign	Cerebellar Abnormalities	Microcephaly	Ventriculomegaly
16–24 Weeks of Gestation				
Nicolaides, et al.[33]	54/54 (100%)	21/20 (95%)	70/53 (62%)	66/57 (86%)
Campbell et al.[65]	26/26 (100%)	26/25 (95%)	26/17 (65%)	26/14 (54%)
Penso, et al.[66]	13/13 (100%)			
Nyberg, et al.[64]				
Retrospective	13/11 (85%)			
Prospective	14/13 (93%)			
Thiagarajah, et al. (current study)	16/16 (100%)	16/16 (100%)	16/11 (69%)	16/10 (63%)
> 24 Weeks of Gestation				
Penso, et al.[66]	11/3 (27%)			
Nyberg, et al.[64]				
Retrospective	18/6 (33%)			
Prospective	5/2 (40%)			
Thiagarajah, et al. (current study)	8/2 (25%)	6†/6 (100%)	8/8 (100%)	8/6 (75%)

* Data are presented as number of cases/number with abnormalities (%).

† The cerebellum could not be visualized adequately in two fetuses.

(Thiagarajah S, et al: Early diagnosis of spina bifida: The value of cranial ultrasound markers. Obstet Gynecol 1990; 76:54.)

mass without structural organization in an area of spina bifida occulta.[45] A subsequent report by Seeds and Powers described and illustrated the early prenatal diagnosis of a familial recurrence of congenital lipomyelomeningocele.[46] Longitudinal

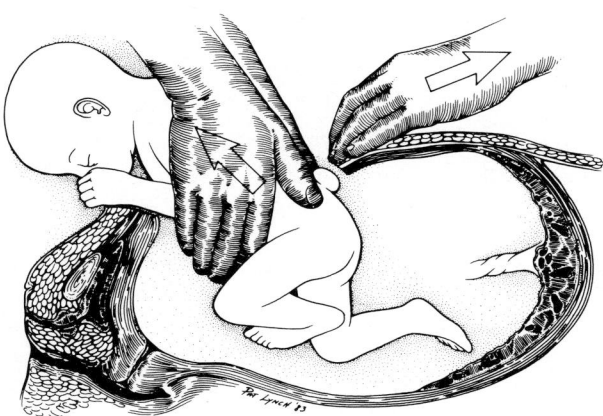

FIGURE 9-28.   C-section for meningomyelocele. Fetus with meningomyelocele as delivered through low transverse uterine incision. Both fetal flanks are grasped, and gentle traction is applied in an outward direction. Assistant retracts edge of uterine incision as body is delivered. (Chervenak FA, Isaacson G, Mahoney MJ, et al: Perinatal management of meningomyelocele. Obstet Gynecol 1984; 63:376.)

and transverse views of the fetal spine detect a deviation from normal in the lumbosacral area at 17 weeks of gestation. Ultrasound images further define a small, echogenic lumbosacral mass (Fig. 9-30).

Early diagnosis and early resection, with untethering of the cord, remain the principles of management. Because the defect is typically covered, vaginal delivery has been suggested, but because the ability to discriminate open and closed neural tube defects by ultrasonography has not been demonstrated, we advise a more conservative approach with elective cesarean delivery at term.

Sacrococcygeal Teratoma

Sacrococcygeal teratomas are tumors that arise from pluripotential embryonic cells of the coccyx and that may mimic a spinal defect. Considered to be the most commonly occurring tumor among neonates, they are reported in 1 in 35,000 births, with about 75% occurring in girls.[47] Four types of sacrococcygeal teratomas are recognized; types 3 and 4 have the highest incidence of malignancy (Figs. 9-31 through 9-33). Most tumors are benign at birth, and the incidence of malignancy increases with increasing age.[48]

(*text continues on page 200*)

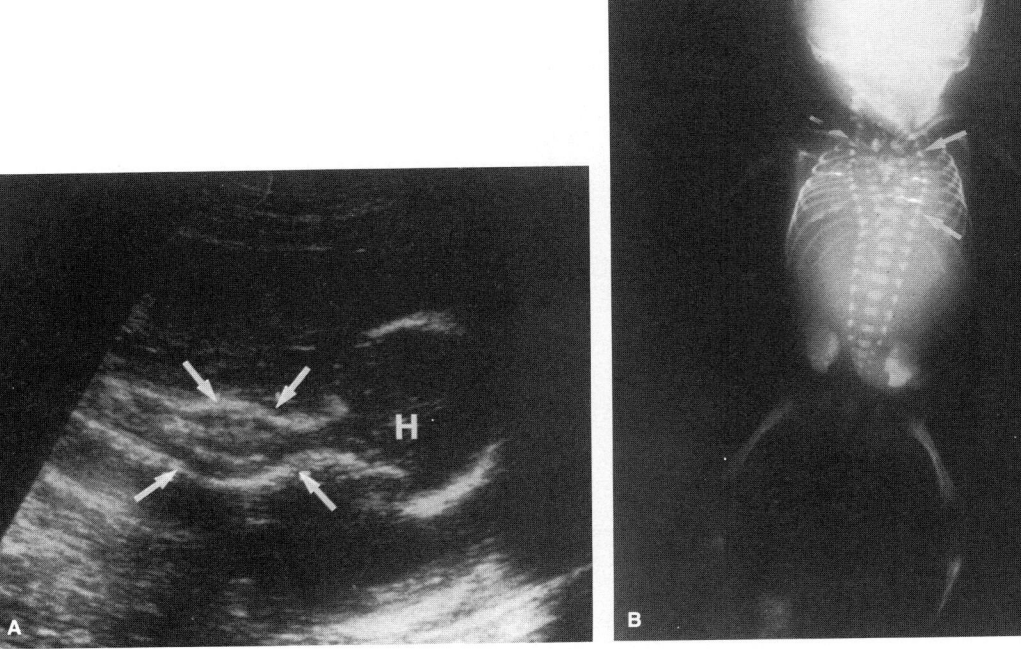

FIGURE 9-29. Diastasis of thoracic spine. **(A)** Longitudinal scan at the level of the vertebral column with diastasis of the bony structures (*arrows*) and a central hypoechogenic area (crest of separation). H, fetal head. **(B)** Radiograph showing uniform vertebral thoracic somatoschisis (*arrows*). (Pachi A, et al: Prenatal sonographic diagnosis of diastematomyelia in a diabetic woman. Prenat Diagn 1992; 12:535.)

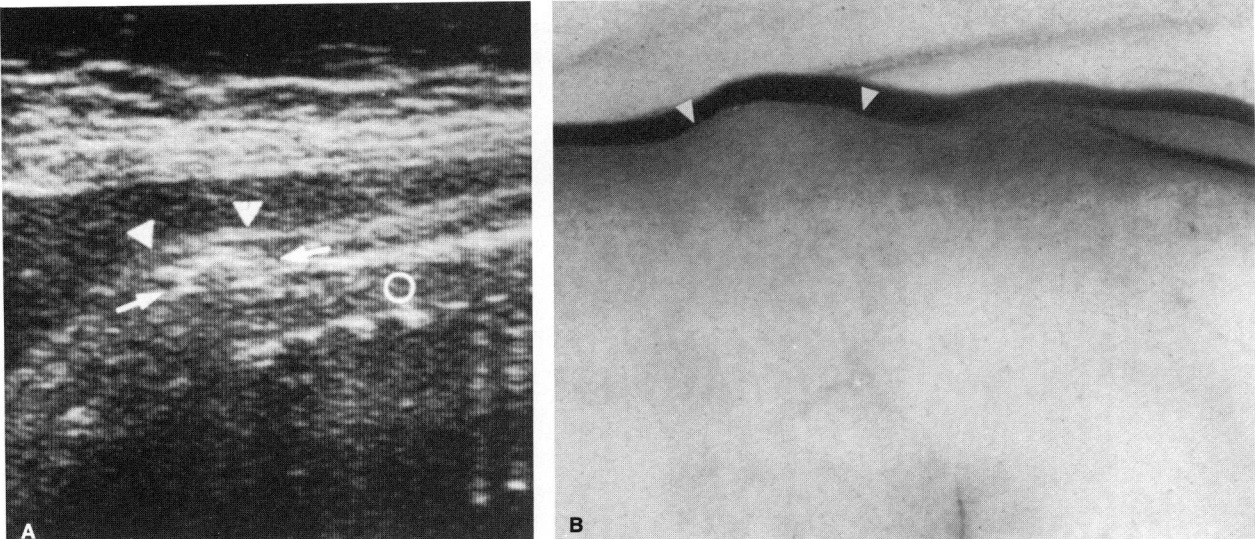

FIGURE 9-30. Lipoma of the spine. **(A)** Longitudinal view of the fetal spine demonstrates an echogenic mass (*arrows*) corresponding to a lipoma, which is a nonshadowing mass dorsal to the spinal canal (*circle*) and below the skin surface (*arrowheads*). **(B)** After birth, a small mass was skin-covered and spongy but not fluctuant (*arrowheads*). (Seeds JW, Powers SK: Early prenatal diagnosis of familial lipomyelomeningocele. Obstet Gynecol 1988; 72:469.)

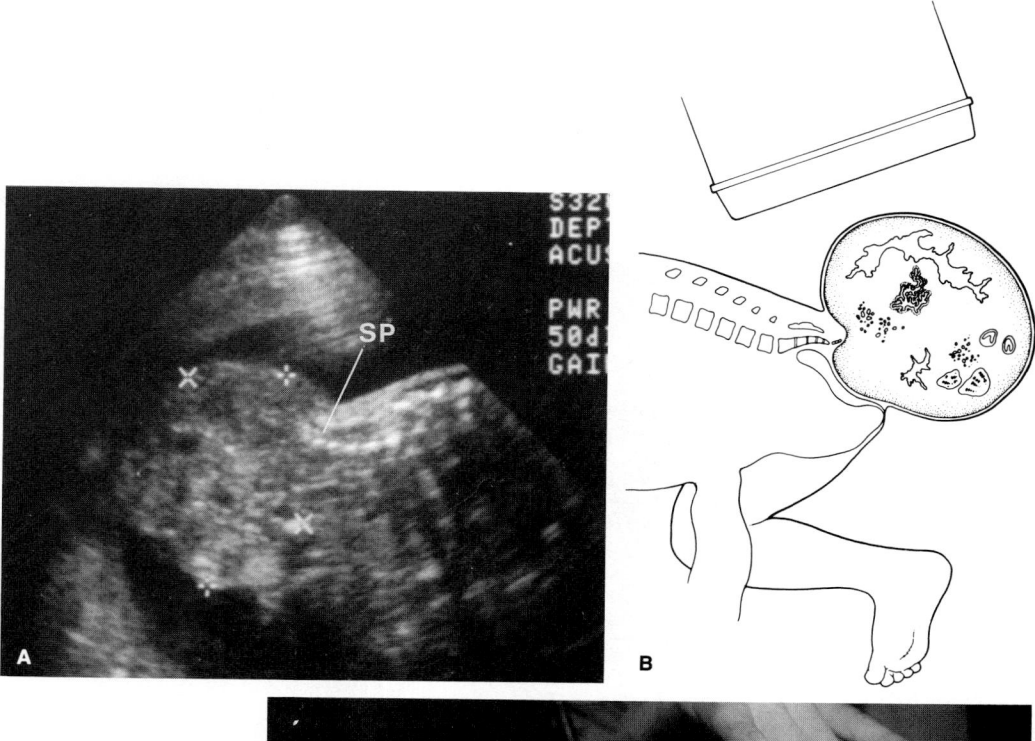

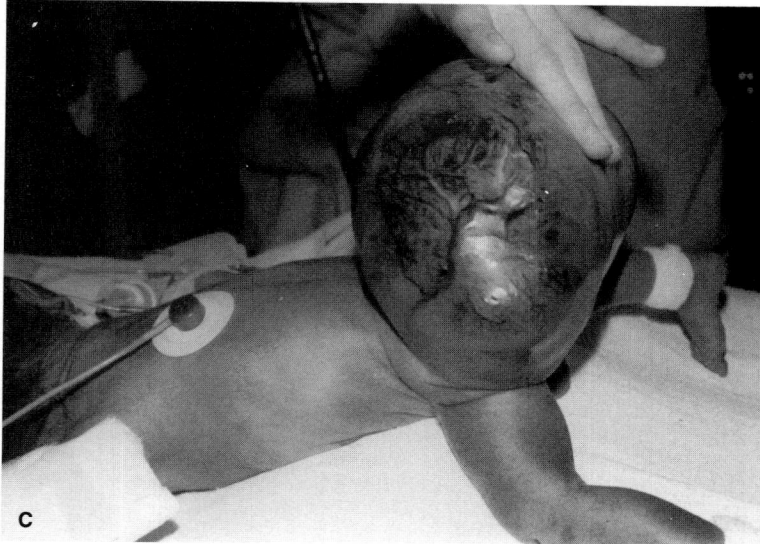

FIGURE 9-31. Sacrococcygeal teratomas. **(A)** Sacrococcygeal teratomas outlined by calipers. SP, spine. **(B)** Fetal sacrococcygeal teratoma. (Chervenak FA, Isaacson G, Lorber J: Anomalies of the Fetal Head, Neck, and Spine: Ultrasound Diagnosis and Management. Philadelphia: WB Saunders, 1988.) **(C)** Neonate with sacrococcygeal teratoma. (Chervenak FA, et al: Diagnosis and management of fetal teratomas. Obstet Gynecol 1985; 66:666.)

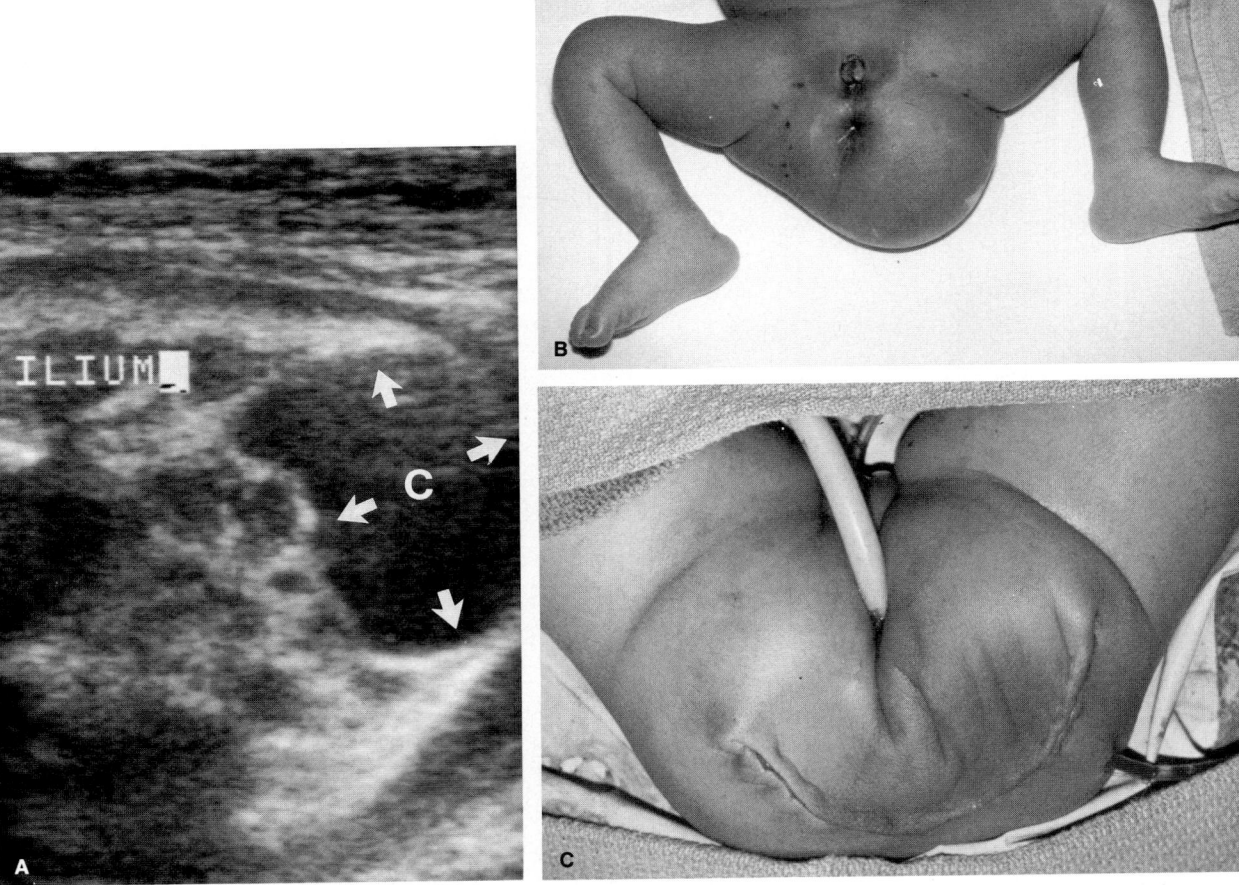

FIGURE 9-32. Cystic sacrococcygeal teratoma. **(A)** Axial scan through the sacrum demonstrates splaying of the sacral elements and a large cystic (C) mass protruding posterior in the midline. (Courtesy of John P. McGahan, MD, Sacramento, CA.) **(B)** Preoperative photograph shows cystic sacrococcygeal teratoma. Part of the cystic mass protruded from inside the fetal pelvis. (Courtesy of Marshall Schwartz, MD, Washington, DC.) **(C)** Postoperative image with rectal tube demonstrates a good cosmetic result after resection of the sacrococcygeal teratoma. (Courtesy of Marshall Schwartz, MD, Washington, DC.)

Sonographically, most sacrococcygeal teratomas are solid or mixed, and only 15% are entirely cystic. The solid areas are composed of tissues of different density (eg, cartilage and liver) and may also include calcific areas of tooth and bone. The cystic components, which frequently have irregular and angular borders, are formed by cavities lined with neural, respiratory, gastrointestinal, and squamous epithelium (see Fig. 9-32).

Anomalies, especially of the musculoskeletal, renal, and nervous systems, have been reported in association with 18% of sacrococcygeal teratomas in newborns. Hydrops, polyhydramnios, and placentomegaly are also commonly associated findings.

Obstetrical management should include elective cesarean delivery after fetal lung maturity has been established to avoid trauma to the mass or dystocia.[49] Aspiration of cystic fluid late in pregnancy to allow vaginal delivery has been reported when the size of the mass exceeded the pelvic capacity.[50] It is advisable that delivery occur in a perinatal center where expert surgical therapy can be started immediately after delivery because delay in surgical

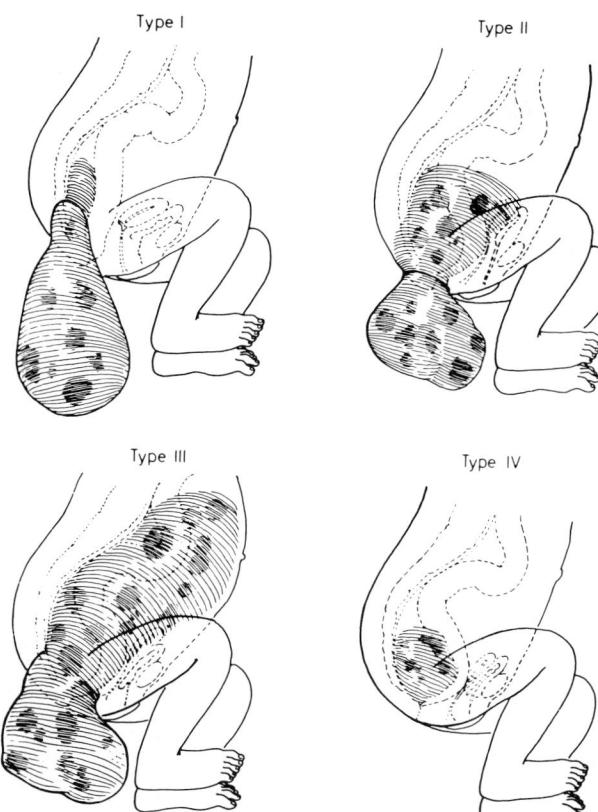

Type I   Type II

Type III   Type IV

FIGURE 9-33. Types of sacrococcygeal teratomas. Sacrococcygeal teratomas may be nearly entirely external or combined internal and external or, as in type III, mainly internal. Those that are mainly external are less commonly malignant; whereas type IV tumors, which are mainly internal, usually have a delayed diagnosis and often are malignant. (Altman RP, et al: Sacrococcygeal teratoma. American Academy of Pediatrics Surgical Section Survey, 1973.)

management can lead to malignant degeneration, pressure necrosis, infection, and hemorrhage in the tumor.[49]

Scoliosis

In its simplest form, scoliosis is a lateral curvature of the spinal column of any cause (see Table 9-10). In the newborn, scoliosis is almost always due to congenital hemivertebra. It is commonly associated with meningomyelocele, but the hemivertebra may be well away from the spina bifida lesion itself (eg, scoliosis of the upper thoracic area with a lumbosacral meningomyelocele).

The fetal skeleton is flexible and subject to strong deformation forces within the uterus. Therefore, the pathologic diagnosis of scoliosis should be made with caution. When gross skeletal defects, including absent ribs or hemivertebra, are detected, associated lateral spinal deflection probably represents true scoliosis.[51] In the absence of such defects, bends in the vertebral column should reach the extreme of 90 degrees and should be demonstrated in serial scans as unchanging before the diagnosis of scoliosis is made (Figs. 9-34 through 9-37).

Fetal scoliosis is associated with a number of congenital abnormalities. In addition to the diagnoses identified in Table 9-10, scoliosis may occur as an isolated defect due to vertebral abnormalities, secondary to arthrogryposis, skeletal dysplasia, and the VACTERL association.[52]

The prognosis for the fetus with abnormal spinal curvature generally is determined from the prognosis of the underlying malformation and is usually poor. Hypoplastic thorax with chest restriction may lead to pulmonary hypoplasia and is a leading cause of death.[53] There is a high frequency of stillborn fetuses and neonatal deaths.

Hemivertebra

During the first trimester, the vertebral body forms from parallel right and left chondrification centers. These centers coalesce during the second fetal month. Aplasia or hydroplasia of one of the two chondrification centers is thought to be the principal cause of hemivertebra.

Sonographically, a hemivertebra may be identified by lateral displacement of the anterior ossification center from the straight-line arrangement of the other anterior ossification centers with or without apparent scoliosis[54,55] (see Fig. 9-36).

Hemivertebra may occur as an isolated entity but may be associated with neural tube defects as well as VATER or VACTERL associations[56] (see Fig. 9-37). A careful study of posterior elements in three perpendicular planes is required before this relatively benign disorder is diagnosed. Amniocentesis for α-fetoprotein and acetylcholinesterase determination should be considered in the search for small neural tube defects.

Although isolated congenital hemivertebra is not a life-threatening malformation, the prenatal diagnosis of this abnormality should raise the index of suspicion for other congenital defects and for orthopedic complications of vertebral body malformations in childhood. Severe scoliosis or kyphoscoliosis can develop later in childhood; therefore, the pediatrician should be alerted to watch for early signs of problems.

A number of other abnormalities of ossification

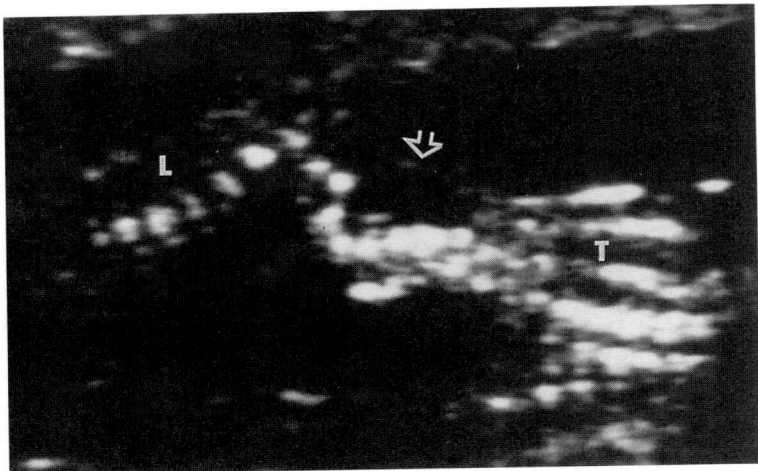

FIGURE 9-34. Amniotic band syndrome. Longitudinal scan of the fetal spine at 19 weeks' gestation showing marked disruption of the spine with kyphoscoliosis involving the thoracolumbar region. A thoracolumbar meningocele (*open arrow*) was also diagnosed. T, upper thoracic vertebra; L, lumbar vertebra. (Harrison LA, Pretorius DH, Budorick NE: Abnormal spinal curvature in the fetus. J Ultrasound Med 1992; 11:473.)

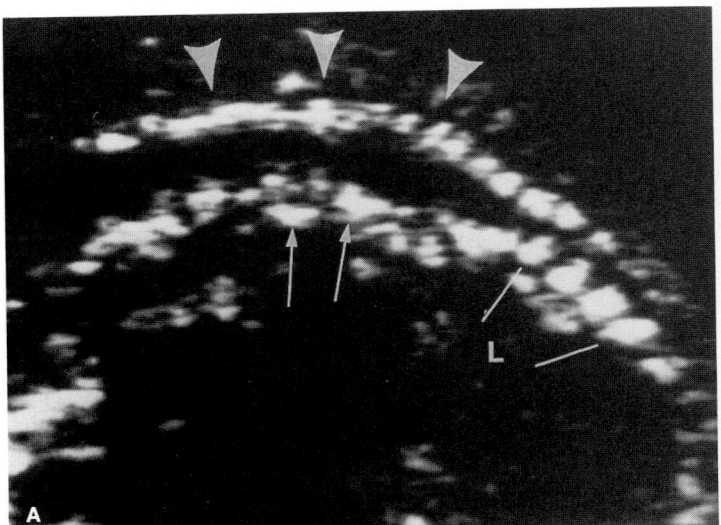

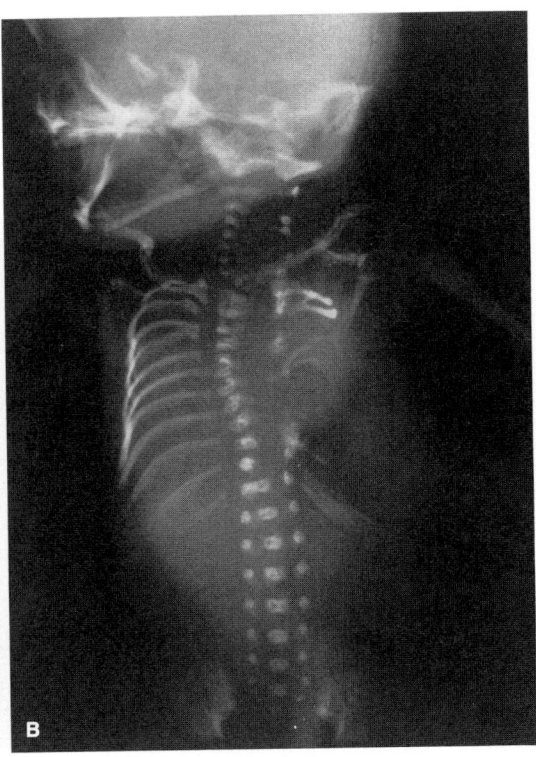

FIGURE 9-35. Spinal scoliosis vertebral anomalies. **(A)** Longitudinal, coronal scan of fetal spine at 18 weeks confirms irregularity of the vertebral bodies and mild scoliosis. Note splaying of the spine at this level (*arrowheads*) and only a few posterior ossification centers on one side of the scoliosis (*long arrows*). L, lumbar spine. **(B)** Postmortem radiograph shows marked thoracic cage deformity with mild thoracic scoliosis. (Harrison LA, Pretorius DH, Budorick NE: Abnormal spinal curvature in the fetus. J Ultrasound Med 1992; 11:473.)

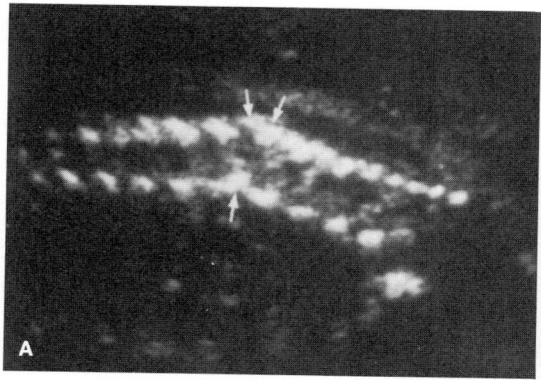
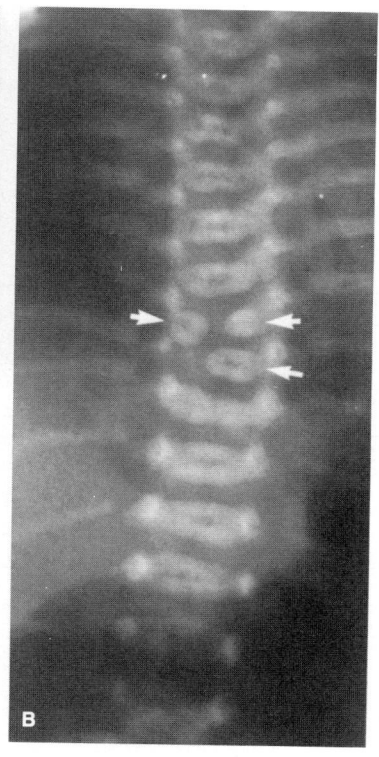

FIGURE 9-36. Hemivertebra thoracic spine (isolated). **(A)** Longitudinal sagittal view of the lower thoracic spine in the late second trimester. Shown are two abnormal ossification centers (*arrows*) of the posterior elements opposite a single ossification center (*single arrow*) consistent with an abnormal vertebra. **(B)** Radiograph at birth showing a vertebral abnormality at T9 involving two ossification centers on one side and one ossification center on the other side. (Benacerraf BR, et al: Prenatal sonographic diagnosis of congenital hemivertebra. J Ultrasound Med 1986; 5:257.)

can take place. These include abnormalities of either the vertebral body or incomplete or maldeveloped secondary ossification centers.

Caudal Regression Syndrome

An embryologic defect during the third week of development may result in a wedge-shaped defect in the posterior-axis caudal blastema. This defect leads to fusion of the early lower limb buds, with absent or incompletely developed intervening caudal structures. This sirenomelic sequence is considered by some to be the most severe form of caudal regression syndrome, a defect occurring in about 1 in 60,000 newborns. It may result in a single umbilical artery arising directly from the aorta, lower limb fusion, imperforate anus, urologic deficits, and lower vertebral and pelvic abnormalities (including agenesis). There is a wide spectrum of severity in this disorder; imperforate anus alone represents its mildest form. Caudal regression syndrome is strongly associated with poorly controlled insulin-dependent diabetes mellitus and monozygotic twin gestation. The relative risk for this rare lesion is increased 200-fold in infants of

diabetic women, but still it has been observed in only 2 per 1000 pregnancies complicated by diabetes mellitus.[57] The potential pitfall of caudal regression is various forms of conjoined twins, who may be separate at the skull base but fused from the lumbosacral spine caudally (see Chapter 20).

In reported cases of caudal regression syndrome, defects included grossly distorted or absent vertebrae beginning at the thoracic level, absent or rudimentary pelvic bones, and asymmetrically shortened limbs. Abnormalities of the abdominal wall and the genitourinary, cardiac, and pulmonary systems also have been identified sonographically.[58,59] Depending on the presence of associated anomalies, the prognosis of caudal regression is poor. In a series of 12 cases of caudal regression syndrome reported by Loewy and colleagues, 5 perinatal deaths occurred and were related to associated anomalies of the renal and cardiorespiratory systems.[59] Because survivors sustain major degrees of neurologic impairment and bladder dysfunction, appropriate counseling and intervention should be performed at the time of diagnosis.

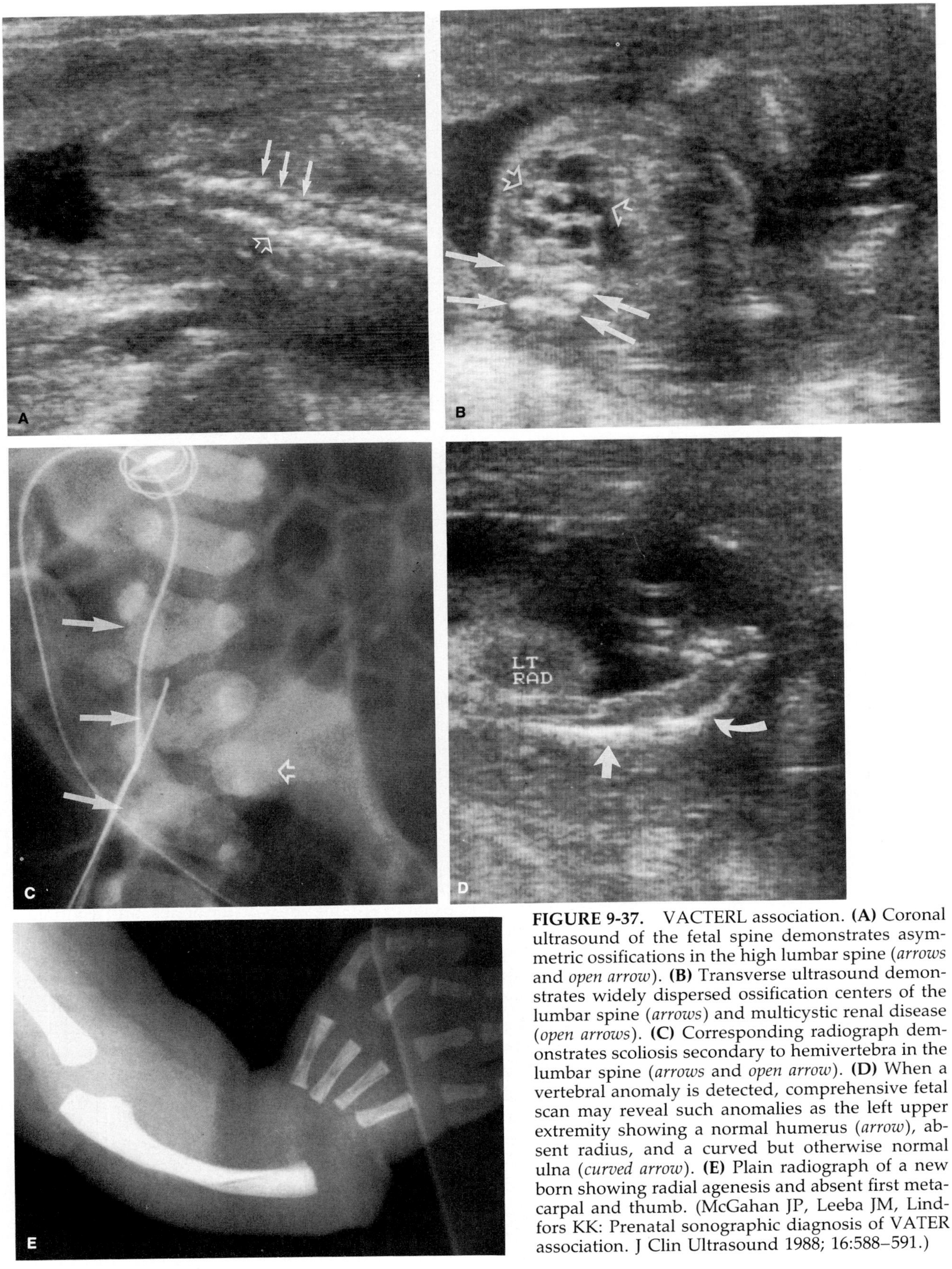

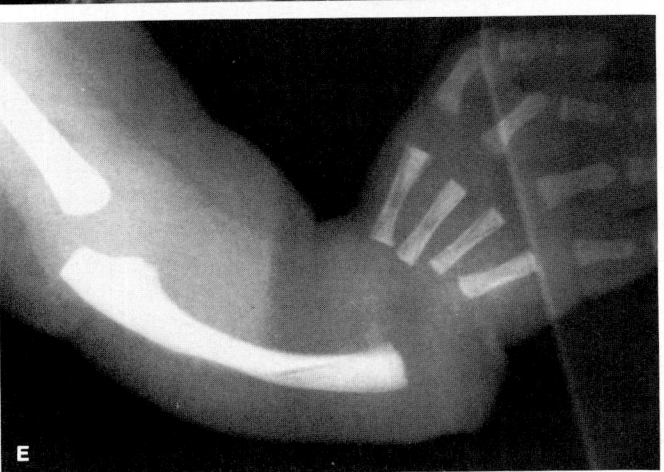

FIGURE 9-37. VACTERL association. **(A)** Coronal ultrasound of the fetal spine demonstrates asymmetric ossifications in the high lumbar spine (*arrows* and *open arrow*). **(B)** Transverse ultrasound demonstrates widely dispersed ossification centers of the lumbar spine (*arrows*) and multicystic renal disease (*open arrows*). **(C)** Corresponding radiograph demonstrates scoliosis secondary to hemivertebra in the lumbar spine (*arrows* and *open arrow*). **(D)** When a vertebral anomaly is detected, comprehensive fetal scan may reveal such anomalies as the left upper extremity showing a normal humerus (*arrow*), absent radius, and a curved but otherwise normal ulna (*curved arrow*). **(E)** Plain radiograph of a newborn showing radial agenesis and absent first metacarpal and thumb. (McGahan JP, Leeba JM, Lindfors KK: Prenatal sonographic diagnosis of VATER association. J Clin Ultrasound 1988; 16:588–591.)

REFERENCES

1. Van der Putte SCJ: The development of the lymphatic system in man. Adv Anat Embryol Cell Biol 1975; 51:3.
2. Chervenak FA, Isaacson G, Blakemore KJ, et al: Fetal cystic hygroma: Cause and natural history. N Engl J Med 1983; 309:822–825.
3. Bernstein HS, Filly RA, Goldberg JD, Golbus MS: Prognosis of fetuses with a cystic hygroma. Prenat Diagn 1991; 11:349–355.
4. Cullen MT, Gabrielli S, Green JJ, et al: Diagnosis and significance of hygroma in the first trimester. Prenat Diagn 1990; 10:643–651.
5. Shulman LP, Emerson DS, Felker RE, et al: High frequency of cytogenetic abnormalities in fetuses with cystic hygroma diagnosed in the first trimester. Obstet Gynecol 1992; 80:80–82.
6. Johnson MP, Johnson A, Holzgreve W, et al: First trimester simple hygroma: Cause and outcome. Am J Obstet Gynecol 1993; 168:156–161.
7. Shaub M, Wilson R, Collea J: Fetal cystic lymphangioma (cystic hygroma) ultrasound findings. Radiology 1976; 121:449.
8. Lee CY, Madrazo BL, Van Dyke DL, Smith J: Prenatal diagnosis of fetal cystic hygromas associated with generalized lymphangiectasia. Henry Ford Hosp Med J 1981; 29:93.
9. Ingraham FD, Swah H: Spina bifida and cranium bifidum. I. A survey of five hundred and forty six cases. N Engl J Med 1943; 228:559.
10. Quinlan RW: A sonographic artifact, fetal hair, mimicking a craniocervical meningocele in pregnancy complicated by hydramnios: A report of two cases. J Reprod Med 1984; 29:354.
11. Fink IJ, Chinn DH, Callen PW: A potential pitfall in the ultrasonographic diagnosis of fetal encephalocele. J Ultrasound Med 1983; 2:313.
12. Saners RC: Atlas of Ultrasonographic Artifacts and Variants. Chicago: Year Book Medical Publishers, 1986: 8.
13. Van Zalen-Sprock MM, van Vugt JMG, van der Harten HJ, van Geijn HP: Cephalocele and cystic hygroma: Diagnosis and differentiation in the first trimester of pregnancy with transvaginal sonography. Report of two cases. Ultrasound Obstet Gynecol 1992; 2:289–292.
14. Graham D, Johnson TR, Winn K, et al: The role of sonography in the prenatal diagnosis and management of encephalocele. J Ultrasound Med 1982; 1:111.
15. Chervenak FA, Isaacson G, Mahoney MJ, et al: Diagnosis and management of fetal cephalocele. Obstet Gynecol 1984; 64:86.
16. Mehta PS, Mehta SJ, Vorherr H: Congenital iodide goiter and hypothyroidism: A review. Obstet Gynecol Surv 1983; 38:237.
17. Wenstrom KD, Weiner CP, Williamson RA, Grant SS: Prenatal diagnosis of fetal hyperthyroidism using funipuncture. Obstet Gynecol 1990; 76:513–517.
18. Gonzalez-Crussi F: Extragonadal teratomas. In Atlas of Tumor Pathology, 2nd series. Bethesda: Armed Forces Institute of Pathology, 1982: 1–198.
19. Teal LN, Angtuaco TL, Jimenez JF, Quirk JG: Fetal teratomas: Antenatal diagnosis and clinical management. J Clin Ultrasound 1988; 16:329–336.
20. Gundry SR, Wesley JR, Klein MD, et al: Cervical teratomas in the newborn. J Pediatr Surg 1983; 18:382.
21. Rosenfeld CR, Coln CD, Duenhoelter JH: Fetal cervical teratoma as a cause of polyhydramnios. Pediatrics 1979; 64:176.
22. Langer JC, Tabb T, Thompson P, et al: Management of prenatally diagnosed tracheal obstruction: Access to the airway in utero prior to delivery. Fetal Diagn Ther 1992; 7:12–16.
23. Levine AB, Alvarez M, Wedgwood J, et al: Contemporary management of a potentially lethal fetal anomaly: A successful perinatal approach to epignathus. Obstet Gynecol 1990; 76:962.
24. McGahan JP, Schneider JM: Fetal neck hemangioendothelioma with secondary hydrops fetalis: Sonographic diagnosis. J Clin Ultrasound 1986; 14:384–388.
25. Benacerraf BR, Frigoletto FD Jr, Laboda LA: Sonographic diagnosis of Down's syndrome in the second trimester. Am J Obstet Gynecol 1985; 153:49–52.
26. Nicolaides KH, Azar G, Snijders RJM, Gosden CM: Fetal nuchal oedema: Associated malformations and chromosomal defects. Fetal Diagn Ther 1992; 7:123–131.
27. Ville Y, Lalondrelle C, Doumerc S, et al: First-trimester diagnosis of nuchal anomalies: Significance and fetal outcome. Ultrasound Obstet Gynecol 1992; 2:314–316.
28. Crane JP, Gray DL: Sonographically measured nuchal skinfold thickness as a screening tool for Down syndrome: Result of a prospective clinical trial. Obstet Gynecol 1991; 77:533.
29. Hrgovic Z, Panitz HG, Kurjak A, Jurkovic D: Contribution to the recognition of iniencephaly on the basis of a new case. J Perinat Med 1989; 17:375.
30. Foderaro AE, Abu-Yousef MM, Benda JA, et al: Antenatal ultrasound diagnosis of iniencephaly. J Clin Ultrasound 1987; 15:550.
31. Meizner I, Bar-Ziv J: Prenatal ultrasonic diagnosis of a rare case of iniencephaly apertus. J Clin Ultrasound 1987; 15:200.
32. Dennis MA, Drose JA, Pretorius DH, Manco-Johnson ML: Normal fetal sacrum simulating spina bifida: "Pseudodysraphism." Radiology 1985; 155:751.
33. Nicolaides KH, Campbell S, Gabbe SG, Guidetti R: Ultrasound screening for spina bifida: Cranial and cerebellar signs. Lancet 1986; 2:72.
34. Lorber J, Ward AM: Spina bifida: A vanishing nightmare? Arch Dis Child 1985; 60:1086.
35. Stein SC, Feldman JG, Friedlander M, Klein RJ: Is

myelomeningocele a disappearing disease? Pediatrics 1982; 69:511.

36. Bell JE, Gordon A, Maloney AFJ: The association of hydrocephalus and Arnold-Chiari malformation with spina bifida in the fetus. Neuropathol Appl Neurobiol 1980; 6:29.

37. McIntosh R: The incidence of congenital malformations: A study of 5964 pregnancies. Pediatrics 1954; 14:505.

38. Ingraham FD, Hamilin H: Spina bifida and cranium bifidum. II. Surgical treatment. N Engl J Med 1943; 228:631.

39. Sharrard WJ, Zachary RB, Lober J: A controlled trial of immediate and delayed closure of spina bifida cystica. Arch Dis Child 1963; 38:18.

40. Lorber J: Ventriculo-cardiac shunts in the first week of life: Results of a controlled trial in the treatment of hydrocephalus in infants born with spina bifida cystica or cranium bifidum. Dev Med Child Neurol 1969; 20:13.

41. Lynch L, Mehalek K, Berkowitz RL: Invasive fetal therapy. In Rodeck CH (ed): Fetal Medicine/1. Oxford, Blackwell Scientific Publications, 1989: 118–52.

42. Luthy DA, Wardinsky T, Shurtleff DB, et al: Cesarean section before the onset of labor and subsequent motor function in infants with meningomyelocele diagnosed antenatally. N Engl J Med 1991; 324:662–666.

43. Silverman FN: Caffey's Pediatric X-ray Diagnosis: An Integrated Teaching Approach. Chicago: Year Book Medical Publishers, 1985: 295–298, 298–300.

44. Dubowitz, W, Lorber J, Zachary RBZ: Lipoma of the cauda equina. Arch Dis Child 1965; 40:207.

45. Seeds JW, Jones FD: Lipomyelomeningocele: Prenatal diagnosis and management. Obstet Gynecol 1986; 67:34S.

46. Seeds JW, Powers SK: Early prenatal diagnosis of familial lipomyelomeningocele. Obstet Gynecol 1988; 72:469.

47. Flake AW, Harrison MR, Adzick NS, et al: Fetal sacrococcygeal teratoma. J Pediatr Surg 1986; 21:563–566.

48. Donnellan WA, Sewnson O: Benign and malignant sacrococcygeal teratomas. Surgery 1968; 64:834–836.

49. Holzgreve W, Miny P, Anderson R, Golbus MS: Experience with 8 cases of prenatally diagnosed sacrococcygeal teratomas. Fetal Ther 1987; 2:88–94.

50. Mintz MC, Minnuti M, Fishman M: Prenatal aspiration of sacrococcygeal teratoma. AJR 1983; 141:367–378.

51. Patten RM, Van Allen M, Mack LA, et al: Limb-body wall complex: In utero sonographic diagnosis of a complicated fetal malformation. AJR 1986; 146:1019.

52. Nyberg DA, Mack LA: The spine and neural tube defects. In Nyberg DA, Mahoney BS, Pretorius DH (eds): Diagnostic Ultrasound of Fetal Anomalies. Chicago, Year Book Medical Publishers, 1990: 192.

53. Harrison LA, Pretorius DH, Budorick NE: Abnormal spinal curvature in the fetus. J Ultrasound Med 1992; 11:473–479.

54. Benacerraf BR, Greene MF, Barss VA: Prenatal sonographic diagnosis of congenital hemivertebrae. J Ultrasound Med 1986; 5:257.

55. Abrams SL, Filly RA: Congenital malformations: Prenatal diagnosis using ultrasonography. Radiology 1985; 155:762.

56. McGahan JP, Leeba JM, Lindfors KK: Prenatal sonographic diagnosis of VATER association. J Clin Ultrasound 1988; 16:588–591.

57. Sonek JD, Gabbe SG, Landon MB, et al: Antenatal diagnosis of sacral agenesis syndrome in a pregnancy complicated by diabetes mellitus. Am J Obstet Gynecol 1990; 162:806–808.

58. Elejalde MM, Elejalde BF: Visualization of the fetal spine: A proposal of a standard to increase reliability. Am J Med Genet 1985; 21:445.

59. Loewy JA, Richards DG, Toi A: In-utero diagnosis of the caudal regression syndrome: Report of three cases. J Clin Ultrasound 1987; 15:469–474.

60. Benacerraf BR, Gelman R, Frigoletto FD: Sonographic identification of second trimester fetuses with Down syndrome. N Engl J Med 1987; 317:1371–1376.

61. Perrella R, Duerinckx AJ, Grant EG: Second-trimester sonographic diagnosis of Down syndrome: Role of femur-length shortening and nuchal fold thickening. AJR 1988; 151:981–985.

62. Schreinemachers DM, Cross PK, Hook EB: Rates of trisomies 21, 18, 13 and other chromosome abnormalities in about 20,000 prenatal studies compared with estimated rates in live births. Hum Genet 1982; 61:318–324.

63. DiMaio MS, Baumgarten A, Greenstein RM, et al: Screening for Down's syndrome in pregnancy by measuring maternal serum alpha-fetoprotein levels. N Engl J Med 1987; 317:342–346.

64. Nyberg DA, Mack LA, Hirsch J, Mahoney BS: Abnormalities of fetal cranial contour in sonographic detection of spina bifida: Evaluation of the "lemon" sign. Radiology 1988; 167:387–392.

65. Campbell J, Gilbert WM, Nicolaides KH, Campbell S: Ultrasound screening for spina bifida: Cranial and cerebellar signs in a high-risk population. Obstet Gynecol 1987; 70:247–250.

66. Penso C, Redline RW, Benacerraf BR: A sonographic sign which predicts which fetuses with hydrocephalus have an associated neural tube defect. J Ultrasound Med 1987; 6:307–311.

John P. McGahan and Manuel Porto:
DIAGNOSTIC OBSTETRICAL ULTRASOUND.
© 1994 J.B. Lippincott Company.

Terry L. Coates   John P. McGahan

Chapter *10*

The Fetal Face

The American Institute of Ultrasound in Medicine has published guidelines for performance of the Antepartum Obstetrical Ultrasound Examination.[1] Within these guidelines are specific recommendations for evaluation of the second- and third-trimester fetus. These official guidelines do not specifically recommend an examination of the fetal face; however, they do state that suspected abnormalities may require a specialized evaluation to permit diagnosis of numerous anomalies that could significantly alter perinatal management.

Fetal facial anomalies may be isolated or may be associated with more complex fetal malformation syndromes, and therefore identification of a facial malformation may suggest a specific diagnosis when found in association with other anomalies.[2] When a fetal anomaly is detected, a careful evaluation of the fetal face may also be useful in contributing to a specific diagnosis. In most cases, a meticulous and time-consuming examination of the face is unnecessary and unlikely to be productive in low-risk obstetrical sonography.[3] However, recent improvements in the resolution of real-time ultrasound equipment and operator technique allow a better survey of the fetal face and should

improve the detection of subtle structural defects and allow a more accurate diagnosis of anomalous pregnancies.[2,3]

EMBRYOLOGY

Facial development begins at about 4 to 5 menstrual weeks and is almost complete by the end of the embryonic period, at about 10 menstrual weeks.[4,5] Therefore, the embryo has acquired all its basic morphologic characteristics before the face has attained adequate size to permit sonographic examination. Although a detailed knowledge of the complex embryogenesis of the facial region is not necessary to diagnose most facial abnormalities,[6] a brief review of normal facial embryology is appropriate in predicting patterns of malformation.

Most malformations of the face originate from anomalous development of the *branchial apparatus, optic vesicles, pharyngeal pouches,* and *facial processes,* as listed by days after fertilization[4,5,7] (Fig. 10-1). By 14 days after fertilization, the early embryo has formed a circular bilaminar disk containing Hen-

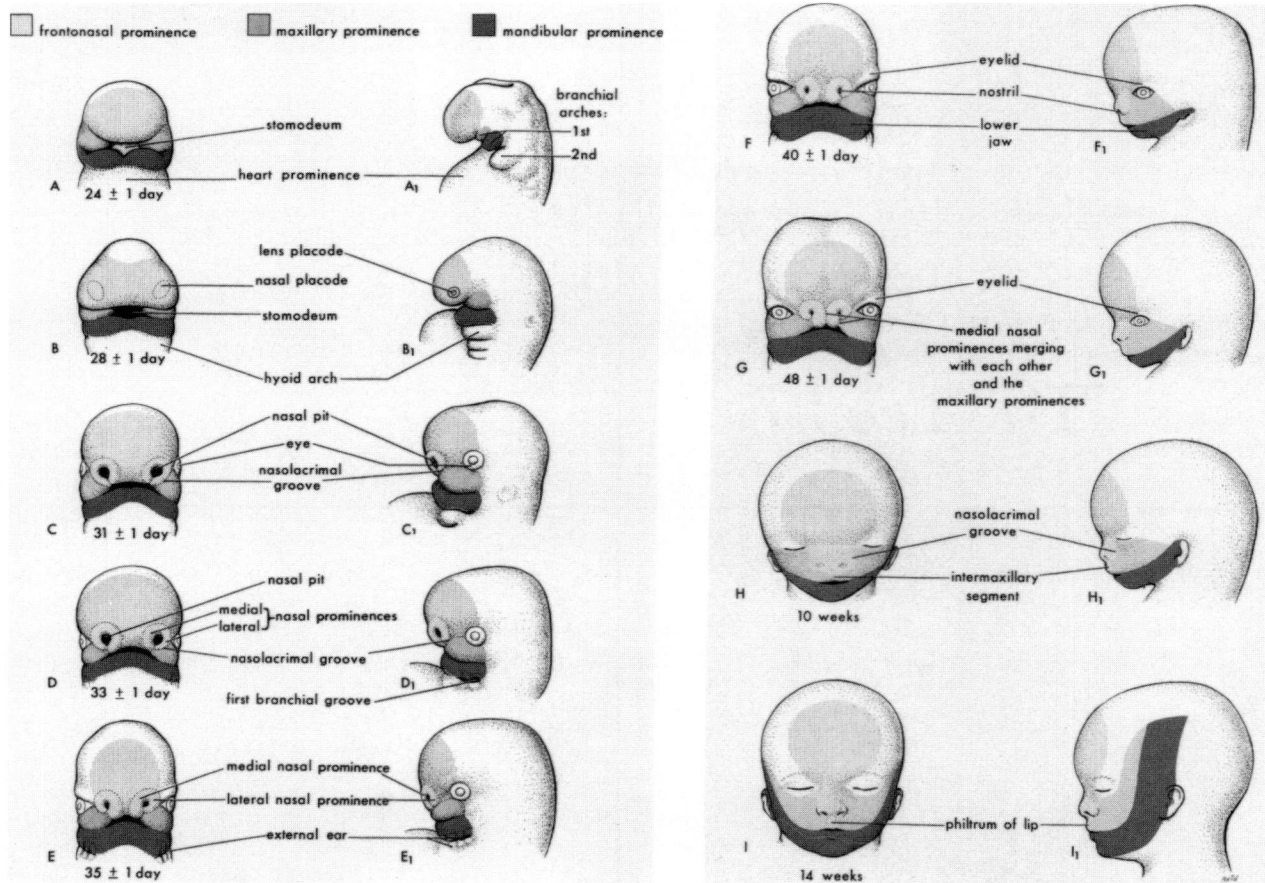

FIGURE 10-1. Embryologic development of the face. Frontal and lateral drawings illustrate progressive stages in the development of the human face. *Hatched area,* frontonasal prominence; *light shaded area,* maxillary prominence; *dark shaded area,* mandibular prominence. (Moore KL: The Developing Human: Clinically Oriented Embryology, 5th ed. Philadelphia: WB Saunders, 1993.)

sen's node. Hensen's node eventually gives rise to many of the primordia of the craniofacial complex.[5] By 21 to 31 days after fertilization, the cranial portion of the embryo develops mesenchymal elevations, which form the facial processes and pharyngeal arches. With the differential growth of these mesodermal masses, the ectodermal grooves soon become obliterated; however, it is along these grooves that facial clefts commonly develop.[5] The maxillary, mandibular, and frontonasal prominences of the facial processes are of great importance because they determine through fusion and differential growth the size of the mandible, upper lip, palate, and nose.[7] At about 24 to 26 days, the branchial arches and optic vesicle (precursor of the eye) make their appearance. Development of the tongue, face, lips, jaws, palate, pharynx, and neck largely involves transformation of the branchial apparatus into adult structures. During the late embryonic period, development of the face is characterized mainly by changes in proportion and relative position of individual structures.[5] The eyes, initially directed laterally, gradually move medially to become directed anteriorly. The nose begins above the orbits as two widely separated nasal placodes, which move medially and inferiorly as the nasal septum thins and the medial nasal folds fuse. The external ears initially develop below the level of the mandible but gradually assume a more cephalic orientation. At about 60 days after fertilization, the embryo has acquired all its basic morphologic characteristics and then enters the fetal period, during which growth and maturation of these primordia continue along with reorganization of the spatial relations between various structures.[5]

OVERVIEW OF ANOMALIES

Although a large number of malformations and syndromes involving the face have been documented, the prevalence figures for many specific anomalies are either unknown or low.[6,8,9] Most of the literature concerning the fetal face has involved small series or case reports. Two prenatal sonographic series, however, have discussed the accuracy of detecting facial abnormalities and the frequency of detection of these anomalies using prenatal ultrasound. Because the data for both these series were obtained during the period of 1980 to 1985, it is likely that technological innovations have improved the accuracy at detecting these abnormalities, but there have been no known recent large series.

Hegge and colleagues detected 17 facial abnormalities in 11 fetuses from 7100 low- and high-risk obstetrical sonographic examinations (0.15%), examined from 20 to 39 weeks of gestation.[10] All affected fetuses had coexistent structural abnormalities, polyhydramnios, or a history of maternal teratogenic exposure. The facial abnormalities detected consisted of absent orbits, single nostril, proboscis, absent nose, hypertelorism, markedly flattened or sunken nose, micrognathia, proptosis, or cleft nose, lip, and palate. Five abnormalities were known to have been missed, including 4 cases of cleft palate (2 with cleft lip) and 1 flattened nose. Coexistent facial abnormalities, however, were identified in 3 of the 5 fetuses, and only in 2 of 5 fetuses were facial abnormalities missed entirely. Pilu and colleagues examined the accuracy of prenatal ultrasound in detecting craniofacial malformations among 223 fetuses between 18 and 40 weeks of gestation, who were at risk for craniofacial malformations.[11] Optimal visualization of the fetal face was not possible on two separate occasions in 11.2% of their targeted high-risk obstetrical population because of an unfavorable position of the fetus, severe oligohydramnios, or maternal obesity. Prenatal ultrasound examinations successfully detected craniofacial malformations in 14 of 18 (78%) fetuses. Fifteen of 18 fetuses (83%) had cranial abnormalities, 12 of 18 (67%) had holoprosencephaly, and 3 others had anencephaly, microcephaly, or hydrocephalus. Anomalies diagnosed sonographically included anophthalmia, median cleft lip or palate, hypotelorism, hypertelorism, micrognathia, proboscis, and absent nasal bridge. Polyhydramnios was present in 11 (61.1%) of 18 cases. Anomalies not detected with prenatal ultrasound included 4 cases with cleft palate, 3 with cleft lip, and 1 with cyclopia. The authors believed that the posterior palate in the fetus was difficult to visualize sonographically because of the acoustic shadow that arises from the surrounding bony structures. There were no false-positive diagnoses. These two studies demonstrate that prenatal ultrasound can be an accurate and reliable tool for the prenatal diagnosis of facial anomalies.

SONOGRAPHIC APPROACH TO THE FETAL FACE

Major features of the fetal face, such as the orbit, forehead, nose, and mouth, can be identified as early as 12 weeks of gestation; however, it is usually not until 16 weeks of gestation that one can observe more detailed facial anatomy.[12] A targeted examination of the face may be particularly useful in pregnancies complicated by polyhydramnios, concomitant extrafacial structural anomalies, a maternal history of teratogen exposure, or a family history of previous craniofacial malformation (eg, facial cleft).[10,11] Detailed facial anatomy, including specific muscles, nerves, and arteries, can be observed.[10,11] Visibility may be limited in the presence of oligohydramnios, maternal obesity, or fetal position, especially the occiput anterior position.[2,11]

The following views for detailed facial anatomy can be obtained:

- Axial views of the orbits, nose, lips, and anterior palate
- Coronal views through the orbits, nose, lips, and anterior portion of the mandible
- Profile view for soft tissues and facial bones
- Views of the ears

Sonographic evaluation of the fetal face is not only useful for the identification of structural abnormalities but also may be helpful in assessing fetal state and behavioral changes. Birnholz and colleagues correlated the presence of eye movements with fetal well-being and also reported the blink reflex in response to an auditory stimulus related to gestational age.[13,14] Fetal vomiting or regurgitation can be identified by watching the fetal mouth, with color flow indicating regurgitation in fetuses with upper gastrointestinal obstruction.[15] Therefore, sonographic evaluation of the fetal face not only identifies facial anomalies that may signify other structural anomalies and chromosomal abnormalities but also may serve as an indicator of fetal well-being and behavioral changes.

This chapter is divided into anatomic regions that correlate with the four different facial views described previously.

Orbit and Periorbital Regions: Axial View

In most cases, an axial view of the orbits allows visualization of the different components of the eyes, including the globe, vitreous body, lens, anterior chamber, extraocular muscles, optic nerve, and hyaloid artery.[16] Documentation of the presence and size of two eyes and of the distance between them probably provides the most useful di-

agnostic information[6,17,18] (Table 10-1). Jeanty and colleagues tabulated normal ultrasound values for ocular biometry throughout pregnancy.[18,19] The axial plane of the orbits is a section parallel but caudal to the section used for the biparietal diameter (Fig. 10-2). The criteria used for this plane include:

- A symmetric image
- Both eyes imaged and of equal diameter
- The largest possible diameter of the eye[18]

Measurements for the orbits have been made and include:

- Ocular diameter (OD), which is measured from the medial to the lateral wall of the bony orbit

TABLE 10-1. Growth of the Ocular Parameters

Age (wks)	Binocular Distance (mm)			Interocular Distance (mm)			Ocular Diameter (mm)		
	5th	50th	95th	5th	50th	95th	5th	50th	95th
11	5	13	20	—	—	—	—	—	—
12	8	15	23	4	9	13	1	3	6
13	10	18	25	5	9	14	2	4	7
14	13	20	28	5	10	14	3	5	8
15	15	22	30	6	10	14	4	6	9
16	17	25	32	6	10	15	5	7	9
17	19	27	34	6	11	15	5	8	10
18	22	29	37	7	11	16	6	9	11
19	24	31	39	7	12	16	7	9	12
20	26	33	41	8	12	17	8	10	13
21	28	35	43	8	13	17	8	11	13
22	30	37	44	9	13	18	9	12	14
23	31	39	46	9	14	18	10	12	15
24	33	41	48	10	14	19	10	13	15
25	35	42	50	10	15	19	11	13	16
26	36	44	51	11	15	20	12	14	16
27	38	45	53	11	16	20	12	14	17
28	39	47	54	12	16	21	13	15	17
29	41	48	56	12	17	21	13	15	18
30	42	50	57	13	17	22	14	16	18
31	43	51	58	13	18	22	14	16	19
32	45	52	60	14	18	23	14	17	19
33	46	53	61	14	19	23	15	17	19
34	47	54	62	15	19	24	15	17	20
35	48	55	63	15	20	24	15	18	20
36	49	56	64	16	20	25	16	18	20
37	50	57	65	16	21	25	16	18	21
38	50	58	65	17	21	26	16	18	21
39	51	59	66	17	22	26	16	19	21
40	52	59	67	18	22	26	16	19	21

(Romero R, Pilu G, Jeanty P, Ghidini A, Hobbins J: Prenatal Diagnosis of Congenital Anomalies. Norwalk CT: Appleton and Lange, 1988: 83.)

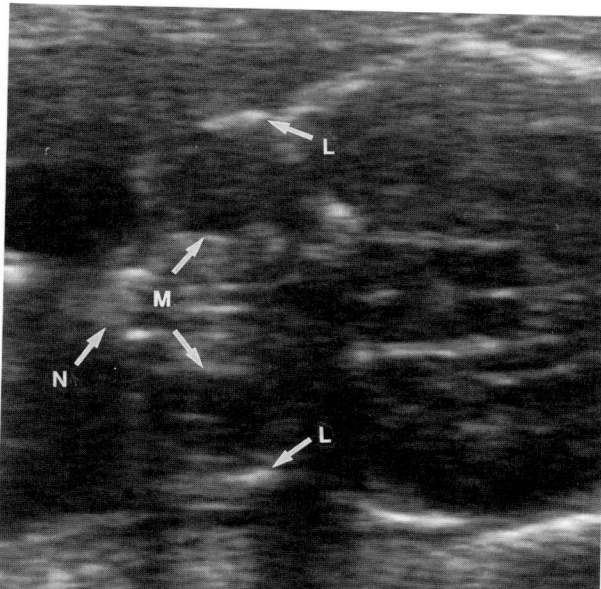

FIGURE 10-2. Axial scan through the level of the normal orbits at 29 menstrual weeks demonstrates the nasal bridge (N), the medial wall of each orbit (M), and lateral wall of each orbit (L). The *ocular diameter* is the distance from the medial (M) to the lateral (L) wall of the orbit and is approximately equal to the *interocular distance,* which is measured from one medial wall to the other. The *binocular distance* is the sum of the two ocular diameters and the interocular distance, or the measurement from one lateral wall to the other lateral wall of the orbit.

• Interocular distance (ID), which is measured from the medial wall of one orbit to the medial wall of the other orbit
• Binocular distance (BD), which is determined by measurement between the lateral orbital rims

These measurements have been tabulated and may be useful in predicting such abnormalities as ocular hypertelorism, ocular hypotelorism, and other orbital abnormalities or, less frequently, may assist in obstetrical dating when there is severe distortion of other biometric parameters.[17–19]

The hyaloid artery, a branch of the main ophthalmic artery, can normally be visualized sonographically in the second trimester of pregnancy (Fig. 10-3). The hyaloid artery appears as an echogenic line coursing through the vitreous of the globe to the posterior surface of the lens. It normally regresses before the middle of the third trimester. Birnholz and Farrel suggested that temporarily delayed regression of the hyaloid artery may occur with trisomy 21 syndrome and other forms of retarded brain development.[20] The following questions may prove useful in the detection of anomalies involving the orbital and periorbital region:

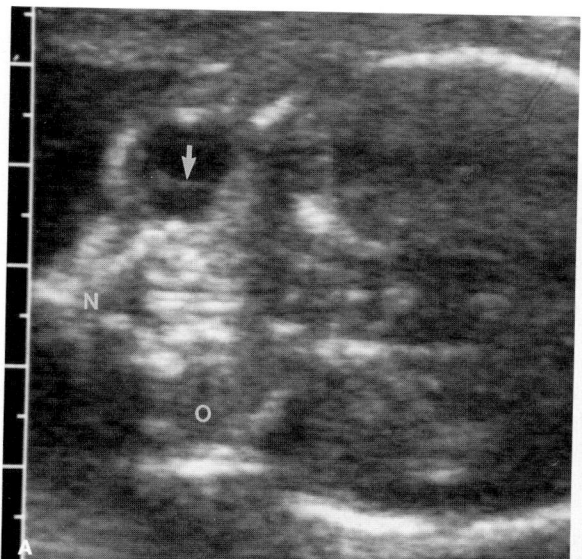

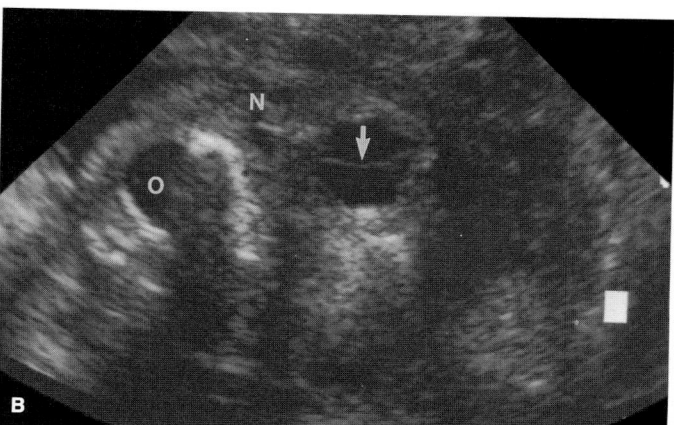

FIGURE 10-3. Fetal orbit hyaloid artery. **(A)** Axial scan through the brain and orbits demonstrates linear echogenic structure running from posterior to anterior within one orbital globe, representing the hyaloid artery in this 20-week fetus. **(B)** Axial transvaginal ultrasound through the face demonstrates the hyaloid artery running posterior to anterior within the globe of the orbit, which is deviated laterally in this first-trimester fetus with anencephaly. N, nose; O, opposite orbit.

1. Is hypotelorism, hypertelorism, microphthalmia, or anophthalmia present?
2. Is a proboscis or cebocephaly present?
3. Are any periorbital masses or intraocular abnormalities present?

Hypotelorism

Clinical Features. The prenatal sonographic diagnosis of a decreased interorbital distance (hypotelorism) has been most commonly associated with holoprosencephaly. Other, less common causes of hypotelorism are listed in Table 10-2.[8,21]

Holoprosencephaly is a complex spectrum of intracranial abnormalities resulting from absent or incomplete median cleavage of the forebrain (prosencephalon) during early embryonic development.[22,23] Holoprosencephaly is categorized as alobar, semilobar, or lobar, depending on the degree of forebrain cleavage[22–25] (see Chapter 8). Alobar holoprosencephaly, the most severe form, is associated with the most severe facial deformities and is characterized by complete absence of cleavage of the forebrain, resulting in a monoventricular cavity and absent midline structures. DeMeyer stated that "the face predicts the brain," and therefore holoprosencephaly is associated with a number of characteristic intracranial and facial abnormalities.[24] These include cyclopia, ethmocephaly, cebocephaly, median cleft lip and palate, lateral cleft lip and palate, bilateral cleft lip, and mild hypotelorism (Fig. 10-4).

TABLE 10-2. Anomalies Associated With Hypotelorism

Common

Holoprosencephaly

Uncommon

Trigonocephaly
Oculodentodigital dysplasia
Microcephaly
Meckel-Gruber syndrome
Williams' syndrome
Maternal phenylketonuria
Myotic dystrophy
Chromosomal aberrations
   Trisomy 13
   Trisomy 21
   18p−
   5p−
   14q+

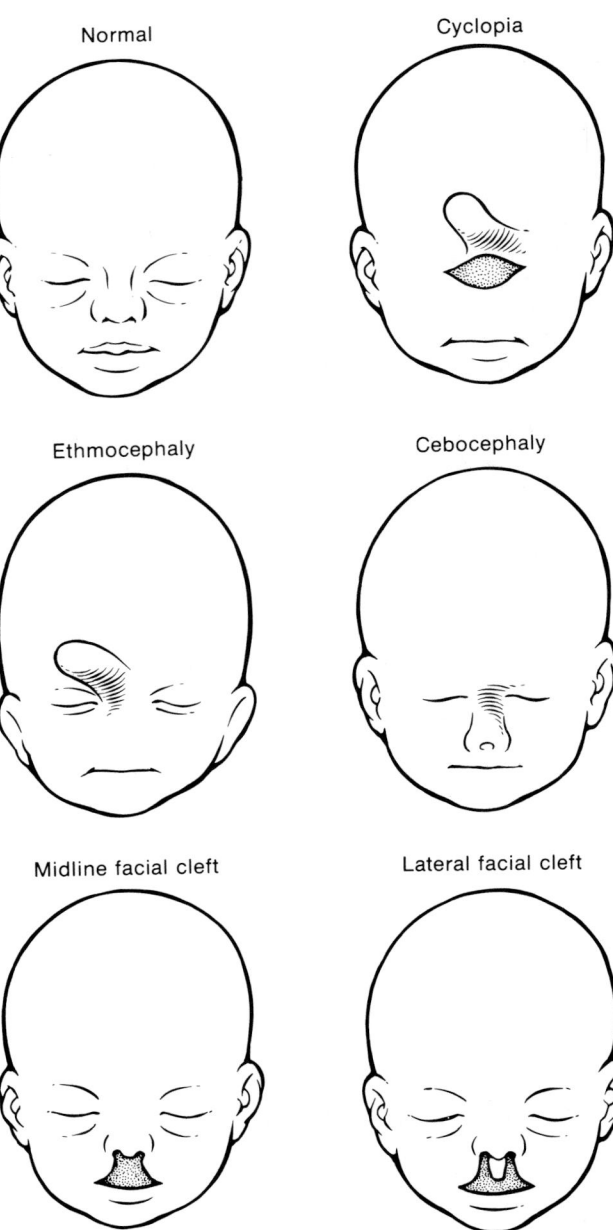

FIGURE 10-4. The variable facial features of holoprosencephaly in contrast to the normal facial features.

Cyclopia: Median orbit with various degrees of ocular fusion, absent nose, proboscis from the lower forehead, absent facial bones, absent philtrum of the upper lip, and low-set ears (Fig. 10-5)
Ethmocephaly: Marked hypotelorism, absent nose with proboscis present at the level of

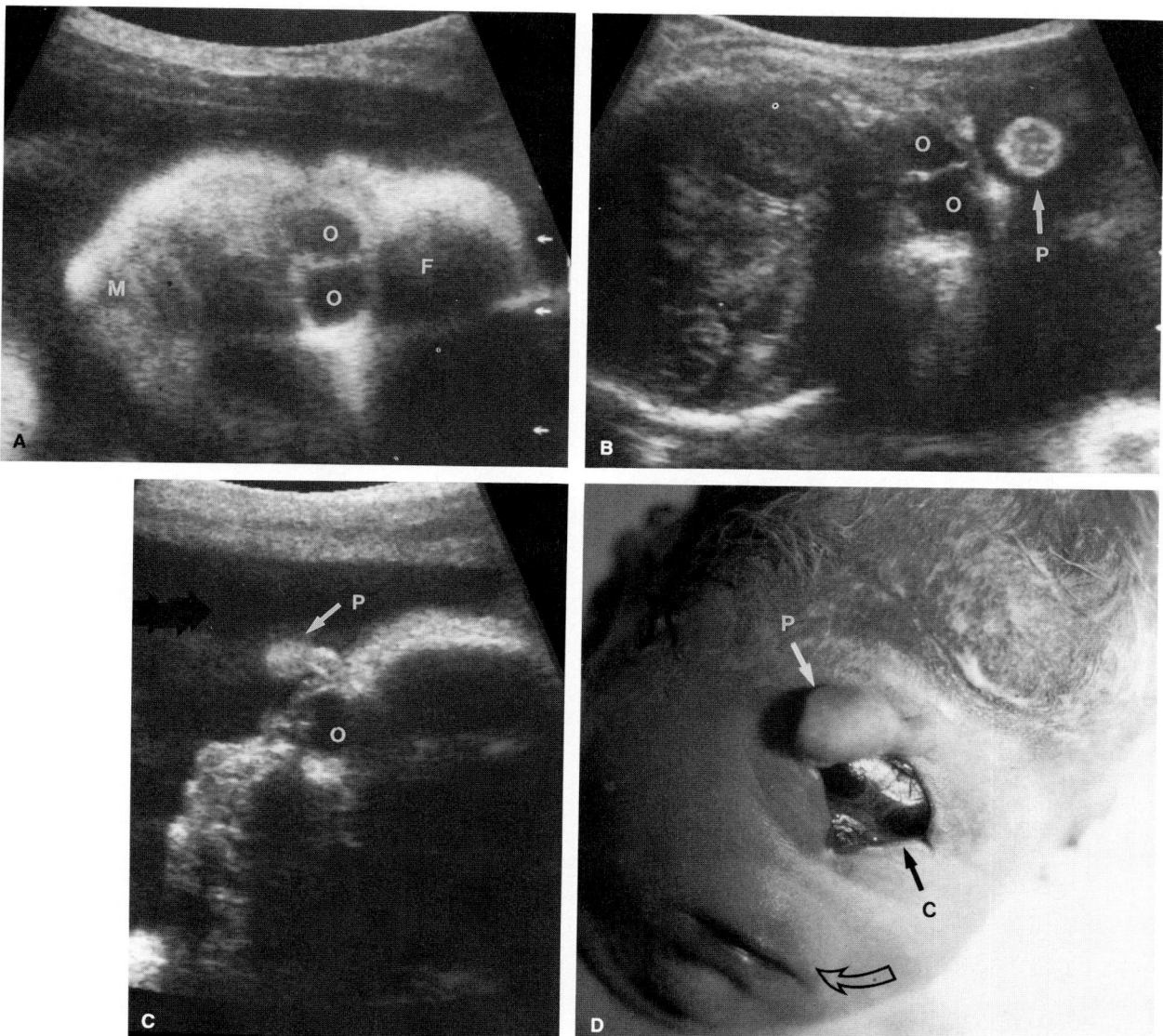

FIGURE 10-5.   Cyclopia. **(A)** In utero coronal ultrasound of the face shows two fused orbits (O). F, forehead; M, mandible. **(B)** Axial ultrasound of the face demonstrates two fused orbits (O) and anteriorly located proboscis (P). **(C)** Midsagittal profile view demonstrates the proboscis (P) above the fused orbits (O). **(D)** Gross specimen shows cyclopia with median fused orbits (C) and the proboscis (P). Note that the normal fold of upper lip, the philtrum, is absent (*open curved arrow*).

the orbits, and low-set, malformed ears (Fig. 10-6)

Cebocephaly: Flat and rudimentary nose, hypotelorism, single flat nostril, and absent philtrum of the upper lip (Fig. 10-7)

Median cleft lip: Mild and subtle hypotelorism, flat nose, and median cleft lip with or without cleft palate

Lateral cleft lip: Unilateral or bilateral lateral cleft lip and palate

In all cases of cyclopia, ethmocephaly, cebocephaly, and hypotelorism with median cleft lip, intracranial features of holoprosencephaly, usually the alobar type, are present.[22,24,26] The converse, however, is not true. DeMeyer reported that 17% of patients with alobar holoprosencephaly had a normal face.[25] The less severe forms of holoprosencephaly (semilobar and lobar types) are often associated with lesser degrees of facial abnormality or no facial deformities.[22]

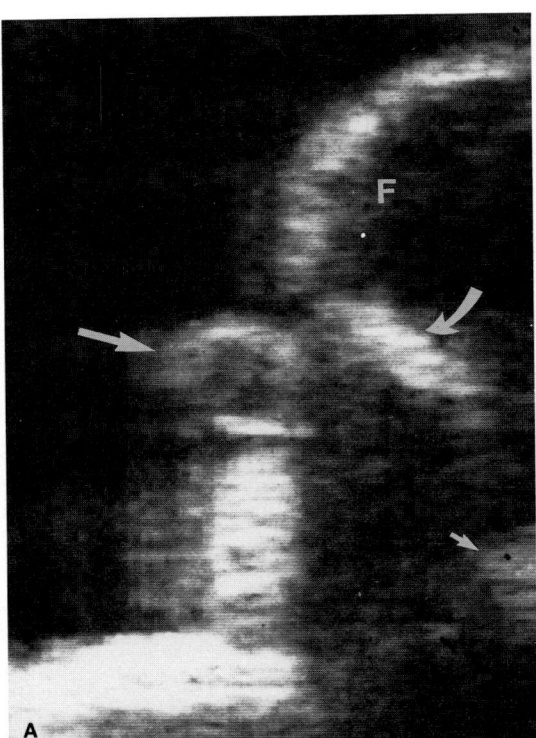
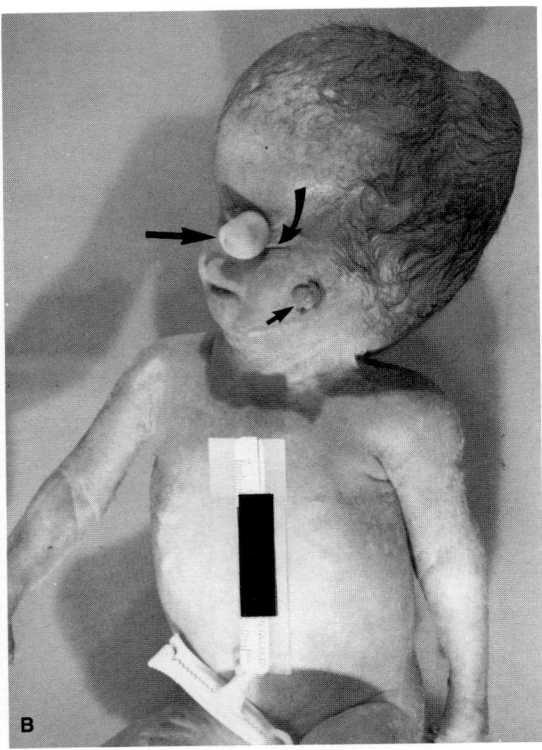

FIGURE 10-6. Ethmocephaly. In utero sagittal ultrasound of the face **(A)** and corresponding gross specimen **(B)** show slit-like orbits (*curved arrows*), prominent forehead (F), and a proboscis (*long straight arrow*). Low-set ears (*short straight arrows*) are also identified on prenatal sonogram. (McGahan JP, Ellis W, Lindfors KK, et al: Congenital cerebrospinal fluid–containing intracranial abnormalities: A sonographic classification. JCU 1988; 16:531–544.)

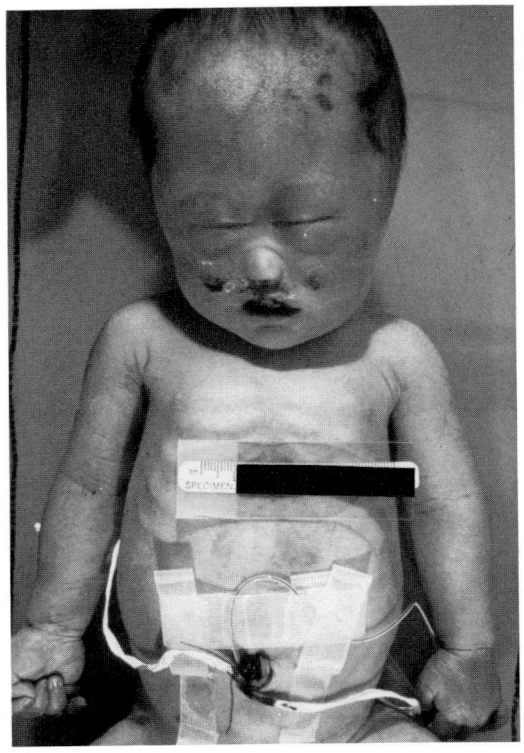

FIGURE 10-7. Cebocephaly. Gross specimen of fetus shows hypotelorism and a flattened nasal bridge. The nose has a single opening. (McGahan JP, Nyberg DA, Mack LA: Sonography of facial features of alobar and semilobar holoprosencephaly. AJR 1990; 154:144–148.)

Sonographic Findings. In a sonographic review of facial features of 27 cases of holoprosencephaly consisting of 22 of the alobar type and 5 of the semilobar type, facial abnormalities were present in 24, and 14 (58%) of these were seen on prenatal sonography.[22] The menstrual age at the time of diagnosis of holoprosencephaly was younger than 24 weeks in 8 cases. Prenatal abnormalities detected by sonography included cyclopia (4 of 5), ethmocephaly (2 of 3), cebocephaly (1 of 3), midline cleft lip (4 of 8), lateral cleft lip (2 of 2), and mild hypotelorism (1 of 3). Chromosomal analysis revealed abnormal karyotype in 13 (50%) of the 26 fetuses in whom it was performed. The most common abnormality was trisomy 13 (7 cases), but other abnormalities included triploidy (XXY), partial chromosomal deletions, and chromosome translocation.

Holoprosencephaly: Associated Anomalies and Prognosis. The extrafacial anomalies associated with holoprosencephaly are numerous and are listed in Table 10-3.[22,23] Extracranial malformations have been identified in about half the fetuses with alobar or semilobar holoprosencephaly. Associated abnormalities in the fetus may be overlooked on prenatal sonography, particularly when there has been a confident prenatal diagnosis of holoprosencephaly and therapeutic options have been chosen, so that the associated findings may be deemed less important.

TABLE 10-3.   Extracranial Malformations Associated With Holoprosencephaly

Abdomen
Renal dysplasia
Omphalocele
Esophageal atresia
Intestinal abnormalities
Bladder exstrophy

Thorax
Pulmonary hypoplasia
Cardiac defects
   Ventricular septal defect
   Atrial septal defect
   Two-chamber heart
   Transposition of great vessels

Other
Meningomyelocele
Polydactyly
Clubfoot

Additional prognostic information regarding the fetus is provided when there is demonstration of facial and extra central nervous system anomalies. Cyclopia and ethmocephaly are uniformly associated with a fatal outcome, and affected infants rarely live beyond the neonatal period, while fetuses with cebocephaly or premaxillary agenesis rarely survive beyond 1 year.[22-24,27-29]

Hypertelorism

Clinical Features. Increased interorbital distance (hypertelorism) may be an isolated *primary* defect or may occur *secondarily* as part of multiple syndromes, many of which are associated with chromosomal abnormalities or may occur as a result of maternal teratogen exposure[9,21,30,31] (Table 10-4). Some of the most commonly associated syndromes or malformations accompanied by *secondary hypertelorism* are:

- Anterior cephalocele
- Median cleft syndrome
- Craniosynostosis (Apert's syndrome, Crouzon's syndrome, Carpenter's syndrome)

The few cases of hypertelorism detected with prenatal sonography have been in association with an anterior or frontal cephalocele[30,31] (Fig. 10-8). Frontonasal cephaloceles are rare and appear to arise from intrinsic calvarial defects, where they project through a defect in the ethmoid, sphenoid, or frontal bone.[31] Frontal cephaloceles may also be associated with other midline facial defects, such as cleft lip and palate.[31] Frontal cephaloceles often displace the orbital globe downward and outward, resulting in hypertelorism.[7] Frontonasal cephaloceles in general are smaller than cephaloceles in other locations. The median cleft face syndrome is characterized by hypertelorism, median clefting of the nose, various degrees of clefting of the lip, maxilla, and palate, a V-shaped anterior hairline, and cranium bifidum occulta.[32] This syndrome is believed to result from arrest of the development, migration, and fusion of nasal maxillary structures, which allows intracranial structures to be displaced inferiorly as an anterior cephalocele.[32]

Sonographic Findings. The sonographic diagnosis of a cephalocele requires the demonstration of a calvarial defect.[31] A frontal cephalocele protruding through a frontal calvarial defect may produce hypertelorism and a mass visible on the sagittal profile view or on axial view through the periorbital region.[6] Visualization of the calvarial defect assists

TABLE 10-4.   Malformations and Syndromes Associated With Hypertelorism

Median Plane Facial Malformations

Median cleft face syndrome
Frontal, ethmoidal, or sphenoidal meningoencephalocele
Frontal, ethmoidal, or sphenoidal (dermolipoma) teratoma
Nasal glioma
Nasofrontal mucocele

Miscellaneous Facial Defects

Proboscis lateralis
Facial clefts other than median
Facial hemangioma
Extra nares

Prominent Skull Dysplasias

Craniosynostosis
    Apert's syndrome
    Crouzon's syndrome
    Carpenter's syndrome
    Pfeiffer's syndrome
    Kleeblattschädel
Thickened skull
    Albers-Schönberg disease
Metopism

Teeth Defects

Rieger's syndrome

Prominent Neurologic and Brain Defects

Hydrocephalus (any type)
Megalencephaly with skull enlargement
Familial neurovisceral lipidosis syndrome
Lissencephaly
Agenesis of the septum pellucidum
Agenesis of the corpus callosum

Chromosomal Anomalies

Wolf's syndrome of 4p−
5p− cri du chat
Various translocations
18p, 18q− Syndromes
Turner's XO syndrome
48,XXXX
49,XXXXY
49,XXXXX
Various trisomies (10, partial 7, 9, 14)

Others

Ocular defects
Cleft lip and/or palate
Prominent skin manifestations
Prominent skeletal manifestations
Sexual organ malformations

Miscellaneous

Hypercalcemia with supravalvular aortic stenosis
Potter's syndrome
Inguinal hernia
Lymphedema and yellow nails
Acquired immunodeficiency syndrome dysmorphism
Noonan's syndrome

(Adapted from, and for more complete list see, Romero R, Pilu G, Jeanty P, et al: Prenatal Diagnosis of Congenital Anomalies. Norwalk CT: Appleton and Lange, 1988: 90–91.)

in distinguishing a cephalocele from other *frontonasal masses,*[6] such as:

- Lacrimal duct cyst
- Orbital duplication
- Facial hemangioma
- Dermoid cysts

Associated Anomalies and Prognosis. Because the list of syndromes associated with hypertelorism is extensive, the detection of hypertelorism in the fetus, at risk for a specific syndrome or in association with other malformations, may provide convincing evidence for its diagnosis. The associated anomalies depend on the underlying malformation syndrome, which characteristically determines the prognosis and reoccurrence risk as well as the prenatal sonographic findings.[30,31] Because nasofrontal cephaloceles are generally smaller than other cephaloceles, they have been observed to have a better prognosis than cephaloceles in other locations. When the cephalocele is associated with major multiple malformation syndromes, such as atelosteogenesis, a generalized chondrodysplasia that itself carries a poor prognosis, a poor outcome can be expected.[31]

Diprosopus

Clinical Features. Diprosopus is an extremely rare form of conjoined twining that consists of a single neck and body and a spectrum of duplication of craniofacial structures, ranging from isolated du-

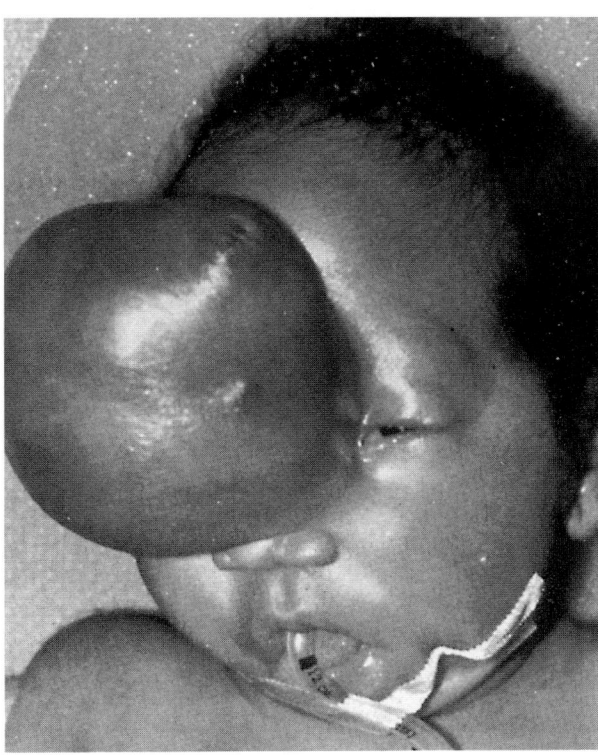

FIGURE 10-8. Hypertelorism with anterior encephalocele. Gross photograph of a large frontonasal cephalocele resulting in hypertelorism. (Nadich TP, Altman NR, Braffman GH, et al: Cephaloceles and related malformations. Am J Neuroradiol 1992; 13:655–690.)

plication of the nose to complete facial duplication. The different types of conjoined twins are presented in Chapter 20. The two median globes may be fused partially, may be separate but share a central orbit, or may occupy completely separate orbits.[33,34]

Sonographic Findings. Diprosopus twins are the rarest variety of symmetric conjoined twins, with less than 30 cases reported in the literature[35,36] (Fig. 10-9). The prenatal sonographic diagnosis of four cases of diprosopus occurred between 20 to 28 weeks of gestation, and a more recent case was diagnosed within the first trimester at 12.5 weeks of gestation. The prenatal sonographic findings include polyhydramnios, hydrocephalus, and partial duplication of the intracranial structures[33–36] (see Fig. 10-9). As with other cases of monozygotic twinning, there is an increased incidence of neural tube defects in association with diprosopus, especially anencephaly.[34] Visualization of duplication of intracranial contents distinguishes this entity

from others, and in the presence of anencephalic fetuses, the characteristic duplication of facial structures is specific for diprosopus.[6] Scans through the level of the orbits and nose should demonstrate three or four orbits and usually more than one nose.

Associated Anomalies and Prognosis. A high incidence of neural tube defects, especially anencephaly, is associated with diprosopus. Each of the reviewed reported cases with diprosopus had a concomitant neural tube defect, including craniorachischisis or a form of spinal dysraphism. Other anomalies identified in addition to the common findings of polyhydramnios, hydrocephalus, and partial duplication of intracranial structures included a diaphragmatic hernia, dextrocardia, and left gastroschisis. The fetal prognosis is extremely poor.[33–36]

Otocephaly

Clinical Features. Otocephaly is a rare disorder of unknown incidence characterized by a spectrum of malformations always associated with agnathia or micrognathia, close-set temporal bones, and abnormal position and development of the auricles.[37] In severe cases, complete failure of neural crest development and crest cell migration occurs, resulting in absence of the eyes and forebrain. Varying degrees of cyclopia, presence of a proboscis, or absence of the mouth may also occur.

Sonographic Findings. The sonographic findings of otocephaly were reported by Cayea and colleagues in a case at 26 weeks of gestation in which no normal facial morphology was evident[37] (Fig. 10-10). The ultrasound findings included an anterior cephalocele protruding in the midline at the level of the forehead, and two obliquely angled soft tissue structures resembling ears were visualized near the midline in the mid-facial region. The orbits and mouth were absent. Polyhydramnios was also observed. A detailed survey of facial structures, including position and location of the auricles, the mandible, and orbits, should aid in achieving the correct diagnosis.

Associated Anomalies and Prognosis. Other anomalies reported in association with otocephaly include alobar holoprosencephaly, hypoplastic tongue, tracheoesophageal fistula, cardiac anomalies, adrenal hypoplasia, and single umbilical artery. Otocephaly is incompatible with life.[37]

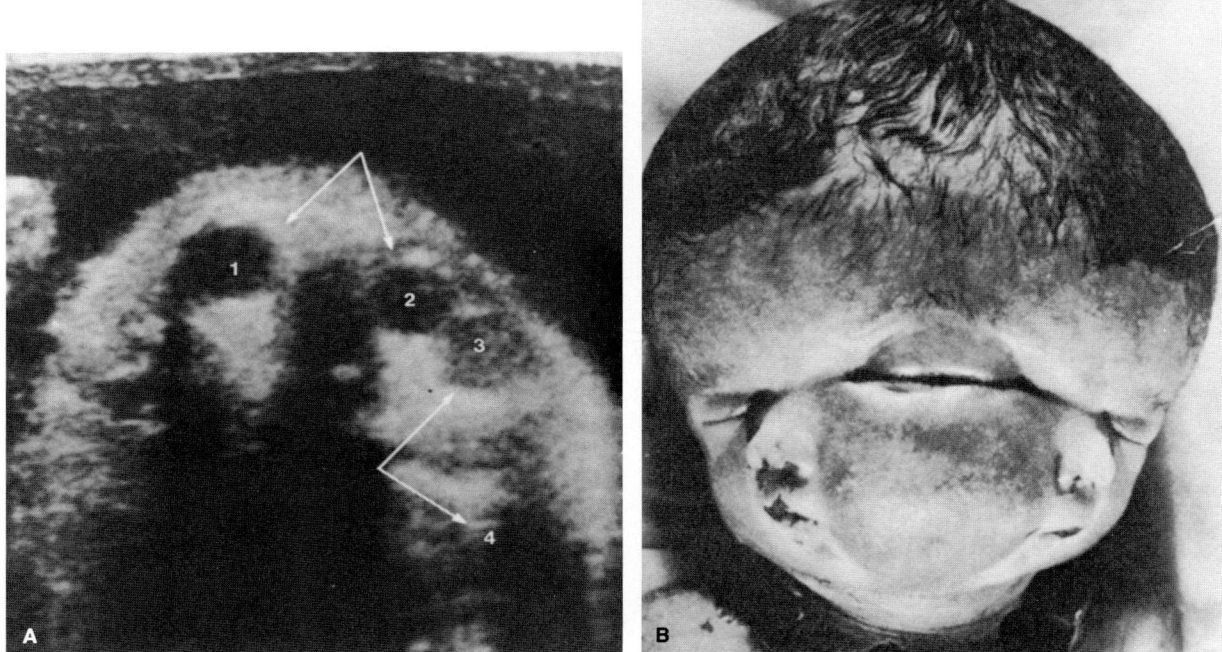

FIGURE 10-9.   Diprosopus. **(A)** Real-time sonogram of the fetal face at 28 weeks of gestation demonstrates four globes (*arrows*). The two median globes (2 and 3) share a single orbit. **(B)** Postmortem photograph at 31 weeks of gestation illustrates the duplication of facial structures with a single large midline orbit. (Okazaki JR, Wilson JL, Holmes SM, et al: Diprosopus: Diagnosis in utero. AJR 1987; 149:147–148.)

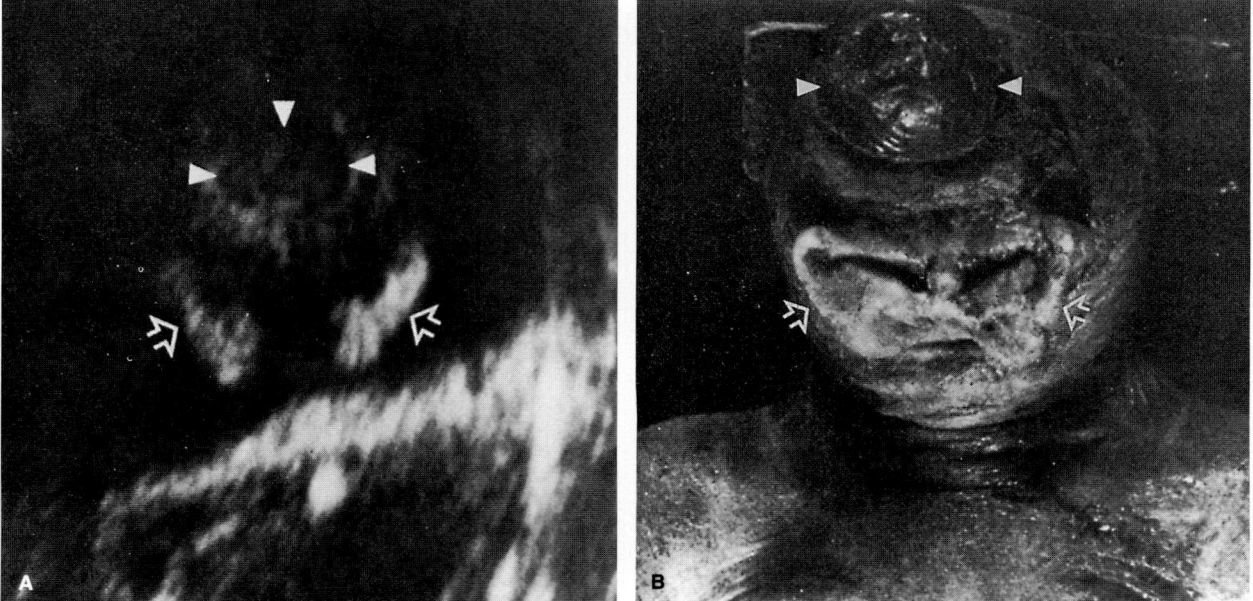

FIGURE 10-10.   Otocephaly. **(A)** Coronal scan of the face demonstrates absence of the eyes with an anterior encephalocele (*arrowheads*) and two soft tissue structures, obliquely positioned near the midline, resembling ears (*open arrows*). **(B)** Postmortem photograph of the 26-week male fetus shows absence of normal facial morphology, midline ears (*open arrows*), and anterior encephalocele (*arrowheads*). (Cayea PD, Bieber FR, Ross MJ, et al: Sonographic findings in otocephaly (synotia). J Ultrasound Med 1985; 4:377–379.)

Microphthalmia and Anophthalmia

Clinical Features. Microphthalmia (decreased orbital size) and anophthalmia (absence of the eye or vestigial eye) are rare disorders. Microphthalmia and anophthalmia are associated with at least 25 syndromes, chromosomal abnormalities (trisomy 13), and intrauterine infection.[8,9,38,39]

Although routine measurement of the intraocular diameter may detect recurrence of these syndromes, it would not be expected to provide more than a low diagnostic yield.[6] Assessment for the presence or absence of microphthalmia may become important when other intracranial abnormalities are present or in the fetus with a familial risk of orbital abnormalities.[39] A detailed survey for other anatomic anomalies and karyotype analysis usually are warranted when an orbital abnormality is detected.

Anophthalmia occurs more rarely than microphthalmia and results from failure of the optic vesical to form.[39] Taybi and Lachman associated anophthalmia with Goldenhar-Gorlin syndrome, trisomy 13, Lenz's syndrome (X-linked microphthalmia), and microphthalmia with digital anomalies.[8] Among these entities, only the Goldenhar-Gorlin syndrome (hemifacial microsomia) has associated ipsilateral ear and facial abnormalities.

Sonographic Findings. Diagnosis of microphthalmia during the second trimester may be considerably more difficult than in the third trimester, unless the orbits are unequivocally small.[6] The ocular diameter increases progressively but not linearly in size during the second and third trimesters; however, the normal global size becomes progressively more variable in the third trimester.[40] The use of ocular measurements and the potential usefulness of nomograms to confirm and recognize an anomaly are emphasized in a case reported by Feldman and colleagues of recurrent Fraser's syndrome.[38] This is an autosomal recessive disorder manifested by cryptophthalmus, usually with microphthalmus or anophthalmus, absence of septum nasi, and ambiguous genitalia.

Prenatal detection of anophthalmia was described in a case with the Goldenhar-Gorlin syndrome[39] (hemifacial microsomia; Fig. 10-11). This is best demonstrated in axial and frontal coronal sections through the expected level of the orbits and is manifested by absence of the globe and often the orbit.

Because of the frequent association between anophthalmia or microphthalmia and other chromosomal, craniofacial, vertebral, and extremity abnormalities, detection of the absence of the globe or severe microphthalmia should prompt a careful search of the fetus for other subtle malformations and consideration of chromosomal analysis.[6]

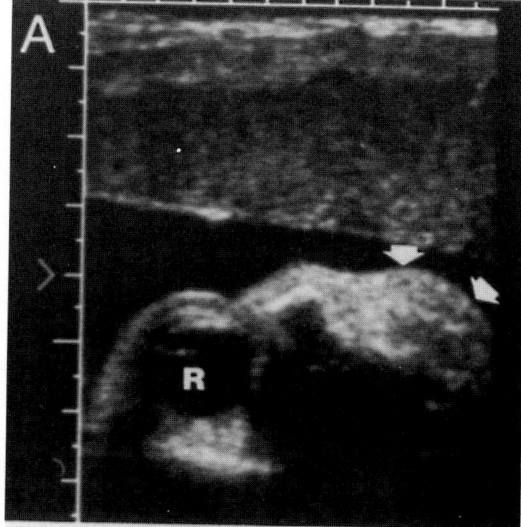

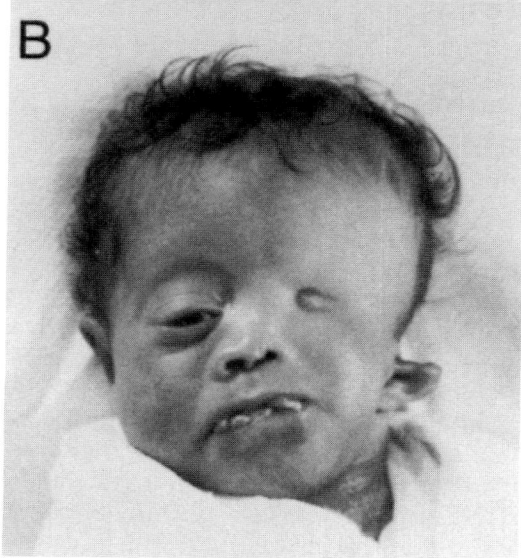

FIGURE 10-11. Goldenhar-Gorlin syndrome (hemifacial microsomia) at 30 weeks of gestation. **(A)** Axial sonogram at the mid-orbital level demonstrates absence of the left orbit (*arrows*). R, right eye. **(B)** Postnatal photograph confirms the prenatal sonographic features, including facial asymmetry with absence of the left orbit and low-set, malformed left ear. The left maxilla and mandible are hypoplastic. (Tamas DE, Mahony BS, Bowie JD, et al: Prenatal sonographic diagnosis of hemifacial microsomia [Goldenhar-Gorlin syndrome]. J Ultrasound Med 1986; 5:461–463.)

Periorbital and Facial Masses

Dacryocystoceles

Clinical Features. *Dacryocystoceles* (lacrimal duct cysts) result from congenital impatency of the distal portion of the nasolacrimal duct leading to cystic dilation of the lacrimal duct.[41] The nasolacrimal duct usually becomes patent by the eighth intrauterine month. Impatency is caused by a thin obstructing mucosal membrane near Hasner's valve, resulting in a dacryocystocele inferomedial to the orbit. About 30% of all newborns have an impatent nasolacrimal duct, but only 2% develop symptomatology. Spontaneous rupture of the obstructing membrane occurs in 78% of cases by 3 months of age and in 91% by 6 months.[41]

The differential diagnosis for periorbital masses includes:

- Dacryocystoceles
- Hemangioma
- Anterior cephalocele
- Teratomas
- Dermoid cyst
- Isolated cystic hygromas
- Soft tissue sarcoma

Hemangiomas

Hemangiomas. Hemangiomas are one of the most common benign neoplasms seen in the neonatal age. Most are cutaneous in origin and remain small and clinically insignificant. Although histologically benign, large, rapidly growing hemangiomas can result in grotesque deformity in the head and neck area and can progressively distort normal structures, resulting in airway or esophageal obstruction, pressure and necrosis of surrounding structures, and obstruction of the auditory canal.[42,43] Periorbital hemangiomas can often be distinguished from other periorbital masses by their characteristic Doppler signal.

Sonographic Findings

Dacryocystoceles. Prenatal sonographic findings of *dacryocystoceles* include the demonstration of a hypoechoic mass in their typical location inferomedial to the fetal globe, without displacement of the globe but with synchronous eye movements[41] (Fig. 10-12). In two reported cases by Davis and colleagues, these cysts measured less than 1.5 cm in diameter and were not evident at 20 to 23 weeks of gestation but became visible at 30 to 33 weeks.[41]

The sonographic features of hypoechoic masses inferomedial to the fetal globe are listed in Table

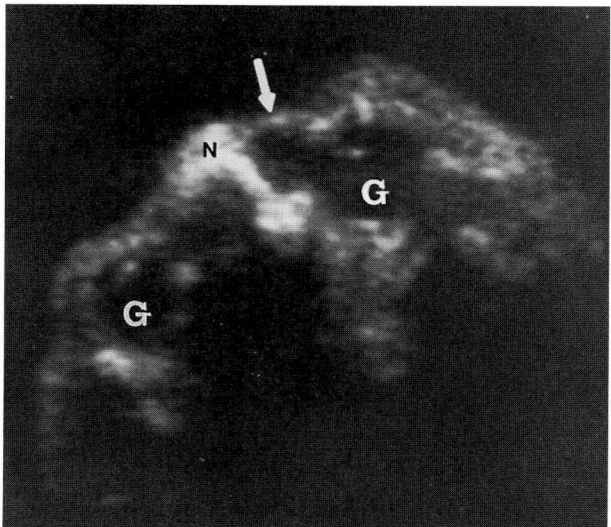

FIGURE 10-12. Dacryocystocele. Slightly oblique axial sonogram in a 33-week fetus demonstrates a small lacrimal duct cyst (dacryocystocele). The hypoechoic mass arose along the inferomedial margin of the orbit adjacent to the nose. The globe is not displaced, and synchronous eye movements were noted. *Arrow,* dacryocystocele; G, orbital globe; N, nasal bridge. (Davis WK, Mahony BS, Carroll BA, et al: Antenatal sonographic detection of benign dacryocystoceles [lacrimal duct cysts]. J Ultrasound Med 1987; 6:461–465.)

10-5 (Figs. 10-13 and 10-14). Each of these is much less common in the perinatal period. The typical location of a dacryocystocele should help to suggest its diagnosis because cephaloceles rarely occur medial to the orbit, often displace the globe downward and outward, are associated with an underlying calvarial defect and often with hydrocephalus. Periorbital dermoid cysts typically occur superolateral to the globe as opposed to inferomedial.

Hemangiomas. Periorbital and facial *hemangiomas* may present as either cystic or solid masses but frequently are at least of the same echogenicity as the placenta or are more echogenic.[42–44] The differential diagnosis for hemangiomas is similar to that for dacryocystoceles (see Table 10-5). Hemangiomas are usually larger, demonstrate well-defined vascular spaces, and exhibit characteristic Doppler signal.[43,44] Whenever a solid facial tumor is detected, one should look for areas of calcification. If gross, they suggest a possibility of a teratoma, whereas small, widely scattered calcifications giving rise to homogeneous echogenicities may suggest a hemangioma.

TABLE 10-5. Differential Diagnosis of Periorbital Masses

Lesion	Location	Sonographic Features
Dacryocystocele	Inferomedial to orbital globe	Hypoechoic mass
Hemangioma	Cutaneous head and neck	Cystic or solid
		Similar or greater echogenicity to placenta
		Characteristic Doppler signal
		Occasionally scattered calcifications
Teratoma	Head and neck	Cystic or solid
	If periorbital, superolateral to orbital globe	Usually complex
		Possibly coarse calcification
Anterior cephalocele	Usually midline	Small
	Projects through ethmoid, sphenoid, or frontal calvarial defect	Displace orbit inferiorly and laterally
		Calvarial defect
		Possibly hydrocephalus

The larger hemangiomas may be more readily diagnosed prenatally. With an increasing detection rate, it is important to be able to differentiate these benign lesions from other, more serious fetal facial cranial and nuchal masses to avoid the possibility of suggesting a therapeutic termination procedure. Early detection is also important with the larger lesions because they may cause hydrops fetalis, dystocia, or fetal injury during labor. Larger hemangiomas may cause platelet sequestration in the neonatal period, and it is valuable to recognize these in advance to observe the child for any hematologic consequences.[43]

Intraocular Abnormalities

Walker-Warburg Syndrome
Clinical Features. Because the eye is an embryologic derivative of the forebrain, fetal and neonatal ocular findings, including fetal eye movement patterns and regression of the hyaloid artery of the eye, may provide useful information about the general pattern of cerebral development and function.[20,45] Walker-Warburg syndrome is a rare autosomal recessive condition characterized by type II lissencephaly with agyria, hydrocephalus, other brain malformations, and eye abnormalities.[46] About half of cases have an occipital cephalocele. The eye abnormalities comprise a wide spectrum of malformations, including severe microphthalmia, anterior and posterior chamber defects including persistent hypoplastic primary vitreous and retinal dysplasia and detachment, corneal clouding, cataracts, and colobomatous malformations.[46,47]

Sonographic Findings. Of the many ocular findings seen postnatally in patients with Walker-Warburg syndrome, only retinal dysplasia was diagnosed antenatally in these prior reports. Farrell and colleagues diagnosed Walker-Warburg syndrome on the basis of the detection of retinal detachment in the setting of a small occipital cephalocele, absent cerebellar vermis, and hydrocephalus[46] (Fig. 10-15). The retinal detachment was not apparent at 30 weeks of gestation, but a subsequent study 2 weeks later revealed an abnormal concentric echogenic ring, which initially was thought to represent an unusually small globe but which on further follow-up at 35 weeks of gestation assumed a conical echogenic appearance attributed to retinal detachment.

Eye Movements. Birnholz reported that normal slow eye movements typically occur by 16 weeks of gestation and rapid eye movements begin at 23 weeks.[45] Rapid eye movements are more frequent between 24 and 35 weeks, after which eye inactivity becomes more common. Birnholz also detected abnormal fetal eye movement patterns in eight fetuses between 16 and 39 weeks of gestation, all of whom had obvious abnormalities of brain structure.[6,45]

Hyaloid Artery. The hyaloid artery originates from the main ophthalmic artery, runs through the center of the eye, and terminates at the posterior surface of the lens.[20] This vessel is seen in fetuses of 20 weeks gestational age or younger and regresses spontaneously at the start of the third trimester. It appears as an echogenic line coursing

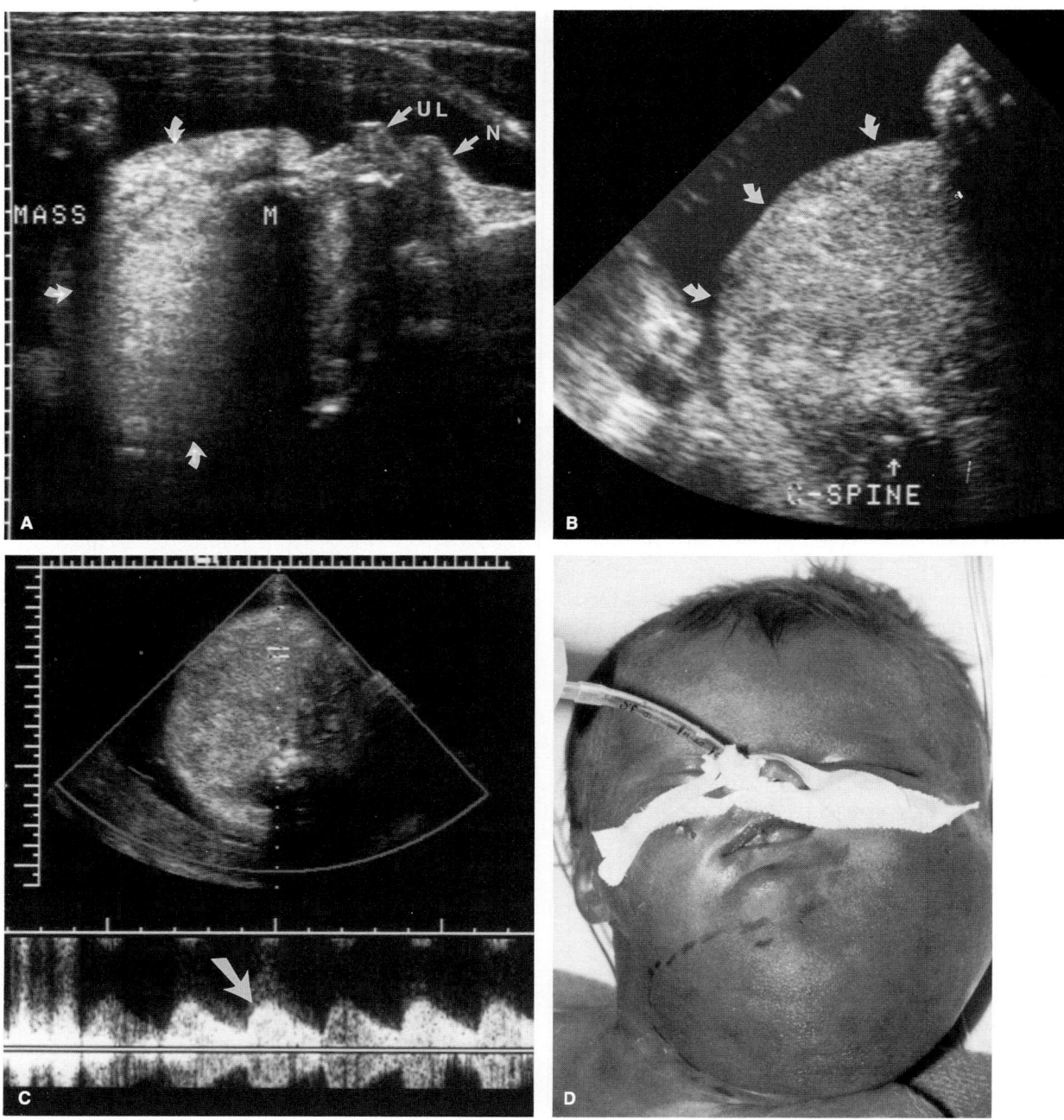

FIGURE 10-13.   Facial hemangioma. **(A)** Profile view through the fetal face demonstrates the nose (N), upper lip (U), mandible (M), and large echogenic mass (*arrows*). **(B)** Axial scan through the mass (*arrows*) demonstrates echogenic appearance of the mass. C-spine, cervical spine posteriorly. **(C)** Doppler cursor placed through the mass demonstrates low-resistance arterial waveform (*arrow*). **(D)** Preoperative photograph of the newborn demonstrates marked deformity of the face and neck due to the large hemangioma. **(D,** Courtesy of Marshall Schwartz, M.D., Children's Hospital, Pittsburgh, PA.)

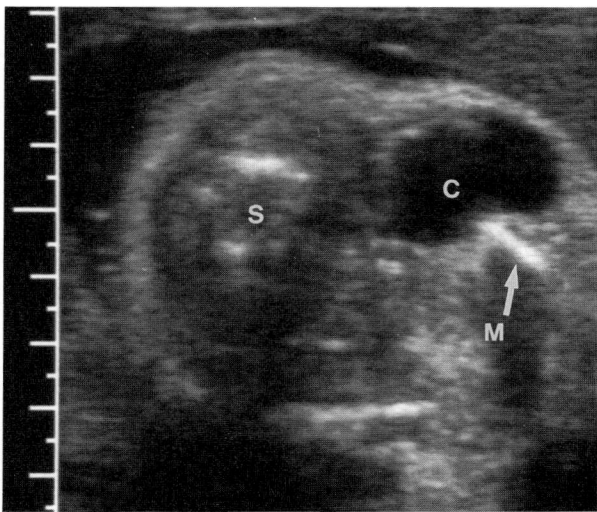

FIGURE 10-14. Isolated cystic hygroma. Axial scan through the fetal face and mandible (M) demonstrates a retromandibular cystic mass (C) that corresponded to a cystic hygroma. S, cervical spine.

centrally through the eye and demonstrates a beaded appearance as it begins to regress. The hyaloid artery remained visible beyond 30 weeks of gestation in 9 of 25 abnormal pregnancies (trisomy 21, microcephaly without chromosomal abnormality, trisomy 13, trisomy 18, fetal alcohol syndrome, and fetal hydantoin syndrome).[20] Delayed hyaloid artery regression may indicate retardation in early third-trimester cerebral development.

Lips, Mouth, and Tongue: Coronal View

Coronal views of the fetal mouth, tongue, and lips, especially the upper lip, provide useful information regarding cleft lip or macroglossia. They are especially useful in the setting of polyhydramnios, concomitant anomalies, or a positive family history when detection of facial clefts, macroglossia, or an unusually shaped mouth may suggest the presence of a specific syndrome.[6,48]

Fetal Regurgitation

A variety of fetal movements often associated with swallowing can be seen normally in utero and should be considered a part of normal fetal activity. This activity is intermittent and is not carried on continuously by the fetus.[15] Detection of fetal regurgitation or vomiting in a setting of otherwise unexplained polyhydramnios may be associated with fetal abnormalities that are most likely high gastrointestinal obstruction, for example, tracheoesophageal fistula or duodenal atresia.[15]

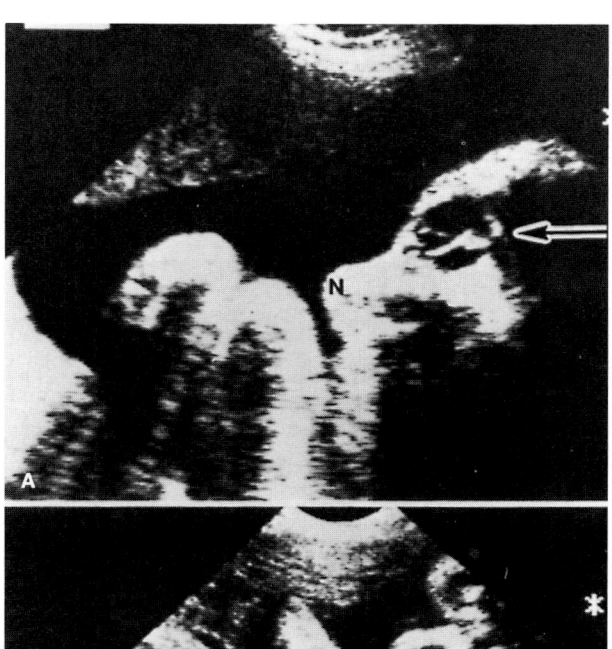

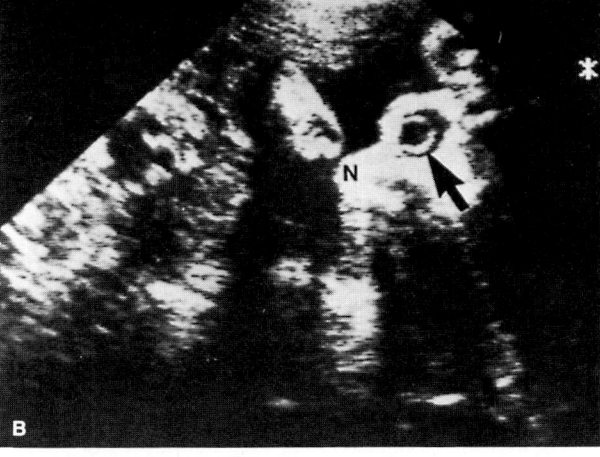

FIGURE 10-15. Walker-Warburg syndrome at 35 weeks of gestation. Semicoronal (**A**) and axial (**B**) views of the right orbit display the detached retina as an echogenic conical structure, with its base toward the lens and its apex pointing posteriorly toward the optic nerve. Hydrocephalus, absence of the cerebellar vermis, and occipital encephalocele were also observed. *Arrow*, detached retina; N, nose. (Farrell SA, Toi A, Leedman ML, et al: Prenatal diagnosis of retinal detachment in Walker-Warburg syndrome. Am J Med Genet 1987; 28:619–624.)

Fetal Lips

The scanning plane that has been proposed for optimal evaluation of the fetal lips is a coronal scan that approximates the frontal plane through the fetal nose, upper and lower lips, and chin (Figs. 10-16 and 10-17). The following questions may prove useful in the detection of abnormalities involving the upper lip and mouth:

1. Is the upper lip cleft?
2. Is the tongue protuberant?
3. Is the mouth widely open or fixed in position?

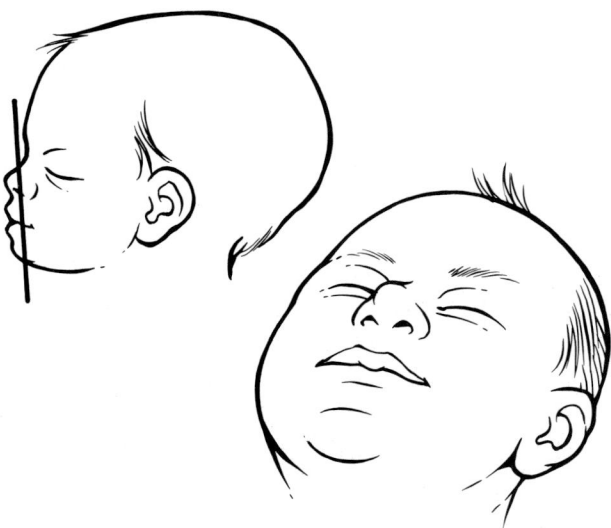

FIGURE 10-16. The approximate frontal plane of section through the upper lip, nose, and chin.

Cleft Lip and Cleft Palate

Clinical Features. Cleft lip and cleft palate are one of the most common congenital malformations of the face and palate. Although often associated, cleft lip and cleft palate are embryologically and etiologically distinct malformations, originate at different times during development, and involve different developmental processes.[4] Cleft lip and cleft palate may be complete or incomplete, unilateral or bilateral, lateral or midline, symmetric or asymmetric.[49] There are two major groups of cleft lip and palate: (1) clefts involving the upper lip and the anterior part of the maxilla, with or without involvement of parts of the remaining hard and soft regions of the palate, and (2) clefts involving the hard and soft regions of the palate.[4]

Cleft lip with or without cleft palate results from failure of fusion of the maxillary prominence with the medial nasal prominence on one or both sides at about the seventh week of development. Cleft

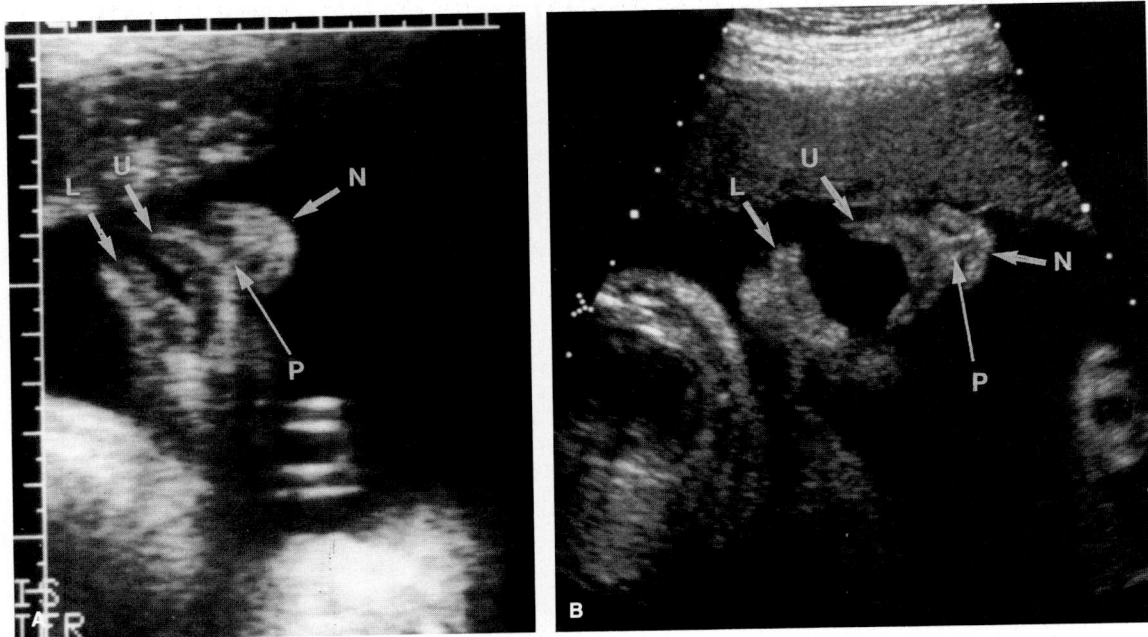

FIGURE 10-17. **(A)** Coronal ultrasound of the lips demonstrates the nose (N), upper lip (U), lower lip (L), and hypoechoic linear region in the midline between the upper lip and the nose corresponding to normal philtrum (P). **(B)** Coronal view of lips with open mouth shows nose (N), upper (U) and lower (L) lips, and the normal philtrum (P).

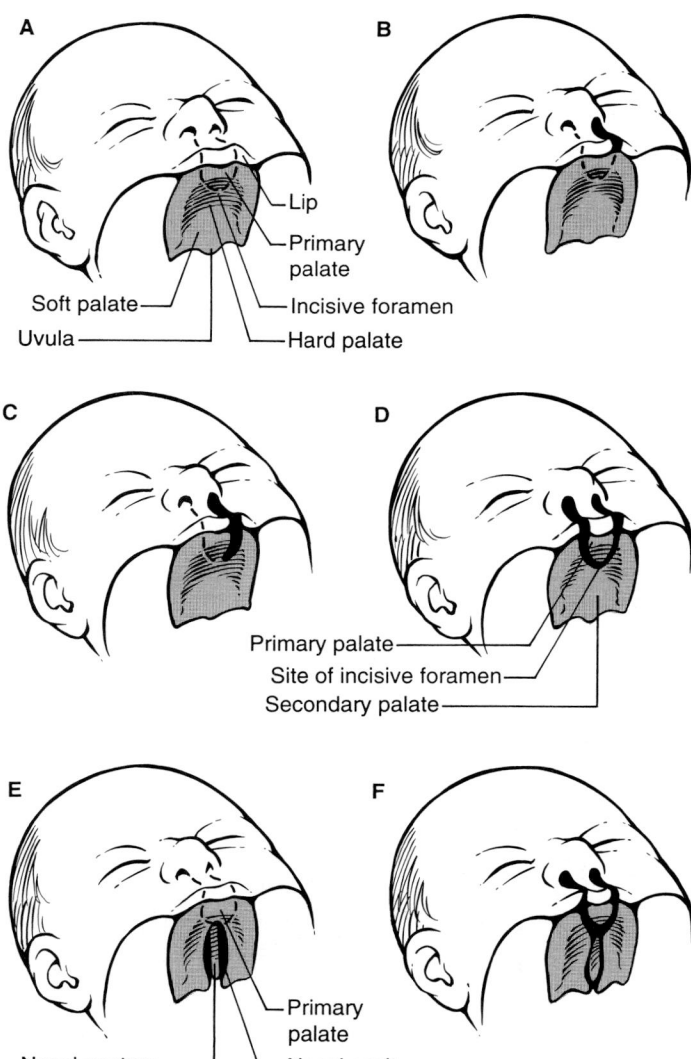

FIGURE 10-18. Various types of cleft lip and cleft palate. **(A)** Normal lip and palate. **(B)** Unilateral cleft lip extending into the nose. **(C)** Complete unilateral cleft of the lip and alveolar process with a unilateral cleft of the anterior or primary palate. **(D)** Bilateral cleft of the lip and alveolar process with bilateral cleft of the anterior palate. **(E)** Isolated cleft palate. **(F)** Bilateral cleft of the lip and alveolar process with bilateral cleft of the anterior and posterior palate. Can also occur with unilateral anterior cleft.

palate results from a failure of the mesenchymal masses in the lateral palatine processes to meet and fuse with each other, with the nasal septum, and/or with the posterior margin of the median palatine process[4,7,49] (Fig. 10-18). Two thirds of those with cleft lip also have cleft palate.[6] The incidence of cleft lip and cleft palate varies widely among various races and geographic locations. The incidence for nonsyndromic cases occurs with a frequency in the range of 1 in 800 for cleft lip with or without cleft palate, 1 in 1300 for cleft lip and cleft palate, and 1 in 2000 for isolated cleft lip or cleft palate.[6] A higher incidence has been reported in the Japanese and certain Native American tribes, whereas African-Americans have a lower incidence. Sixty to 80% of affected infants are males.[4] The incidence is slightly higher with increasing maternal age.[7]

At least 100 syndromes are associated with cleft lip and palate.[8,9,21] In most cases, the cause is idiopathic, and syndromes probably account for less than 10% of all cases[6] (Table 10-6). In those cases not associated with a syndrome, the cause is most likely a multifactorial combination of environmental and genetic factors with a threshold effect.[6] The incidence is increased in those with an affected close relative and in certain chromosomal syndromes, particularly trisomy 13 and 18.[49] The recurrence risk is 4% with one affected sibling, 4% with one affected parent, 9% with two affected siblings, and 17% with one affected sibling and one affected parent.[6,21]

TABLE 10-6.   Some Common Associations, Malformations, and Syndromes Associated With Cleft Lip and Palate

Familial

Chromosomal Abnormalities

Trisomy 13
Trisomy 18
Trisomy 21
XXXXY Syndrome
Various translocations
Triploidy

Autosomal Dominant, Autosomal Recessive, and X-Linked Cleft Syndromes

Multiple syndromes

Nongenetic Cleft Syndromes

Amniotic band syndrome
Anencephaly
Congenital heart disease
Holoprosencephaly
Encephaloceles
Median cleft face syndrome
Congenital oral teratoma

(For a more complete list, see Romero R, Pilu G, Jeanty P, et al: Prenatal Diagnosis of Congenital Anomalies. Norwalk CT: Appleton and Lange, 1988.)

The likelihood of having cleft lip or cleft palate in association with multiple malformations or a syndrome depends on the associated malformations or syndrome. For example, in one study, 15% of newborns with cleft lip had other abnormalities.

Dividing this according to subtype, 27% of those with isolated cleft palate had associated abnormalities, 14% of those with cleft lip combined with cleft palate had associated abnormalities, and 8% of those with isolated cleft lip had associated abnormalities.[50] Most isolated cleft lips and palates can be repaired with good cosmetic results, but the severity of the cleft lip and palate influences the repair. Associated anomalies may be difficult to detect sonographically; frequently, however, the other anomalies tend to be more conspicuous then the facial cleft. Chromosomal analysis may be offered once a cleft is detected because of the potential for chromosomal abnormalities and associated anomalies. Even if the antenatal detection of a facial cleft is an isolated malformation, prepartum knowledge of the cleft may help to prepare the parents psychologically for the visually disturbing deformity at birth, particularly if a treatment plan has been discussed.

Sonographic Findings

Normal. Sonographic screening of the face is accomplished best with coronal images. After about 16 weeks of gestation, normal hypoechoic orbicularis oris muscles of the lip can be visualized in continuity with the lips and nose. Subtle changes in transducer angulation from the coronal plane permit sequential scans through the soft tissues of the lips, chin, alveolar ridge, and nose. Fetal positioning, maternal body habitus, and oligohydramnios can interfere with obtaining the optimal images of these landmarks.

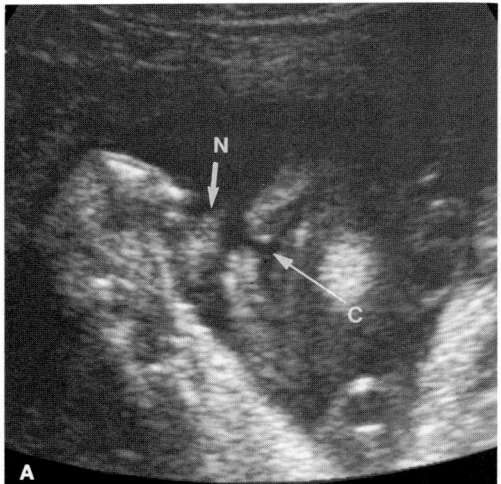
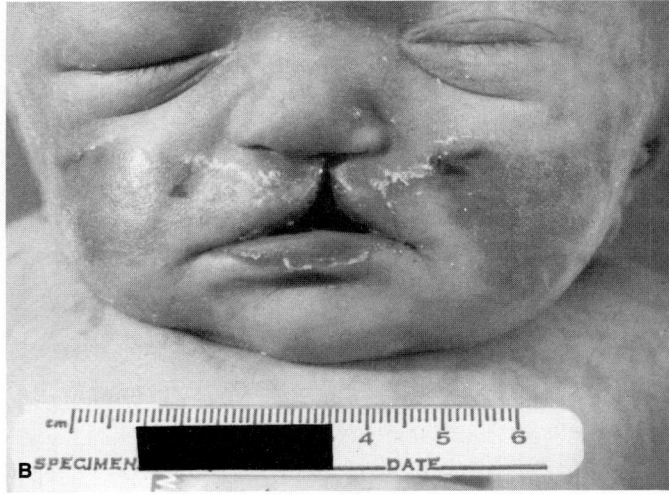

FIGURE 10-19.   Lateral cleft lip. **(A)** Coronal scan through the nose (N) demonstrates a small, hypoechoic region lateral to the midline in the upper lip, which extends to the nares (N) and corresponds to a lateral cleft lip (C). **(B)** Specimen from another fetus demonstrates typical findings of isolated lateral cleft lip extending lateral of midline in the upper lip to the nares.

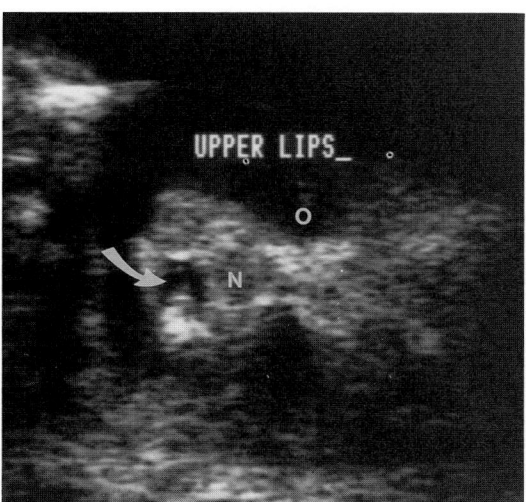

FIGURE 10-20. Lateral cleft lip plus palate. Coronal ultrasound through the maxilla demonstrates a larger defect (*curved arrows*) lateral to midline corresponding to a cleft lip and cleft palate. N, nose; O, orbit.

TABLE 10-7. Differential Diagnosis of Cleft Lip and Palate

Type of Cleft	Comment
Normal philtrum	Normal finding
Lateral cleft lip and/or palate	Most common craniofacial malformation
	Common embryologic paramedian locations
	Left lateral more common
Midline cleft	Rare
	Associated primarily with median cleft face syndrome or holoprosencephaly
Amniotic band syndrome	Bizarre facial clefts
	Not in embryologic paramedian or median distributions

Pitfalls. A false-positive diagnosis of a cleft lip can be made when visualization of the normal philtrum (midline groove of the upper lip) or frenulum labii superioris is confused for a cleft (see Fig. 10-17 and Table 10-7).

Lateral Cleft Lip and Palate. Most clefts detected prenatally with ultrasound are not subtle and tend to be large. Typical ultrasound features include an anechoic region in the upper lip just lateral to the midline, which extends to the nares (Fig. 10-19). Often with larger lateral abnormalities, the defect appears to be midline. The sensitivity with which smaller defects are detected is not known. Parasagittal and sagittal profile views may assist in identifying premaxillary protrusion, which may be the first or primary clue to the presence of a facial abnormality and so can permit early prenatal identification of bilateral cleft lip and cleft palate.[51,52]

In about 25% of cases, only the lip is cleft; in 50% there is combined clefting of the lip and palate (Fig. 10-20); and in less than 25%, there is clefting of the palate only[53] (see Fig. 10-18). Cleft lip is bilateral in 20% of cases and may be asymmetric in 70% of these cases.

Bilateral Cleft Lip and Palate. A demonstration of premaxillary protrusion is a primary clue to the presence of a facial abnormality permitting earlier prenatal identification of bilateral cleft lip and cleft palate.[54] Premaxillary protrusion occurs only with bilateral complete cleft lip and palate (Figs. 10-21

and 10-22). The perinasal echogenic mass represents protruding bone and alveolar structures within the premaxillary protrusion. The mass typically is inferior to the nose, irregular in shape, and of similar echogenicity to bone and alveolar structures. A soft tissue mass protruding outward and

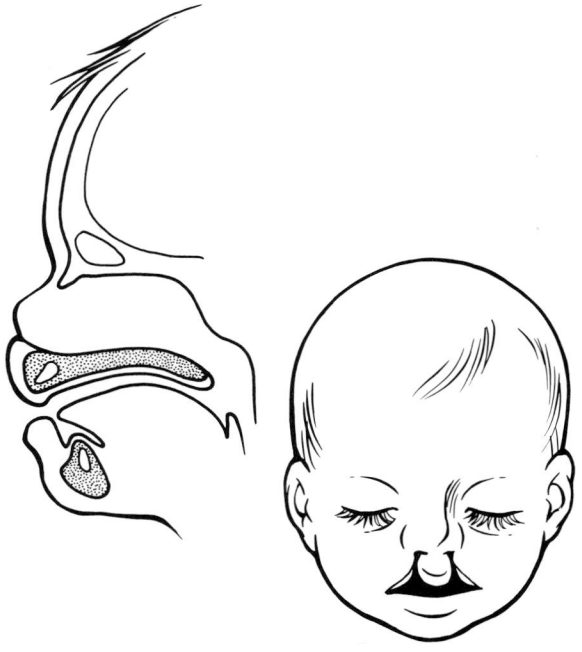

FIGURE 10-21. Bilateral complete cleft lip and palate. Frontal and sagittal views demonstrating the position of the protruding premaxillary mass. The echogenic mass seen on prenatal sonography is related in part to the alveolar bone and teeth, which have migrated anteriorly.

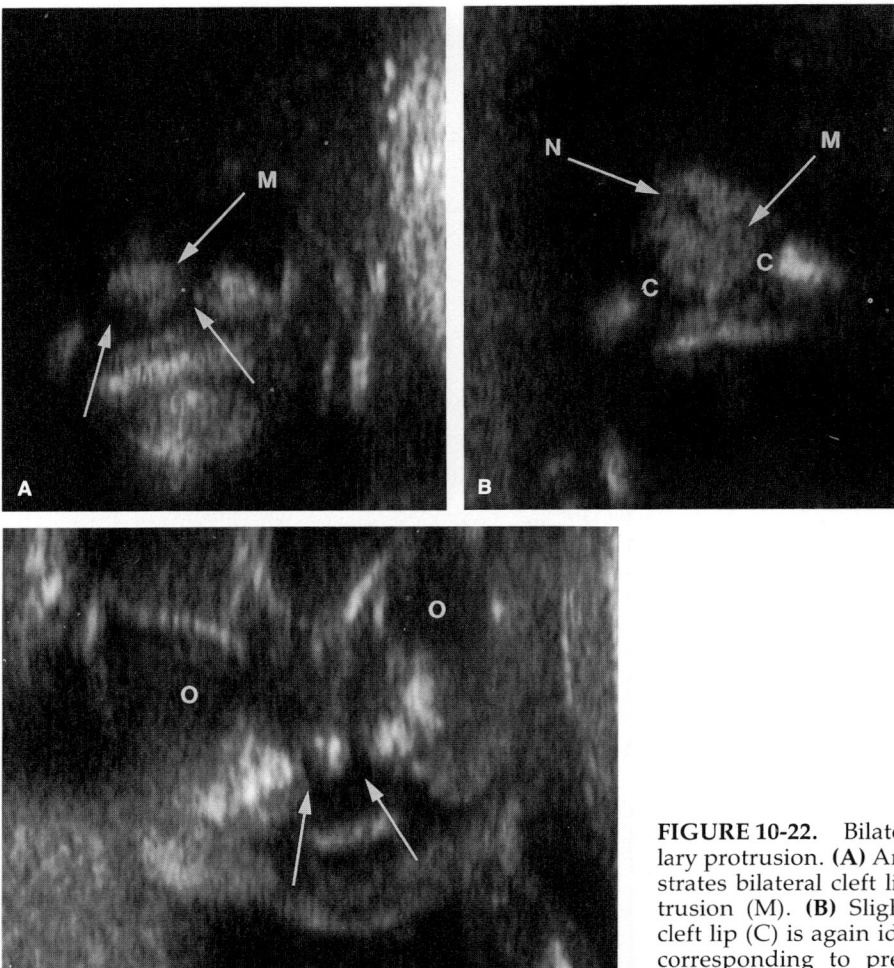

FIGURE 10-22. Bilateral cleft lip and palate—premaxillary protrusion. **(A)** Anterior coronal ultrasound demonstrates bilateral cleft lip (*arrows*) with premaxillary protrusion (M). **(B)** Slightly more posterior, the bilateral cleft lip (C) is again identified, and echogenic mass (M) corresponding to premaxillary protrusion is demonstrated. N, nose. **(C)** Scan slightly posterior demonstrates the clefts extending into the anterior hard palate (*arrows*). O, orbit.

upward from the upper lip on sagittal views of the face may also be seen in some fetuses with premaxillary protrusion. This soft tissue component correlates with an everted upper lip.[52,54] The perinatal echogenic mass appears most prominent during the second trimester at a time when the cleft itself is small and often difficult to detect. The mass may become less prominent with advancing gestational age.[54] The differential diagnosis for *premaxillary protrusion* includes:

- Anterior cephalocele
- Hemangioma
- Teratoma
- Enlarged, protruding tongue
- Proboscis (associated with holoprosencephaly)

Premaxillary protrusion should be distinguished from these masses by its position, size, and sonographic appearance because only premaxillary protrusion contains an echogenic bone component within the mass.[52]

Cleft Palate. Antenatal detection of cleft lip and palate has been well documented in the literature, but antenatal detection of cleft palate has been reported only in one case with Pierre Robin's syndrome.[55]

Cleft palate is much more difficult to observe and diagnose sonographically, and isolated cleft palate is frequently missed on prenatal sonograms because of shadowing from facial bones. If a cleft lip is detected, coronal frontal scans obtained more posteriorly may demonstrate incomplete formation of the maxillary ridge, indicating cleft palate.[6] Suggestive features of cleft palate include findings of associated cleft lip, maxillary interruption, and increased tongue excursion.[49] Cleft lip is easier to visualize sonographically than cleft palate, and since the fetal face is not always easily visualized, ancillary signs of this diagnosis become important. A small, absent, or transiently visualized fetal stomach and polyhydramnios may be sonographic clues that the fetus has cleft palate. These findings are related to impaired fetal swallowing, but the diagnosis is not made unless the cleft is observed because these ancillary signs may alternatively result from any proximal gastrointestinal tract obstruction from an anatomic or functional cause.

Median Cleft Lip. When a cleft is detected, one should attempt to distinguish midline clefts from lateral clefts because the two forms of clefting are distinct pathologic entities (see Figs. 10-19 and 10-20). The median cleft lip is the rare form and occurs primarily in association with two syndromes: the median cleft face syndrome (frontonasal dysplasia) and the holoprosencephaly complex.[8] The median cleft lip is caused by the incomplete merging of the two medial nasal prominences in the midline. This anomaly is usually accompanied by a deep groove between the right and left sides of the nose.[7]

Associated Findings and Prognosis. The causes of cleft lip and/or cleft palate are multifactorial and include syndromes, autosomal trisomies, and teratogens. Most cases of cleft lip and cleft palate diagnosed prenatally have been detected as a manifestation of a syndrome.[56–58]

In a study by Kraus and colleagues, a 60% incidence of associated anomalies was found, most commonly clubfoot and polydactyly.[59] It is estimated that 14% of surviving patients with cleft lip with or without cleft palate and 55% of survivors with only cleft palate have a broader syndrome or complex. Trisomy 13, which occurs in about 1 in 6000 births, is associated with cleft lip and cleft palate or isolated cleft palate in 60% of cases. Other common features of trisomy 13 include the holoprosencephaly complex with distinct facial features. Trisomy 13 is also associated with cystic kidneys, encephalocele, polydactyly, and cardiac structural defects[6,21,57] (see Chapter 21). In trisomy 18, which occurs in about 1 in 3000 births, 40% of cases have cleft lip and/or cleft palate.[6,57] Both these trisomies are associated with poor prognosis. Cleft lip and/or cleft palate also occurs in about

0.5% of cases with trisomy 21 and in 30% of triploidy cases.[6] When a cleft lip and/or cleft palate is detected prenatally, a thorough search for other anomalies should be undertaken and may warrant chromosomal analysis.

Marked progress has been made in the structural and functional repair of isolated cleft lip and palate. This has been through a team approach that combines plastic surgeons, orthodontists, prosthodontists, speech pathologists, social workers, psychologists, and parents.[51] Mental retardation is no more frequent in these newborns, but eustachian tube dysfunction and hearing impairment are common, as are associated defects.

Amniotic Band Syndrome

Clinical Features. The amniotic band syndrome, also known as the amniotic band disruption complex or limb body wall complex, is a common, nonrecurrent cause of various fetal malformations involving the craniofacial region, limbs, and trunk. It is estimated to occur in 1 in 1200 live births.[60] The malformations range from mild deformities to severe anomalies that are incompatible with postnatal life. Bizarre facial clefts, fissures, or slash defects in nonembryologic distributions are common. The pathogenesis is thought to be related to rupture of the amnion, with subsequent entrapment and entanglement of the fetus by fibrous mesodermic bands that emanate from the chorionic side of the amnion. The fetal head, trunk, and extremities may be involved individually or in combination, with entrapment of fetal parts by the bands causing lymphedema, amputation, or slash defects in nonembryologic distributions.[60,61] The facial defects probably result from fetal swallowing of the fibrous bands.[61] The swallowed portion of the band most likely tethers the unswallowed portion, which then cuts across the face in a random fashion producing the bizarre slash defects of the face or mandible. The prognosis for the amniotic band syndrome varies depending on the level and degree of fetal entrapment, ranging from death secondary to disruption of the umbilical cord or discordant anencephaly to minor facial clefts, lymphedema, or extremity amputations.[60,62]

Sonographic Findings. Detection of bizarre facial clefts in unusual locations warrants a careful search for other manifestations of the amniotic band syndrome[63] (Fig. 10-23). These include asymmetric encephalocele, gastropleuroschisis, asymmetric amputations, and focal constrictions with

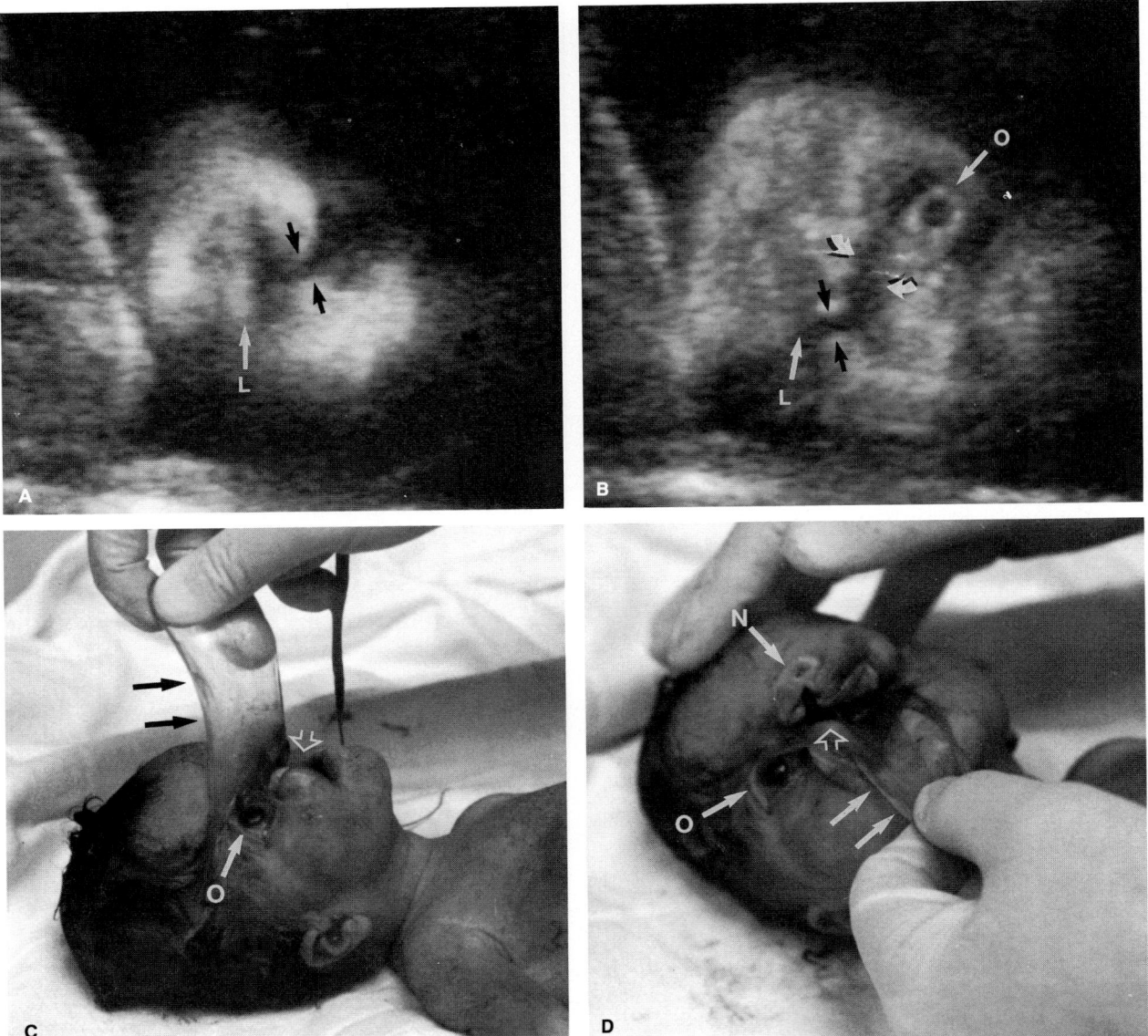

FIGURE 10-23.   Facial clefts with the amniotic band syndrome. **(A)** Anterior coronal ultrasound of the face demonstrates large, asymmetric defect in the upper lip (*black arrows*). L, lower lip. **(B)** Another semicoronal view shows defect (*arrows*) in the upper lip extending across the face (*curved arrows*) into the orbit (O). L, lower lip. **(C,D)** Postmortem photographs illustrate the bizarre facial clefts and slash defects in nonembryologic distributions indicative of the amniotic band syndrome. Some of the facial defects result from fetal swallowing of the fibrous bands. O, orbit; N, nose; *open arrowhead*, cleft; *white and black arrows*, fibrous amniotic bands.

distal lymphedema.[60,63] A search for the amniotic bands themselves also should be made. Visualization of the fibrous bands attached to the fetus, with characteristic deformities and restriction of motion, is diagnostic of the amniotic band syndrome. Identification of a band is not necessary to make the diagnosis, and a diagnosis of amniotic band syndrome should never be made on observation of

these bands in the absence of fetal deformities because several types of membranes may be seen in normal pregnancies.[60]

Macroglossia
Clinical Features.   Prenatal sonography frequently demonstrates normal fetal tongue movement. Macroglossia is rare but can be seen in at least 20

syndromes described by Taybi and Lachman[8] and Smith.[9] The most common cause for an enlarged tongue prenatally is the *Beckwith-Wiedemann syndrome.* This syndrome is more common in females and usually occurs sporadically but may occur as an autosomal dominant trait with incomplete penetrance and variable expressivity.[9,64] Others have suggested multifactorial inheritance as an explanation for familial recurrences.[64] This condition is most commonly associated with somatic macrosomia, macroglossia, gigantism, and omphalocele. Other commonly present abnormalities include variable visceromegaly, such as hepatomegaly, renal hyperplasia and dysplasia, distinctive horizontal earlobe creases, prolonged neonatal hypoglycemia, and increased incidence of intraabdominal malignancies, such as Wilms' tumor and hepatoblastoma.[64-66] Macroglossia is the most frequent anomaly present and occurs in 97.5% of cases, whereas 60% have other anomalies.[66]

Macroglossia has also been reported in a rare case of *congenital ichthyosis (harlequin fetus).*[48] Mild and moderately severe forms of ichthyosis are relatively common disorders, but the harlequin fetus represents a rare, severe, and dramatic form of this disorder. It is associated with high perinatal mortality, thick fissured skin, marked ectropion (eyelid eversion), eclabium (eversion of the lips), and flexion deformities. The disorder may be inherited as an autosomal recessive trait.

Sonographic Findings

Beckwith-Wiedemann Syndrome. Sonographic detection of an enlarged and protuberant tongue has permitted the prenatal diagnosis of Beckwith-Wiedemann syndrome, especially when associated with large-for-gestational-age measurements, polyhydramnios, visceromegaly, or omphalocele[66] (Fig. 10-24). A detailed evaluation of the fetal face, especially the fetal facial profile, is important when there is a positive family history.

The prenatal diagnosis of the Beckwith-Wiedemann syndrome based on the detection of macroglossia has been reported in only two cases.[64,66] Cobellis and colleagues were the first to report the prenatal diagnosis of macroglossia at 30 menstrual weeks in a large-for-gestational-age fetus and in a family at risk for the syndrome.[66] Shah and Metlay did not demonstrate evidence of macroglossia in a fetus who had multiple serial ultrasound examinations between 16 and 39 menstrual weeks, but examination of the neonate did demonstrate a large and protuberant tongue.[64] The diagnosis of the Beckwith-Wiedemann syndrome was made at 26

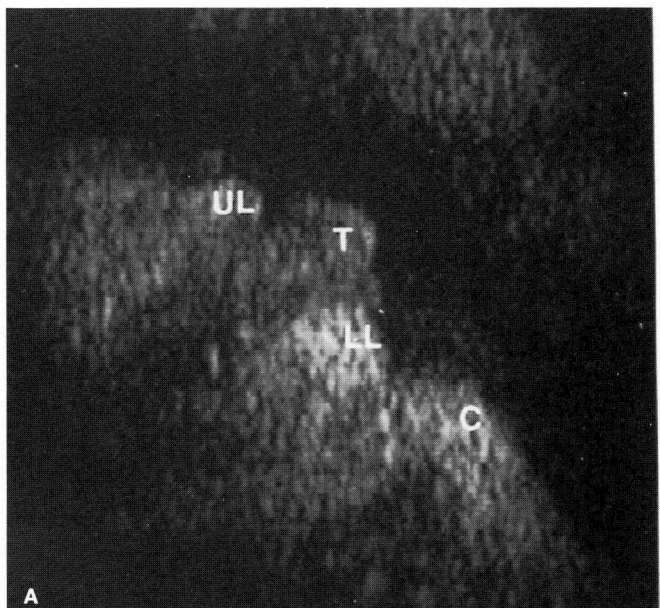 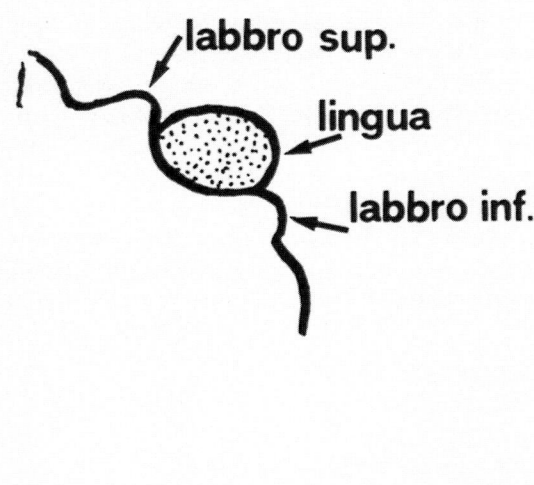

FIGURE 10-24. Macroglossia. Sagittal sonogram **(A)** and corresponding drawing **(B)** of the mouth show a protuberant tongue extending through the open mouth in this 30-week fetus with the Beckwith-Wiedemann syndrome. UL, upper lip (labbro sup); T, enlarged tongue (lingua); LL, lower lip (labbro inf); C, chin. (Cobellis G, Iannoto P, Stabile M, et al: Prenatal ultrasound diagnosis of macroglossia in the Wiedemann-Beckwith syndrome. Prenat Diagn 1988; 8:79–81.)

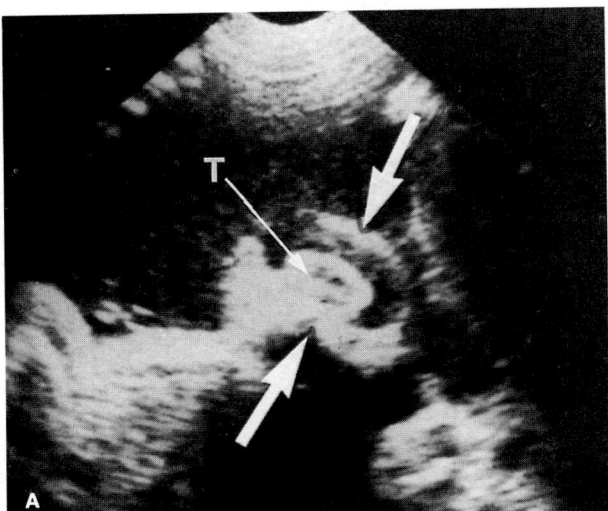
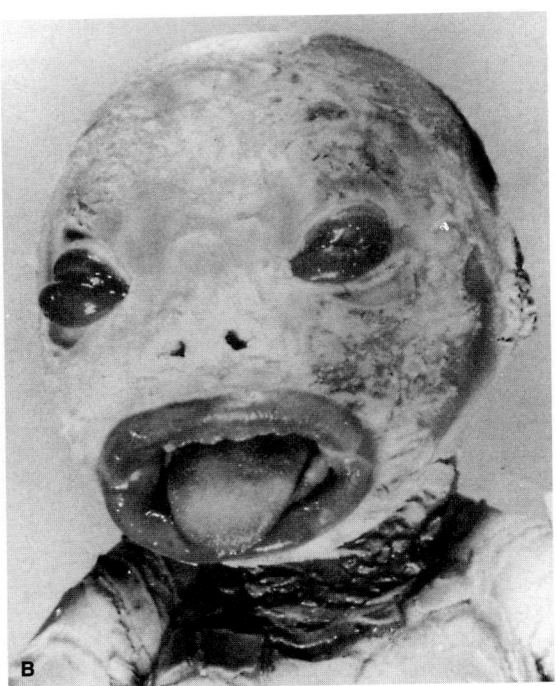

FIGURE 10-25. Congenital ichthyosis (harlequin fetus). **(A)** Coronal view of the fetal face at 31 weeks of gestation demonstrates large, thickened lips (*arrows*) and a protuberant tongue (T). **(B)** Postmortem photograph demonstrates the grotesque, clown-like appearance with marked ectropion and eclabium, absent nose, and widely opened mouth. (Meizner I: Prenatal ultrasonic features in a rare case of congenital ichthyosis (harlequin fetus). J Clin Ultrasound 1992; 20:132–134.)

menstrual weeks and was based on the presence of omphalocele, fetal macrosomia, and polyhydramnios. The fetal facial profile appeared normal at 26 menstrual weeks. Macroglossia may be a late sonographic feature.[66] Placental enlargement is another manifestation of the Beckwith-Wiedemann syndrome.[64] The anomalies associated with the Beckwith-Wiedemann syndrome, such as visceromegaly and omphalocele, most commonly occur in entities other than the Beckwith-Wiedemann syndrome. Macroglossia might occur with the following disorders:[6,67]

- Congenital ichthyosis
- Mucopolysaccharide syndromes
- Athyrotic hypothyroidism
- Chromosomal abnormalities

The differential diagnosis for macroglossia includes:

- Anterior cephalocele
- Tumors of the tongue
- Epignathus

Occasionally, an anterior cephalocele may extend through the ethmoid sinuses into the mouth and resemble an enlarged tongue.[6] Epignathus is a pharyngeal teratoma that extends through the mouth and is explained in more detail in the next section.

Harlequin Fetus. The prenatal sonographic diagnosis of marked eclabium (eversion of the lips) and macroglossia has been reported in two cases of the rare disorder congenital ichthyosis[48,68] (*harlequin fetus;* Fig. 10-25). The sonographic signs leading to prenatal diagnosis of harlequin fetus may include widely open mouth, marked eclabium and ectropion, hypoplastic nose, macroglossia, lack of fetal breathing movements, edematous-like limbs, and intrauterine membranes.[48,68]

Facial Profile View

The fetal profile is optimally demonstrated with the mid-sagittal view of the face (Fig. 10-26). When evaluating the facial profile, the following questions may prove useful in the detection of facial anomalies:

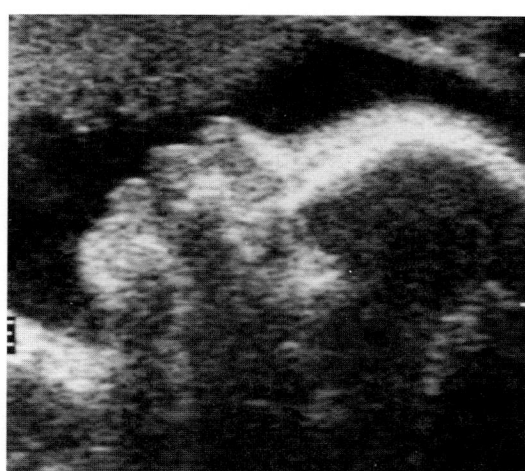

FIGURE 10-26. The normal mid-sagittal facial profile view. Note the echogenic nasal bridge, the normal maxilla, and the normally formed mandible.

1. Is the nose flattened or the nasal bridge absent?
2. Is the chin abnormally small?
3. Is an abnormal mass present?

The mid-sagittal view may reveal large facial or neck masses as well as more subtle abnormalities, including abnormal or absent nose, micrognathia, enlarged tongue, or absent nasal bridge.[6] The profile view aids in demonstrating most large masses, including epignathus, anterior cephaloceles, cervical teratomas, and hemangiomas. Parasagittal scans may be necessary to detect small tumors that do not extend to the midline, as may be the case with some facial hemangiomas or sarcomas. The sagittal view also assists in the diagnosis of bilateral cleft lip and cleft palate, with a small premaxillary protrusion, and the proboscis associated with the holoprosencephaly complex.

Routine mid-sagittal images of the face may be especially helpful in pregnancies complicated by a family history of facial abnormalities, the presence of other anomalies or polyhydramnios, and maternal teratogen exposure. Hegge and colleagues diagnosed the fetal warfarin syndrome at 20 menstrual weeks based on visualization of a sunken nose in a fetus whose mother had a history of warfarin (Coumadin) use.[10] They also detected a markedly flattened nose in a fetus with Conradi's syndrome (chondrodysplasia punctata) and in a case of thanatophoric dwarfism.

To our knowledge, the normal and abnormal profiles of the fetal forehead, nose, and chin have not been well defined. Pilu and colleagues re-

ported a case with Pierre Robin's syndrome in which a mid-sagittal facial view at 23 weeks of gestation was interpreted as normal; however, a similar view at 35 weeks demonstrated marked micrognathia.[69] Unequivocal facial deformity of a fetus at risk for a specific syndrome allows confirmation of a diagnosis and permits accurate diagnosis. Normal sonographic findings, however, do not absolutely exclude an affected fetus because the reliability of sonography in detecting a syndrome depends on severity of expression in the fetus. For example, there is great variability in the degree of micrognathia and facial clefting in the autosomal dominant mandibulofacial dysostosis (Treacher Collins syndrome).[70] Abnormalities seen on a facial profile view may assist in accurate diagnosis in multiple malformation syndromes, even in the absence of genetic or teratogen risk.[6] Benson and colleagues reported a case of Nager acrofacial dysostosis syndrome, a rare syndrome characterized by mandibulofacial dysostosis and upper limb radial defects in which a fetus at 30 weeks of gestation demonstrated severe micrognathia, polyhydramnios, malformed ear, and severely shortened and deformed upper extremities[71] (Fig. 10-27). The profile view may also assist in the detection of absence of the nasal bridge and frontal bossing, especially in cases with multiple malformations.[6] These findings are nonspecific, however, and may be seen in association with many different syndromes.[6,8,9] One must be careful when scanning in the parasagittal axis because hypoplasia of the nasal bridge and mandibular hypoplasia may be simulated (Fig. 10-28).

Epignathus

Clinical Features. Epignathus is a rare pharyngeal teratoma that arises from the palate in the region of Rathke's pouch. Epignathus generally extends through the mouth and creates an anterior mass that varies greatly in size and texture. There is no known genetic risk or predisposing factor. When an epignathus is identified antenatally, fetal surveillance with sonography and bioelective monitoring is indicated. If there is no evidence of hydropic change, perinatal management usually involves planned cesarean section to avoid dystocia and fetal trauma, with immediate establishment of an airway followed by surgical excision. Survival rates are only about 30% to 40%.[72-74]

Sonographic Findings. Demonstration of a variable-size complex cystic and solid mass adjacent to the anterior portion of the face should suggest the possible diagnosis of epignathus (Fig. 10-29). Of

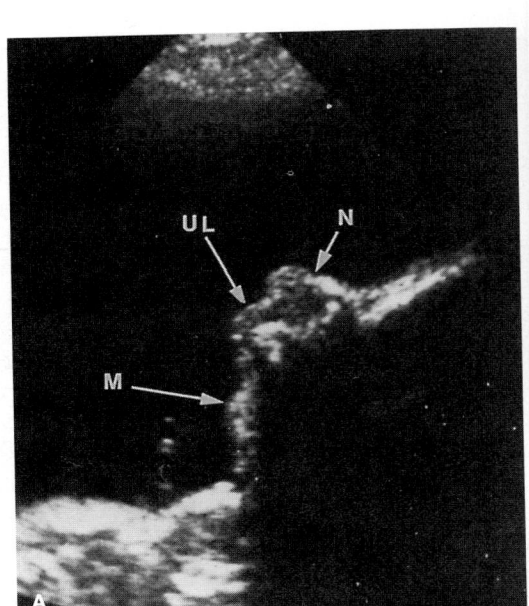 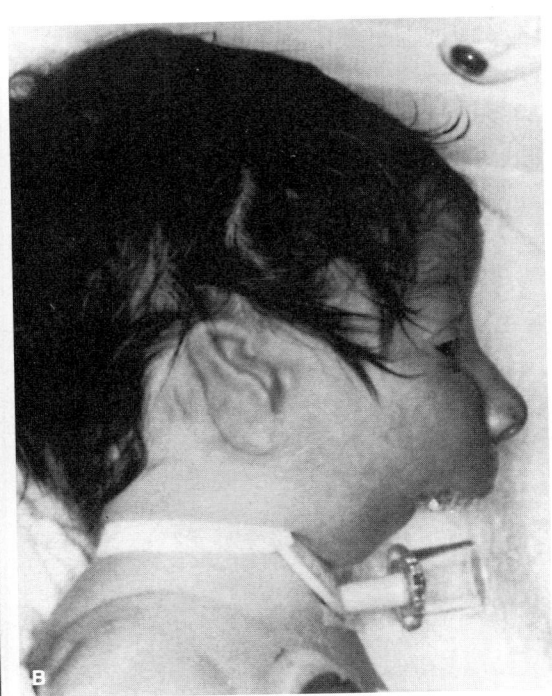

FIGURE 10-27.   Micrognathia with Nager acrofacial dysostosis syndrome. **(A)** Sagittal sonogram of the face demonstrates marked micrognathia (M). Other images showed polyhydramnios, marked extremity shortening, four digits on the hand, and deformed external ear. N, nose; UL, upper lip. **(B)** Postnatal lateral view of the face demonstrates marked micrognathia, dysplastic external ear, and absence of external auditory canal. (Benson CB, Pober BR, Hirsh MP, et al: Sonography of Nagar acrofacial dysostosis syndrome in utero. J Ultrasound Med 1988; 7:163–176.)

the six reported prenatally detected cases of epignathus, the earliest diagnosis was made at 21 weeks of gestation.[72,73,75–78] These masses were generally large, ranging from about 6 to 12 cm in diameter. One case demonstrated calcification within the mass.[72] Variable neck posturing may also occur, as was demonstrated in one case with noticeable hyperextension of the head.[78]

Associated Anomalies and Prognosis. Concomitant polyhydramnios has been detected in all reported cases, presumably because of obstruction of the fetal oropharynx causing a failure of fetal swallowing. Polyhydramnios may also occur secondary to high-output cardiac failure and hydrops fetalis in the presence of a large and vascular epignathus. None of the cases detected prenatally survived the neonatal period. The prognosis is improved in cases of relatively small tumors, in which survival after postnatal surgical resection has been reported.[74]

Fetal Ears

Routine sonographic examination of the fetal external ears rarely provides any useful information in the absence of other or obvious abnormalities. Low-set ears and malformation of the external ear may occur as a manifestation of more than 85 syndromes listed by Smith.[9] On prenatal sonographic examination, anatomic detail of at least one external ear is usually visible when amniotic fluid outlines the ear structure.[79] Fetal positioning, maternal obesity, and oligohydramnios frequently limit visibility of one or both ears.

Few sonographic reports have documented abnormalities of the fetal external ear despite the large number of potential causes for malformations, probably as a result of the lack of routine surveying of the ears.[39,71,79–81] In most cases, the deformities are either gross or occur as a part of a syndrome with more obvious sonographic findings.

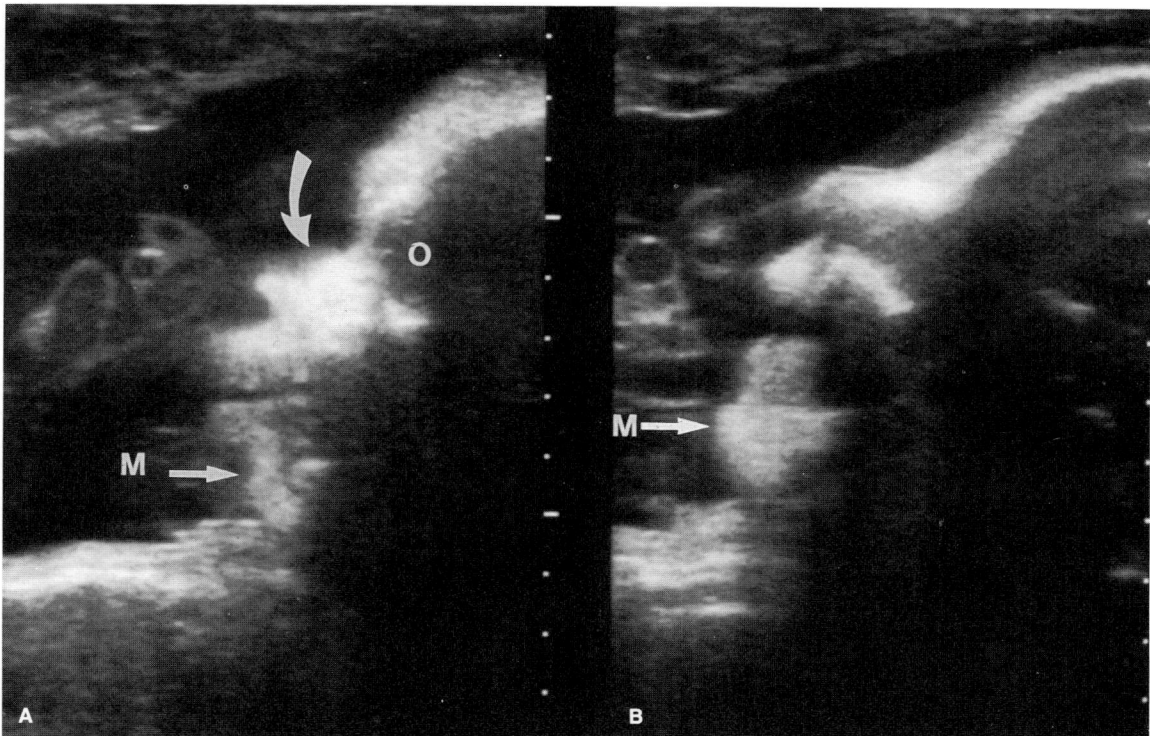

FIGURE 10-28.   Off-axis (parasagittal) profile view—pseudomandibular hypoplasia. **(A)** Parasagittal view demonstrates apparent mandibular hypoplasia (M) and hypoplasia of the nasal bone (*arrow*) when scanning off to one side of the face. This mistake may be avoided by noting that the scanning is off-axis through the orbit (O). **(B)** When moving the scanning plane to the true midline, we note the normal nasal bridge, the maxilla, and the normally developed mandible (M).

Coronal and parasagittal views of the fetal external ear may prove useful in the detection of anomalies involving the ear and allow the physician to answer the following questions:

1. Are the ears obviously deformed?
2. Are the ears low-set or of abnormal size?

Birnholz reported edema of the fetal external ear in hydrops fetalis, thickened ear in diabetic macrosomia, prominent mid-helix in thanatophoric dwarfism and osteogenesis imperfecta, and rounded pinnae in achondrogenesis.[79] The prenatal diagnosis in each of these cases was not made on the basis of the ear findings.

Pitfalls

Fink and colleagues described a potential pitfall in which a prominent external ear could be mistaken for a rare parietal cephalocele.[82] This error can be avoided by documenting the characteristic external ear anatomy in the absence of a calvarial defect.

Sonography

The diagnosis of low-set ears depends on obtaining the exact horizontal section that shows the corner of the orbit and the point where the helix of the ear meets the cranium. Normally, the helix meets the cranium above this point.[80] This may be difficult except in obvious cases; therefore, a coronal view demonstrating the position of the ear relative to the mandible and neck may prove more useful in diagnosing low-set ears.

Birnholz and Farrell found a linear relation between the maximal normal fetal ear length and gestational age: ear length (mm) = 1.1011 × gestational age (wk) − 9.5089.[83] Abnormally short ears were defined as more than 1.5 standard deviations less than the age-corrected mean. Abnormally short ears were found in three fetuses with trisomy 13, three with trisomy 18, and about half of those with trisomy 21. On the basis of these data, Birnholz and Farrell suggest that ear length be determined in any pregnancy with a risk or suspicion of a chromosomal disorder or when a fetal anom-

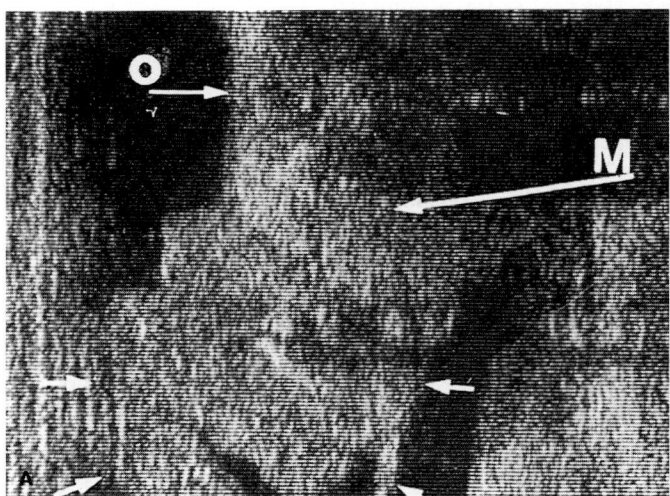

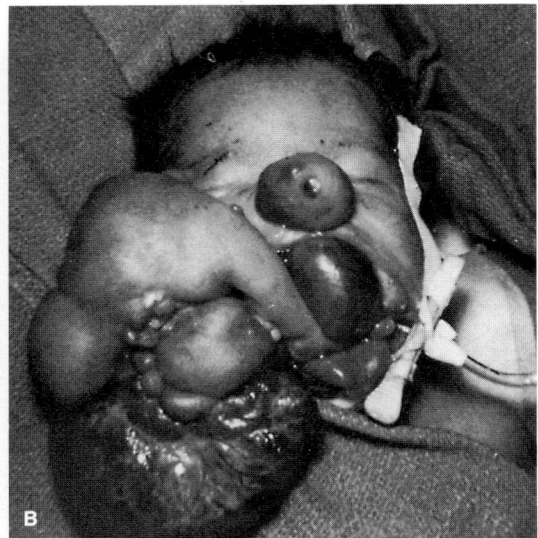

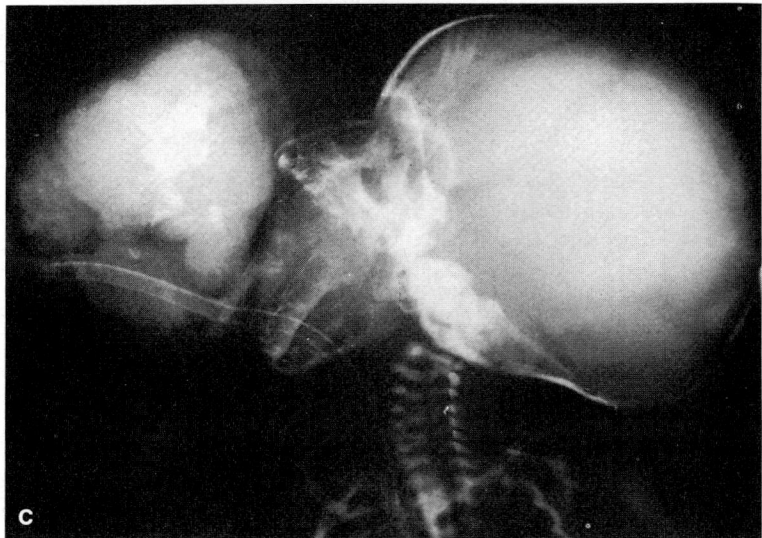

FIGURE 10-29. Epignathus. **(A)** Coronal sonogram of a fetus at 32 weeks of gestation with a mainly solid mass, with a few cystic components, arising in the region of the mouth (M) and extending to the right (outlined by *arrows*). O, orbit. **(B)** Large mass arising from the palate, obstructing the mouth opening and nostril of the neonate. **(C)** Lateral radiograph demonstrates the relation of the mass to the skull and calcifications within the mass. O, orbit; M, mouth area; mouth not visualized. (Chervenak FA, Tortora M, Moya FR, et al: Antenatal sonographic diagnosis of epignathus. J Ultrasound Med 1984; 3:235–237.)

aly is detected. Targeted examination of the fetal ears may rarely provide useful information that enables a specific prenatal diagnosis or suggests a chromosomal abnormality when other structural anomalies have been detected.

REFERENCES

1. Leopold GR: Editorial: Antepartum obstetrical ultrasound examination guidelines. J Ultrasound Med 1986; 5:241.
2. Benacerraf BR, Frigoletto FD Jr, Bieber FR: The fetal face: Ultrasound examination. Radiology 1984; 153:495.
3. Mahony BS, Nyberg DA: The fetal face. In Chervenak FA, Issacson GC, Campbell S (eds): Ultrasound in Obstetrics and Gynecology, 1st ed. Chicago: Little, Brown, 1993: 859.
4. Moore KL: The Developing Human: Clinically Oriented Embryology, 4th ed. Toronto: WB Saunders, 1988: 170.
5. Stewart RE: Craniofacial malformations: Clinical and genetic considerations. Pediatr Clin North Am 1978; 25(3):485.
6. Mahony BS, Hegge FN: The face and neck. In Mahony BS, Nyberg DA, Pretorius DH (eds): Diagnostic Ultrasound of Fetal Anomalies: Text and Atlas. Chicago: Year Book, 1990: 203.
7. Sadler TW: Head and neck. In Langman's Medical

Embryology, 6th ed. Baltimore: Williams & Wilkins, 1990: 297.

8. Taybi H, Lachman RS: Radiology of Syndromes, Metabolic Disorders, and Skeletal Dysplasias, 3rd ed. Chicago: Year Book, 1990.

9. Smith DW: Recognizable Patterns of Human Malformation, 3rd ed. Philadelphia: WB Saunders, 1982.

10. Hegge FN, Prescott GH, Watson PT: Fetal facial abnormalities identified during obstetric sonography. J Ultrasound Med 1986; 5:679.

11. Pilu G, Reece EA, Romero R, et al: Prenatal diagnosis of craniofacial malformations with ultrasonography. Am J Obstet Gynecol 1986: 45.

12. Escobar LF, Bixler D, Padilla LM, et al: Fetal craniofacial morphometrics: In utero evaluation at 16 weeks gestation. Obstet Gynecol 1988; 72:674.

13. Birnholz JC: The development of human fetal eye movement patterns. Science 1981; 72:674.

14. Birnholz JC, Benacerraf BR: The development of human fetal hearing. Science 1983; 222:516.

15. Bowie JD, Clair MR: Fetal swallowing and regurgitation: Observation of normal and abnormal activity. Radiology 1982; 144:877.

16. Jeanty P, Romero R, Staudach A, Hobbins JC: Facial anatomy of the fetus. J Ultrasound Med 1986; 5:607.

17. Mayden K, Tortora RD, Berkowitz RL, et al: Orbital diameters: A new parameter for prenatal diagnosis and dating. Am J Obstet Gynecol 1992; 144:289.

18. Jeanty P, Cantraine F, Cousaert MS, et al: The binocular distance: A new way to estimate fetal age. J Ultrasound Med 1984; 3:241.

19. Jeanty P, Dramaix-Wilmet M, Van Fansbeke D, et al: Fetal ocular biometry by ultrasound. Radiology 1982; 143:513.

20. Birnholz JC, Farrel EE: Fetal hyaloid artery: Timing of regression with US. Radiology 1988; 166:781.

21. Romero R, Pilu G, Jeanty P, et al: Prenatal Diagnosis of Congenital Anomalies. Norwalk, CT: Appleton and Lange, 1988.

22. McGahan JP, Nyberg DA, Mack LA: Sonography of facial features of alobar and semilobar holoprosencephaly. AJR 1990; 154:143.

23. Nyberg DA, Mack LA, Bronstein A, et al: Holoprosencephaly: Prenatal sonographic diagnosis. AJR 1987; 149:1051.

24. DeMeyer W, Zeman W, Palmer CG: The face predicts the brain: Diagnostic significance of median facial anomalies for holoprosencephaly (arhinencephaly). Pediatrics 1964; 34:256.

25. De Meyer W: Classification of cerebral malformations. Birth Defects 1971; 7:78.

26. Filly RA, Chinn DH, Callen PW: Alobar holoprosencephaly: Ultrasonographic prenatal diagnosis. Radiology 1984; 151:455.

27. Greene MF, Benacerraf BR, Frigoletto FD Jr: Reliable criteria for the prenatal sonographic diagnosis of alobar holoprosencephaly. Am J Obstet Gynecol 1987; 236:47.

28. Schinzel A, Savoldelli G, Briner J, Schmid W: Prena-

tal ultrasonographic diagnosis of holoprosencephaly two cases of cebocephaly and two of cyclopia. Arch Gynecol 1984; 236:47.

29. Pilu F, Romero R, Rizzo N, et al: Criteria for the prenatal diagnosis of holoprosencephaly. Am J Perinatol 1987; 4(1):41.

30. Chervenak FA, Tortora M, Mayden K, et al: Antenatal diagnosis of median cleft face syndrome: Sonographic demonstration of cleft lip and hypertelorism. Am J Obstet Gynecol 1984; 149:94.

31. Chervenak FA, Isaacson G, Rosenberg JC, Kardon NB: Antenatal diagnosis of frontal cephalocele in a fetus with atelosteogenesis. J Ultrasound Med 1986; 5:111.

32. DeMeyer W: The median cleft face syndrome. Neurology 1967; 17:961.

33. Strauss S, Tamarkin M, Englegerg S, et al: Prenatal sonographic appearance of diprosopus. J Ultrasound Med 1987; 6:93.

34. Plazaki JR, Wilson JL, Holmes SM, Vandermark LL: Diprosopus: Diagnosis in utero. AJR 1987; 149:147.

35. Fontanarosa M, Bagnoli G, Ciolini P, et al: First trimester sonographic diagnosis of diprosopus twins with craniorachischisis. J Clin Ultrasound 1992; 20:69.

36. Chervenak FA, Pinto MM, Heller CI, et al: Obstetric significance of fetal craniofacial duplication: A case report. J Reprod Med 1985; 30:74.

37. Cayea PD, Bieber FR, Ross MJ, et al: Sonographic findings in otocephaly (synotia). J Ultrasound Med 1985; 4:377.

38. Feldman E, Shalev E, Weiner E, et al: Microphthalmia—prenatal ultrasonic diagnosis: A case report. Prenat Diagn 1985; 5:205.

39. Tamas DE, Mahony BS, Bowie JD, et al: Prenatal sonographic diagnosis of hemifacial microsomia (Goldenhar-Gorlin syndrome). J Ultrasound Med 1986; 5:461.

40. Birnholz JC: Ultrasonic fetal ophthalmology. Early Hum Dev 1985; 12:199.

41. Davis WK, Mahony BS, Carroll BA, Bowie JD: Antenatal sonographic detection of benign dacrocystoceles (lacrimal duct cysts). J Ultrasound Med 1987; 6:461.

42. Meizner I, Bar-Ziv J, Holcberg G, Katz M: In utero prenatal diagnosis of fetal facial tumor-hemangioma. J Clin Ultrasound 1985; 13:435.

43. Pennell RG, Baltarowich OH: Prenatal sonographic diagnosis of a fetal facial hemangioma. J Ultrasound Med 1986; 5:525.

44. Lasser D, Preis O, Dor N, et al: Antenatal diagnosis of giant cystic cavernous hemangioma by Doppler velocimetry. Obstet Gynecol 1988; 72:476.

45. Birnholz JC: Fetal eye movement pattern. Science 1981; 213:679.

46. Farrell SA, Toi A, Leadman ML, et al: Prenatal diagnosis of retinal detachment in Walker-Warburg syndrome. Am J Med Genet 1987; 28:619.

47. Maynor CH, Hertzberg BS, Ellington KS: Antenatal

sonographic features of Walker-Warburg syndrome: Value of endovaginal sonography. 1992; 11:301.

48. Meizner I: Prenatal ultrasonic features in a rare case of congenital ichthyosis (harlequin fetus). J Clin Ultrasound 1992; 20:132.

49. Bundy AL, Saltzman DH, Emerson D, et al: Sonographic features associated with cleft palate. J Clin Ultrasound 1986; 14:486.

50. Greene JC, Vermillion JR, Hays S: Utilization of birth certificates in epidemiologic studies of cleft lip and palate. Cleft Palate J 1965; 2:141.

51. Seeds JW, Cefalo RC: Technique of early sonographic diagnosis of bilateral cleft lip and palate. Obstet Gynecol 1983; 62:2S.

52. Nyberg DA, Mahony BS, Kramer D: Paranasal echogenic mass: Sonographic sign of bilateral complete cleft lip and palate before 20 menstrual weeks. Obstet Ultrasound 1992; 184:757.

53. Gorlin RJ, Cervenka J, Pruzansky S: Facial clefting and its syndromes. Birth Defects 1971; 7:3.

54. Nyberg DA, Hegge FN, Kramer D, et al: Premaxillary protrusion: A sonographic clue to bilateral cleft lip and palate. J Ultrasound Med 1993; 12:331.

55. Meizner I, Katz M, Bar-ziv J, Insler V: Prenatal sonographic detection of fetal facial malformations. Isr J Med Sci 1987; 23:881.

56. Benacerraf BR, Miller WA, Frigoletto D Jr: Sonographic detection of fetuses with trisomies 13 and 18: Accuracy and limitations. Am J Obstet Gynecol 1988; 158:404.

57. Saltzman DH, Benacerraf BR, Frigoletto FD: Diagnosis and management of fetal facial clefts. Am J Obstet Gynecol 1986; 155:377.

58. Benacerraf BR, Frigoletto FD, Greene MF: Abnormal facial features and extremities in human trisomy syndromes: Prenatal US appearance. Radiology 1986; 159:243.

59. Kraus BS, Kitamura H, Ooe T: Malformations associated with cleft lip and palate in human embryos and fetuses. Am J Obstet Gynecol 1963; 86:321.

60. Burton DJ, Filly RA: Sonographic diagnosis of the amniotic band syndrome. AJR 1991; 156:555.

61. Fiske CE, Filly RA, Golbus MS: Prenatal ultrasound diagnosis of amniotic band syndrome. J Ultrasound Med 1982; 1:45.

62. Kalousek DK, Bamforth S: Amnion rupture sequence in previable fetuses. Am J Med Genet 1988; 31:63.

63. Mahony BS, Filly RA, Gallen PW, Golbus MS: The amniotic band syndrome: Antenatal sonographic diagnosis and potential pitfalls. Am J Obstet Gynecol 1985; 152:63.

64. Shah YG, Metlay L: Prenatal ultrasound diagnosis of Beckwith-Wiedemann syndrome. J Clin Ultrasound 1990; 18:597.

65. Koontz WL, Shaw LA, Lavery JP: Antenatal sonographic appearance of Beckwith-Wiedemann syndrome. J Clin Ultrasound 1986; 14:57.

66. Cobellis G, Iannoto P, Stabile M, et al: Short communication: Prenatal ultrasound diagnosis of macroglossia in the Wiedemann-Beckwith syndrome. Prenat Diagn 1988; 8:79.

67. Zanetti B, Signori E, Consolaro, et al: Congenital fibrosarcoma of the tongue. Z Kinderchir 1982; 35:7.

68. Mihalko M, Lindfors KK, Grix AW, et al: Prenatal sonographic diagnosis of harlequin ichthyosis. AJR 1989; 153:827.

69. Pilu G, Romero R, Reece EA, et al: The prenatal diagnosis of Robin anomalad. Am J Obstet Gynecol 1986; 154:630.

70. Meizner I, Carmi R, Katz M: Prenatal ultrasonic diagnosis of mandibulofacial dysostosis (Treacher Collins syndrome). J Clin Ultrasound 1991; 19:124.

71. Benson CB, Pober BR, Hirsh MP, Doubilet PM: Sonography of nager acrofacial dysostosis syndrome in utero. J Ultrasound Med 1988; 7:163.

72. Chervenak FA, Tortora M, Moya F, Hobbins JC: Antenatal sonographic diagnosis of epignathus. J Ultrasound Med 1984; 3:235.

73. Holmgren G, Rydnert J: Male fetus with epignathus originating from the ethmoidal sinus. Eur J Obstet Gynecol Reprod Biol 1987; 24:69.

74. Alter AD, Cove JK: Congenital nasopharyngeal teratoma: Report of a case and review of the literature. J Pediatr Surg 1987; 22:179.

75. Chervenak FA, Issacson G, Touloukian R, et al: Diagnosis and management of fetal teratomas. Obstet Gynecol 1985; 66:666.

76. Kang KW, Hissong SL, Langer A: Prenatal ultrasound diagnosis of epignathus. J Clin Ultrasound 1978; 6:330.

77. Kaplan C, Perlmutter S, Molinoff S: Epignathus with placental hydrops. Arch Pathol Lab Med 1980; 104:374.

78. Teal LN, Angtuaco TL, Jimenez JF, et al: Fetal teratomas: Antenatal diagnosis and clinical management. J Clin Ultrasound 1988; 16:329.

79. Birnholz JC: The fetal external ear. Radiology 1983; 147:819.

80. Hill LM, Thomas ML, Peterson CS: The ultrasonic detection of apert syndrome. J Ultrasound Med 1987; 6:601.

81. McGahan JP, Ellis W, Lindfors KK, et al: Congenital cerebrospinal fluid containing intracranial abnormalities: A sonographic classification. JCU 1988; 16:531.

82. Fink IJ, Chinn DH, Callen PW: A potential pitfall in the ultrasonographic diagnosis of fetal encephalocele. J Ultrasound Med 1983; 2:313.

83. Birnholz JC, Farrell EE: Fetal ear length. Pediatrics 1988; 81:555.

John P. McGahan and Manuel Porto:
DIAGNOSTIC OBSTETRICAL ULTRASOUND.
© 1994 J.B. Lippincott Company.

Ruth B. Goldstein

Chapter *11*

The Fetal Thorax

A number of important abnormal conditions of the fetal thorax can be detected using antenatal sonography. Published guidelines for the second- and third-trimester obstetrical sonogram recommend, at a minimum, a relatively limited examination of the fetal chest, which includes a four-chamber view of the heart.[1] Obtaining this view in each sonogram has had an important benefit in greatly increasing prenatal detection of noncardiac fetal thoracic malformations as well. This chapter focuses on antenatal detection of fetal chest abnormalities using ultrasound, with an emphasis on differential diagnosis, characteristic and distinguishing features, and associated malformations.

EMBRYOLOGY

Many sonographically detectable pulmonary malformations can be linked to the interruption of normal developmental sequences. During the first 5 weeks of gestation, the lung buds grow out of the ventral aspect of the primitive foregut. If these buds do not form, lung agenesis results. The trachea and esophagus become separated by the fifth gestational week. Buds from the early trachea form and penetrate the mesenchymal masses destined to become the lungs. An abnormal budding of a segment of the tracheobronchial tree may result in formation of a bronchogenic cyst. Through a series of divisions and budding, bronchi give rise to bronchioles, and each terminal bronchiole later gives rise to a number of alveolar ducts and alveoli. By 16 weeks, the formation of the bronchial tree is essentially complete. Insults to the lung before this time result in fewer than expected bronchi.

Between 16 and 24 weeks, there is a dramatic increase in the number and complexity of airspaces, large blood vessels, and capillaries. Insults to the lungs during this phase result in smaller airways and in a reduction in the number and size of acini.

After 24 weeks, terminal sacs and alveoli continue to develop and mature, and the number and complexity of the airspaces is further increased. If an abnormality could be removed or interrupted before this stage, the normal process of airspace maturation might be renewed, and fetal surgery has been performed for this purpose. The number of alveoli continues to grow during childhood, after which alveolar expansion becomes the major means of lung growth until adolescence.[2]

NORMAL ANATOMY

Bones and Subcutaneous Tissues of the Thorax

The fetal thoracic cavity is bell-shaped and bordered by the clavicles at the apex and the smooth, hypoechoic diaphragm inferiorly (Fig. 11-1). The chest wall is lean and made up of skin, muscles, and little fat. The ribs, smoothly marginated and regularly spaced, form the lateral boundaries and extend anteriorly more than halfway around the thorax from their dorsal attachments (Fig. 11-2). Recall that the ribs also extend inferiorly to the upper abdomen.

Intrathoracic Contents

On a four-chamber view, the heart occupies about one third of the thoracic volume, and most of the cardiac volume is located in the left anterior quadrant of the chest on an axial plane at the level of the four-chamber view[3] (Fig. 11-3). On this image, no abdominal viscera should be visualized. With real-time imaging, mediastinal and pulmonary vessels can be easily appreciated: pulmonary veins (see Fig. 11-3) can be followed to the left atrium, confirming normal venous connections to the heart.

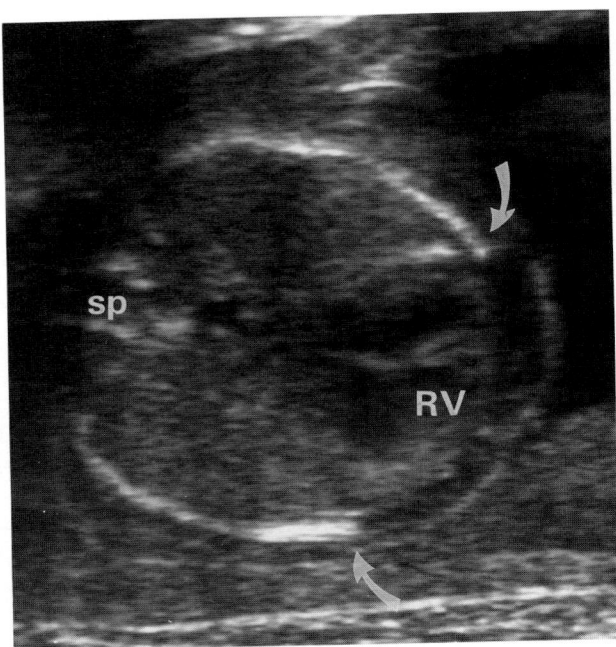

FIGURE 11-2. Transverse view of the normal fetal chest. The smoothly marginated ribs extend anteriorly more than halfway around the thorax (*curved arrow*). RV, right ventricle; sp, spine.

The fetal thymus is usually not distinguishable unless large pleural effusions are present.

Normal fetal lungs are homogeneous in echotexture, and echogenicity may be greater than, less than, or equal to the echogenicity of the liver (see

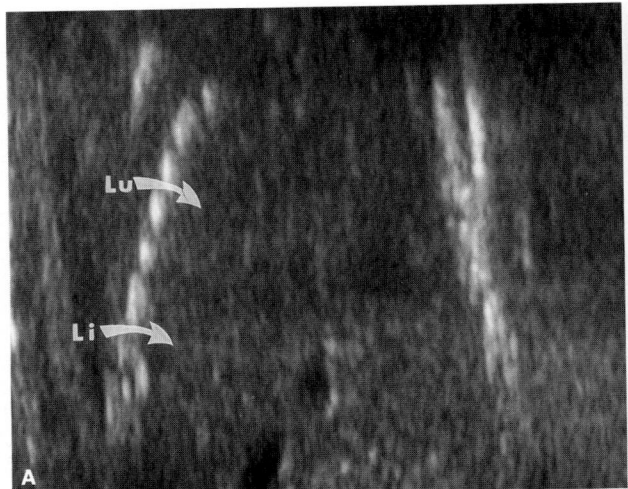

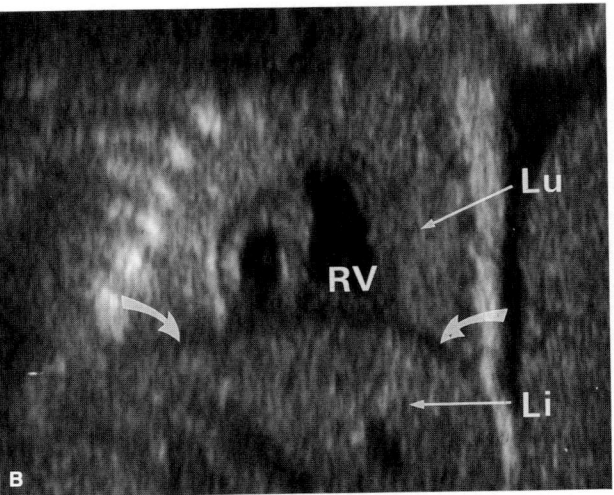

FIGURE 11-1.   Normal fetal chest. **(A)** Coronal view. Lu, lung; Li, liver. **(B)** The hypoechoic muscular diaphragm (*curved arrows*) separates the lungs (Lu) from the abdominal contents. Li, liver; RV, right ventricle.

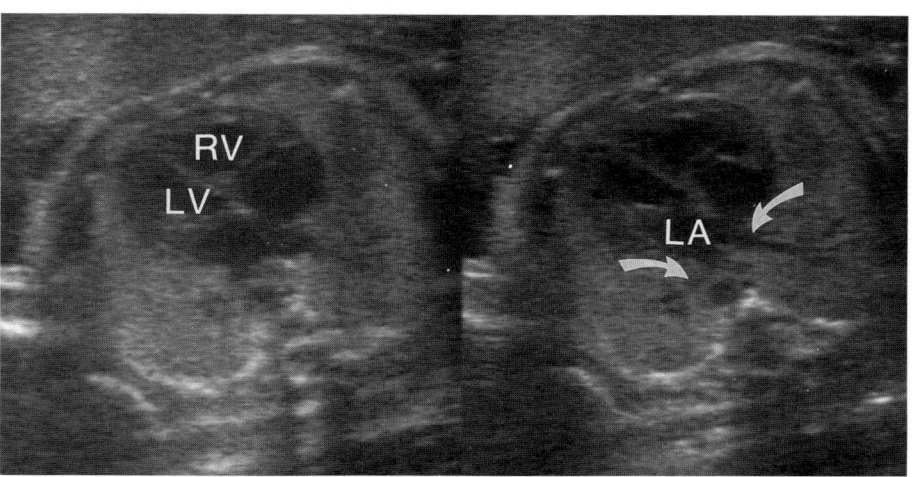

FIGURE 11-3. Axial views of the normal fetal chest. Note that the heart occupies about one third of the volume of the normal chest, and most of the cardiac volume lies within the left anterior quadrant of the chest on the axial plane. RV, right ventricle; LV, left ventricle; LA, left atrium. *Curved arrows* indicate the normal pulmonary veins draining into the left atrium.

Fig. 11-1*B*). Some investigators have found that the lungs become progressively more echogenic than the liver as gestation progresses, but there is too much variability in lung echogenicity during development to use echogenicity as a reliable predictor of lung maturity.[4]

PITFALLS IN ULTRASOUND EXAMINATION

False Diagnosis of a Diaphragmatic Hernia

Oblique images of the chest and abdomen may include abdominal viscera in the heart. This may be misleading, causing the examiner to misinterpret normal findings as abnormal (ie, false diagnosis of a diaphragmatic hernia; Fig. 11-4).

Ribs and the Abdomen

As noted previously, when scanning the chest, the ribs may extend inferiorly into the upper abdomen. Therefore, observation of the ribs and the abdominal structures in the same transverse plane should not be misinterpreted as abnormal.

Pseudo Skin Thickening

Examiners should interpret the thickening of subcutaneous tissue of the middle upper chest cautiously. This is especially true on images that include the scapula because the fetal tissues in this region may normally appear somewhat thicker than those of the abdomen or scalp (Fig. 11-5).

PULMONARY HYPOPLASIA

Pulmonary hypoplasia, pathologically defined as an absolute decrease in lung volume or weight for gestational age, remains an important source of postnatal morbidity and mortality. Four factors are most important for normal lung development: adequate gestational duration for lung maturation, adequate amniotic fluid volume, adequate intrathoracic space, and adequate fetal breathing movements.[5,6] The pathogenesis of pulmonary hypoplasia is often obscure, but experiments confirm that both distention of the lung with lung fluid and fetal respiratory movements are necessary for normal lung growth. Fetal conditions that adversely influence any of these factors and therefore compromise lung growth can be grouped into several major categories (Table 11-1).

Thoracic space can be compromised by a skeletal dysplasia (small thorax) or an intrathoracic mass that compresses the developing lung and functionally reduces thoracic space available for lung expansion and growth. Similarly, depressed fetal breathing movements due to a severe neurologic defect, and experimental sectioning of the phrenic nerve in animals, result in pulmonary hypoplasia. Finally, it is well known that severe prolonged oligohydramnios, either through chest compression or reduction of fluid within the fetal lung, is almost always associated with pulmonary hypoplasia. In many cases, multiple factors may be operative.

Although it would be ideal for obstetrical management and parental counseling to be able to relate observed sonographic abnormality to the degree of the pulmonary deficiency expected, un-

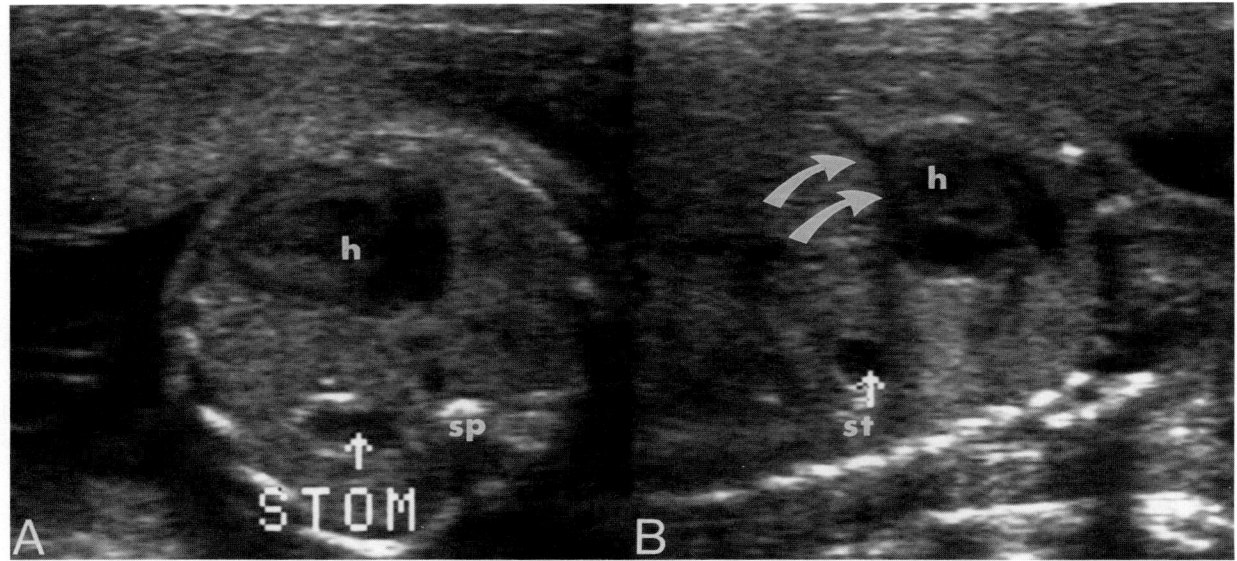

FIGURE 11-4. Potentially confusing image of the normal fetal chest. **(A)** Oblique scanning through the chest may produce a misleading image in which the stomach (stom) is imaged on the same plane as the heart (h). sp, spine. **(B)** Sagittal image confirms the infradiaphragmatic location of the stomach. *Curved arrows*, diaphragm; st, stomach; h, heart.

fortunately this is not always possible. The onset of the insult is often not known, and abnormalities that may interfere with normal pulmonary development (eg, oligohydramnios, chest masses) can vary in severity during gestation. Nevertheless, concern about potentially significant postnatal re-

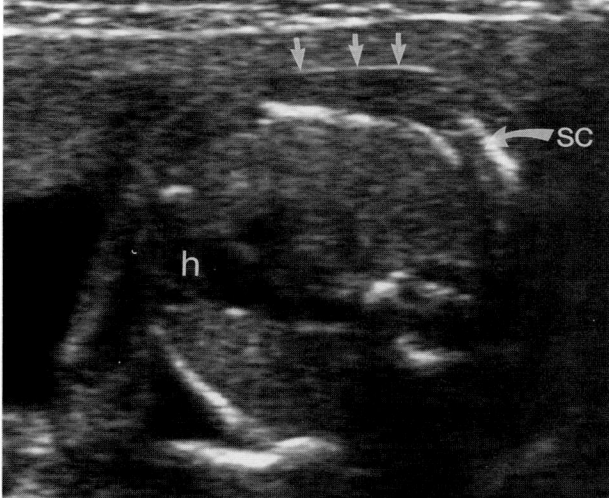

FIGURE 11-5. Normal fetal chest. Examiner should interpret thickening of the subcutaneous tissue of the mid- to upper chest (*short arrows*) cautiously because these tissues normally appear somewhat thicker than the subcutaneous tissues of the abdomen or scalp. sc, scapula; h, heart.

spiratory compromise is warranted in any pregnancy affected by prolonged oligohydramnios or a large space-occupying fetal chest lesion.

Thoracic Circumference

Numerous investigators have attempted to correlate the degree of pulmonary maturity with sonographic observations in the fetal chest. Unfortunately, predictions of lung maturity based on observations, such as pulmonary echogenicity, coarsening of the lung echotexture, and progressive increase in sound transmission, have largely been unsuccessful.[4,7] Other methods for sonographic estimation of lung growth are more reliable, especially in the setting of oligohydramnios. Thoracic size and growth have been correlated

**TABLE 11-1.   Some Causes
of Fetal Pulmonary Hypoplasia**

Prolonged oligohydramnios
Skeletal dysplasia (small thorax)
Neurologic (decreased breathing movements)
Chest mass (lung compression)
Large hydrothorax (lung compression)
Chromosomal abnormality

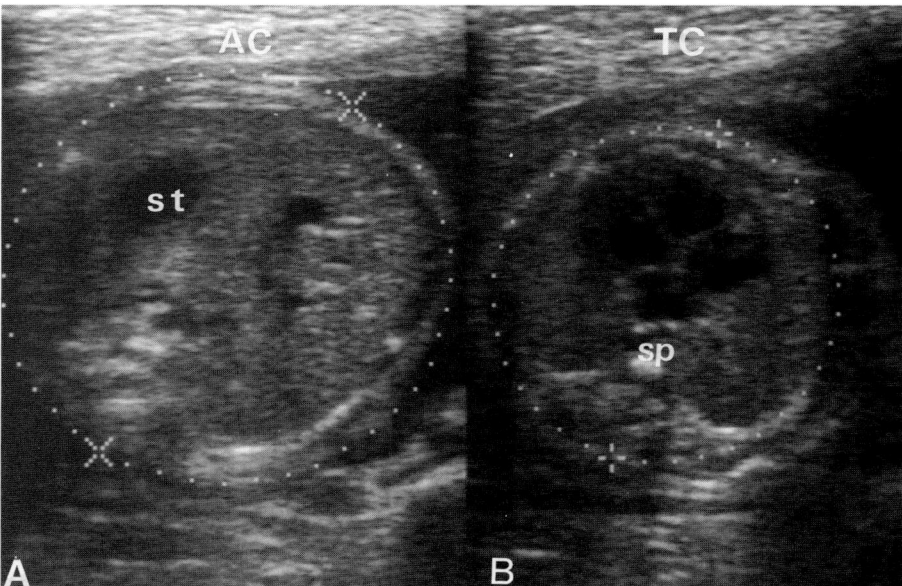

FIGURE 11-6. Normal thoracic and abdominal circumference measurements. **(A)** Abdominal circumference (AC). st, stomach. **(B)** Thoracic circumference (TC) obtained on an axial plane with the four-chamber view of the heart as indicated. sp, spine.

with normal pulmonary development. A correlation between pulmonary hypoplasia and a small thoracic circumference (TC) has been demonstrated[8,9] with fairly high sensitivities (80% or more), specificities (80%–90%), and normal and abnormal predictive values (85%–90%). TC is measured on an axial plane of the chest that includes the four-chamber view of the heart (Fig. 11-6). The subcutaneous tissues are generally not included in the measurement, or only minimally so, to avoid overestimating chest size in the fetus with integumentary edema or a bone dysplasia associated with redundant skinfold (Table 11-2).

Biometric Parameter Ratios
The rate of growth of the fetal TC is linear between 16 and 40 weeks of gestation, similar to other biometric parameters, including abdominal circumference (AC), head circumference (HC), and femur length (FL). Therefore, the ratio of TC to AC, HC, or FL is fairly constant, and these ratios may, in some clinical settings, function as useful gestational age–independent parameters. The TC/AC ratio appears to have the smallest variability in normal fetuses[10] and has been shown to be greater than 0.80 (mean: 0.89,[10] 0.85[11]) in nearly all normal pregnancies beyond 20 weeks.[12] D'Alton and coworkers reported a 75% sensitivity and 100% specificity using the TC/AC ratio for the prediction of neonatal death from pulmonary disease after pre-

mature rupture of membranes in otherwise normal fetuses[12] (Table 11-3).

Unfortunately, predictors of lung maturity based on the size of the thorax are far from perfect. For example, when the chest is expanded by a pulmonary mass or hydrothorax (causing pulmonary hypoplasia), the size of the fetal thorax does not reflect lung growth. Measurement of *lung lengths* may also be sensitive for the detection of pulmonary hypoplasia,[13] but these measurements have been less extensively investigated. Finally, two points regarding the judgment of adequate lung growth should be emphasized:

1. During routine scanning, initial evaluation of chest size is usually based on nonobjective criteria that include an overall subjective assessment of the size of the heart relative to the thorax. If the heart appears too large for the thorax, and the thorax is suspected to be small, the examiner may use measurements of the heart and thorax in conjunction with published normograms to determine whether the chest is small (ie, normal heart size) or the heart is enlarged.[14]

2. Despite the work of many qualified investigators, amniocentesis accompanied by analysis of lecithin/sphingomyelin ratios and phosphatidylglycerol remains the most reliable method for the important determination of fetal lung maturity.

TABLE 11-2. Fetal Thoracic Circumference Measurements*

Gestational Age (wk)	No.	Predictive Percentiles								
		2.5	5	10	25	50	75	90	95	97.5
16	6	5.9	6.4	7.0	8.0	9.1	10.3	11.3	11.9	12.4
17	22	6.8	7.3	7.9	8.9	10.0	11.2	12.2	12.8	13.3
18	31	7.7	8.2	8.8	9.8	11.0	12.1	13.1	13.7	14.2
19	21	8.6	9.1	9.7	10.7	11.9	13.0	14.0	14.6	15.1
20	20	9.5	10.0	10.6	11.7	12.8	13.9	15.0	15.5	16.0
21	30	10.4	11.0	11.6	12.6	13.7	14.8	15.8	16.4	16.9
22	18	11.3	11.9	12.5	13.5	14.6	15.7	16.7	17.3	17.8
23	21	12.2	12.8	13.4	14.4	15.5	16.6	17.6	18.2	18.8
24	27	13.2	13.7	14.3	15.3	16.4	17.5	18.5	19.1	19.7
25	20	14.1	14.6	15.2	16.2	17.3	18.4	19.4	20.0	20.6
26	25	15.0	15.5	16.1	17.1	18.2	19.3	20.3	21.0	21.5
27	24	15.9	16.4	17.0	18.0	19.1	20.2	21.3	21.9	22.4
28	24	16.8	17.3	17.9	18.9	20.0	21.2	22.2	22.8	23.3
29	24	17.7	18.2	18.8	19.8	21.0	22.1	23.1	23.7	24.2
30	27	18.6	19.1	19.7	20.7	21.9	23.0	24.0	24.6	25.1
31	24	19.5	20.0	20.6	21.6	22.8	23.9	24.9	25.5	26.0
32	28	20.4	20.9	21.5	22.6	23.7	24.8	25.8	26.4	26.9
33	27	21.3	21.8	22.5	23.5	24.6	25.7	26.7	27.3	27.8
34	25	22.2	22.8	23.4	24.4	25.5	26.6	27.6	28.2	28.7
35	20	23.1	23.7	24.3	25.3	26.4	27.5	28.5	29.1	29.6
36	23	24.0	24.6	25.2	26.2	27.3	28.4	29.4	30.0	30.6
37	22	24.9	25.5	26.1	27.1	28.2	29.3	30.3	30.9	31.5
38	21	25.9	26.4	27.0	28.0	29.1	30.2	31.2	31.9	32.4
39	7	26.8	27.3	27.9	28.9	30.0	31.1	32.2	32.8	33.3
40	6	27.7	28.2	28.8	29.8	30.9	32.1	33.1	33.7	34.2

* Measurements in centimeters.

(Chitkara U, Rosenberg J, Chervenak FA, et al: Prenatal sonographic assessment of the fetal thorax: Normal values. Am J Obstet Gynecol 1987; 156:1069–1074.)

TABLE 11-3. Mean Values With Standard Deviations for Various Thoracic Ratios

Ratio	Mean Predicted Value	Standard Deviation (n = 543)
TC/AC*	0.89	0.06
TC/HC*	0.80	0.12
TC/HL	4.31	0.36
TC/FL	4.03	0.33

* Ratios did not vary significantly with gestational age.

TC, thoracic circumference; AC, abdominal circumference; HC, head circumference; HL, humerus length; FL, femur length.

(Chitkara U, Rosenberg J, Chervenak FA, et al: Prenatal sonographic assessment of the fetal thorax: Normal values. Am J Obstet Gynecol 1987; 156:1069–1074.)

FETAL THORACIC MALFORMATION

If a fetal chest abnormality is observed on the sonogram, the examiner can be somewhat comforted by the fact that a relatively limited number of thoracic malformations have been observed prenatally. Bony thoracic abnormalities usually manifest as an abnormally small or misshapen thorax. The latter is often due to primary skeletal dysplasia (usually with abnormal ribs; Figs. 11-7 and 11-8) or pulmonary hypoplasia secondary to nonpulmonary factors (eg, severe and prolonged oligohydramnios, severe fetal neurologic disorder).

Intrathoracic abnormalities include hydrothorax, masses of the lung or mediastinum, and diaphragmatic hernias. Among masses observed

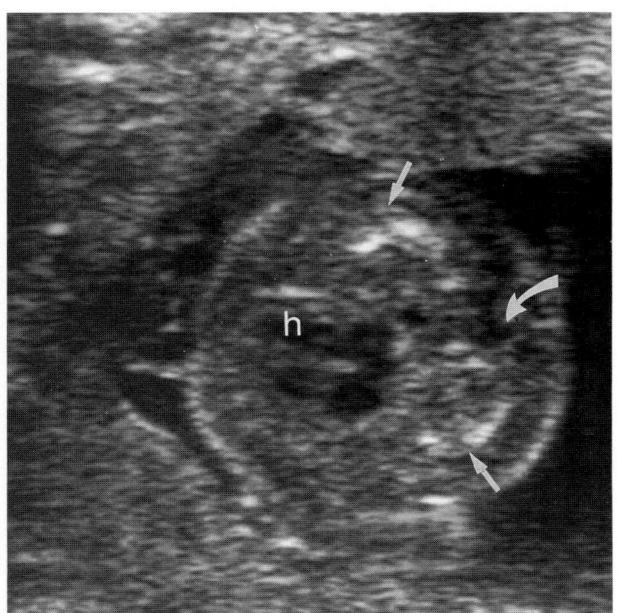

FIGURE 11-7. Axial image through the chest of the fetus with achondrogenesis demonstrates short, irregular ribs (*arrows*). Note the poorly ossified spine (*curved arrow*). h, heart.

within the fetal chest, congenital diaphragmatic hernia (CDH) is the most common, followed by cystadenomatoid malformation (CAM), pulmonary sequestration, bronchogenic cyst, bronchial atresia, and the mass-like appearance of the lungs that results from upper respiratory tract atresias. All these anomalies may be associated with life-threatening pulmonary hypoplasia, mediastinal

shift, and hydrops. Although it may not always be possible to make a specific diagnosis antenatally, diagnostic consideration can be prioritized based on the location and sonographic characteristics of the lesion and associated malformations.

Poor prognostic indicators that may be observed sonographically in association with intrathoracic abnormalities, regardless of origin, are the presence of hydrops and concomitant malformations. In addition, larger pulmonary lesions and CDH are generally more likely to be associated with significant, life-threatening pulmonary hypoplasia. Marked mediastinal shift probably contributes to the development of hydrops by impeding venous return or cardiac output, or both.

The natural history, associated malformations, and characteristic sonographic appearances of these intrathoracic abnormalities are discussed next.

Abnormal Subcutaneous Tissues of the Fetal Chest

The most common cause of diffuse thickening of the subcutaneous tissues is integumentary edema associated with hydrops or lymphangiectasia. Recall that redundant skinfold may be associated with a bone dysplasia (eg, thanatophoric dysplasia), and fetuses affected by neurologic disorders, such as Pena Shokeir, often have skin thickening. As previously noted, the fetal tissues in the region of the scapula may normally appear somewhat thicker than those of the abdomen or scalp (see Fig. 11-5).

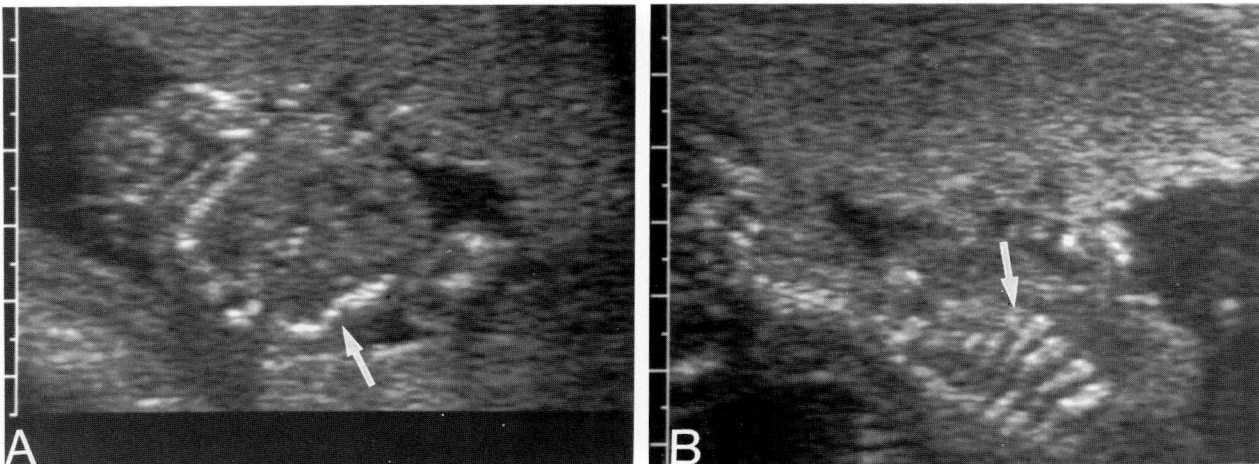

FIGURE 11-8. Fetus with osteogenesis imperfecta. **(A)** Note the irregular contour of the rib due to fracture (*arrow*). **(B)** Coronal view demonstrates rib fractures (*arrow*).

TABLE 11-4. Abnormal Subcutaneous Tissues of the Fetal Chest

Integumentary edema (hydrops)
Cystic hygroma (lymphangioma)
Hamartoma[15]
Hemangioma[16]
Fetal breasts[17]
Thoracic myelomeningocele

Masses of the subcutaneous tissue of the chest are rare and include hemangiomas, lymphangiomas (cystic hygromas), teratomas, hamartomas, and thoracic myelomeningoceles (Table 11-4). With the exception of the last, these masses may be difficult to distinguish antenatally. Hamartoma of the chest wall arises from the ribs and has been detected prenatally as an intrathoracic, highly echogenic, heterogeneous mass with calcifications, associated with pleural effusion.[15]

Intrathoracic Masses

The origin of an intrathoracic mass is nearly always pulmonary, subdiaphragmatic (CDH), or mediastinal. These masses are important not only because they frequently require surgical removal postnatally but also because of their potential to cause pulmonary hypoplasia or hydrops. Masses in the mediastinum are rare, but fetal goiter, cystic hygroma, teratoma (pericardial), and fetal thoracic neuroblastoma[18] have been observed prenatally and are listed in Table 11-5.

Intrathoracic masses are detected on the sonogram as a result of altered lung echogenicity and mediastinal shift; they may appear cystic, solid, or mixed, and most are unilateral.

Unilateral Fetal Chest Masses

Three lesions constitute most unilateral fetal chest masses: CDH, CAM, and pulmonary sequestra-

TABLE 11-5. Rare Fetal Mediastinal Masses

Mass	Helpful Differential Points
Fetal goiter	Originating anterior from the neck
Cystic hygroma	Cystic with septations
Teratoma	Pericardial in origin
Neuroblastoma	More common posteriorly

TABLE 11-6. Differential Diagnosis of Fetal Chest Masses*

Cystic
CAM
Bronchogenic cyst
CDH
Enteric cyst[19]
Mediastinal meningocele[20]

Cystic and Solid
CAM
Enteric cyst
Teratoma (pericardial)
CDH
Possibly sequestration (cystic lesions not described antenatally)

Solid
CAM (microcystic)
Sequestration
Bronchial atresia
Brochogenic cyst with obstructed bronchus
CDH (bowel and/or liver)

CAM, congenital cystadenomatoid malformation; CDH, congenital diaphragmatic hernia.

tion. Bronchogenic cysts, unilateral bronchial atresia, and stenosis are rarer but have been detected in the fetus. The latter lesions are detected because an obstructed bronchus prevents normal efflux of fetal lung fluid, causing the lung to become distended and appear mass-like on the sonogram. Because chest masses in the fetus may be cystic, solid, or mixed, there is considerable overlap in their presentations, and the sonographic appearances are often nonspecific, but characteristic features may be helpful in prioritizing the differential diagnosis (Table 11-6).

Congenital Cystadenomatoid Malformation

Congenital cystadenomatoid malformation is described pathologically as a hamartoma or focal dysplasia of the lung, and it accounts for about 25% of congenital lung lesions.[21-24] It is speculated that this malformation results from an early embryonic insult (before 10 weeks of gestation) because the bronchial system within the lesion is poorly developed. It is thought to occur from a failure of the endodermal bronchiolar epithelium to induce surrounding mesenchyme to form normal bronchopulmonary segments. Stocker and associates described three pathologic categories of CAM:

Type I—macrocystic, with cysts 2 to 10 cm in diameter

Type II—medium-size cysts

Type III—microcystic, with cysts 0.3 to 0.5 cm in diameter[21]

Associated renal and chromosomal anomalies, especially with type II CAM, were reported by Stocker and colleagues but were not confirmed by some investigators.[25,26] Chromosomal analysis, as well as careful fetal survey, is recommended when a suspected CAM is detected in the fetus. Lungs with CAM lack bronchi, but most of these lesions communicate with the tracheobronchial tree. Postnatally (air trapping), and possibly prenatally, CAM may become obstructed due to the absence of cartilaginous bronchi within the lesion.[27] Most of these lesions are unilateral, and the CAM usually involves one lobe or segment (usually the lower lobe). On rare occasions, it may be bilateral, or a single whole lung may be involved.[28] Arterial and venous connections are typically normal (although rare cases with a systemic arterial supply have been reported).[29] There is no known risk of recurrence.

CAM has been associated with ipsilateral or bilateral pulmonary hypoplasia and hydrops. Although hydrops fetalis is nearly always associated

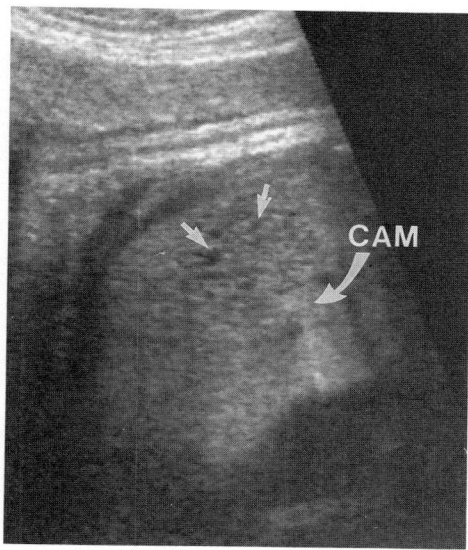

FIGURE 11-10. Type III microcystic adenomatoid malformation (CAM). High-resolution scanning demonstrates tiny cysts (*small arrows*) within this large, right-sided lesion.

with a poor prognosis, in utero resolution of hydrops in a fetus with CAM has been reported.[30,31] CAM may be associated with polyhydramnios, possibly resulting from compression of the fetal esophagus impairing fetal swallowing or compression of the heart and mediastinal vessels. Lung fluid produced in the CAM also may contribute to polyhydramnios.

Sonographic appearances range from a multicystic mass (Fig. 11-9) to a solid pulmonary lesion (Fig. 11-10) with mass effect and mediastinal shift. The differential diagnosis includes pulmonary sequestration, bronchogenic cyst, bronchial atresia, and neurenteric cyst. Calcifications are not observed in CAM. Type III lesions appear solid on the sonogram due to reflections from the walls of many tiny cysts (similar to infantile polycystic kidney disease). Although it was initially suggested that fetuses with solid-appearing lesions (ie, type III) had a poorer outcome than those with macrocystic forms, experience at my institution and other centers suggests that prognosis is not related to the size of the cysts.[32,33] Regardless of type, outcome of affected fetuses is poorer when the chest mass is large and associated with hydrops or polyhydramnios.[34]

Most patients with isolated small or moderate-sized CAM who survive after birth are asymptomatic during the neonatal period. In these cases, the lesions are amenable to surgical correction, and

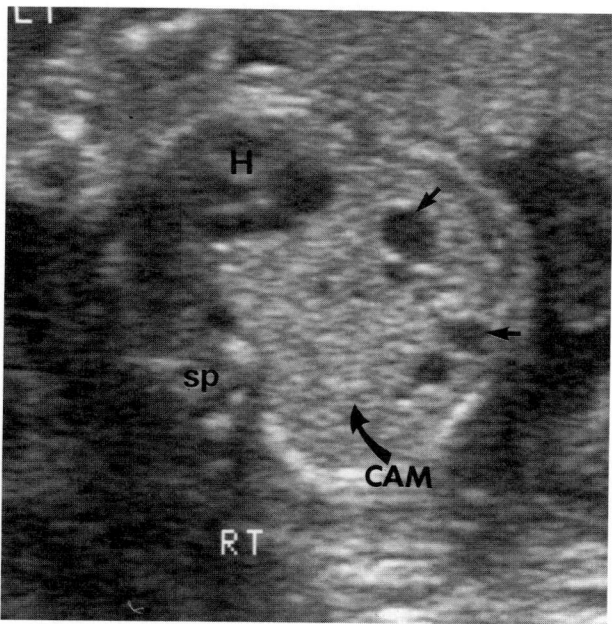

FIGURE 11-9. Type II cystic adenomatoid malformation (CAM). Largely echogenic, right-sided lesion with discrete, medium-sized cyst (*straight arrows*) displaces the heart to the left. H, heart; sp, spine.

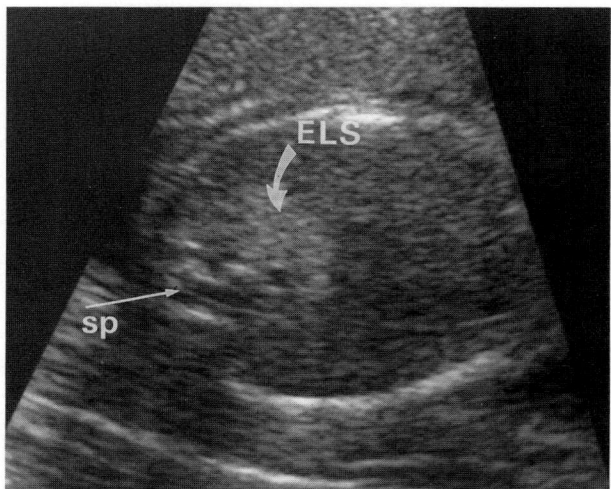

FIGURE 11-11. Extralobar pulmonary sequestration (ELS). A small, well-circumscribed left basal mass appears homogeneous and echogenic. sp, spine.

survival is good.[23] In some cases, macrocystic lesions in the fetus are drained percutaneously in utero, but this is rarely curative because fluid often reaccumulates.[34,35] When the cysts are large and associated with hydrops, successful surgical resection in the fetus (in utero) has been accomplished.[36]

Bronchopulmonary Foregut Malformation

Because the bronchial tree arises from the primitive foregut, there is a close association between malformations of these two systems. Pulmonary sequestrations, bronchogenic cysts, and enteric and neurenteric cysts are considered within the spectrum of bronchopulmonary foregut malformations.

Pulmonary Sequestration. A pulmonary sequestration is a mass of pulmonary tissue separated from its normal bronchial and vascular connections and supplied by systemic arteries. Two forms of sequestrations have been described: intralobar and extralobar. Both are supplied by an anomalous systemic artery from the thoracic or abdominal aorta. An intralobar sequestration (ILS) shares a common pleural investment with the rest of the lung but is separated from the bronchial tree. Venous drainage of an ILS is usually to the pulmonary veins. Postnatally, cysts may be found in the bronchiectatic form of ILS, but to my knowledge, cysts have not been observed in sequestrations detected in the fetus. Overall, about 25% of pulmonary sequestrations detected in children and adults are extralobar, but for reasons that are unclear, most pulmonary sequestrations detected in fetuses are extralobar.[37]

An extralobar sequestration (ELS) is anatomically and physiologically separate from the rest of the lung. It is invested by a pleural envelope separate from the rest of the lung, and venous drainage is through systemic veins, often the hemiazygous or portal veins. ELS most likely represents an accessory lung bud from the foregut. Ninety percent are left-sided and are found in a posterior, basal location in the costophrenic sulcus; 5% occur below the diaphragm. Lymphatic dilation within the ELS is common. Interestingly, focal areas with microscopic features of type II CAM can be found within 15% to 25% of ELS cases.[38] The incidence of concomitant anomalies is increased in association with ELS (but not ILS), and anomalies are reported to occur in 15% to 60% of cases and include diaphragmatic hernia, cardiac defects, gastric duplications, and other foregut communications.[39,40]

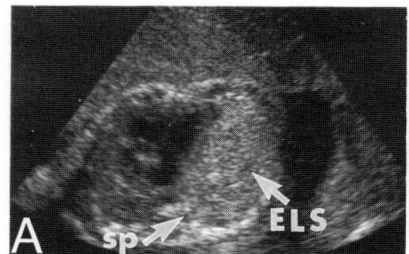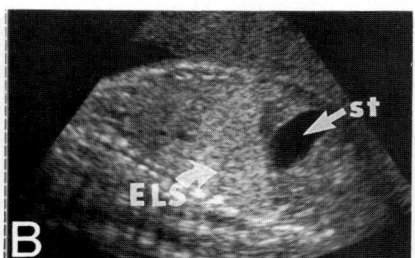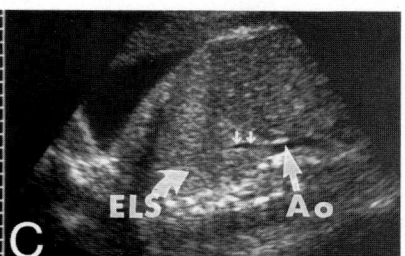

FIGURE 11-12. Extralobar pulmonary sequestrations (ELS). **(A)** Axial view of the chest demonstrates a left lower-lobe echogenic mass displacing the heart and mediastinal structures to the right. sp, spine. **(B)** Longitudinal view of the same fetus demonstrates the triangular echogenic mass (ELS) above the diaphragm. st, stomach. **(C)** Another longitudinal view demonstrates the ELS with the systemic feeding vessel (*small arrows*) from the aorta (Ao).

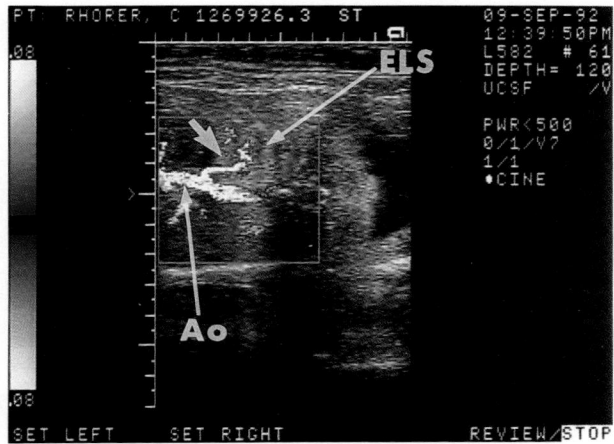

FIGURE 11-13. Color flow Doppler image demonstrates the feeding systemic vessel (*small arrow*) to the extralobar sequestration (ELS). Ao, aorta.

Sometimes a lobe or entire lung may communicate through a fistula with the esophagus or stomach, and at least one fetus with a bronchioesophageal communication within a sequestration has been described prenatally.[41] In this case, the abnormality detected was a large, echogenic mass secondary to the bronchioesophageal communication (obstructed lung) and associated with mediastinal shift.

Sonographically, a fetal pulmonary sequestration appears as a homogeneous, echogenic lung

mass (Fig. 11-11). Sequestrations often cause mediastinal shift and, when large enough, have been associated with fetal hydrops. Color Doppler has been used to identify the feeding vessel from the abdominal aorta (Figs. 11-12 and 11-13). If such a vessel can be demonstrated, the diagnostic considerations overwhelmingly favor pulmonary sequestration (as opposed to CAM, CDH, or bronchial atresia). Occasionally, a lobar-appearing mass, later proved to be an ELS, is associated with a large, ipsilateral tension hydrothorax (Fig. 11-14). Some authors have speculated that this tension hydrothorax results from torsion of the ELS on a pedicle or its small attachment to the lung, mediastinum, or diaphragm.[42]

Regressing Fetal Chest Masses. Recent evidence suggests that there is a great deal of variability in the natural history of CAMs and sequestrations. The potential for a chest mass to spontaneously regress in utero greatly impacts on the counseling offered to parents of an affected fetus. It is true that some fetuses with large lesions develop irreversible pulmonary hypoplasia or hydrops and die. In an important fraction of others, however, even those with bulky CAMs and pulmonary sequestrations, several investigators have reported significant diminution in size or apparent disappearance during gestation (Table 11-7). Postnatally, the neonates may be clinically well, obviating the need for neonatal resection or any surgery at

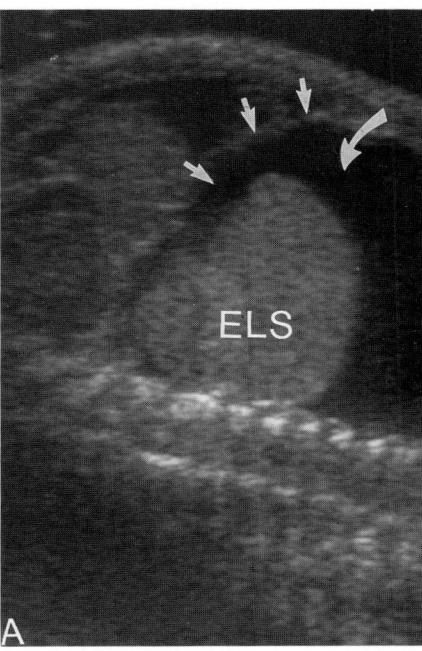
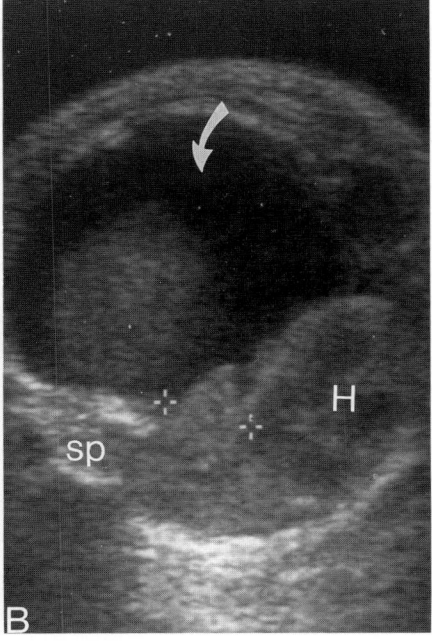

FIGURE 11-14. Extralobar pulmonary sequestration (ELS) associated with hydrothorax. **(A)** Echogenic lobar-appearing mass associated with a large hydrothorax (*curved arrow*) and inverted diaphragm (*small arrows*), indicating tension hydrothorax. **(B)** Axial view of the chest demonstrates large tension hydrothorax (*curved arrow*), producing mediastinal shift and displacement of the heart (H) to the right. Calipers indicate compressed, normal lung. sp, spine.

TABLE 11-7. Characteristics of Fetal Chest Masses That Regress During Gestation

Both congenital cystadenomatoid malformations and pulmonary sequestrations may regress
Chest masses may first show improvement at 22 to 37 weeks of gestation (wide range) by:
    Decreasing in absolute or relative size
    Becoming less echogenic
    Decreasing in mediastinal shift

Note: Some fetal chest masses may not begin to regress until the third trimester.

all. MacGillivray reported on a series of nine large fetal pulmonary lesions (three CAMs and six sequestrations) that spontaneously decreased in size or disappeared during gestation.[31] Budorick and coworkers reported 14 fetuses with chest masses, 5 of whom demonstrated regression during gestation.[33] Among the latter group of regressing lesions, all three types of CAM and a pulmonary sequestration were represented. The observations of regressing fetal pulmonary masses may be in keeping with findings from surgical studies, in which sequestrations appear as incidental findings in 1% to 2% of all patients undergoing pulmonary resection.[43]

Unfortunately, we are not able to predict which lesions are likely to spontaneously regress, and management decisions are further complicated by the fact that those destined to regress may not do so until the third trimester.

Bronchogenic Cysts. Bronchogenic cysts are bronchopulmonary foregut malformations thought to originate from abnormal budding of the ventral diverticulum of the foregut. Therefore, they probably develop between the 26th and 40th day of life. They are usually found in the anterior mediastinum but can occur within the lung substance and generally do not communicate with the bronchial lumen. Prenatal detection is rare but has been accomplished by observing a single unilocular pulmonary cyst[44] or an echogenic, distended lung obstructed by a small bronchogenic cyst.[45] Bronchogenic cysts are not usually associated with other congenital anomalies.[24,46]

Enteric and Neurenteric Cysts. Simple duplication of the esophagus is a rare form of foregut duplication and probably originates in the fourth gestational week. If the cyst is attached dorsally to the spine, the malformation is referred to as a neuren-

teric cyst. Neurenteric cysts are the rarest of bronchopulmonary foregut malformations and are thought to originate from incomplete separation of the foregut and notochord. They are invariably associated with spinal dysraphism that includes hemivertebrae, thoracic myelomeningocele, and absent vertebra. They may also communicate with bowel below the diaphragm through a diaphragmatic defect. Although a cyst within the thorax is a relatively nonspecific observation, when associated with a thoracic spinal dysraphism, a neurenteric cyst should be strongly considered.

Bronchial Atresia

Atresia of the segmental, lobar, or main-stem bronchus is thought to occur secondary to a vascular accident during development. The bronchi distal to the atresia are usually normal in number. It is speculated that the insult occurs after the 15th week of gestation (when bronchial branching is complete) because an earlier insult would be more likely to result in lung agenesis. This abnormality has been detected in the fetus sonographically as a large echogenic fetal lung mass (presumably the fluid-filled lung distal to the bronchial obstruction). A dilated fluid-filled bronchus may also be observed. The abnormality may not be visible before 24 weeks of gestation.[47] Other fetal and neonatal pulmonary lesions, such as lobar emphysema[48] and CAM,[49] have also been associated with bronchial atresia, raising speculation that lobar emphysema and CAM may be linked in some way to the insult causing the bronchial atresia or to the bronchial obstruction itself.

Congenital Diaphragmatic Hernia (Right- and Left-Sided)

The most common location of CDH is posterolateral on the left side (85%–90%)[50]; unilateral (97%) CDH occurs in about 1 in 3000 births. Posterolateral hernias are thought to result from incomplete fusion of the pleuroperitoneal membrane at 6 to 10 weeks of gestation. The size of the defects in the diaphragm are variable, and in 1% to 2% of cases, the diaphragm is completely absent.[51] Associated malformations occur in more than 25% of cases, including most notably cardiac defects (9%–23%),[52,53] neural tube defects (28%), spinal defects, trisomies (trisomy 21 and 18, in 4%), and certain well-defined syndromes.[54–56]

Mediastinal shift is one of the first abnormalities observed on the sonogram (Fig. 11-15). If a fluid-filled stomach cannot be detected below the diaphragm, CDH should be strongly considered in

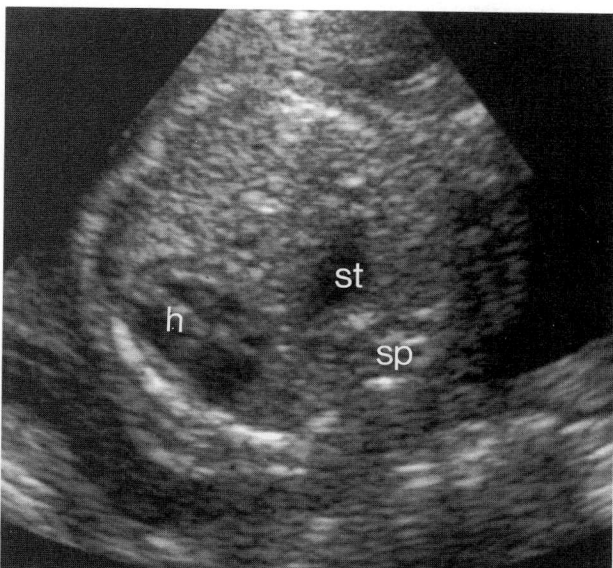

FIGURE 11-15. Left congenital diaphragmatic hernia. Axial view of the chest demonstrates the stomach (st) posterolateral to the heart (h) within the chest, causing significant mediastinal shift. sp, spine.

the differential diagnosis of a chest mass. An intrathoracic stomach and peristalsis of the herniated small bowel are helpful in confirming that the chest mass is a hernia. The herniated viscera nearly always include the stomach and bowel; in large defects, the spleen, left kidney, and left lobe of the liver may herniate as well.

Prognosis is guarded, with overall mortality of fetuses with CDH higher than 70% (about 10% lower in fetuses without cardiac defects). Poorer prognostic sonographic observations include a large defect, dilated intrathoracic stomach, antenatal detection before 25 weeks of gestation, intrathoracic liver, hydrops, and the presence of associated malformations (Table 11-8).

Although the defect in the diaphragm can be repaired postnatally, some degree of pulmonary

TABLE 11-8. Poor Prognostic Indicators for Left Congenital Diaphragmatic Hernia

Large defect
Dilated intrathoracic stomach
Diagnosis before 25 menstrual weeks
Intrathoracic liver
Hydrops
Other malformations

hypoplasia is nearly always present in these fetuses and is the leading cause of perinatal mortality. Morphometric analyses of neonates with CDH confirm an arrest in pulmonary development (reduced number of alveoli and pulmonary vessels), and infants dying of a large CDH usually have lungs that weigh 15% to 40% of the expected weight. Most investigators believe that compression of the developing lung by the herniated viscera interrupts normal pulmonary development. Despite improved postnatal care and extracorporeal membrane oxygenation, pulmonary hypoplasia and persistent fetal circulation remain important causes of neonatal mortality among newborns with CDH. As a result, surgical correction of CDH has been attempted in utero to promote lung development, but thus far survival rates have been poor.

Right-sided posterolateral hernias are much less common than those on the left. The right lobe of the liver most commonly herniates; the small bowel and kidney herniate less commonly. Surprisingly, right-sided hernias are less conspicuous and therefore more difficult to detect with sonography than those on the left (Fig. 11-16). The presence of a solid right-sided chest mass displacing the heart to the left is usually the first sign of a right-sided CDH. Associated ipsilateral pleural effusions (which represent herniated peritoneal sac and ascites) can be associated.[57] A helpful observation is a small, single cystic structure within the right-sided mass that is the gallbladder (see Fig. 11-16). Unlike in left-sided hernias, the fetal stomach is usually below the diaphragm.

Anteromedial hernias are the rarest form of hernia, occurring in 1 in 100,000. They are found in the retrosternal area (Morgagni's foramen) and are thought to result from malformation of the septum transversum. A defect in the pericardium may be associated that allows the viscera to herniate into the pericardium, or the heart into the peritoneal cavity. Associated malformations are common, and chromosomal abnormalities, mental retardation, and heart defects are found in more than half of cases.

Eventrations of the diaphragm are much rarer diaphragmatic defects (5%) that are characterized by thinning of the diaphragm, which results in upward migration of viscera and shift of the heart and mediastinum. A fetal diaphragmatic eventration may be sonographically indistinguishable from a bona fide hernia. Unilateral eventration may be associated with Beckwith-Wiedemann syndrome and is frequently associated with chromo-

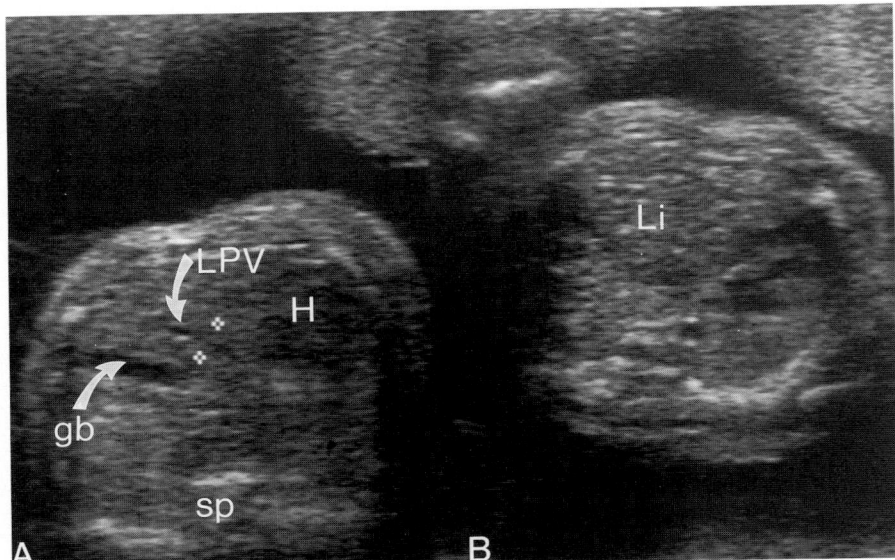

FIGURE 11-16. Two images of a fetus with a right congenital diaphragmatic hernia. Axial views of the chest demonstrate a mass within the right hemithorax displacing the heart (H) to the left. The gallbladder (gb) and left portal vein (LPV) can also be seen within this mass. Right-sided hernias tend to be less conspicuous on sonographic images compared with left-sided lesions. sp, spine; Li, liver.

somal abnormalities, especially trisomies 13, 14, 15, and 18. Bilateral eventrations have been associated with toxoplasmosis, cytomegalovirus, arthrogryposis, and other syndromes.

Bilateral Chest Masses

Bilateral fetal chest masses most commonly reflect enlarged, echogenic lungs due to stenosis or atresia of the upper respiratory tract (eg, laryngeal or tracheal atresia). Laryngeal atresia is more common, and tracheal agenesis is associated with laryngeal atresia in 40% of cases. The cause of this defect is not known, but it is speculated that the insult occurs at 5 to 7 weeks of gestation. Mortality is extremely high, with no survivors among fetuses in whom the diagnosis was made prenatally.

Although the antenatal sonographic findings

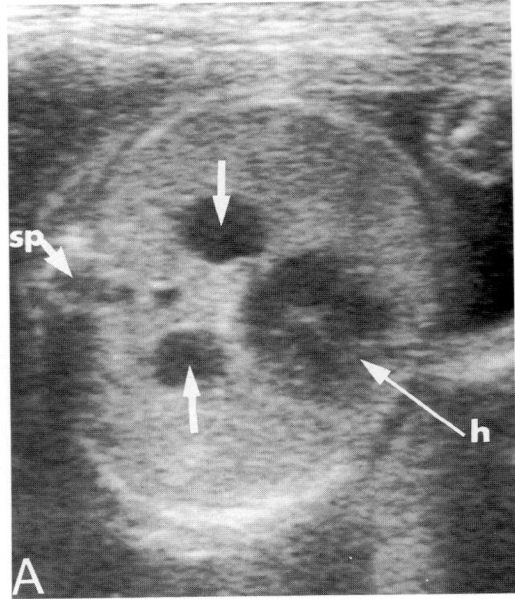

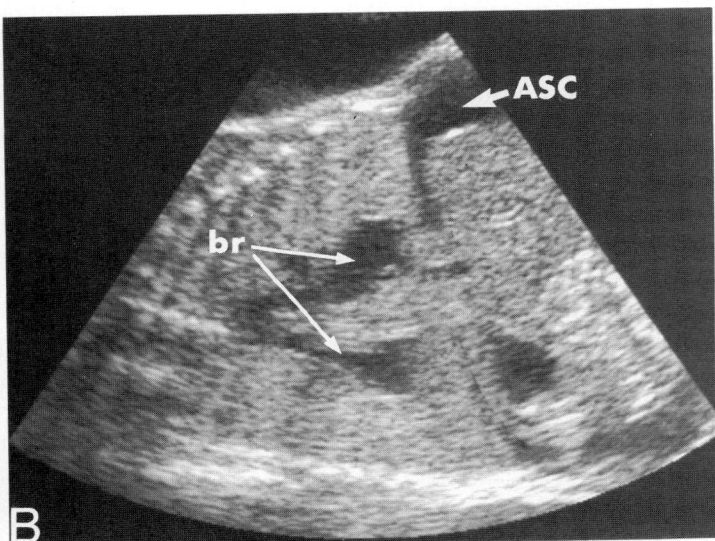

FIGURE 11-17. Tracheal atresia. **(A)** Axial view of the chest demonstrates symmetrically positioned cystic areas (*straight arrows*) within the echogenic lungs. The heart (h) is midline. sp, spine. **(B)** Coronal view of the chest of the same fetus demonstrates that these cystic areas are fluid-filled, dilated bronchi (br). Also note the mass effect of the distended lungs causing flattening of the diaphragms and ascites (ASC).

TABLE 11-9.   Differential Diagnosis of Bilateral Chest Masses

Laryngeal or tracheal atresia
Bilateral congenital cystadenomatoid malformations (rare)
Bilateral congenital diaphragmatic hernia

TABLE 11-10.   Fetal Chest Masses: Narrowing the Differential Diagnosis

Solid and left lower lobe usually indicates pulmonary sequestration
Discernible cysts suggest CAM (also consider CDH)
Right lung involvement most likely indicates CAM; if solid, also consider sequestration
Bilateral solid masses indicate upper respiratory tract atresia
Vascular supply (CAM fed by pulmonary artery, extralobar sequestration fed by vessel from aorta)
Presence of calcifications (hamartoma, neuroblastoma, or CDH with meconium peritonitis)

CAM, congenital cystadenomatoid malformation; CDH, congenital diaphragmatic hernia.

have been described in only a few fetuses with upper respiratory tract atresia, the sonographic findings are impressively similar: bilateral, enlarged echogenic lungs associated with ascites with or without hydrops[58-60] (Fig. 11-17). Symmetrically positioned tubular anechoic structures reflecting the mucus-filled bronchi have also been observed. The lungs are enlarged due to retention of lung fluid, and their increased echogenicity is likely due to reflections from the multiple tiny fluid-filled spaces within them. In contradistinction to the hypoplastic lungs often present in fetuses with other chest masses, lungs associated with laryngotracheal atresia are histologically normal or hyperplastic.[61] Ascites and hydrops are attributed to the cardiomediastinal compression by the enlarged lungs. Although the defect occurs early, sonographic detection may not be possible before 20 weeks of gestation.[60]

The differential diagnosis in these fetuses is limited. Rarely, CAM may be bilateral, but it is unlikely that the appearance would be so symmetric. A centrally placed mass, such as a bronchogenic cyst or teratoma, could conceivably obstruct the trachea and produce this appearance, although this has not been described. Finally, bilateral diaphragmatic hernias can result in bilateral chest masses, but it is expected that the mass effect would not be evenly distributed in both hemithoraces (Table 11-9).

Approach to a Fetus With a Chest Mass

Although a specific diagnosis cannot always be made before birth, sonographic characteristics of the mass can often help to narrow the diagnostic considerations (Table 11-10). For example, a mass that is predominantly cystic is statistically most likely to be a CAM, but CDH or a bronchogenic or enteric cyst should also be considered. Normal infradiaphragmatic anatomy usually excludes a CDH. If the thoracic spine is dysraphic, neurenteric cyst is most likely. A completely solid lesion may be a CAM, sequestration, or obstructed lung or segment. Because sequestration occurs most commonly in the basilar portion of the left lower lobe, a solid lesion in the right upper lobe is more likely to be a CAM or is less likely due to bronchial atresia or stenosis. If an anomalous artery directly from the aorta feeding the solid mass is observed, regardless of side, pulmonary sequestration is most likely. Mixed cystic and solid lesions are usually CAM, but a teratoma or CDH should be strongly considered.

PLEURAL EFFUSIONS

Fetal hydrothorax may be isolated but in most cases is associated with one of a broad spectrum of maternal and fetal disorders, including immune and nonimmune anemia; fetal chromosomal (especially trisomy 21 and 45,XO), cardiac, and metabolic abnormalities; pulmonary masses; and abnormalities of the placenta and umbilical cord (Table 11-11).

In many cases, a detailed anatomic survey of the fetus and karyotype testing suggest the origin of the hydrothorax, but a specific cause cannot always be determined. Poor prognostic signs are bilaterality (Fig. 11-18), associated hydrops, and

TABLE 11-11.   Causes of Pleural Effusion

Idiopathic primary chylothorax
Hydrops fetalis (multiple causes)
Abnormal karyotype—mostly 45,XO, trisomy 21
Lung mass (ie, sequestration, congenital diaphragmatic hernia

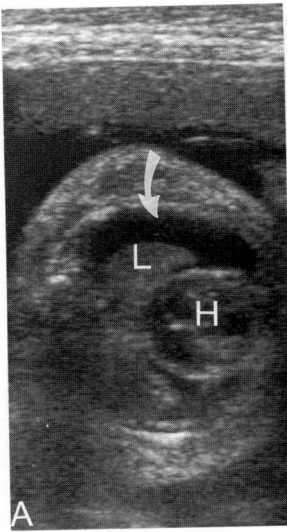
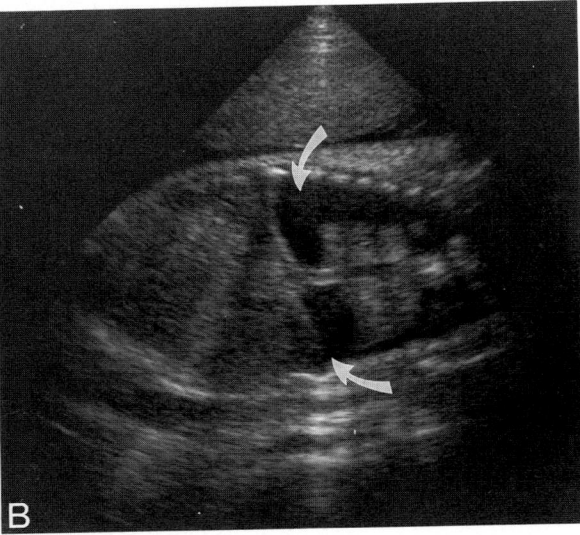

FIGURE 11-18. Fetal hydrothorax associated with hydrops. **(A)** Axial view of the chest demonstrates small, compressed lungs (L) surrounded by bilateral, moderate-sized hydrothoraces (*curved arrow*). Note the integumentary edema. H, heart. **(B)** Coronal view of the same fetus demonstrates bilateral hydrothoraces (*curved arrows*) with somewhat flattened diaphragms.

abnormal karyotype. Longaker and colleagues reported a 53% mortality rate for fetuses with antenatally detected hydrothorax.[62] Fetal pleural effusions may resolve spontaneously in utero,[62–64] and this is more likely if the effusion is unilateral, small, and unassociated with hydrops or other malformations.

Most isolated or primary hydrothoraces are chylous in origin. The cause is unknown.[65–69] It is more common in boys and usually unilateral, although a small fraction are bilateral.[66] In the newborn, chylothorax is the most frequent cause of isolated pleural effusion leading to respiratory distress,[65,66] and respiratory insufficiency associated with pleural effusions in the newborn is associated with a 15% to 25% mortality.[67–68] The diagnosis of chylous effusion in the feeding infant or adult is based on the milky appearance of aspirated chest fluid, which contains chylomicrons. In contradistinction, chest aspirates in the fetus are generally clear and straw-colored, and chylomicrons are not found (the fetus is fasting). A large number of lymphocytes is found in the fluid of fetal chylous effusions.

Sonographically, pleural effusions appear as anechoic fluid collections in the fetal chest that conform to the normal chest and diaphragmatic contour. When the effusions are large, hydrothorax may be associated with bulging of the chest and flattening or inversion of the diaphragm[70] (see Figs. 11-14 and 11-18). It is nearly impossible to distinguish primary from secondary pleural effusions in the fetus based solely on the appearance of the fluid.[65–68,71] Sonographic features that suggest

that the pleural effusion is a primary fetal chylothorax include the following:

1. The pleural effusion is an isolated finding;
2. The effusion occurs first as an isolated finding and is later followed by the development of other signs of hydrops fetalis; or
3. The size of the effusion is disproportionately large compared with other effusions (least reliable option).

Because fetal hydrothorax is associated with a poor outcome and significantly increased risk of pulmonary hypoplasia, aspiration and catheter drainage of large effusions have been accomplished antenatally with moderate success.[67,71] Best results have been obtained in fetuses with unilateral effusions and no evidence of hydrops at the time of catheter placement.[72,73] It may be helpful to perform in utero thoracentesis just before delivery to improve ventilation in the immediate postpartum period.[74] Postnatally, these effusions are treated with chest tube drainage for days to weeks, and in a series of cases diagnosed at birth, the condition eventually resolved, with normal outcome in almost all cases.[65,69]

REFERENCES

1. AIUM: Guidelines for performance of the abdominal and retroperitoneal, and the antepartum and obstetrical, ultrasound examination. J Ultrasound Med 1991; 10:576–578.

2. Hislop AA, Wigglesworth JS, Desai R: Alveolar development in the human fetus and infant. Early Hum Dev 1986; 13:1–11.
3. Comstock CH: Normal fetal heart axis and position. Obstet Gynecol 1987; 70:255–259.
4. Fried AM, Loh FK, Umer MA, et al: Echogenicity of fetal lung: Relation to fetal age and maturity. AJR 1985; 145:591–594.
5. Harrison MR, Jester JA, Ross NA: Correction of congenital diaphragmatic hernia in utero. I. The model: Intrathoracic balloon produces fatal pulmonary hypoplasia. Surgery 1980; 88:174–182.
6. Harrison MR, Bressack MA, Chung AM, et al: Correction of congenital diaphragmatic hernia in utero. II. Simulated correction permits fetal lung growth with survival at birth. Surgery 1980; 88:260–268.
7. Gayea PD, Grant DC, Doubilet PM, Jones TB: Prediction of fetal lung maturity: Inaccuracy of study using conventional ultrasound instruments. Radiology 1985; 155:473–475.
8. Nimrod C, Davies D, Iwanicki S, et al: Ultrasound prediction of pulmonary hypoplasia. Obstet Gynecol 1986; 68:495–497.
9. DeVore GR, Horenstein J, Platt LD: Fetal echocardiography: Assessment of cardiothoracic disproportion—A new technique for the diagnosis of thoracic hypoplasia. Am J Obstet Gynecol 1986; 155:1066–1071.
10. Chitkara U, Rosenberg J, Chervenak FA, et al: Prenatal sonographic assessment of the fetal thorax: Normal values. Am J Obstet Gynecol 1987; 156:1069–1074.
11. Vintzileos AM, Campbell WA, Rodis JF, et al: Comparison of six different ultrasonographic methods for predicting lethal fetal pulmonary hypoplasia. Am J Obstet Gynecol 1989; 161:606–612.
12. D'Alton M, Mercer B, Riddick E, Dudley D: Serial thoracic versus abdominal circumference ratios for the prediction of pulmonary hypoplasia in premature rupture of the membranes remote from term. Am J Obstet Gynecol 1992; 166:658–663.
13. Roberts AB, Mitchell JM: Direct ultrasonographic measurement of fetal lung length in normal pregnancies and pregnancies complicated by prolonged rupture of membranes. Am J Obstet Gynecol 1990; 163:1560–1566.
14. Jordan HVF: Cardiac size during prenatal development. Obstet Gynecol 1987; 69:854–858.
15. Brar MK, Cubberley DA, Baty BJ, Branch DW: Chest wall hamartoma in a fetus. J Ultrasound Med 1988; 7:217–220.
16. Smith LG Jr, Carpenter RJ Jr, Gonsoulin W, et al: Prenatal diagnosis of a chest wall mass with ultrasonography and Doppler velocimetry: A case report. Am J Obstet Gynecol 1990; 163:567–569.
17. Bezzi M, Mitchell DG, Kurtz AB, et al: Prominent fetal breasts: A normal variant. J Ultrasound Med 1987; 6:655–658.
18. De Filippi G, Canestri G, Bosio U, et al: Thoracic neuroblastoma: Antenatal demonstration in a case

19. with unusual postnatal radiographic findings. Br J Radiol 1986; 59:704–706.
19. Spock A, Schneider S, Baylin GJ: Mediastinal gastric cysts: A case report and review of English literature. Am Rev Respir Dis 1966; 94:97–103.
20. Knochel JQ, Lee TG, Melendez MG, Henderson SC: Fetal anomalies involving the thorax and abdomen. Radiol Clin North Am 1982; 20:297–310.
21. Stocker JT, Madewell JE, Drake RM: Congenital cystic adenomatoid malformation of the lung. Hum Pathol 1977; 8:155–171.
22. Van Dijk C, Wagenvoort CA: The various types of congenital adenomatoid malformations of the lung. J Pathol 1973; 110:131–134.
23. Wolf SA, Hertzler JH, Philippart AI: Cystic adenomatoid dysplasia of the lung. J Pediatr Surg 1980; 15:925–930.
24. Fraser RG, Pare JAP: Pulmonary abnormalities of developmental origin. In Diagnosis of Disease of the Chest, 2nd ed. Philadelphia: WB Saunders, 1977: 602–628.
25. Bale PM: Congenital cystic malformation of the lung. Am J Clin Pathol 1979; 71:411–420.
26. Oster AG, Fortune DW: Congenital cystic adenomatoid malformation of the lung. Am J Clin Pathol 1978; 70:595–604.
27. Fine C, Adzick NS, Doubilet PM: Decreasing size of a congenital cystic adenomatoid malformation in utero. J Ultrasound Med 1988; 7:405–408.
28. Morcos SF, Lobb MO: The antenatal diagnosis by ultrasonography of type III congenital cystic adenomatoid malformation of the lung. Br J Obstet Gynaecol 1986; 93:1002–1005.
29. Miller RK, Sieber WK, Yunis EJ: Congenital adenomatoid malformations of the lung: A report of 17 cases, and review of the literature. Pathol Annu 1980; 15:387–407.
30. Glaves J, Baker JL: Spontaneous resolution of maternal polyhydramnios in congenital cystic adenomatoid malformation of the lung. Br J Obstet Gynaecol 1983; 90:1065–1068.
31. MacGillivray TE, Adzick S, Goldstein RB, Harrison MR: Disappearing fetal lung lesions. J Pediatr Surg 1993; 28:1321–1325.
32. Kuller AJ, Yankowitz J, Goldberg JD, et al: Outcome of antenatally diagnosed cystic adenomatoid malformation. Am J Obstet Gynecol 1992; 167:1038–1041.
33. Budorick NE, Pretorius DH, Leopold GR, Stamm ER: Spontaneous improvement of intrathoracic masses diagnosed in utero. J Ultrasound Med 1992; 11:653–662.
34. Adzick NS, Harrison MR, Glick PL: Fetal cystic adenomatoid malformation: Prenatal diagnosis and natural history. J Pediatr Surg 1985; 20:483–488.
35. Clark SL, Vitale DJ, Minton SD, et al: Successful fetal therapy for cystic adenomatoid malformation associated with second trimester hydrops. Am J Obstet Gynecol 1987; 157:294–297.
36. Harrison MR, Adzick NS, Jennings R, et al: Antena-

tal intervention for congenital cystic adenomatoid malformation. Lancet 1990; 336:965–967.

37. Maulik D, Robinson L, Daily D, et al: Prenatal sonographic depiction of intralobar pulmonary sequestration. J Ultrasound Med 1987; 6:703–706.

38. Rosado-de-Christenson ML, Stocker JT: Congenital cystic adenomatoid malformation. Radiographics 1991; 11:865–886.

39. Ryckman PC, Rosenkrantz JG: Thoracic surgical problems in infancy and childhood. Surg Clin North Am 1985; 65:1423–1454.

40. Savic B, Birtel FJ, Tholen W, et al: Lung sequestration: Report of seven cases and review of 540 published cases. Thorax 1979; 34:96–101.

41. Siffring PA, Forrest TS, Hill WC, Crick MP: Prenatal sonographic diagnosis of bronchopulmonary foregut malformations. J Ultrasound Med 1989; 8:277–280.

42. Hernanz-Schulman M, Stein SM, Neblett WW, et al: Pulmonary sequestration: Diagnosis with color Doppler sonography and a new theory of associated hydrothorax. Radiology 1991; 180:818–821.

43. Carter R: Pulmonary sequestration. Ann Thorac Surg 1969; 7:68–88.

44. Albright EB, Crane JP, Schackelford GD: Prenatal diagnosis of a bronchogenic cyst. J Ultrasound Med 1988; 7:91–95.

45. Young G, L'Heureux PR, Krueckenberg ST, Swanson DA: Mediastinal bronchogenic cyst: Prenatal sonographic diagnosis. AJR 1989; 152:125–127.

46. Dumontier C, Graviss ER, Silberstein MJ, McAlister WH: Bronchogenic cysts in children. Clin Radiol 1985; 36:431–436.

47. McAlister WH, Wright JR Jr, Crane JP: Main-stem bronchial atresia: Intrauterine sonographic diagnosis. AJR 1987; 148:364–366.

48. Mendoza A, Wolf P, Edwards DK, et al: Prenatal ultrasonic diagnosis of cystic adenomatoid malformation of the lung. Arch Pathol Med 1986; 110:402–404.

49. Cachia R, Sobornya RE: Congenital cystic adenomatoid malformation of the lung with bronchial atresia. Hum Pathol 1981; 12:947–950.

50. Schumacher RE, Farrell PM: Congenital diaphragmatic hernia: A major remaining challenge in neonatal respiratory care. Perinatol Neonatol 1985; 9(4):29–44.

51. Wenstrom KD, Weiner CP, Hanson JW: A five-year statewide experience with congenital diaphragmatic hernia. Am J Obstet Gynecol 1991; 165:838–842.

52. Greenwood RD, Rosenthal A, Nadas AS: Cardiovascular abnormalities associated with congenital diaphragmatic hernia. Pediatrics 1976; 57:92–97.

53. David TJ, Illingsworth CA: Diaphragmatic hernia in the southwest of England. J Med Genet 1976; 13:253–262.

54. Nakayama DK, Harrison MR, Chinn DH, et al: Prenatal diagnosis and natural history of the fetus with a congenital diaphragmatic hernia: Initial clinical experience. J Pediatr Surg 1985; 20:118–124.

55. Puri P, Gorman F: Lethal nonpulmonary anomalies associated with congenital surgery. J Pediatr Surg 1984; 19:29–32.

56. Sharland GK, Lockhart SM, Heward AJ, Allan D: Prognosis in fetal diaphragmatic hernia. Am J Obstet Gynecol 1992; 166:9–13.

57. Gilsanz V, Emons D, Hansmann M, et al: Hydrothorax, ascites and right diaphragmatic hernia. Radiology 1986; 158:243–246.

58. Watson WJ, Thorp JM, Miller RC, et al: Prenatal diagnosis of laryngeal atresia. Am J Obstet Gynecol 1990; 163:1456–1457.

59. Dolkart LA, Reimers FT, Wertheimer IS, Wilson BO: Prenatal diagnosis of laryngeal atresia. J Ultrasound Med 1992; 11:496–498.

60. Weston MJ, Porter HJ, Berry PJ, Andrews HS: Ultrasonographic prenatal diagnosis of upper respiratory tract atresia. J Ultrasound Med 1992; 11:673–675.

61. Silver MM, Thurston WA, Patrick JE: Perinatal pulmonary hyperplasia due to laryngeal atresia. Hum Pathol 1988; 19:110–113.

62. Longaker MT, Laberge JM, Dansereau J, et al: Primary fetal hydrothorax: Natural history and management. J Pediatr Surg 1989; 24:573–576.

63. Pjipers L, Reuss A, Stewart PA, Wladimiroff JW: Noninvasive management of isolated bilateral fetal hydrothorax. Am J Obstet Gynecol 1989; 161:330–332.

64. Estroff JA, Parad RB, Frigoletto FD Jr, Benacerraf BR: The natural history of isolated fetal hydrothorax. Ultrasound Obstet Gynecol 1992; 2:162–165.

65. Vain NE, Swarner OW, Cha CC: Neonatal chylothorax: A report and discussion of nine consecutive cases. J Pediatr Surg 1980; 15:261–265.

66. Chernick V, Reed MH: Pneumothorax and chylothorax in the neonatal period. J Pediatr 1970; 76:624–632.

67. Petres RE, Redwine FO, Cruikshank DP: Congenital bilateral chylothorax: Antepartum diagnosis and successful intrauterine surgical management. JAMA 1982; 248:1360–1361.

68. Lange IR, Manning FA: Antenatal diagnosis of congenital pleural effusion. Am J Obstet Gynecol 1981; 140:839–840.

69. Broadman RF: Congenital chylothorax. NY State J Med 1975; 75:553–557.

70. Mahony BS, Filly RA, Callen PW, et al: Severe nonimmune hydrops fetalis: Sonographic evaluation. Radiology 1984; 151:757–761.

71. Benacerraf BR, Frigoletto FD: Mid-trimester fetal thoracentesis. J Clin Ultrasound 1985; 13:202–204.

72. Blott M, Nicolaides KH, Greenough A: Pleuroamniotic shunting for decompression of fetal pleural effusions. Obstet Gynecol 1988; 71:798–800.

73. Rodeck CH, Fisk NM, Fraser DI, Nicolini U: Long-term in utero drainage of fetal hydrothorax. N Engl J Med 1988; 319:1135–1138.

74. Seeds JW, Bowes WA: Results of treatment of severe fetal hydrothorax with bilateral pleuroamniotic catheters. Obstet Gynecol 1986; 68:577–580.

John P. McGahan and Manuel Porto:
DIAGNOSTIC OBSTETRICAL ULTRASOUND.
© 1994 J.B. Lippincott Company.

John P. McGahan   Beryl R. Benacerraf

Chapter *12*

Real-Time Examination of the Fetal Heart

Congenital heart disease is one of the more common congenital anomalies, estimated to be present in just less than 1% of all live births.[1,2] Although noncardiac fetal malformations have been diagnosed for over a decade, only recently has increased attention been given to ultrasound assessment of the fetal heart and thorax. Prenatal diagnosis of congenital heart disease is especially important when considering that fetal cardiac malformations often have a high associated rate of morbidity and mortality in both the fetus and the neonate. The American Institute of Ultrasound in Medicine recently published guidelines that for the first time recommend a four-chamber view of the fetal heart as a standardized part of the antenatal obstetrical examination during the second and third trimesters of pregnancy.[3] Complete examination of the fetal heart includes use of high-resolution real-time ultrasound examination of the heart in several anatomic planes, M-mode sonography, pulsed Doppler ultrasound, and color flow mapping. The emphasis of this chapter is on recogni-

tion of fetal cardiac abnormalities that may be detected by real-time ultrasound examination of the fetal heart.

INDICATIONS

A number of fetuses are at high risk for congenital heart disease. Risk factors may be divided into two separate groups: (1) fetal risk factors and (2) maternal or familial risk factors[4,5] (Table 12-1). Although the risk of congenital heart disease in a neonate is 8 in 1000, this risk increases up to 12% if a parent has congenital heart disease.[6] In situations in which any fetal anomaly is detected, careful scrutiny and examination of the fetal heart should be performed because there is a high risk of associated cardiac malformations in these cases[7] (Table 12-2). Some syndromes associated with specific cardiac abnormalities are listed in Table 12-3. Likewise, certain chromosomal abnormalities are associated with specific cardiac malformations[8] (Table 12-4).

**TABLE 12-1.   Risk Factors
for Congenital Heart Disease**

Fetal Risk Factors

Extracardiac anomalies
Chromosomal abnormality
Fetal cardiac arrhythmia
   Heart block
   Premature atrial or ventricular contractions
   Tachycardia (> 200 beats/min)
   Bradycardia
Nonimmune hydrops fetalis
Question of cardiac anomaly on prior ultrasound
Intrauterine growth retardation
Polyhydramnios

Maternal/Familial Risk Factors

Congenital heart disease
   Sibling
   Maternal
   Paternal
Teratogenic exposures
   Alcohol
   Lithium carbonate
   Progestins
   Amphetamines
   Anticonvulsants
   Others
Maternal disorders
   Diabetes mellitus
   Collagen vascular disease
   Phenylketonuria
Maternal infections
   Rubella
   Toxoplasmosis
   Coxsackievirus
   Cytomegalovirus
   Mumps
Familial syndromes

(Adapted from Copel JA, Pilu G, Green J, et al: Fetal echocardiographic screening for congenital heart disease: The importance of the four-chamber view. Am J Obstet Gynecol 1987; 157:648, and Schmidt KG, Silverman NH: Evaluation of the fetal heart by ultrasound. In Callen PW [ed]: Ultrasonography in Obstetrics and Gynecology, 2nd ed. Philadelphia: WB Saunders, 1988:165.)

TECHNIQUE AND NORMAL ANATOMY

When evaluating the fetal heart, the fetal position should be documented. Then, the stomach side and the relation of the suprahepatic portion of the inferior vena cava to the right atrium should be noted. Fetal cardiac malposition is extremely complex. For more detail, refer to an excellent review of malposition of the heart in a chapter by Van Praagh and colleagues.[9]

The ten cardiac segments may be greatly simplified into three main cardiac segments that are diagnostically important: (1) the visceroatrial situs, which is important in localization of the atrium; (2) the ventricular loop, which is important in diagnosing the relation of the ventricles to the atrium; and (3) the truncus arteriosus, which is important for diagnostic understanding of the relation between the great arteries and the ventricle.

Visceroatrial situs abnormalities may be divided into three separate types:

Situs solitus is the normal, noninverted type in which there is a normal visceral situs with the stomach to the left. The morphologic right atrium is right-sided and the morphologic left atrium is left-sided.

Situs inversus is the exact mirror image of situs solitus. The stomach is to the left, but the morphologic right atrium is left-sided, and the morphologic left atrium is right-sided in an inverted anatomic pattern.

**TABLE 12-2.   Systemic Malformations
Associated With Congenital Heart Disease**

Central nervous system
   Hydrocephalus
   Dandy-Walker syndrome
   Agenesis of corpus callosum
   Meckel-Gruber syndrome
   Microcephaly
   Holoprosencephaly
Mediastinum
   Tracheoesophageal fistula
   Esophageal atresia
Gastrointestinal
   Duodenal atresia
   Jejunal atresia
   Anorectal anomalies
   Imperforate anus
Ventral wall
   Omphalocele
   Ectopic cordis
Diaphragmatic hernia
Genitourinary
   Renal agenesis
   Horseshoe kidney
   Renal dysplasia

(Adapted from Copel JA, Pilu G, Kleinman CS: Congenital heart disease and extracardiac anomalies: Associations and indications for fetal echocardiography. Am J Obstet Gynecol 1986; 154:1121–1132.)

TABLE 12-3.   Syndromes Associated
With Congenital Heart Disease

Syndrome	Cardiac Malformation
Beckwith-Wiedemann	ASD, VSD
DiGeorge's	Aortic arch abnormalities, VSD
Hurler's	Cardiomyopathy
Goldenhar's	Tetralogy of Fallot
Ellis-van Creveld syndrome	VSD, ASD
Holt-Oram	VSD, ASD
Noonan's	Pulmonary stenosis, VSD, ASD, cardiomyopathy
Pierre Robin's	ASD
Williams'	Supravalvular aortic stenosis

ASD, atrial septal defect; VSD, ventricular septal defect.

(Modified by permission of Copel JA, Pilu G, Kleinman CS: Congenital heart disease and extracardiac anomalies: Associations and indications for fetal echocardiography. Am J Obstet Gynecol 1986; 154:1121–1132, and Nyberg DA, Emerson DS: Cardiac malformations. In Nyberg DA, Mahony BS, Pretorius DH [eds]: Diagnostic Ultrasound of Fetal Anomalies: Text and Atlas. Chicago: Year Book Medical Publishers, 1990:300–341.)

TABLE 12-4.   Chromosomal Syndromes
Associated With Congenital Heart Disease

Chromosomal Abnormality	Cardiac Malformation
Trisomy 21 (Down's)	VSD, ASD, AVC
Trisomy 18 (Edward's)	VSD, DORV, AVC
Trisomy 13 (Patau's)	VSD, DORV, Tetralogy of Fallot
45,X (Turner's)	CO, BAV
4p− (Cri du Chat)	VSD
4p− (Wolf's)	ASD
XXY (Klinefelter's)	VSD

ASD, atrial septal defect; AVC, atrial ventricular canal; DOVR, double-outlet right ventricle; VSD, ventricular septal defect; CO, coarctation of aorta; BAV, bicuspid aortic valve.

(Adapted from Copel JA, Pilu G, Kleinman CS: Congenital heart disease and extracardiac anomalies: Associations and indications for fetal echocardiography. Am J Obstet Gynecol 1986, 154:1121–1132, and Nyberg DA, Emerson DS: Cardiac malformations. In Nyberg DA, Mahony BS, Pretorius DH [ed]: Diagnostic Ultrasound of Fetal Anomalies: Text and Atlas. Chicago: Year Book Medical Publishers, 1990: 300–341.)

Situs ambiguous is an anatomically indeterminate type of visceral situs in which the liver is usually located in the midline with the stomach located either to the left or the right. This has been typically divided into what can be thought of as the *asplenia* syndrome and the *polysplenia* syndrome. Asplenia syndrome is often thought morphologically to be two right atria. Although this is not completely true, it is important to recognize this abnormality because most of these fetuses present with severe cyanosis as a newborn from congenital heart disease. Alternatively, *polysplenia*, often thought of as bilateral left-sidedness, usually presents with less severe cardiac problems (Table 12-5).

The relation of the atria to the ventricle may be important to recognize prenatally. Anatomically, the right atrium may open into the right ventricle in a normal or concordant relation, or it may be discordant, with the right atrium opening into the left ventricle. Furthermore, there may be other abnormalities of the relation of the atria to the ventricles, including abnormal positions of the tricuspid valve within the right ventricle, such as occur with Ebstein's anomaly.

Finally, an abnormal relation of the outflow tracts may be diagnosed prenatally. The most common abnormality of this type is transposition of the great vessels in which the right ventricle gives rise to the aorta and the left ventricle supplies the pulmonary artery.

Four-Chamber View of the Heart

After determining that the heart is located within the left side of the chest, the fetal thoracic spine is identified and a scan is obtained transverse to the

TABLE 12-5.   Classification
of Visceroatrial Situs and Associated
Congenital Heart Disease (CHD)

Situs Solitus

Thoracic and abdominal viscera in normal position
Levocardia—less than 1% incidence of CHD
Dextrocardia—95% incidence of CHD

Situs Inversus

Thoracic and abdominal viscera completely inverted
Levocardia—extremely rare with greater than 95% incidence of CHD
Dextrocardia—about 5% incidence of CHD

Situs Ambiguous

Liver midline
Asplenia—95% incidence of CHD
Polysplenia—about 75% incidence of CHD

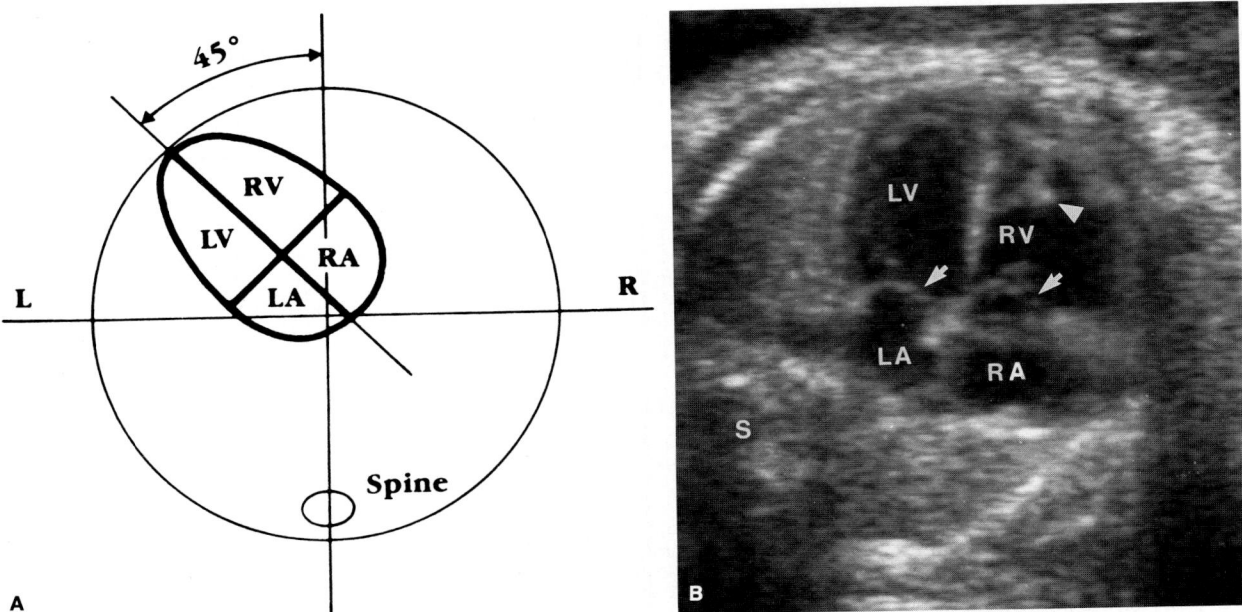

FIGURE 12-1. **(A)** Schematic drawing through normal fetal thorax shows four cardiac chambers. A line drawn through interventricular septum will transverse a plane about 45 degrees with a line drawn between fetal spine and sternum. (Comstock CH: Normal fetal heart axis and position. Obstet Gynecol 1987; 70:255.) **(B)** Magnified sonogram of fetal heart and thorax shows four chambers. Note trabeculated appearance of muscles of right ventricle (*arrowhead*) and atrioventricular valves (*arrows*). LV, left ventricle; RV, right ventricle; RA, right atrium; LA, left atrium; S, spine. (McGahan JP: Sonography of the fetal heart: Findings on the four-chamber view. AJR 1991; 156:547.)

thorax to obtain a four-chamber view of the heart (Fig. 12-1). Anatomically, the right ventricle is behind the sternum, and the left ventricle is inferior and to the left of the right ventricle. Differential points in identification of the right and left ventricles are given in Table 12-6.[10] Generally, the right and left ventricles maintain about a 1:1 ratio as identified on sonograms during diastole at the atrial ventricular valve region. This may be assessed on real-time ultrasound, and if precise measurements are to be made, documentation may be done with M-mode ultrasound. M-mode biventricular measurements obtained during ventricular diastole are compared with the thoracic circumference and may be helpful to predict cardiomegaly or pulmonary hypoplasia[11] (Fig. 12-2). Regardless of the fetal position, the interventricular septum transverses a plane of about 35 to 45 degrees with a

TABLE 12-6.   Identification of Right and Left Ventricles From the Four-Chamber View

View	Right Ventricle	Left Ventricle
Position within thorax	Right ventricle retrosternal	Left heart border, same side as stomach
Flap of foramen ovale	—	Present within left atrium
Insertion of atrioventricular valve leaflets on interventricular septum	Tricuspid valve is inserted lower than mitral	Mitral is inserted higher than tricuspid
Muscle	Thicker moderator band	—

(Modified from Devore GR: The prenatal diagnosis of congenital heart disease: A practical approach for the fetal sonographer. JCU 1985; 13:229.)

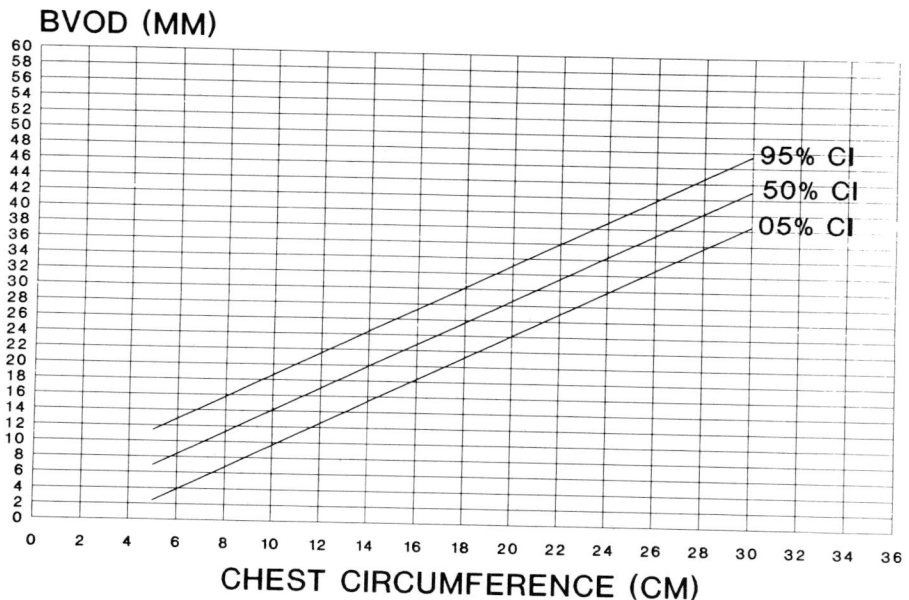

FIGURE 12-2. Confidence-limit (CI) graph for M-mode biventricular outer dimension (BVOD). Mean, 95%, and 5% confidence limits for individual predictions of the biventricular outer dimensions regressed against chest circumference. (DeVore GR, Siassi B, Platt LD: Fetal echocardiography. IV. M-mode assessment of ventricular size and contractility during the second and third trimesters of pregnancy in the normal fetus. Am J Obstet Gynecol 1984; 150:981.)

line drawn between the spine and the sternum (see Fig. 12-1). The heart should occupy about one third of the fetal thorax.

Specific heart chambers can be identified as follows:

The *right atrium* may be identified when scanning in different anatomic planes and noting the hepatic veins, inferior vena cava,

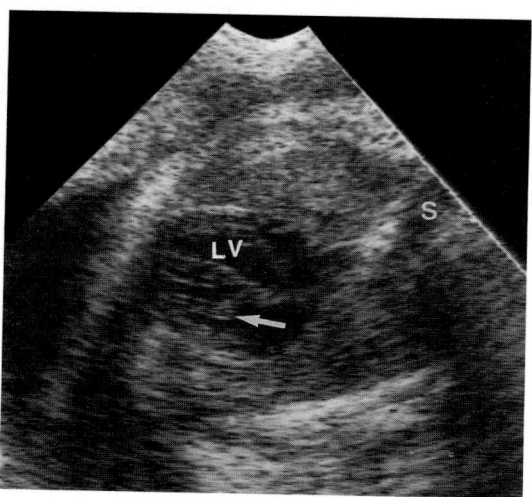

FIGURE 12-3. Four-chamber view of the heart demonstrates thick moderator band (*arrow*), which is an anatomic marker for the right ventricle. LV, left ventricle; S, spine.

and superior vena cava draining into that structure. The foramen ovale is noted opening from the right atrium into the left atrium.

The *left atrium* is posterior in location in comparison to the right atrium, with the foramen ovale opening into this chamber. The position of the spine is noted, with the left atrium lying close to the vertebral column.

The right atrium drains into the *right ventricle*. The right ventricle is retrosternal in location, with the tricuspid valve lower in position within the right ventricle than the mitral valve is within the left ventricle. There is also a large echogenic structure lying within the right ventricle, the muscular moderator band (Fig. 12-3). The right ventricle lies retrosternal in location.

The left atrium drains into the *left ventricle*. Papillary muscles are identified within the left ventricle. Echogenic bright spots may be identified within the left ventricle. These are thought to be attachments of the papillary muscles and are not abnormal (Fig. 12-4). The mitral valve is in a higher location within the left ventricle than the tricuspid is within the right ventricle. The apex of the heart and the interventricular septum are just cephalad to the fetal stomach.

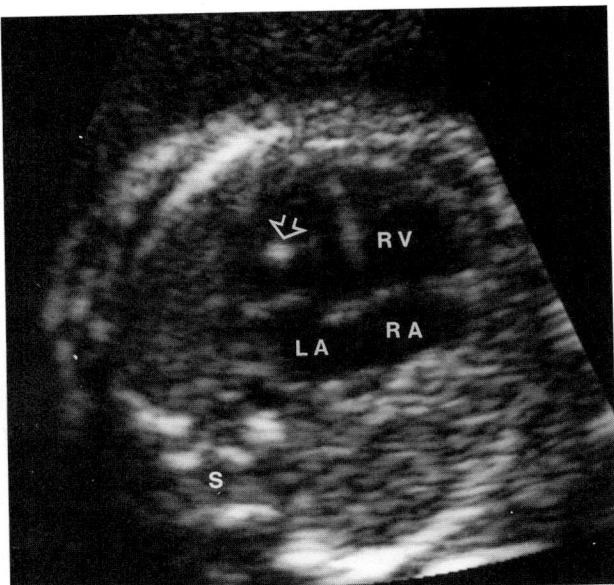

FIGURE 12-4. Normal papillary muscle on four-chamber view of heart. Bright echogenic focus (*arrow*) within left ventricle probably corresponds to a papillary muscle and is a normal finding. LA, left atrium; RA, right atrium; RV, right ventricle; S, spine. (Courtesy of D. Nyberg, Seattle, WA. McGahan JP: Sonography of the fetal heart: Findings on the four-chamber view. AJR 1991; 156:547.)

Long Axis View of the Heart

In most fetuses, the interventricular septum lies perpendicular to the transducer beam. The relation of the aorta to the left ventricle is best evaluated by the left ventricular long axis view of the fetal heart. This view is obtained by rotating the transducer from the four-chamber view into a plane angled from the fetal stomach toward the right shoulder of the fetus (Fig. 12-5). This view is helpful to evaluate the relation of the proximal aortic arch exiting the left ventricle to the right pulmonary artery lying inferior to it.

Pulmonary Outflow Tract

Once the aortic outflow tract is identified (described previously), the transducer is "rocked" into nearly a straight sagittal plane. This view identifies the main pulmonary artery exiting the right ventricle perpendicular to the ascending aorta. This crisscross relation is the result of normal rotation of the great vessels early in embryogenesis (Fig. 12-6). If the pulmonary artery and aorta are parallel rather than forming this criss-cross, there is a rotational abnormality of the great vessel, most commonly transposition of the great vessels.

Short Axis View of the Heart

With the fetus in the supine position, the short axis of the outflow tracts can be identified by directing the transducer parallel to the spine and moving to the left side of the fetus (Fig. 12-7). In this view, a circular structure is identified (aorta) with a similar-size vessel draping over it (pulmonary artery). Lateral to the aorta, the tricuspid valve leaflets can be observed opening and closing. Within the aorta and the pulmonary artery, movement of the valves can be observed. The pulmonary artery bifurcates near the spine.[10]

Other Views

When the apex of the heart is parallel to the transducer beam, the *five-chamber view* of the heart may be identified. This view is obtained by moving slightly more cranial from the four-chamber view of the heart in such a way that the aortic root is identified in the center of the heart. Also, the *longitudinal view* of the aortic arch can be obtained when the transducer is positioned so that a parasagittal scan through a right anterior approach or a left posterior approach can identify the aortic arch and the descending aorta. In this longitudinal view of the aortic arch, the great vessels are identified originating from the aortic arch.[10] A view of the ductus arteriosus entering into the descending aorta can be obtained by moving the transducer slightly from this anatomic plane (Fig. 12-8).

Ultrasound Pitfalls in Examination of the Fetal Heart

Pitfalls that are normally encountered during an examination of the fetal heart include:

> *Septation within the right atrium.* Normally, there is a valve where the inferior vena cava and the coronary sinus empty into the right atrium. This may appear as a septation within the right atrium. Another potential explanation of septation within the right atrium is the small remnants of the valve of the sinus venosus, called Chiari's network. In any case, these are normal structures and should not be mistaken for abnormal folds within the right atrium[12] (Fig. 12-9).

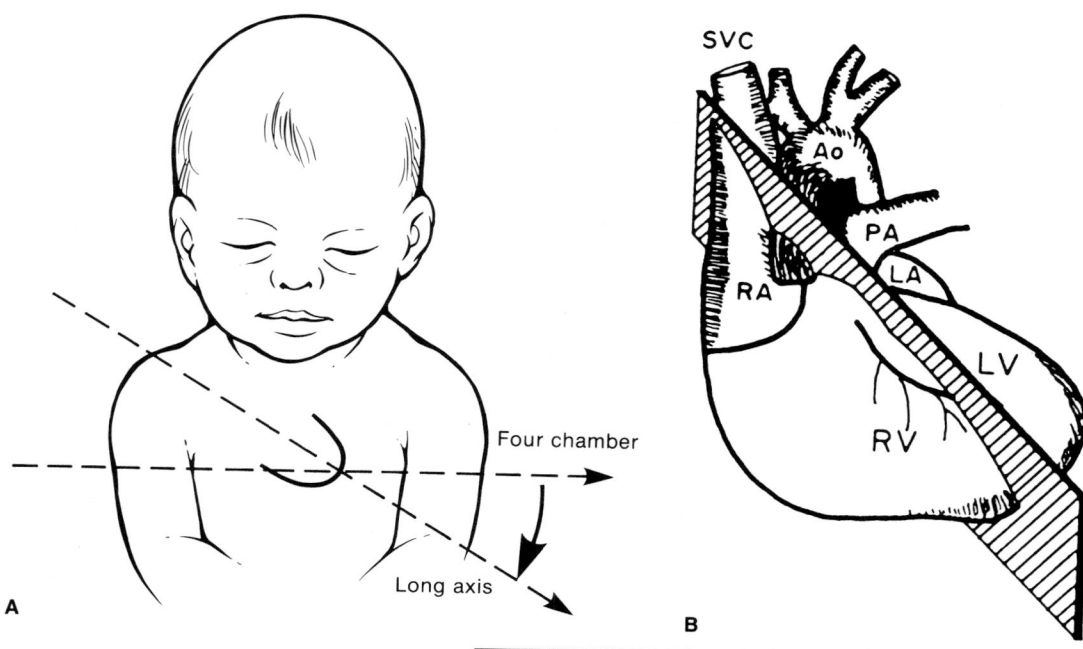

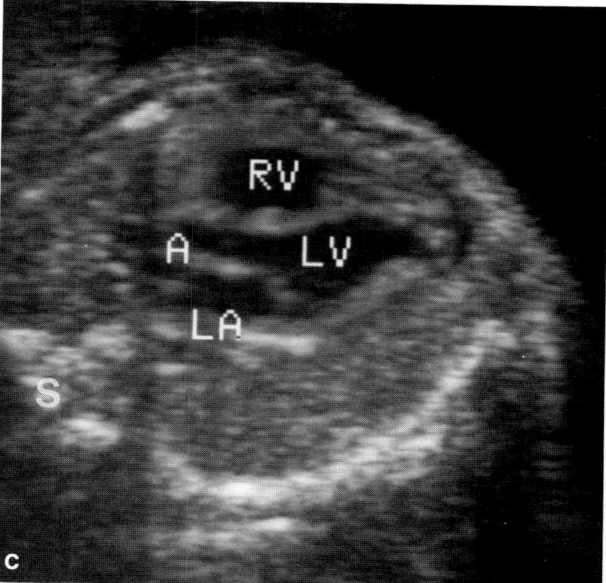

FIGURE 12-5. **(A)** Long axis view of heart. Changing from the four-chamber view of the heart to a more oblique scan plane, angling from the fetal left upper quadrant and abdomen to the right shoulder, provides the correct anatomic plane for the long axis view of the heart. **(B)** Anatomic drawing shows the plane used to obtain the long axis view of the heart through the left ventricle and the aortic outflow tract. (DeVore GR: The prenatal diagnosis of congenital heart disease: A practical approach for the fetal sonographer. JCU 1985; 13:229.) **(C)** Sonogram shows normal left ventricle long axis view of the heart with an aorta (A) originating from the left ventricle (LV). LA, left atrium; RV, right ventricle; S, spine. (McGahan JP: Sonography of the fetal heart: Findings on the four-chamber view. AJR 1991; 156:547.)

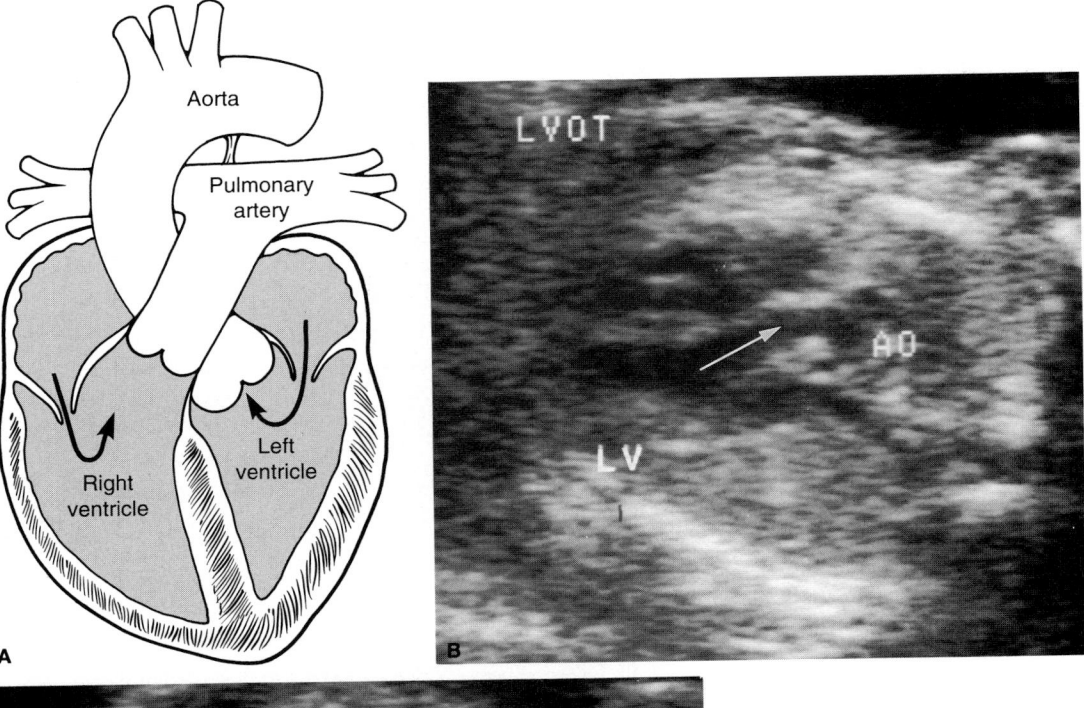

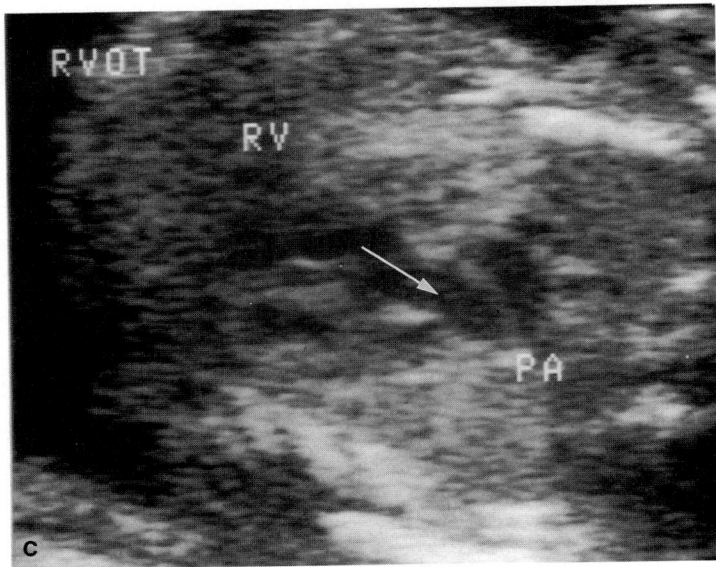

FIGURE 12-6. Crisscross relation of outflow tracts. **(A)** Pulmonary artery crosses the aorta in their normal perpendicular relation. **(B)** Ultrasound shows the left ventricular outflow tract (LVOT) with the aorta (AO) exiting (*arrow*) the left ventricle (LV). **(C)** Ultrasound shows the right ventricular outflow tract (RVOT) with the pulmonary artery (PA) exiting (*arrow*) the right ventricle (RV). This is identified by slight rotation of the transducer, demonstrating the RVOT crossing nearly perpendicular to the LVOT. (Courtesy of Dr. Eugenio Gersovich, Sacramento, CA.)

Bright spot within the ventricle. An echogenic bright spot most commonly is seen within the left ventricle (see Fig. 12-4) but also has been observed within the right ventricle.[12,13] Various theories have been proposed about the cause of this bright spot, including that it is papillary muscle, echogenic cordae tendinea, or the junction of the papillary muscle with the cordae tendinea. In any case, the bright spot is normally 2 to 3 mm in size, is brighter than the rest of the cardiac structures, and can be considered a normal variant. Occasionally, another bright spot may be observed at the apex of the right ventricle or within the ventricular wall. This is probably caused by the echogenic focus of the overlying rib or sternum[12] (Fig. 12-10).

Pseudo ventricular septal defect (VSD). The membranous portion of the ventricular

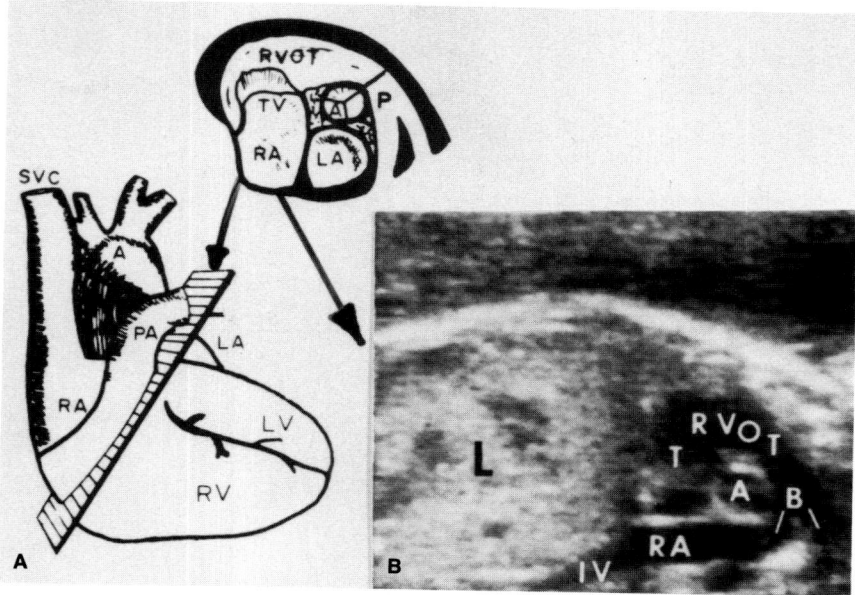

FIGURE 12-7. Short axis views through the fetal heart at the level of the tricuspid and mitral valves and the aortic and pulmonic outflow tracts. **(A)** The schematic illustrates the planes through the fetal heart from which the following images were obtained. **(B)** The right ventricular outflow tract (RVOT) drapes over the aorta (A) and bifurcates (B) into the right and left pulmonary arteries (*white lines*). RV, right ventricle; LV, left ventricle; RA, right atrium; LA, left atrium; SVC, superior vena cava. (Devore GR: The prenatal diagnosis of congenital heart disease: A practical approach for the fetal sonographer. JCU 1985; 13:229.)

septum is located just below the atrial ventricular valves and is normally very thin. It may be so thin that it appears to be a small VSD (Fig. 12-11). Color flow imaging may be helpful to further ascertain if it is in fact a defect in that portion of the ventricular septum.

Pseudo atrial septal defect (ASD). Because of the rapid movement of both the septum primum and the septum secundum, these structures may not be visualized during a frozen or single-frame image and thus may appear to be an ASD. Review of the real-time images may better demonstrate normal motion of the foramen ovale (Fig. 12-12).

Pseudo pericardial effusion. The normal hypoechoic myocardium should not be mistaken for a pericardial effusion (Fig.

(*text continues on page 270*)

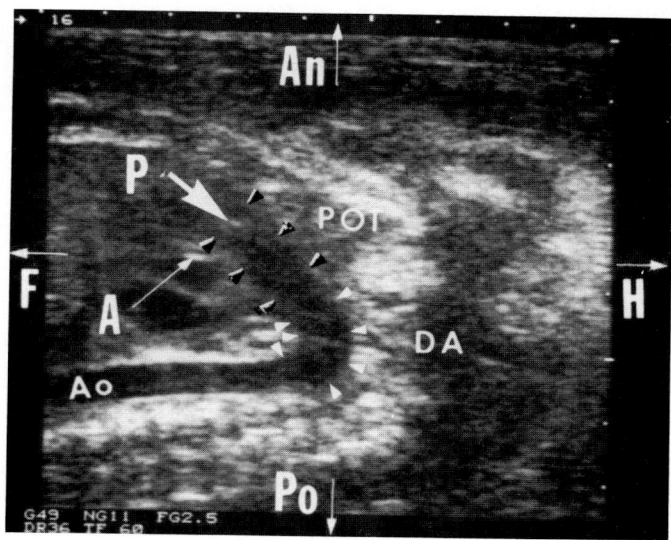

FIGURE 12-8. Imaging of the ductus arteriosus (DA). The transducer is directed parallel to spine. The DA can be followed from the pulmonary valve (P) to the descending aorta (Ao). Unlike the arch of the aorta, which looks like a cane, the ductal-aortic image has the appearance of a hockey stick. POT, pulmonary outflow tract; A, aortic valve; *black arrows*, pulmonary outflow tract; *white arrows*, DA; AN, anterior chest wall; Po, posterior; F, fetal feet; H, fetal head. (DeVore GR: The prenatal diagnosis of congenital heart disease: A practical approach for the fetal sonographer. JCU 1985; 13:229.)

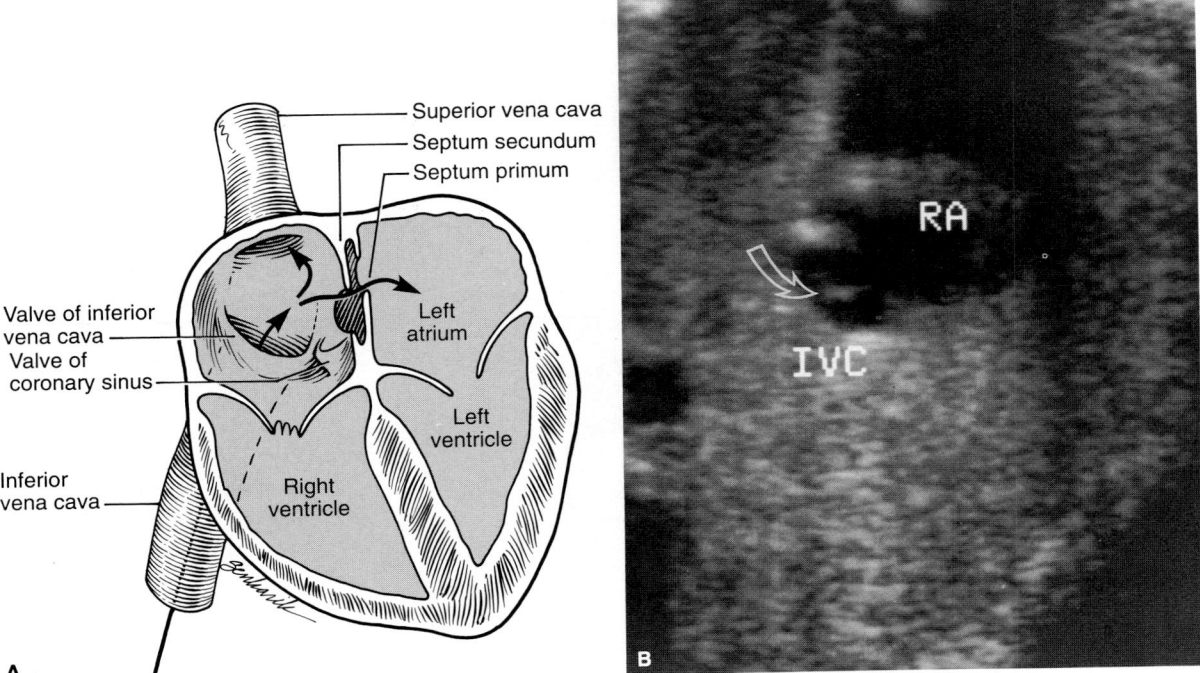

FIGURE 12-9. **(A)** The valve of the inferior vena cava and the valve of the coronary sinus draining into the right atrium and their relationship to the atrial septum. **(B)** The small valve of the inferior vena cava (IVC) may be identified within the right atrium (RA). This should not be mistaken for an abnormal fold within the right atrium.

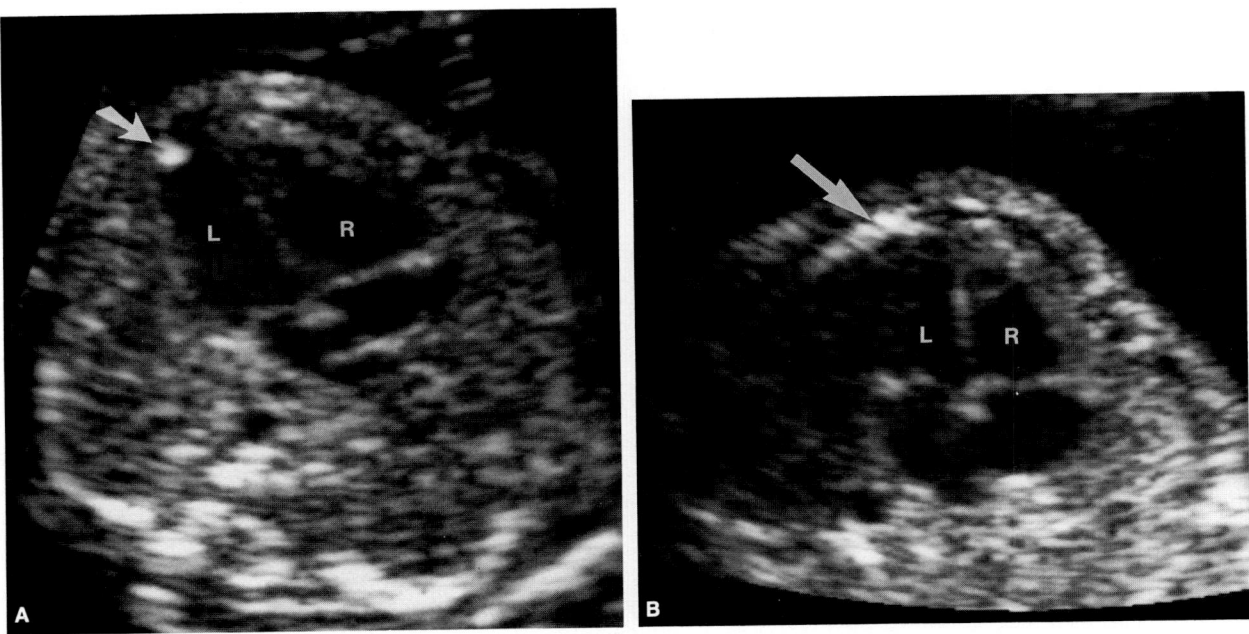

FIGURE 12-10. Sonogram of echogenic focus at edge of the myocardium. **(A)** Four-chamber view shows small echogenic focus (*arrow*) at apex of left ventricle (L). **(B)** If the transducer is rotated into a plane that shows a longer section of rib (*arrow*), this pitfall can be recognized. R, right ventricle. (Brown DL, DiSalvo DN, Frates MC, et al: Sonography of the fetal heart: Normal variants and pitfalls. AJR 1993; 160:1251–1255.)

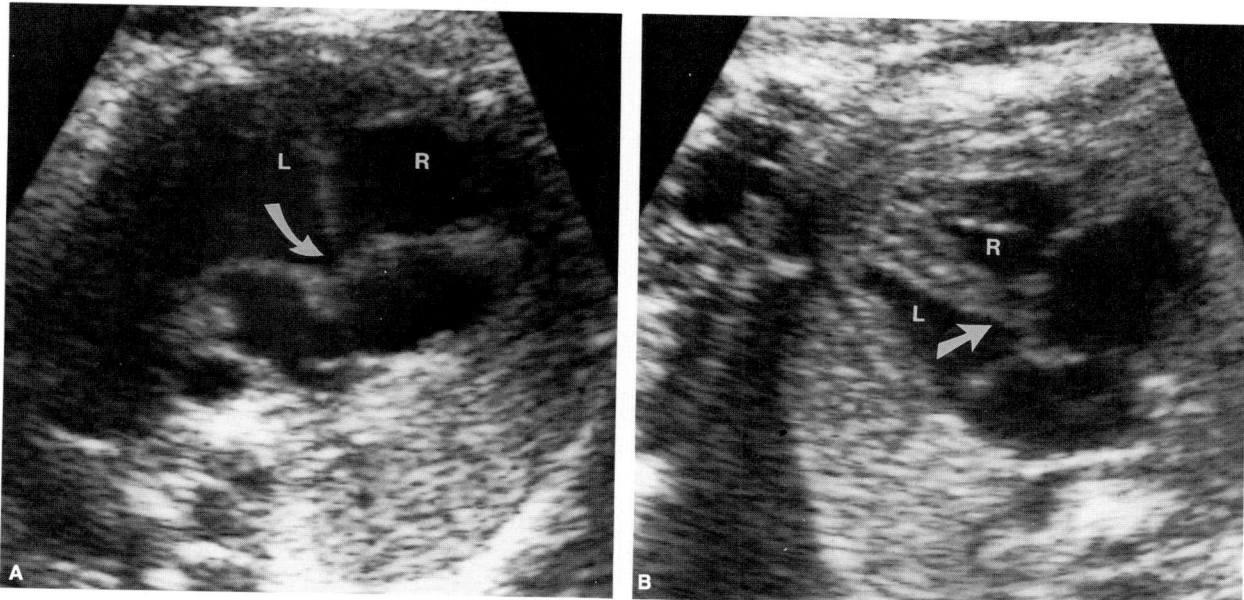

FIGURE 12-11. Sonograms of pseudoventricular septal defect. **(A)** On this four-chamber view (where septum is parallel to ultrasound beam), a defect in ventricular septum (*arrow*) appears to be present. **(B)** This can be recognized as an artifact by scanning same portion of septum from a different orientation, ideally with ultrasound beam more perpendicular to septum (as in this image), showing continuity (*arrow*) of septum (color flow may confirm intact ventricular septum). L, left ventricle; R, right ventricle. (Brown DL, DiSalvo DN, Frates MC, et al: Sonography of the fetal heart: Normal variants and pitfalls. AJR 1993; 160:1251–1255.)

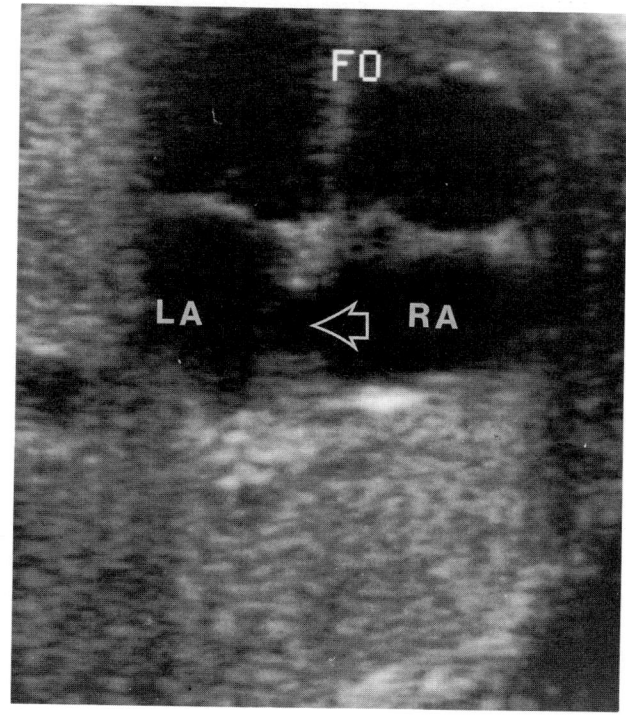

FIGURE 12-12. Pseudo atrial septal defect. Magnified four-chamber view of the heart with the ultrasound transducer angled parallel to the thin, rapidly moving portions of the foramen ovale, which may appear as an atrial septal defect (*arrow*). Scanning perpendicular to the atrial septum may be helpful to document the normal foramen ovale. RA, right atrium; LA, left atrium. (See diagram of Figure 12-9*A*.)

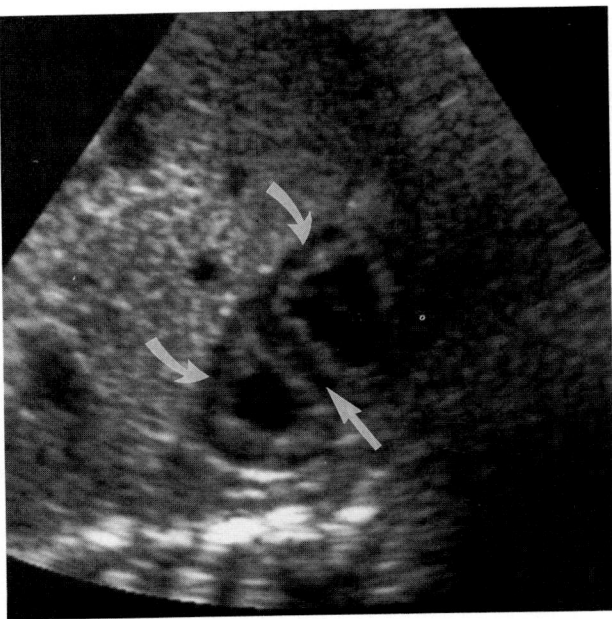

FIGURE 12-13. Pseudo pericardial effusion. On short axis view, the normal peripheral hypoechoic part of myocardium (*curved arrows*) can be distinguished from true pericardial fluid by observing its continuation into ventricular septum (*straight arrow*). (Brown DL, DiSalvo DN, Frates MC, et al: Sonography of the fetal heart: Normal variants and pitfalls. AJR 1993; 160:1251–1255.)

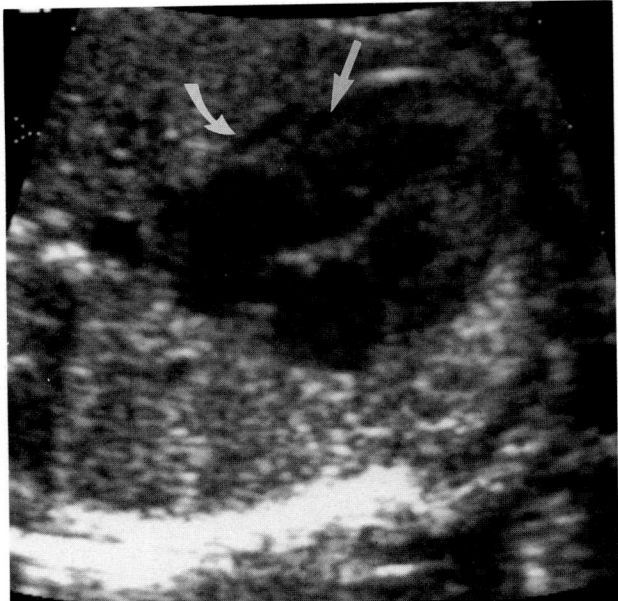

FIGURE 12-14. Normal pericardial fluid. A trace of pericardial fluid (*curved arrow*) is seen in this four-chamber view of a normal fetus. Fluid is peripheral to myocardium, which itself can be relatively hypoechoic peripherally (*straight arrow*). Note that fluid does not surround entire heart but is seen adjacent to a small segment of heart. (Brown DL, DiSalvo DN, Frates MC, et al: Sonography of the fetal heart: Normal variants and pitfalls. AJR 1993; 160:1251–1255.)

TABLE 12-7.   Fetal Cardiac Deaths

Cardiac Abnormality	Incidence (%)*
Hypoplastic left ventricle	29
Coarctation of the aorta	10
Transposition of the great vessels	8.5
Pulmonic stenosis or pulmonic atresia	7.5
Tetralogy of Fallot	6
Truncus arteriosus	3
Ventricular septal defect	2
Atrial ventricular canal	1
Tricuspid atresia	0.5

* This table details the percentage of different cardiac abnormalities identified in newborns who died within the first month of life. Data were collected from 1967 through 1978 at the University of Minnesota.

(Modified from Moller JH, Neal WA: Incidence of cardiac malformations. In Heart Disease in Infancy. New York: Appleton-Century-Crofts, 1981: 1–13.)

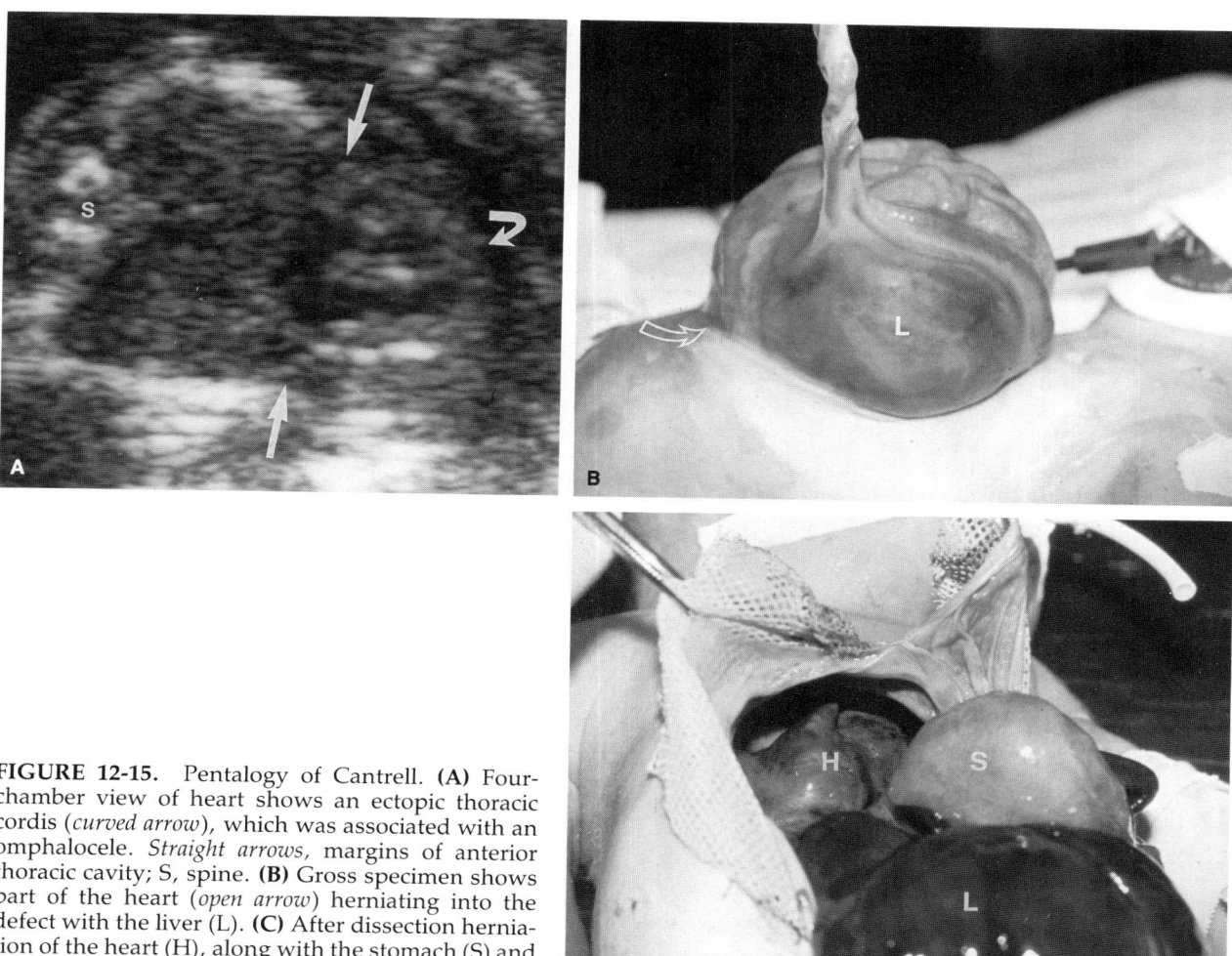

FIGURE 12-15. Pentalogy of Cantrell. **(A)** Four-chamber view of heart shows an ectopic thoracic cordis (*curved arrow*), which was associated with an omphalocele. *Straight arrows,* margins of anterior thoracic cavity; S, spine. **(B)** Gross specimen shows part of the heart (*open arrow*) herniating into the defect with the liver (L). **(C)** After dissection herniation of the heart (H), along with the stomach (S) and liver (L), into the defect is more clearly defined.

TABLE 12-8.   Classification of Ectopic Cordis

Isolated
Pentalogy of Cantrell
   Omphalocele
   Ectopic cordis
   Diaphragmatic defect
   Pericardial defect
   Intrinsic cardiac abnormality

12-13). The myocardium of the ventricles during systole may appear hypoechoic and may be mistaken for a pericardial effusion.[14] Normally, a small amount of pericardial fluid may be observed around the cardiac ventricles. This fluid is observed more prominently during ventricular systole[12,15] (Fig. 12-14).

DETECTION OF CARDIAC ANOMALIES

Four-Chamber View

Controversy exists about the exact number of cardiac malformations that may be diagnosed on a four-chamber view of the heart. The percentage varies from about 63%[16] to as high as 96%.[4] Our personal experience indicates that the former, or lower, percentage is most accurate. A review of the autopsy series of newborns from the University of Minnesota indicates that the more common cardiac anomalies, such as hypoplastic left ventricle, pulmonic atresia, large VSDs, atrioventricular canal, and tricuspid atresia, may be detected on a four-

TABLE 12-9.   Potential Causes of Fetal Cardiomegaly

Hydrops
   Immune
   Nonimmune
Increased flow
   Arteriovenous malformations
   Vein of Galen aneurysm
   Hemangioma of the liver
Intrinsic cardiac anomaly
   Ebstein's anomaly (tricuspid valve abnormality)
   Other isolated valve stenoses with intact septum (rare)
Cardiomyopathy
Cardiac tumor
   Rhabdomyoma

TABLE 12-10.   Congenital Anomalies Detected In Utero Because of an Abnormal Four-Chamber View of the Heart

Are the ventricular chambers about equal in size?

Hypoplastic left ventricle
Hypoplastic right ventricle
Hypoplastic aortic arch
Aortic stenosis
Coarctation of the aorta (simple)
Coarctation of the aorta (complex)
Subaortic stenosis
Ostium primum defect
Single ventricle
Double outlet of right ventricle
Ebstein's anomaly

Is there a septal defect?

Atrial septal defect
Endocardial cushion defect
Ventricular septal defect
   Simple
   Tetralogy of Fallot
   Truncus arteriosus
   Double-outlet right ventricle

Is there an abnormal relation of the atrioventricular valve position?

Ebstein's anomaly

Is there an abnormality of the endocardium or myocardium?

Focal increased thickness (see Table 12-13)
Focal valvular atresia
Diffuse increased thickness
   Cardiomyopathy
Focal masses
   Rhabdomyoma

(Adapted from Devore GR: The prenatal diagnosis of congenital heart disease: A practical approach for the fetal sonographer. JCU 1985; 13:229, and McGahan JP: Sonography of the fetal heart: Findings on the four-chamber view. AJR 1991; 156:547.)

chamber view of the heart (Table 12-7). When performing a four-chamber view, six questions may be asked. The first two questions are often helpful in detecting intrathoracic extracardiac disease.[17]

1. *Is the heart in normal position?* The heart may be used as a normal anatomic marker for extracardiac intrathoracic abnormalities. For instance, a large pulmonary cystadenomatoid malformation or a diaphragmatic hernia displaces the heart into an abnormal location. In this case, the four-chamber view may be used as an anatomic marker for extracardiac intrathoracic abnormalities (see Chapter 11). The heart also may lay in an ectopic location, a

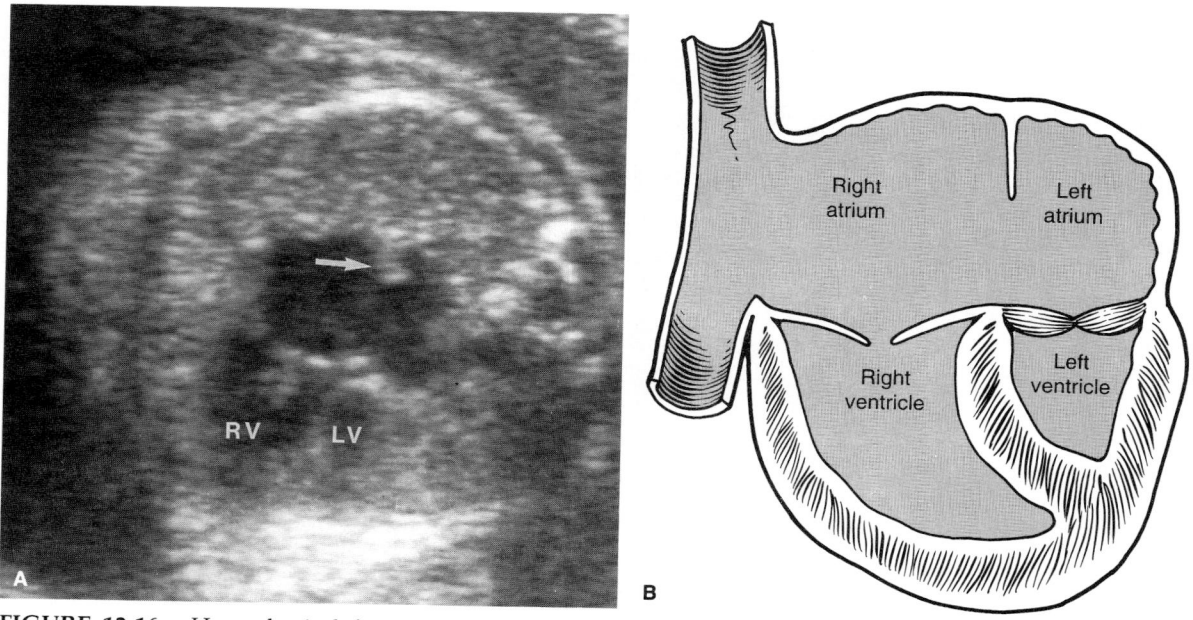

FIGURE 12-16. Hypoplastic left ventricle. **(A)** Attempted four-chamber view of the heart demonstrates a hypoplastic left ventricle (LV) and a small remnant of the atrial septum (*arrow*). RV, right ventricle. **(B)** Corresponding diagram demonstrates hypoplastic left ventricle and atretic mitral valve, an associated atrial septal defect, and a large right ventricle. The atretic aorta is not illustrated. (Modified from McGahan JP, Coy M, Parrish MD, Brant WE: Sonographic spectrum of fetal cardiac hypoplasia. J Ultrasound Med 1991; 10:539.)

condition called *thoracic ectopia cordis*.[18] Ectopic cordis may be an isolated abnormality, or it may be associated with a more complex abnormality, such as pentalogy of Cantrell (Fig. 12-15; Table 12-8).

2. *Is the heart normal in size in comparison to the fetal thorax?* The four-chamber view of the heart may be used to assess fetal cardiothoracic disproportion. Such measurements may be obtained from real-time images but are more accurately obtained from M-mode ultrasound. Standard measurements of the ratio of the cardiac biventricular outer dimensions to the chest circumference obtained by real-time M-mode measurements have been tabulated throughout pregnancy (see Fig. 12-2). These may be helpful to predict cardiomegaly (Table 12-9) or may be used as an indirect measure of fetal pulmonary hypoplasia.[19]

Four of the six questions are important for in utero assessment of intrinsic cardiac malformations. Previous cardiac anomalies have been detected in utero because of abnormal four-chamber views of the heart and are listed with the specific questions in Table 12-10.[17]

3. *Are the ventricle chambers about equal in size?* In general, the right and left ventricle should be about equal in size when studying the four-chamber view of the heart.[17] This is most accurately seen when an M-mode sonogram is obtained during diastole of the atrioventricular valve region. However, real-time examination can be also used as a rough estimate of ventricular chamber size.

Most common anomalies can be classified as either hypoplasia of the left ventricle or hypoplasia of the right ventricle. Hypoplastic left ventricle is usually called the *hypoplastic left heart syndrome*.[20] This syndrome may comprise a spectrum of findings, including underdevelopment of the aorta, aortic valve, left ventricle, or mitral valve and an intact ventricular septum (Fig. 12-16; Table 12-11).

TABLE 12-11. Possible Causes of Left Ventricle Being Smaller Than Right Ventricle

- Hypoplastic left ventricle
- Coarctation of the aorta
- Hypoplastic aortic arch

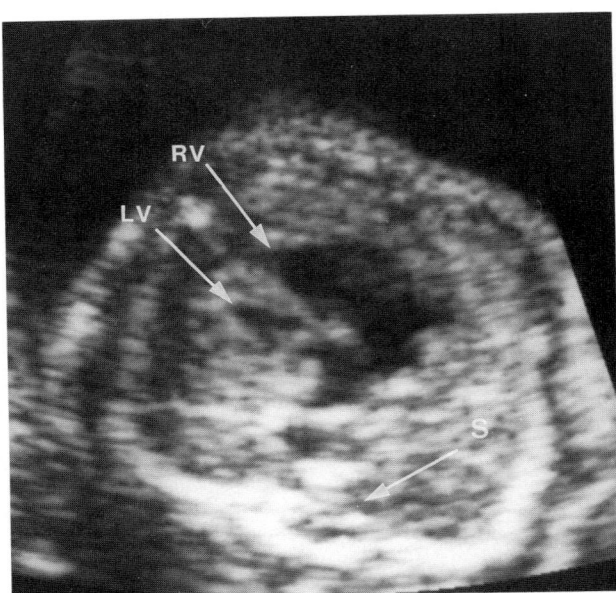

FIGURE 12-17.   Coarctation of the aorta. Discrepancy in size between the left ventricle (LV) and the right ventricle (RV) may be a clue to decreased blood flow through the left ventricle, as in this case of coarctation of the aorta. S, spine.

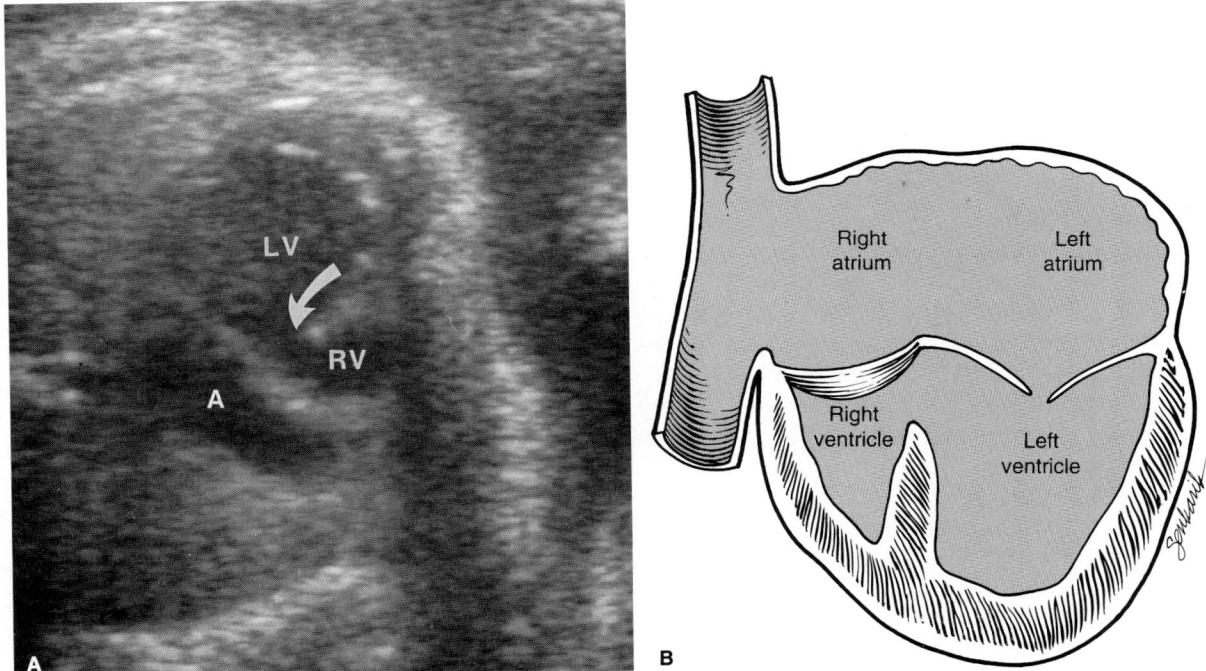

FIGURE 12-18.   Tricuspid atresia with ventricular septal defect. **(A)** Four-chamber view of the heart demonstrates a common atrium (A), an enlarged left ventricle (LV), a hypoplastic right ventricle (RV), and a ventricular septal defect (*curved arrow*). **(B)** Corresponding drawing. (Modified from McGahan JP, Choy M, Parrish MD, Brant WE: Sonographic spectrum of fetal cardiac hypoplasia. J Ultrasound Med 1991; 10:539.)

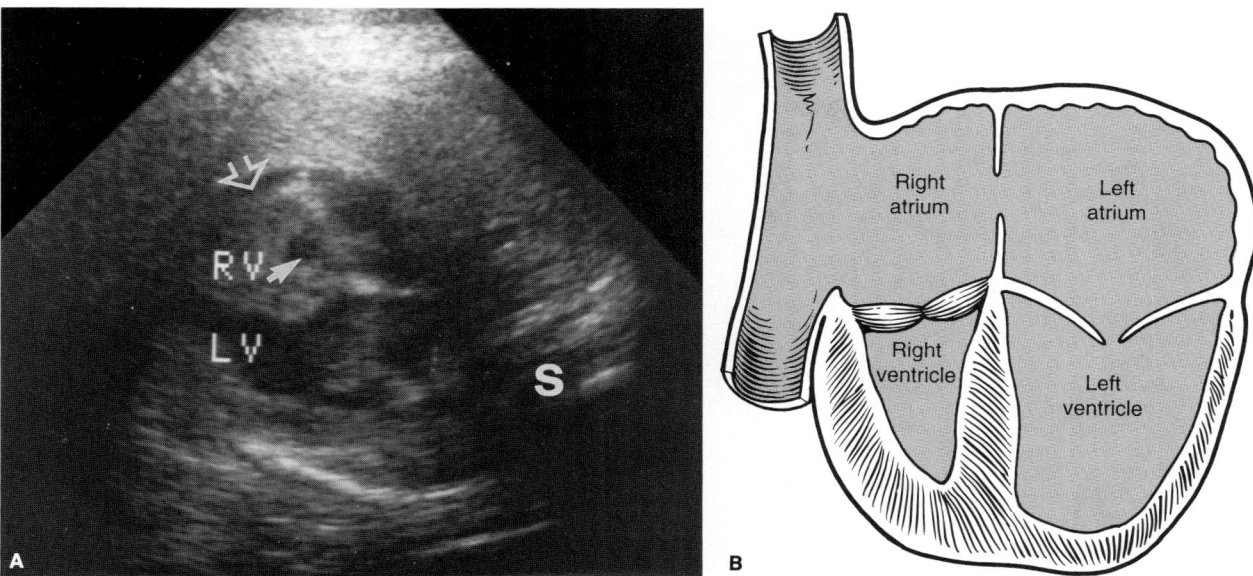

FIGURE 12-19. Hypoplastic right ventricle. **(A)** Attempted four-chamber view of the heart demonstrates a hypoplastic right ventricle (RV) with marked thickening of the right ventricular wall (*open arrow*). LV, left ventricle; S, spine. **(B)** Diagram demonstrates hypoplastic right ventricle, atretic tricuspid valve, atrial septal defect, and a large left ventricle. The atretic pulmonary outflow is not illustrated. (Modified from McGahan JP, Choy M, Parrish MD, Brant WE: Sonographic spectrum of fetal cardiac hypoplasia. J Ultrasound Med 1991; 10:539.)

Likewise, the only clue to an abnormality of the aortic arch may be the discrepancy in size between the left and right ventricles. For instance, in coarctation of the aorta, blood flowing from the left ventricle is decreased and is shunted from the right ventricle into the ductus and the descending aorta. Because the blood flow in the left ventricle is decreased, there is resultant underdevelopment of the left ventricle, and thus the left ventricle is smaller than the right ventricle (Fig. 12-17).

Considerably more confusion concerns the diagnosis of hypoplasia of the right ventricle. This may be considered either one of two anomalies: pulmonary atresia or tricuspid atresia with or with-

TABLE 12-12. Possible Causes of Right Ventricle Being Smaller Than Left Ventricle

• Pulmonary atresia, with or without ventricular septal defect
• Tricuspid atresia, with or without ventricular septal defect
• Aortic stenosis or insufficiency (left ventricle enlarged)

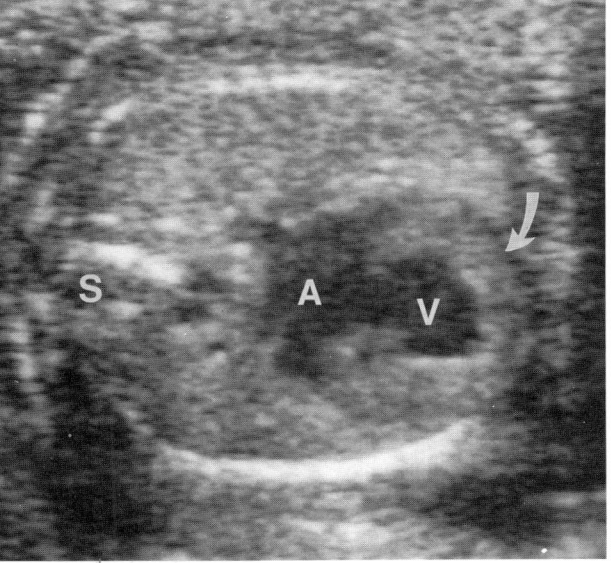

FIGURE 12-20. Two-chamber heart. Four-chamber view of heart shows a single atrium or an atrial septal defect with a common atrium (A) that empties into a single ventricle (V). Note thickening of wall of ventricular chamber (*curved arrow*). S, spine.

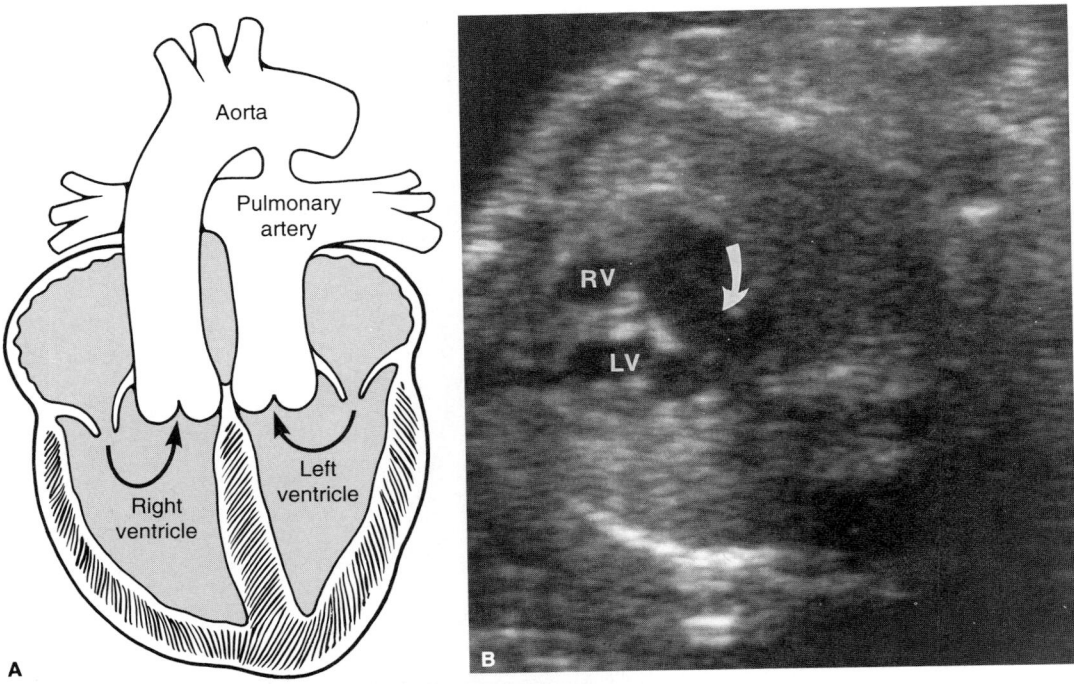

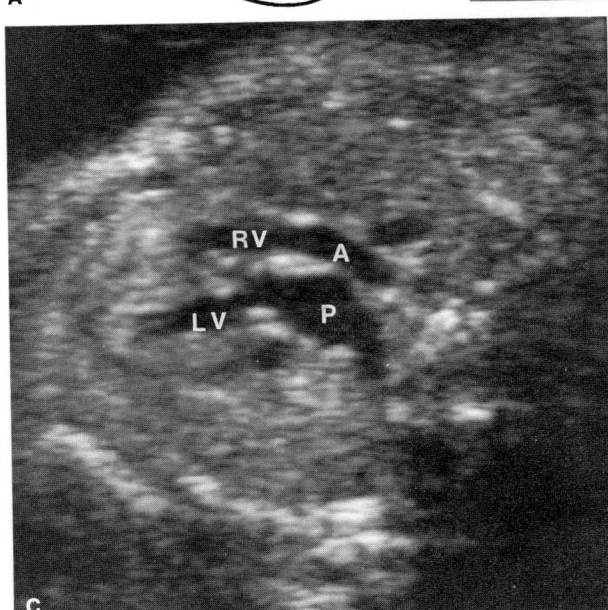

FIGURE 12-21. Transposition of great arteries. **(A)** Transposition of great vessels, with aorta originating from right ventricle and pulmonary artery originating from left ventricle. There may be an accompanying septal defect, and the aorta and the pulmonary artery are parallel rather than perpendicular. (See Figure 12-6.) **(B)** Four-chamber view demonstrates a large atrial septal defect (*curved arrow*). RV, right ventricle; LV, left ventricle. **(C)** A more cephalic view shows the parallel course of aorta (A) and pulmonary artery (P) rather than the normal perpendicular course of these vessels. RV, right ventricle; LV, left ventricle. (McGahan JP, Nyberg DA, Emerson SD: Cardiac malformations. In Nyberg DA, Mahoney BS, Pretorius DH [eds]: Diagnostic Ultrasound of Fetal Anomalies: Text and Atlas. Chicago: Year Book Medical Publishers, 1990: 300–341.)

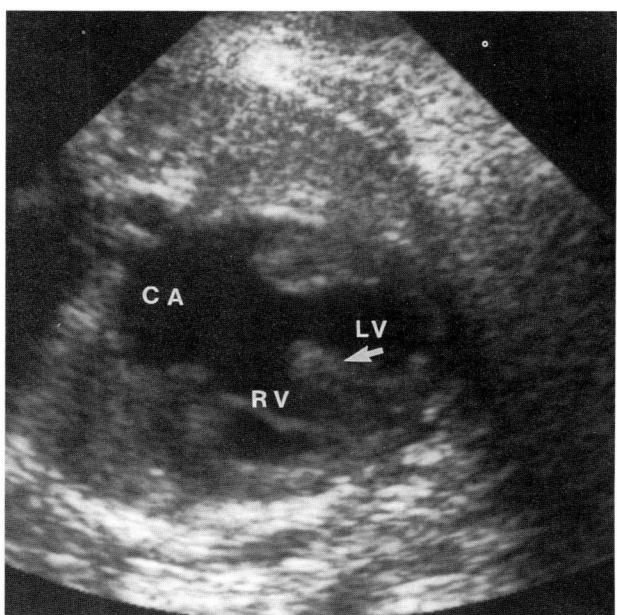

FIGURE 12-22. Large endocardial cushion defect resulting in a common atrium (CA) and absence of the upper portion of the ventricular septum, with only the lower portion of the ventricular septum identified (*arrow*). RV, right ventricle; LV, left ventricle.

out an intact ventricular septum (Fig. 12-18). Usually, severe hypoplasia of the right ventricle is associated with pulmonary atresia and intact ventricular septum, while the amount of hypoplasia of the right ventricle varies with tricuspid atresia when a VSD is present. The degree of hypoplasia of the right ventricle depends on the size of the tricuspid or pulmonary atresia and is inversely dependent on the size of the VSD[17,20] (Fig. 12-19). Typical causes of the right ventricle being smaller than the left ventricle are listed in Table 12-12. In some situations, two atria may enter into a single ventricle. Alternatively, there may be complete absence of both the atrial and ventricular septa, resulting in a common atria and a common ventricle, the so-called two-chamber heart (Fig. 12-20).

4. *Is there a septal defect?* Septal defects may be divided into three basic types: ASD, atrioventricular canal, and VSD.

ASD can be further divided into ostium primum and ostium secundum defects. Ostium secundum defects are located high in the atrial septum, while ostium primum defects are low in the septum and often are associated with an abnormality of the atrioventricular valve. Small defects may be difficult to detect in utero, while large defects may be identified (Figs. 12-16 and 12-21).

An atrioventricular canal defect is more easily recognized in utero with complete absence of the endocardial cushion (Fig. 12-22).

A VSD may be small or large. Smaller defects occur in the membranous portion of the ventricular septum. Larger defects involve larger portions of the ventricular septum and are more easily detectable (see Fig. 12-18). Large VSDs are often associated with other intrinsic cardiac abnormalities (Fig. 12-23). A small VSD may be overlooked on in utero scanning, and a careful scanning of the entire ventricular septum is needed to detect these defects (see Fig. 12-18). Color flow imaging allows easier recognition of the small defects (see Chapter 13). An ASD, VSD, or endocardial cushion defect noted on a four-chamber view should prompt a more complete cardiac examination.

5. *Are the atrioventricular valves in normal position?* A right-sided abnormality of the atrioventricular valve position is usually associated with malformations of the tricuspid valve in which the septal leaflet is displaced into the cavity of the right ventricle. This is called *Ebstein's anomaly.* Sonographically, this results in a large right atrium and a fairly characteristic appearance (Fig. 12-24). Similar enlargement of the right atrium can result from tricuspid dysplasia, with regurgitation not occurring with displacement of the tricuspid valve.[20]

6. *Is there an abnormality of the endocardium or myocardium?* Focal increased thickening of the endocardium or myocardium is usually associated with isolated valvular atresia or severe stenosis. This is illustrated in a case of pulmonary atresia

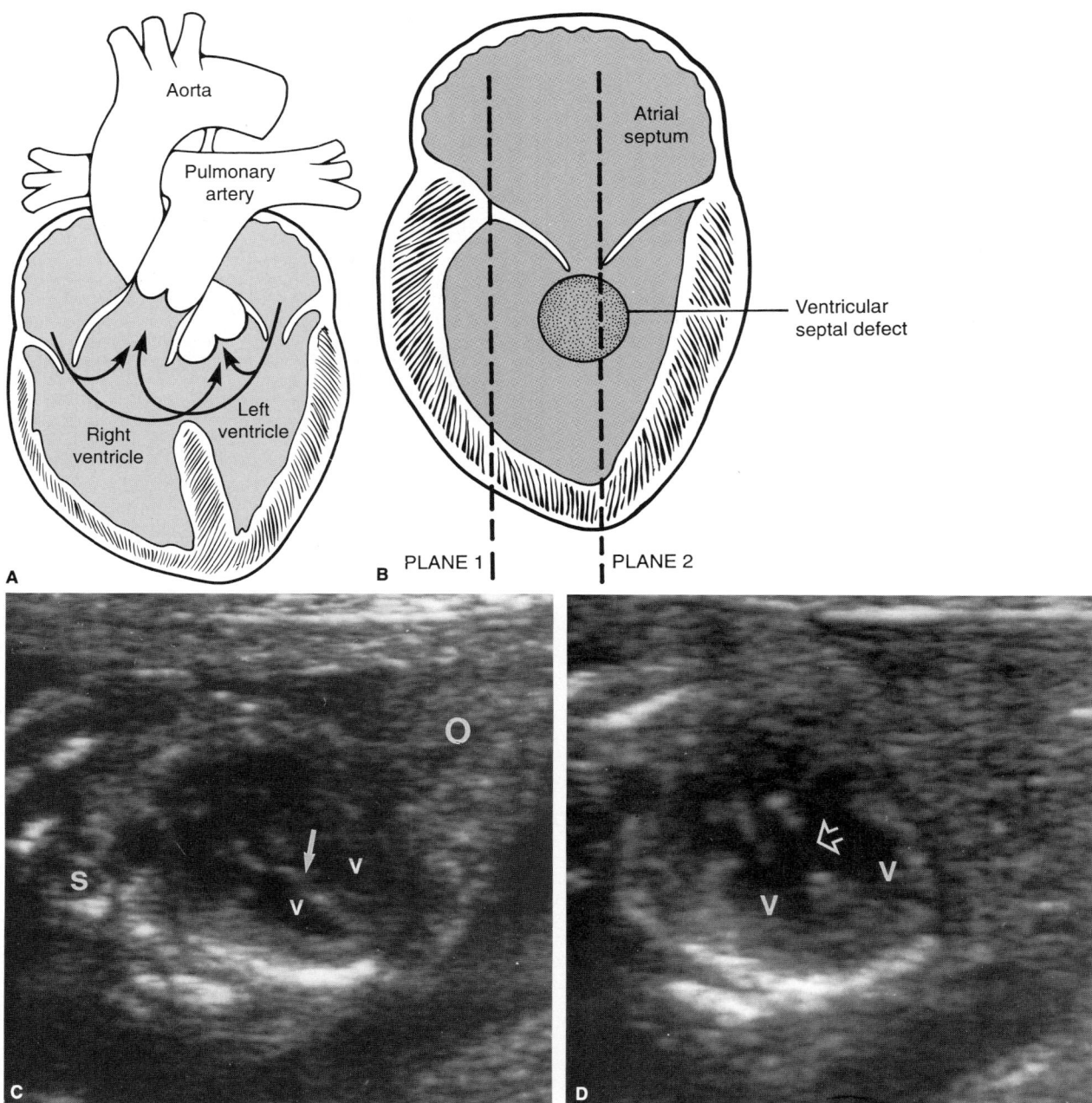

FIGURE 12-23.   **(A)** Ventricular septal defect. **(B)** Complete scanning of ventricular septum is needed to exclude ventricular septal defects. In this diagram, scanning through the ventricular septum in plane 1 would appear normal. Scanning in plane 2 would optimally visualize the defect. **(C)** In this four-chamber view of the heart in a fetus with an omphalocele (O) and transposition of the great vessels, the ventricular septum appears intact (*arrow*) while scanning through plane 1. S, spine; V, ventricle. **(D)** By obtaining plane 2 scan through interventricular septum, a large ventricular septal defect (*open arrow*) is identified between the two ventricles (V). (McGahan JP: Sonography of the fetal heart: Findings on the four-chamber view. AJR 1991; 156:547.)

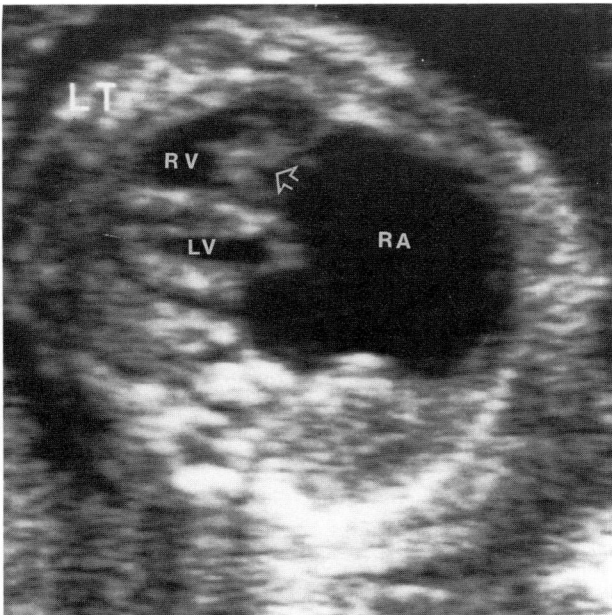

FIGURE 12-24. Ebstein's anomaly. Attempted four-chamber view of heart shows marked dilation of right atrium (RA) and inferior displacement of tricuspid leaflet (*open arrow*) into right ventricle (RV). LV, left ventricle.

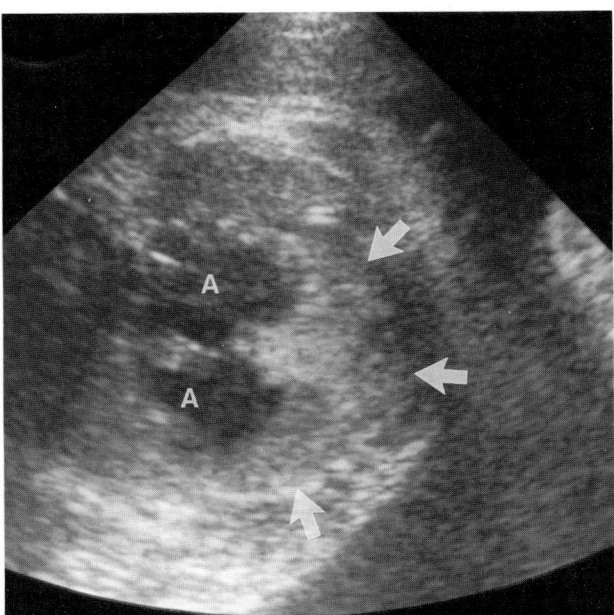

FIGURE 12-25. Diffuse myocardial thickening. Four-chamber view of the heart demonstrates diffuse ventricular myocardial and interventricular septal thickening (*arrows*) secondary to cardiac rhabdomyoma and diffuse cardiomyopathy. A, atria. (Coates T, McGahan JP, et al: Fetal cardiac tachycardia and cardiac hypertrophy secondary to diffuse cardiac rhabdomyoma. J Ultrasound Med [in press].)

with an intact ventricular septum and hypertrophy of the right ventricle (see Fig. 12-19).

Most commonly, diffuse thickening of the heart muscle is associated with cardiomyopathy. A rare cause is represented in Figure 12-25 in which there are multiple cardiac rhabdomyomas that cause outflow obstruction and, therefore, diffuse hypertrophy of the cardiac myometrium. Causes of increased endocardial or myocardial thickness are listed in Table 12-13.

Increased echogenicity within the ventricles is usually associated with a cardiac tumor. The most common in utero cardiac tumor is a cardiac rhabdomyoma, which is often secondary to tuberous sclerosis.[17,21] This tumor should be distinguished from the normal echogenic focus usually observed within the left ventricle (see Fig. 12-4). Tumors are much larger, usually show mildly increased echogenicity, and usually are close to the ventricular wall (Fig. 12-26). Possible cardiac tumors are listed in Table 12-14. The four-chamber view of the heart may be used to detect other abnormalities. For instance, recognition of a pericardial effusion may be a clue to systemic disorders, such as fetal hydrops. Causes of possible fluid around the heart are included in Table 12-15.

Aortic and Pulmonary Outflow Tracts

A number of other significant fetal cardiac malformations can be detected with an examination of the fetal cardiac outflow tracts in addition to a four-chamber view of the heart.[16,22] These include transposition of the great arteries, tetralogy of Fallot, and truncus arteriosus. In fact, about 85% of all cardiac abnormalities may be diagnosed routinely obtaining a four-chamber view of the heart and

TABLE 12-13. Causes of Increased Thickness of the Endocardium or Myocardium

Focal

Critical valve disease
Cardiac tumor
Normal—bright spot of papillary muscle

Diffuse

Cardiomyopathy
    Endocardial fibroelastosis
    Glycogen storage disease
    Hypertrophic cardiomyopathy
Cardiac tumor

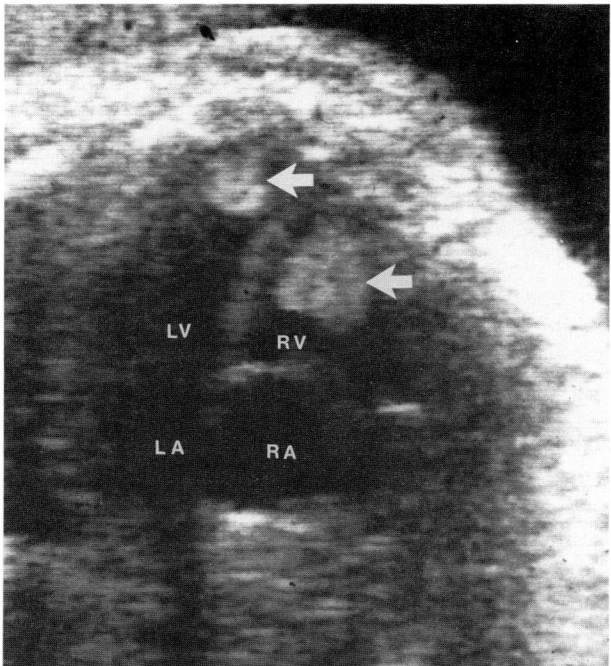

FIGURE 12-26. Cardiac rhabdomyomas. Four-chamber view of fetal heart shows echogenic masses (*arrows*) in both ventricles corresponding to cardiac rhabdomyomas. This fetus was documented to have tuberous sclerosis. LV, left ventricle; RV, right ventricle; LA, left atrium; RA, right atrium. (McGahan JP: Sonography of the fetal heart: Findings on the four-chamber view. AJR 1991; 156:547.)

examining outflow tracts.[16] Potential pitfalls still exist in this schema, including missed diagnosis of ASD, small VSD, isolated valvular stenosis, coarctation of the aorta, and total anomalous pulmonary venous return. When reviewing the data from the University of Minnesota series, however, abnormalities that most often present within the first days to first month of life should be detected with the combination of the four-chamber view of the

TABLE 12-14.   Possible Causes of Fetal and Newborn Cardiac Tumors

Uncommon

Rhabdomyoma (may be associated with tuberous sclerosis)

Extremely Rare

Teratoma
Fibroma
Myxoma
Hemangioma

TABLE 12-15.   Possible Causes of Fluid Around the Heart

- Pericardial effusion
- Pleural effusion
- Variant—hypoechoic myocardium
- Normal—pericardial fluid identified during diastole

heart and outflow tract views[16] (see Tables 12-7 and 12-10).

Three questions should be asked when evaluating the relation of the great arteries to the right and left ventricles:

1. *Is there a normal crisscross relation of the pulmonary artery and aorta?* If this relation does not exist, and the aorta and pulmonary artery lie parallel rather than crisscross, this may be a clue to diagnosis of double outlet of the right ventricle or transposition of the great vessels (see Figs. 12-6 and 12-21). In transposition, the pulmonary artery is noted to rise from the left ventricle and to bifurcate.
2. *Is there a discrepancy in size of the aorta and main pulmonary artery?* The assessment of the relation of the sizes of these two vessels is helpful in diagnosing such abnormalities as tetralogy of Fallot, in which the aortic root is larger than the atretic pulmonary artery.[22] Likewise, in truncus arteriosus, one large or common trunk is identified rather than a separate aorta and pulmonary artery. Causes of increased and decreased aortic diameter are listed in Table 12-16. Aortic measurements

TABLE 12-16.   Causes of Increased and Decreased Aortic Diameter

Increased Aortic Diameter

Common
  Tetralogy of Fallot
Less common
  Truncus arteriosus (common trunk)
Very uncommon
  Hypoplastic left ventricle with transposition

Decreased Aortic Diameter

Common
  Hypoplastic left ventricle
Uncommon
  Coarctation of the aorta

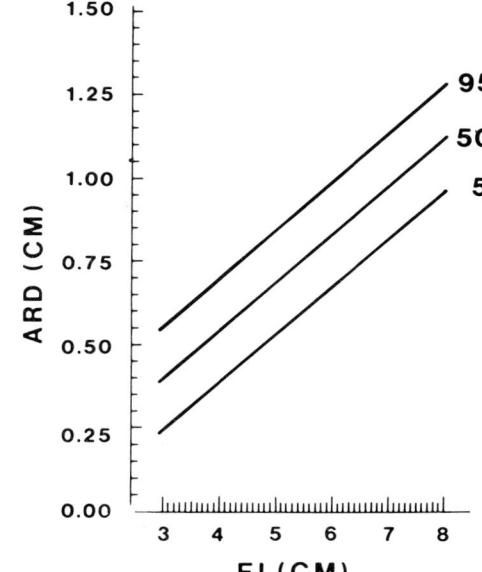

FIGURE 12-27. Aortic root to femur length dimensions. Aortic root dimensions expressed in centimeters compared with the 5th, 50th, and 95th percentiles of the femoral length expressed in centimeters. (DeVore GR: Cardiac imaging. In Sabbagha RE [ed]: Ultrasound Applied to Obstetrics and Gynecology, 2nd ed. Philadelphia: JB Lippincott, 1987: 347.)

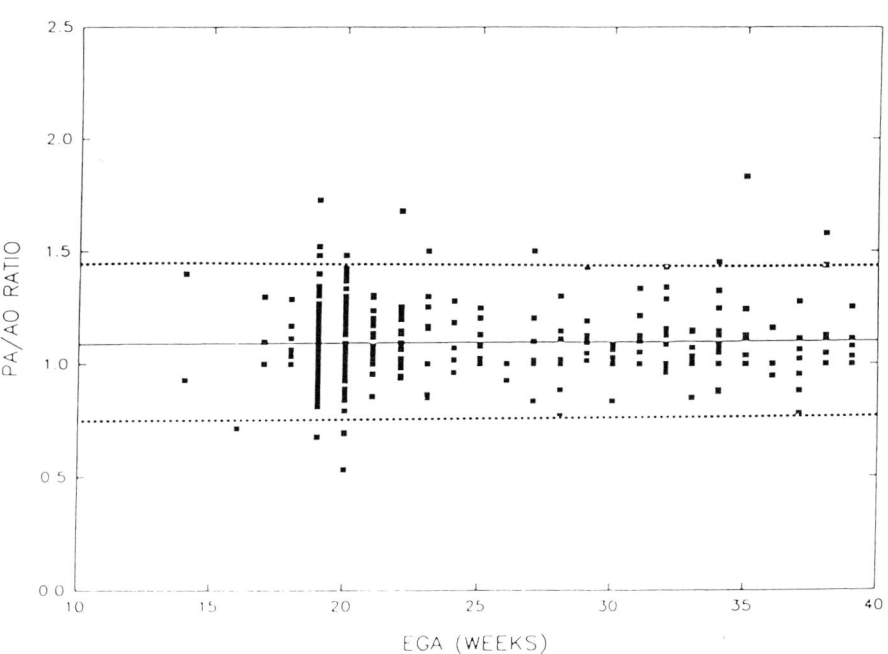

FIGURE 12-28. Pulmonary artery to aortic dimensions. The root of the pulmonary artery compared with the aorta contains a constant relation of nearly 1.09 to 1, with a standard deviation of 0.75 to 1.45 throughout pregnancy. (Comstock CH, Riggs T, Lee W, Kirk J: Pulmonary-to-aorta diameter ratio in the normal and abnormal fetal heart. Am J Obstet Gynecol 1991; 165:1038.)

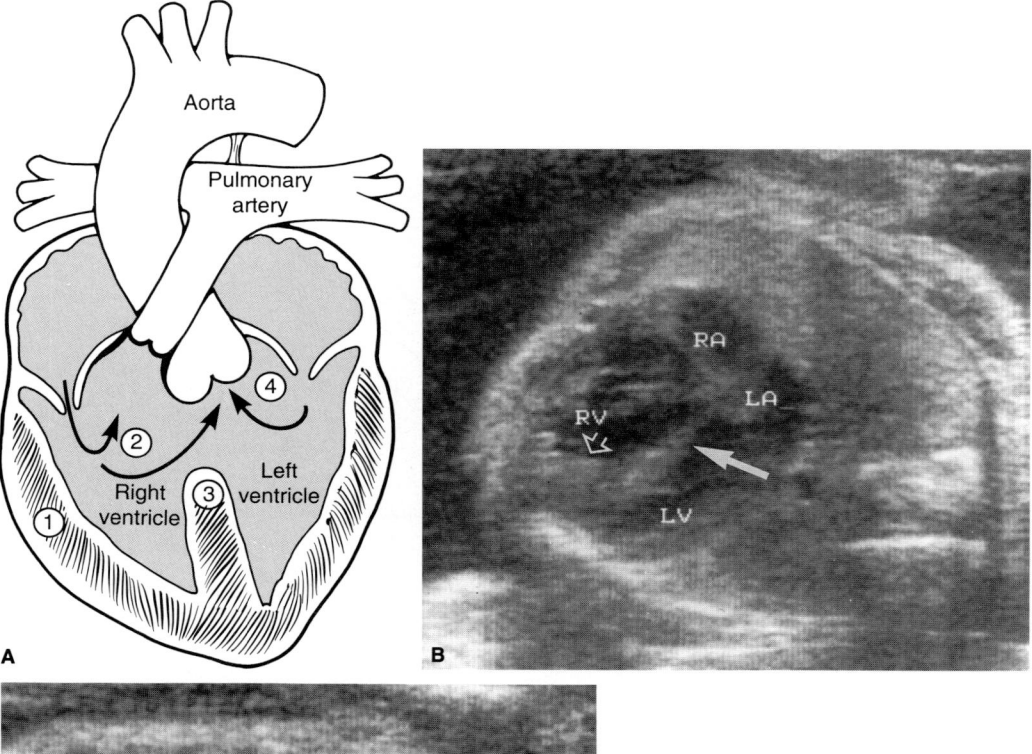

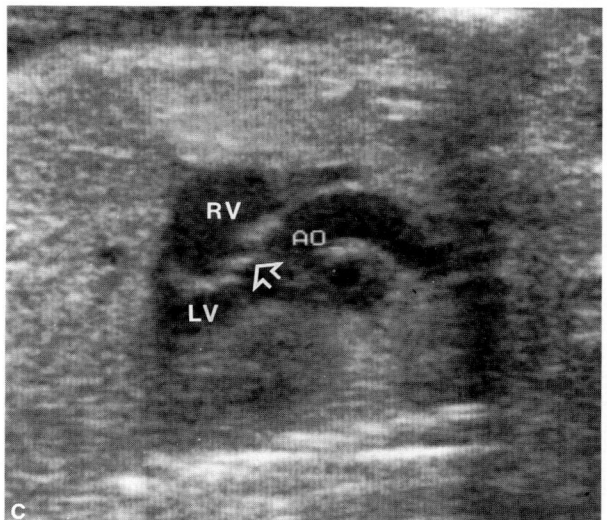

FIGURE 12-29. Tetralogy of Fallot. **(A)** Components of tetralogy of Fallot, including (1) right ventricular hypertrophy, (2) subpulmonic stenosis, (3) ventricular septal defect, and (4) overriding aorta. **(B)** Four-chamber view of heart shows right ventricular hypertrophy (*open arrow*) and slightly increased size of right ventricle (RV) as compared with left ventricle (LV). However, ventricular septum appears intact (*solid arrow*). RA, right atrium; LA, left atrium. **(C)** Long axis view of heart shows a dilated aortic root (AO) overriding interventricular septum (*open arrow*). Ventricular septal defect was not appreciated. RV, right ventricle; LV, left ventricle. (McGahan JP: Sonography of the fetal heart: Findings on the four-chamber view. AJR 1991; 156:547.)

TABLE 12-17. Causes of Aorta Overriding the Ventricular Septum

Common

Tetralogy of Fallot

Uncommon

Pulmonary atresia with ventricular septal defect

Rare

Truncus arteriosus
Double-outlet right ventricle

and femoral length measurements have been tabulated throughout pregnancy, as has the size ratio of the aorta to the main pulmonary artery (Figs. 12-27 and 12-28).

3. *Is the aorta or pulmonary artery in normal relation to the ventricular septum?* The aorta overrides the ventricular septum in tetralogy of Fallot; therefore, this is an important clue to diagnosis (Fig. 12-29). Causes of an aorta overriding the ventricular septum are given in Table 12-17.

ACKNOWLEDGMENTS

Special thanks to Deborah Hoang and Barbara Dyer for preparation of this chapter.

REFERENCES

1. Allan LD, Crawford DC, Chita SK, Tynan MJ: Prenatal screening for congenital heart disease. Br Med J 1986; 292:1717.
2. Moller JH, Neal WA: Incidence of cardiac malformations. In Heart Disease in Infancy. New York: Appleton-Century-Crofts, 1981: 1–13.
3. AIUM guidelines. J Ultrasound Med 1991; 10:576.
4. Copel JA, Pilu G, Green J, et al: Fetal echocardiographic screening for congenital heart disease: The importance of the four-chamber view. Am J Obstet Gynecol 1987; 157:648.
5. Schmidt KG, Silverman NH: Evaluation of the fetal heart by ultrasound. In Callen PW (ed): Ultrasonography in Obstetrics and Gynecology, 2nd ed. Philadelphia: WB Saunders, 1988: 165.
6. Benacerraf BR, Sanders SP: Fetal echocardiography. Radiol Clin North Am 1990; 28:131.
7. McGahan JP, Nyberg DA, Mack LA: Sonography of facial features of alobar and semilobar holoprosencephaly. AJR 1990; 154:143.
8. Copel JA, Pilu G, Kleinman CS: Congenital heart disease and extracardiac anomalies: Associations and indications for fetal echocardiography. Am J Obstet Gynecol 1986; 154:1121–1132.
9. Van Praagh R, Weinberg PM, Smith SD, et al: Malpositions of the heart. In Adams FH, Emmanouilides GC, Riemenschneider TA (eds): Moss' Heart Disease in Infants, Children, and Adolescents, 4th ed. Baltimore: Williams and Wilkins, 1989: 530.
10. DeVore GR: The prenatal diagnosis of congenital heart disease: A practical approach for the fetal sonographer. JCU 1985; 13:229.
11. DeVore GR, Siassi B, Platt LD: Fetal echocardiography. IV. M-mode assessment of ventricular size and contractility during the second and third trimesters of pregnancy in the normal fetus. Am J Obstet Gynecol 1984; 150:981.
12. Brown DL, DiSalvo DN, Frates MC, et al: Sonography of the fetal heart: Normal variants and pitfalls. Am J Radiol 1993; 160:1251–1255.
13. Levy DW, Mintz MC: The left ventricular echogenic focus: A normal finding. AJR 1988; 150:85.
14. Brown DL, Cartier MS, Emerson DS, et al: The peripheral hypoechoic rim of the fetal heart. J Ultrasound Med 1989; 149:529.
15. Jeanty P, Romero R, Hobbins JC: Fetal pericardial fluid: A normal finding of the second half of gestation. Am J Obstet Gynecol 1984; 149:529.
16. Bromley B, Estroff JA, Sanders SP, et al: Fetal echocardiography accuracy: Accuracy and limitations in a population at high and low risk for heart defects. Am J Obstet Gynecol 1992; 166:1473.
17. McGahan JP: Sonography of the fetal heart: Findings on the four-chamber view. AJR 1991; 156:547.
18. Wicks JD, Levine MD, Mettler FA: Intrauterine sonography of thoracic ectopia cordis. AJR 1981; 137:619.
19. DeVore GR, Horenstein J, Platt LD: Fetal echocardiography. VI. Assessment of cardiothoracic disproportion: A new technique for the diagnosis of thoracic hypoplasia. Am J Obstet Gynecol 1986; 155:1066.
20. McGahan JP, Choy M, Parrish MD, Brant WE: Sonographic spectrum of fetal cardiac hypoplasia. J Ultrasound Med 1991; 10:539.
21. Coates T, McGahan JP: Fetal cardiac rhabdomyomas presenting as diffuse myocardial thickening. J Ultrasound Med (in press).
22. DeVore GR: The aortic and pulmonary outflow tract screening examination in the human fetus. J Ultrasound Med 1992; 11:345.

John P. McGahan and Manuel Porto:
DIAGNOSTIC OBSTETRICAL ULTRASOUND.
© 1994 J.B. Lippincott Company.

Greggory R. DeVore

Chapter *13*

The Role of Color Doppler in the Screening Examination of the Fetal Heart

The introduction of color Doppler for use in examination of the fetal heart was first reported in 1987.[1,2] Subsequent studies have confirmed its value in the identification of structural malformations of the cardiovascular system.[3-16] Although some may think that color Doppler is only for the consultative fetal sonologist, I would like to suggest that it has a role during the "screening" examination of the four-chamber and outflow tract views of the heart. The reason for this is the different types of information real-time and color Doppler ultrasound provide. Real-time identifies anatomy that includes the ventricular septum and walls, the size of the atrial and ventricular chambers, and the size and orientation of the aortic and pulmonic outflow tracts.[16] However, it does not provide information regarding the presence and direction of blood flow. When one considers the pathophysiology of congenital heart disease, it is important to realize that most structural defects of the heart have flow abnormalities that may mani-

fest earlier than defects identified from the real-time image. Color Doppler may also assist the examiner to elucidate the significance of suspicious pathology identified with real-time ultrasound. The purpose of this chapter is to illustrate these principles.

INTERPRETING THE COLOR DOPPLER IMAGE

Using the Doppler principle, the direction and velocity of a moving object (blood) can be detected (Fig. 13-1). Conventionally, if the Doppler shift is toward the transducer, the color is displayed in red. If it is away from the transducer, it is displayed in blue. Increasing velocity results in lighter shades of red or blue. Disturbed flow can be identified with a variance tag. If the velocity of blood flow exceeds the ability of the Doppler device to

FIGURE 13-1. Color Doppler display illustrates the four-chamber view of the fetal heart during diastole and systole. The ultrasound beam is directed from the top of the image with the flow of blood parallel to the ultrasound beam. The color bar illustrates blood flow toward the transducer (*orange*). As the flow velocity increases (*arrow*), the color becomes lighter (*yellow*). The *black* represents no flow. The *blue* represents flow of blood away from the transducer, with lighter shades representing increased flow velocity (*arrow*). The *green* side bar is the variance tag that identifies disturbed flow. During ventricular diastole, both ventricles fill with blood (*orange*). During systole, color should only be observed along the interventricular septum of the left ventricle.

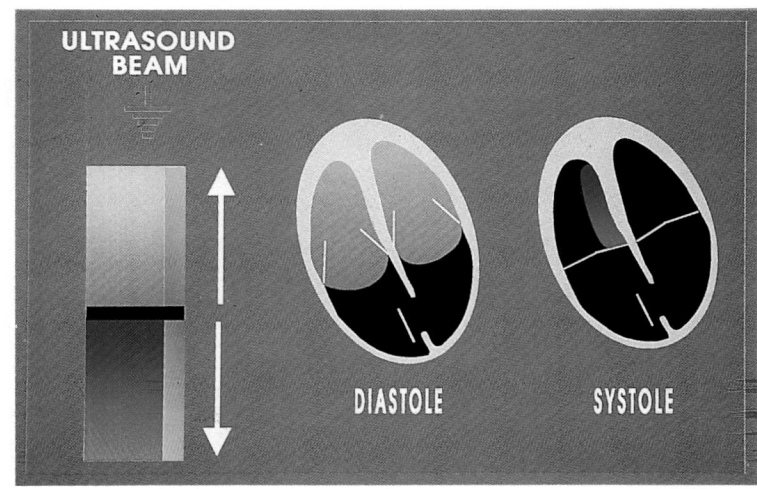

record the Doppler shift, "aliasing" occurs in which an opposite color appears in place of the expected color (ie, red instead of blue or blue instead of red). This occurs when the maximal velocity (Nyquist's limit) settings are too low or when the there is pathology due to increased velocity of blood (Fig. 13-2).

SCREENING FOUR-CHAMBER VIEW

Color Doppler examination provides additional information regarding flow across the interventricular and interatrial septa, tricuspid and mitral valve regurgitation, and abnormal intracardiac flow. Optimal imaging of the four-chamber view occurs when the ventricular septum is oriented tangential or parallel to the ultrasound beam (Fig. 13-3).

Diastole

In the normal fetal heart, both ventricular chambers fill with a single color during ventricular diastole. If the maximal velocity setting is too low, aliasing occurs (see Fig. 13-2). The low setting, however, has the benefit of identifying lower-velocity flow along the endocardium, which clearly outlines the atrial and ventricular septa (Fig. 13-4). By adjusting the baseline, the aliasing can be converted to one color, which has the appearance of a "color ventriculogram" (Fig. 13-5).

(*text continues on page 286*)

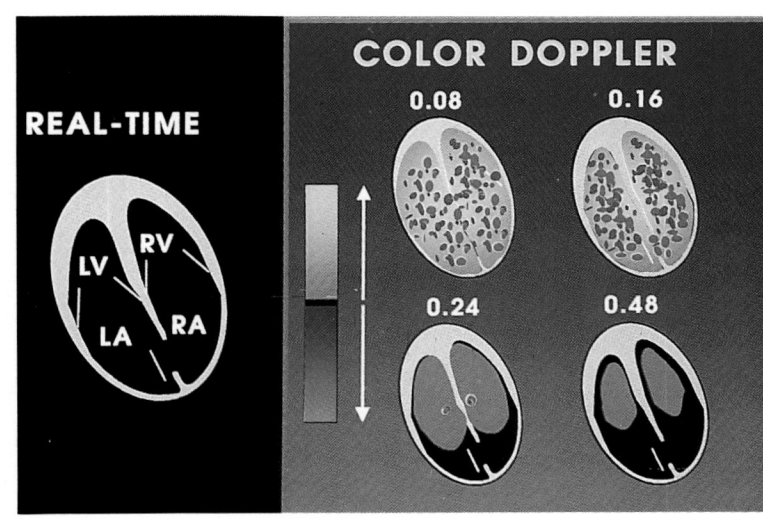

FIGURE 13-2. Aliasing of color. This illustrates the four-chamber view in which the maximal velocity is increased progressively from a low setting (0.06 M/sec) to a higher setting (0.48 M/sec). At lower settings, aliasing occurs, but it disappears at higher settings. The advantage of lower maximal velocity settings is that flow along the ventricular walls and septum is identified.

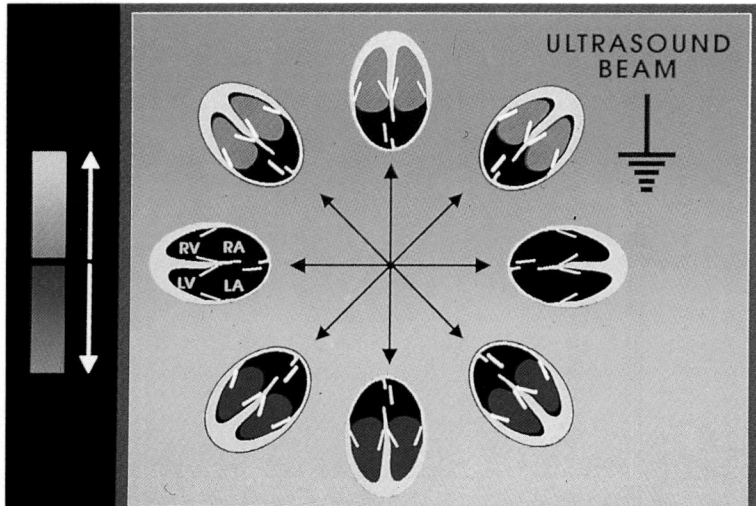

FIGURE 13-3. Color schematic of the effect of the position of the heart as it relates to optimal color Doppler imaging. When the four-chamber view is perpendicular to the ultrasound beam (*arrow*), minimal to no color Doppler is observed at velocity settings appropriate for ventricular flow. However, as the heart approaches a parallel orientation to the ultrasound beam, color Doppler is displayed optimally. The schematic illustrates color Doppler with the flow of blood toward (*red*) or away from the transducer (*blue*). RA, right atrium; LA, left atrium; RV, right ventricle; LV, left ventricle. (DeVore GR: The use of color Doppler imaging to examine the fetal heart: Normal and pathologic anatomy. In Jaffe R, Warsof SL [eds]: Color Doppler Imaging in Obstetrics and Gynecology. New York: McGraw-Hill, 1992: 121–154.)

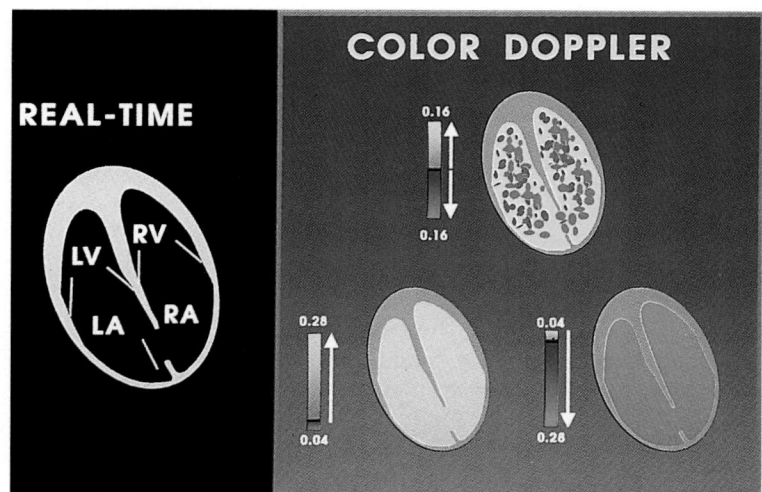

FIGURE 13-4. Color ventriculogram. Adjusting the color baseline to create a color ventriculogram enables the examiner to image flow along the interatrial and interventricular septum using lower maximal velocity settings. Because aliasing may make the image difficult to interpret, changing the baseline to the top or the bottom of the velocity scale creates a color ventriculogram.

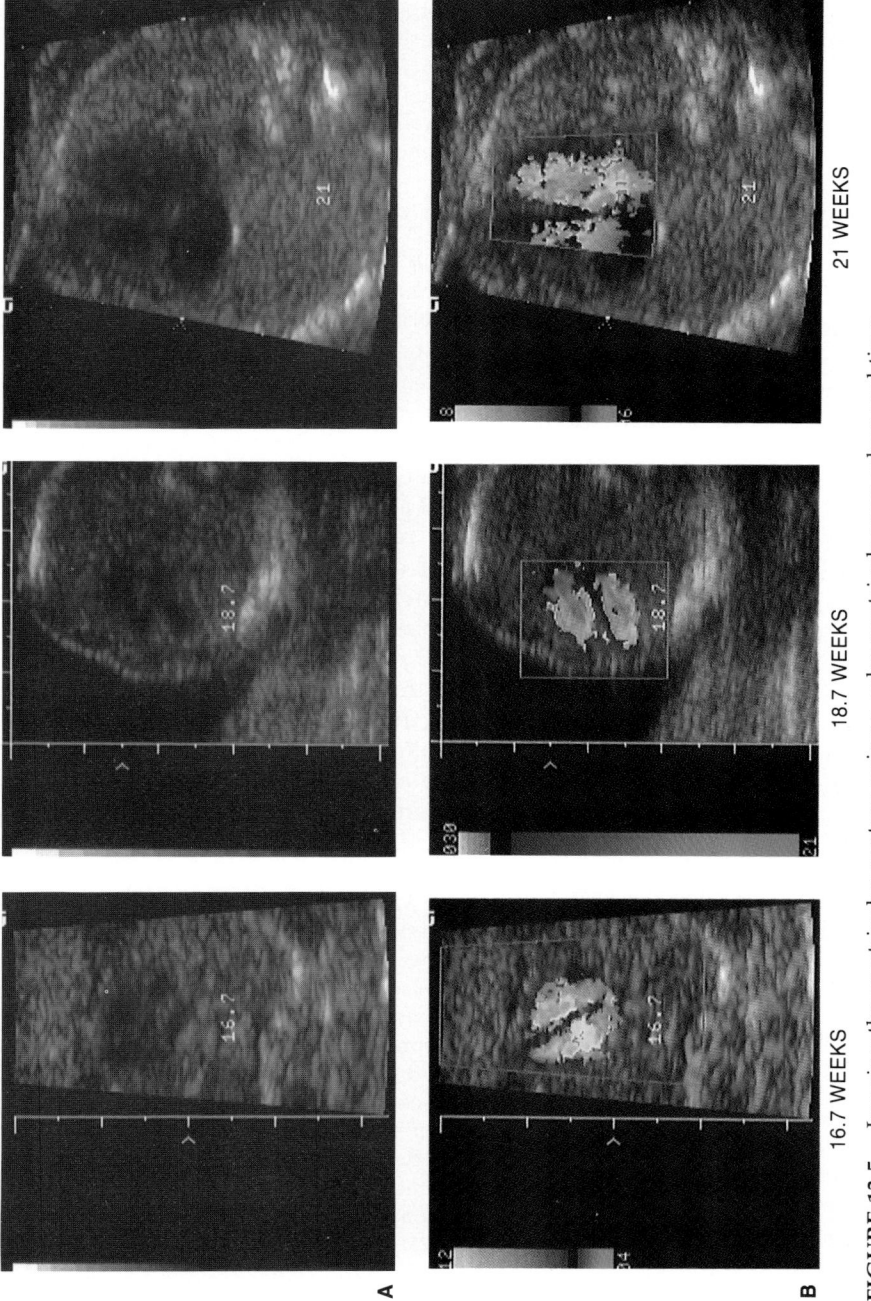

16.7 WEEKS   18.7 WEEKS   21 WEEKS

A

B

FIGURE 13-5. Imaging the ventricular septum using a color ventriculogram when real-time imaging is inadequate. **(A)** Three patients are represented in whom the real-time image does not clearly identify the interventricular or interatrial septum during the second trimester of pregnancy. **(B)** Color Doppler, using the technique described in Figure 13-4, clearly identifies the interatrial and interventricular septa.

Systole

In the normal fetal heart, color Doppler identifies flow along the left border of the interventricular septum as blood exits the left ventricle. No flow of blood should be observed along the ventricular septum of the right ventricle nor across the mitral or tricuspid valves into the atrial chambers (Fig. 13-6).

COLOR DOPPLER IMAGING OF THE FOUR-CHAMBER VIEW

Ventricular Septal Defects

When there is a ventricular septal defect, color Doppler identifies flow of blood across the septum. When examining the ventricular septum, it is important to use the following sequence for identifying whether a ventricular septal defect is present:

1. Evaluate the septum first in real-time with the axis of the septum parallel or tangential to the ultrasound beam. A ventricular septal defect may be present if an abrupt break appears in the septum (Fig. 13-7).
2. Activate the color Doppler and determine whether color fills the area where the break is suspected (see Fig. 13-7).
3. Angle the transducer so that the septum is identified in another angle, and attempt to replicate the defect with real-time and color Doppler (see Fig. 13-7).
4. If color crosses the septum, be sure that it is present in multiple cycles of diastole, systole, or both (Fig. 13-8).

Case 1. A patient was referred for diagnostic ultrasound at 17 weeks of gestation. Examination of the four-chamber view was difficult because of maternal obesity, and a clear image could not be obtained. Activation of the color Doppler demonstrated a ventricular septal and atrial septal defect (Fig. 13-9). Because of the increased risk for chromosomal aneuploidy, amniocentesis was offered to the patient. Trisomy 21 was subsequently diagnosed.

Case 2. A 42-year-old patient was referred at 32 weeks of gestation because of a concern for intrauterine growth retardation. She had refused genetic amniocentesis in the second trimester. Ultrasound demonstrated the head circumference and femur length to be appropriate for gestational age. The abdomen, however, was less than the 1st percentile, with abnormal head circumference/abdominal circumference and femur length/abdominal circumference ratios. Real-time initially demonstrated a normal four-chamber view; however, activation of the color Doppler demonstrated flow across the ventricular septum, suggesting a ventricular septal defect (Fig. 13-10). Further examination of the heart demonstrated the ventricular septal defect in real-time, which was higher in the septum. Percutaneous blood sampling was performed, and trisomy 18 was diagnosed.

Atrioventricular Valve Regurgitation

Tricuspid Regurgitation

Tricuspid regurgitation is the most common form of atrioventricular valve regurgitation in the fetus. It has been observed in the following conditions: increased pulmonary resistance (pulmonary stenosis or atresia, pulmonary hypertension, constriction of the ductus arteriosus from indomethacin); abnormal tricuspid valve (Ebstein's anomaly); and fetal anemia (Rh isoimmunization). Unless tricuspid regurgitation is holosystolic and has been present for some time, the real-time image of the four-chamber view is usually not altered. Color Doppler, however, is an efficient method to screen for tricuspid regurgitation. To accomplish this, the maximal velocity setting should be increased to filter out low flow within the atrial chambers. When tricuspid regurgitation is present, simultaneous flow can be observed along the left side of the interventricular septum during ventricular systole (Fig. 13-11).

Case 3. A patient was referred during the second trimester for advanced maternal age. After genetic counseling, she chose not to undergo amniocentesis because she would not terminate the pregnancy. The patient was informed that if the ultrasound examination were normal, her risk for fetal trisomy would decrease, but if it were abnormal it would increase. Measurements of the head, abdomen, and femur were consistent with 16.8 weeks gestational age. Real-time examination demonstrated no evidence of ventricular disproportion. Color Doppler demonstrated significant tricuspid regurgitation (Fig. 13-12). The patient consented to an amniocentesis, which demonstrated trisomy 13. The patient continued the pregnancy but, owing to the lethality of this condition, emergency cesarean section for fetal distress was averted.

Mitral Regurgitation

Mitral regurgitation is uncommon in the fetus. I have observed it with structural malformations of

(*text continues on page 293*)

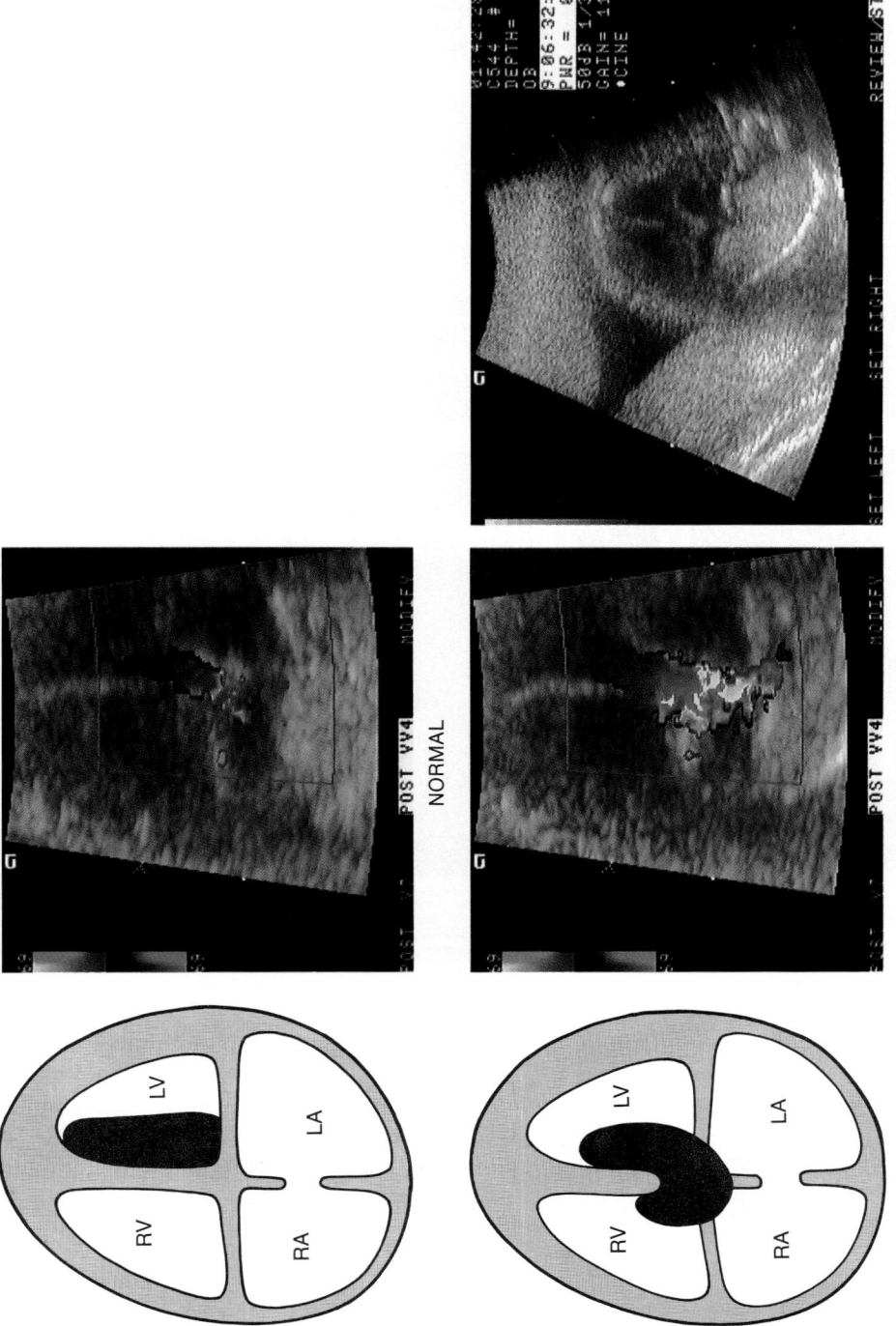

FIGURE 13-6. Normal and abnormal flow along the interventricular septum. In the normal four-chamber view, flow may be identified along the interventricular septum as it exits the left ventricle (*upper panel*). However, when there is a ventricular septal defect located between the atrioventricular valves and the aortic outflow tract associated with pulmonary atresia or stenosis, blood leaving the right ventricle may exit through the ventricular septal defect at the level of the aorta (color Doppler VSD). The real-time image identifies the ventricular septal defect straddling the aorta. This fetus had tetralogy of Fallot. RA, right atrium; LA, left atrium; RV, right ventricle; LV, left ventricle.

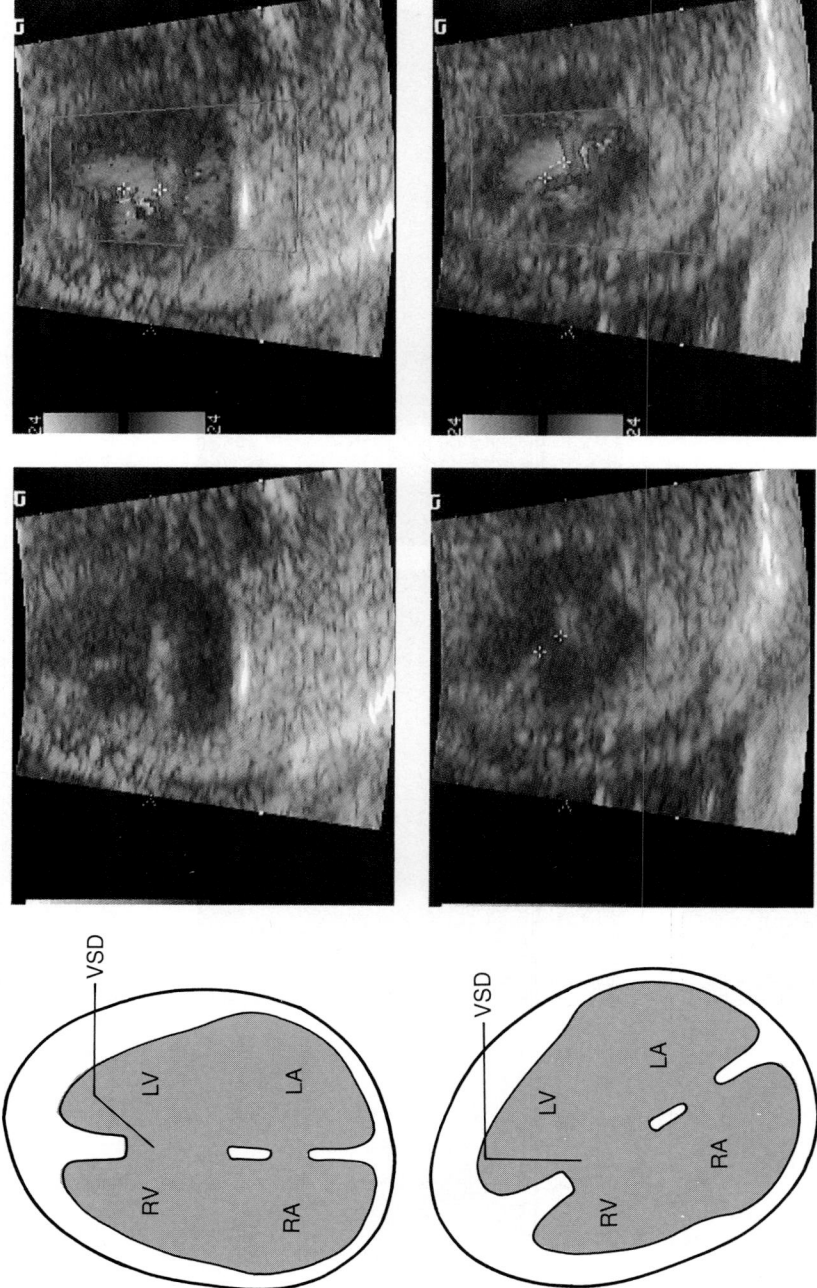

FIGURE 13-7. Identification of a ventricular septal defect. The upper panel demonstrates the real-time and color Doppler images of the heart with the septum parallel to the ultrasound beam. The real-time image suggests a break in the ventricular septum and is confirmed with the color Doppler, which demonstrates blood flowing along the interventricular septum of the left ventricle (*blue*) into the right ventricle (*red*). The lower panel demonstrates the same findings as the upper panel except that the septum is oriented tangential to the ultrasound beam. The size of the ventricular septal defect is measured (**) and is 2 mm. RA, right atrium; LA, left atrium; RV, right ventricle; LV, left ventricle.

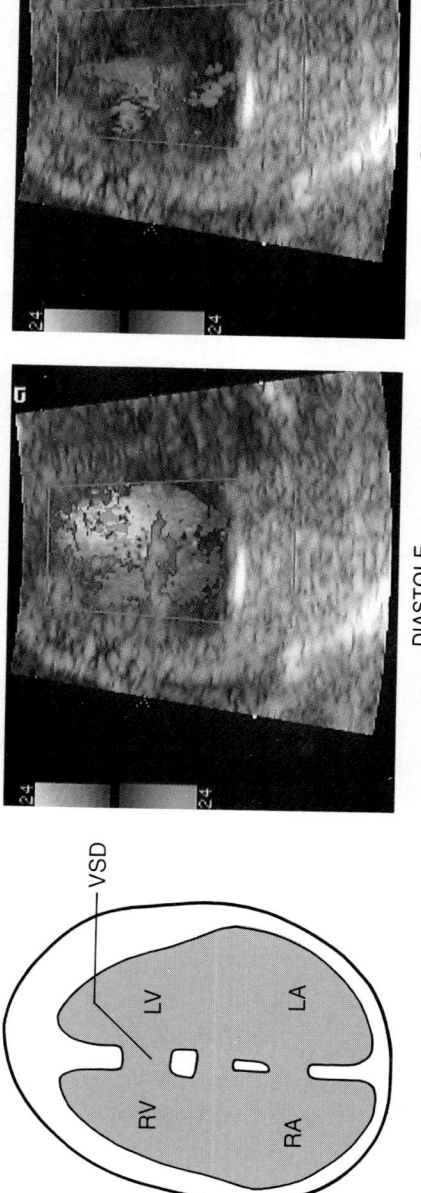

FIGURE 13-8. Color Doppler of a ventricular septal defect during diastole and systole. Flow across the ventricular septal defect can be observed during diastole and is represented as a filling defect. During systole, flow can be observed crossing the septum (*blue*) and flowing back into the right ventricle (*red*). RA, right atrium; LA, left atrium; RV, right ventricle; LV, left ventricle.

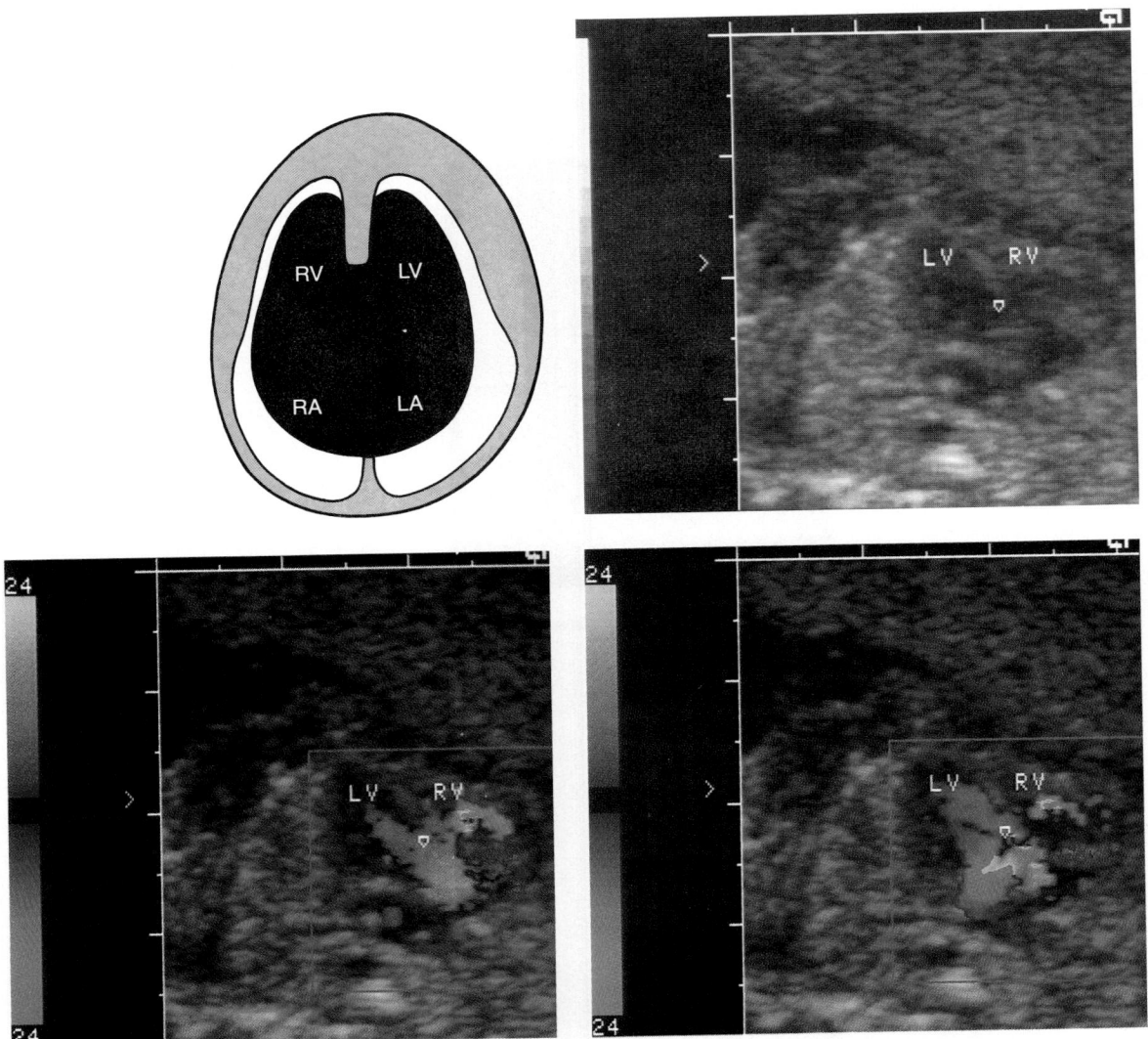

FIGURE 13-9.   Atrioventricular septal defect in a fetus with trisomy 21. It is difficult to identify the interatrial and interventricular septum in a second-trimester fetus using real-time. The color identifies the defect during diastole (*left*) and systole (*right*). RA, right atrium; LA, left atrium; RV, right ventricle; LV, left ventricle. (DeVore GR: The use of color Doppler imaging to examine the fetal heart: Normal and pathologic anatomy. In Jaffe R, Warsof SL [eds]: Color Doppler Imaging in Obstetrics and Gynecology. New York: McGraw-Hill, 1992: 121–154.)

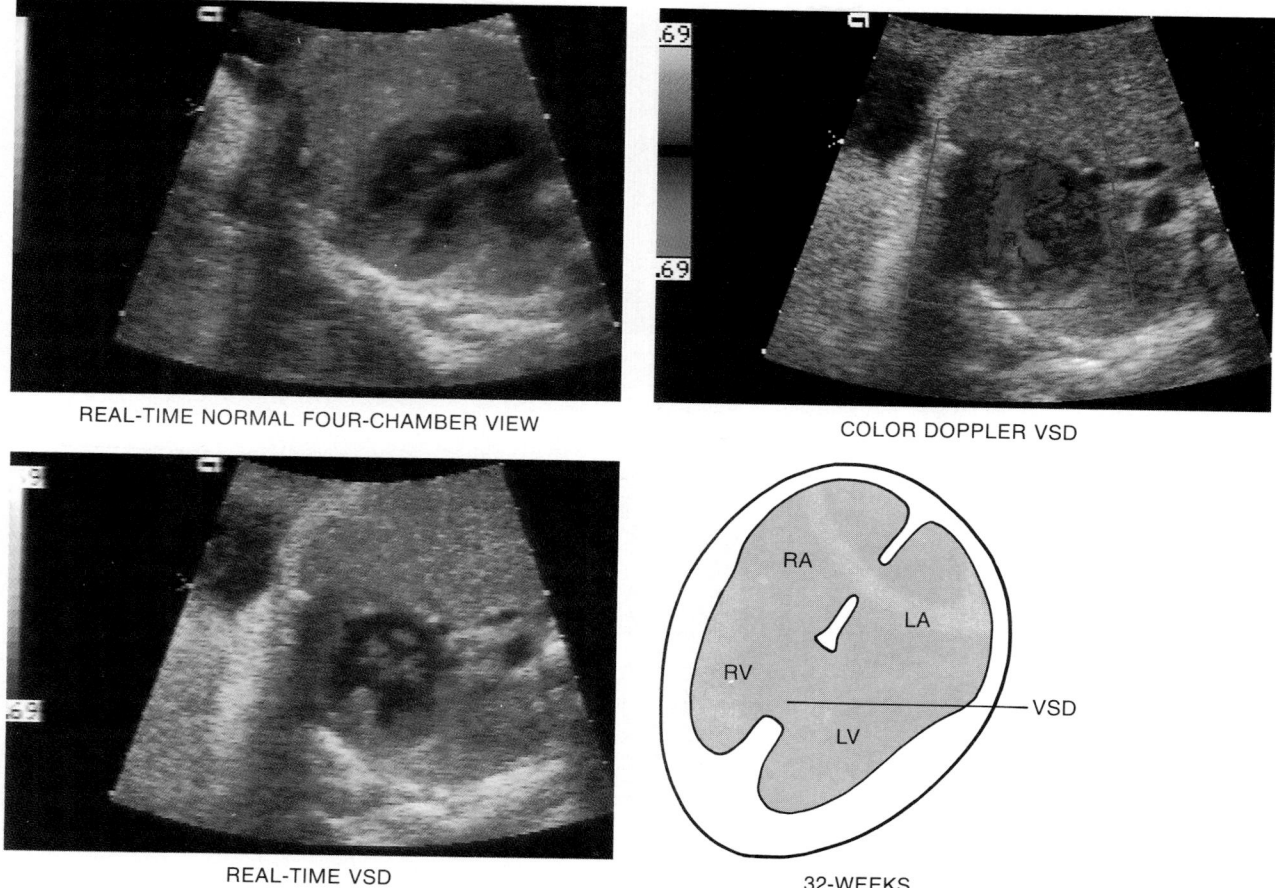

REAL-TIME NORMAL FOUR-CHAMBER VIEW

COLOR DOPPLER VSD

REAL-TIME VSD

32-WEEKS

FIGURE 13-10.   Ventricular septal defect in a fetus with trisomy 18. The four-chamber view demonstrates no evidence of a ventricular septal defect. However, color Doppler suggests flow across the septum. When the heart is imaged at a lower plane, the ventricular septal defect is identified. RA, right atrium; LA, left atrium; RV, right ventricle; LV, left ventricle.

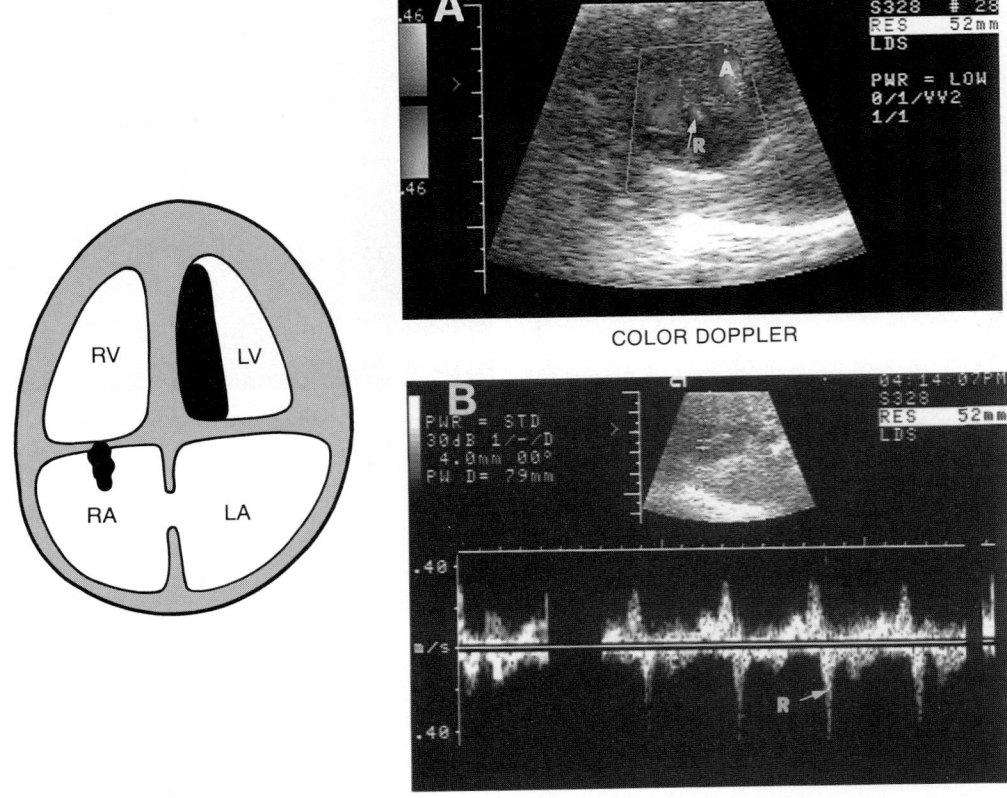

COLOR DOPPLER

PULSED DOPPLER

FIGURE 13-11.   Tricuspid regurgitation. Color Doppler demonstrates a flash within the right atrium consistent with tricuspid regurgitation (R). This coincides with blood leaving along the left ventricle during systole (A). The pulsed Doppler confirms the tricuspid regurgitation (R), which occurs early in the systolic cycle. RA, right atrium; LA, left atrium; RV, right ventricle; LV, left ventricle.

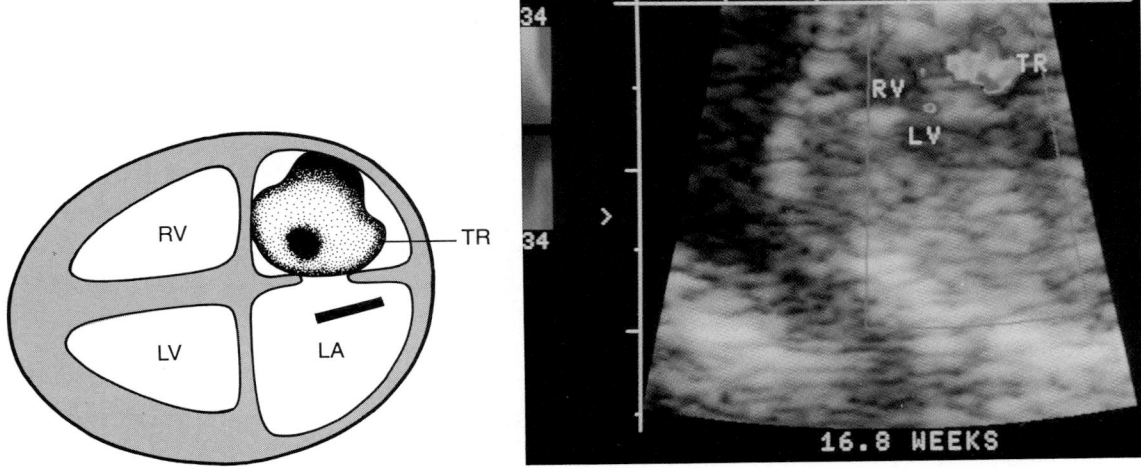

FIGURE 13-12.   Tricuspid regurgitation in a fetus with trisomy 13. The real-time four-chamber view was difficult to identify at 16.8 weeks of gestation. Color Doppler, however, identified abnormal flow within the right atrium. This represented holosystolic tricuspid regurgitation. TR, tricuspid regurgitation; LA, left atrium; RV, right ventricle; LV, left ventricle. (DeVore GR: The use of color Doppler imaging to examine the fetal heart: Normal and pathologic anatomy. In Jaffe R, Warsof SL [eds]: Color Doppler Imaging in Obstetrics and Gynecology. New York: McGraw-Hill, 1992: 121–154.)

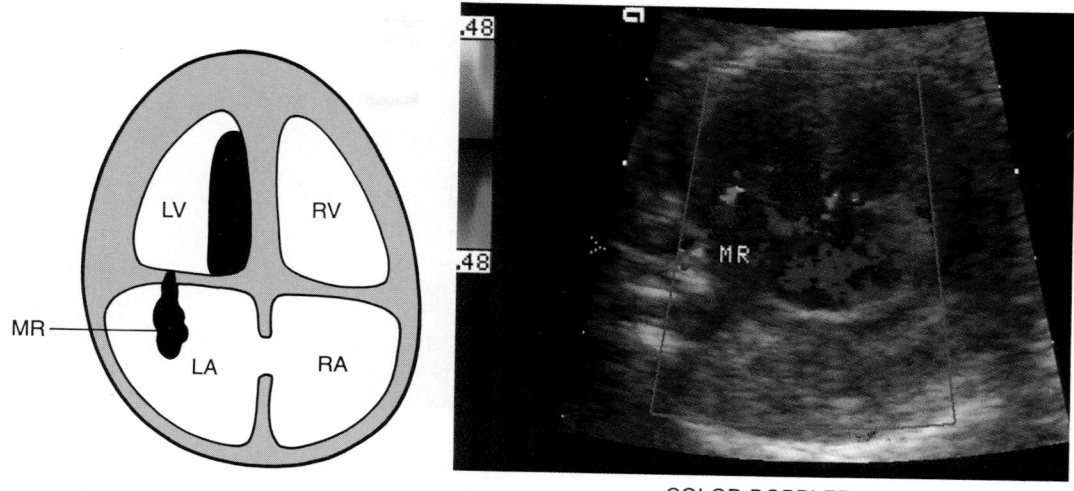

COLOR DOPPLER

FIGURE 13-13.   Mitral regurgitation in a fetus with severe placental dysfunction. During ventricular systole, blood can be observed flowing from the left ventricle into the left atrium. The mitral regurgitation is observed along the lateral aspect of the atrial wall. Flow can be observed along the interventricular septum leaving the left ventricle. MR, mitral regurgitation; RA, right atrium; LA, left atrium; RV, right ventricle; LV, left ventricle.

the aortic valve (aortic stenosis), fetal aneuploidy, and severe placental dysfunction. When mitral valve regurgitation is identified with color Doppler, it should be confirmed with pulsed Doppler as described previously.

Case 4. A 35-year-old patient was referred for diagnostic ultrasound. She had undergone a second-trimester ultrasound and genetic amniocentesis, which placed her at 30 weeks of gestation. Measurements of the head, abdomen, and femur demonstrated a 7-week lag in growth. The amniotic fluid was absent. Examination of the four-chamber view with real-time demonstrated bilateral pericardial effusions. Color Doppler demonstrated tricuspid and mitral valve regurgitation (Fig. 13-13). The newborn died shortly after birth from severe cardiovascular and renal failure secondary to severe in utero asphyxiation.

Case 5. A 36-year-old patient was referred for diagnostic ultrasound and genetic amniocentesis. Ultrasound examination demonstrated normal measurements of the head, abdomen, and femur for 16 weeks of gestation. Examination of the fetal heart with real-time demonstrated a normal four-chamber view. Color Doppler, however, demonstrated tricuspid and mitral valve regurgitation (Fig. 13-14). No other structural malformations were present. The fetal karyotype was trisomy 21.

COLOR DOPPLER IMAGING OF THE OUTFLOW TRACTS

Irrespective of the view used to examine the outflow tracts, information regarding abnormalities can be readily identified using color Doppler.[17,18] The two most common types of abnormality identified are valvular stenosis and retrograde flow from the ductus arteriosus into the aortic isthmus (ie, hypoplastic left ventricle).

Case 6. A 32-year-old patient was referred for assessment of fetal growth at 26 weeks of gestation. Real-time examination of the fetal heart demonstrated a normal four-chamber view with normal M-mode measurements. Examination of the outflow tracts, using a previously described technique,[17] suggested no evidence of transposition, nor was there evidence of underdevelopment of the aortic or pulmonary outflow tracts. Color Doppler ultrasound, however, demonstrated turbulent flow with aliasing distal to the aortic valve (Fig. 13-15). This was consistent with aortic stenosis. After delivery, moderate aortic stenosis was confirmed. The interesting finding with this patient was that, unlike other fetuses with aortic stenosis in which left ventricular wall hypertrophy or changes in ventricular chamber dimensions are identified with real-time, these findings were not present at the time of the in utero diagnosis of aortic stenosis using color Doppler.

(*text continues on page 296*)

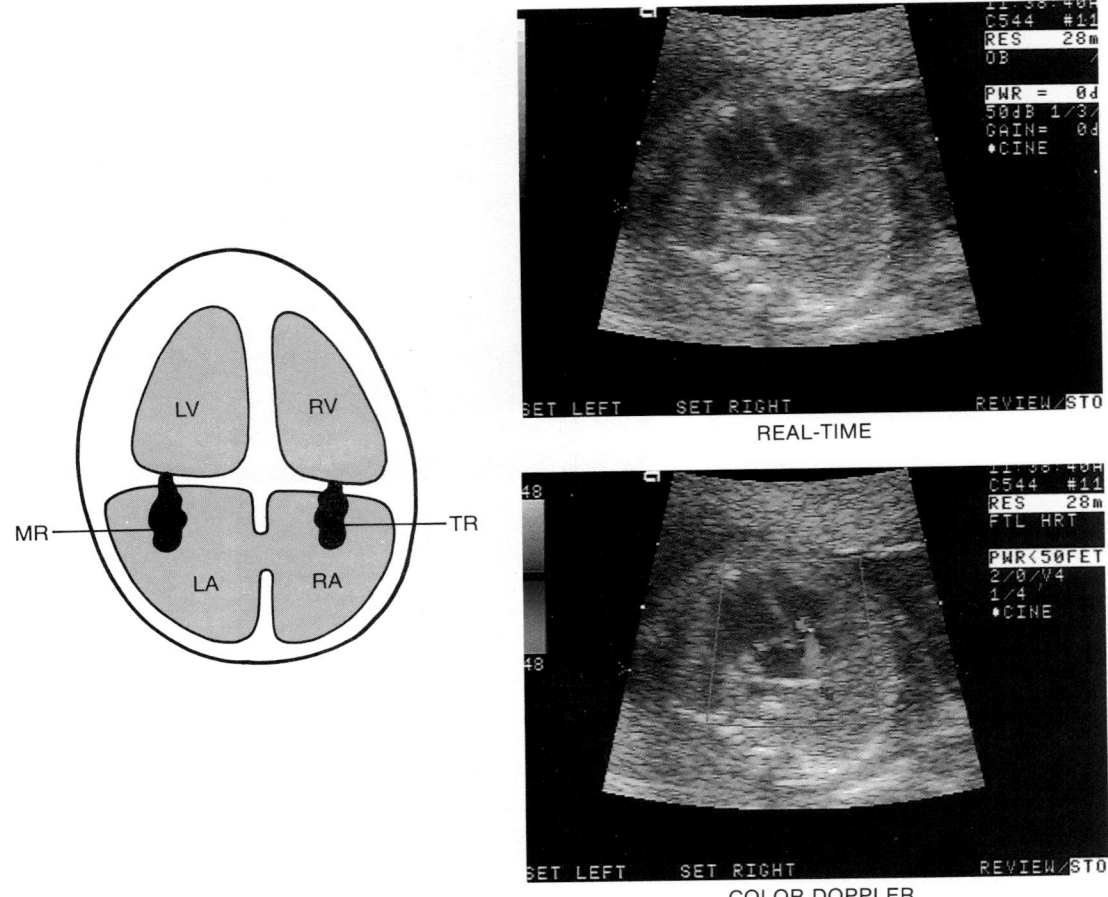

FIGURE 13-14.   Mitral and tricuspid regurgitation during the second trimester. The real-time image of the four-chamber view is normal. However, when the color Doppler is activated, tricuspid and mitral regurgitation are observed. MR, mitral regurgitation; TR, tricuspid regurgitation; RA, right atrium; LA, left atrium; RV, right ventricle; LV, left ventricle.

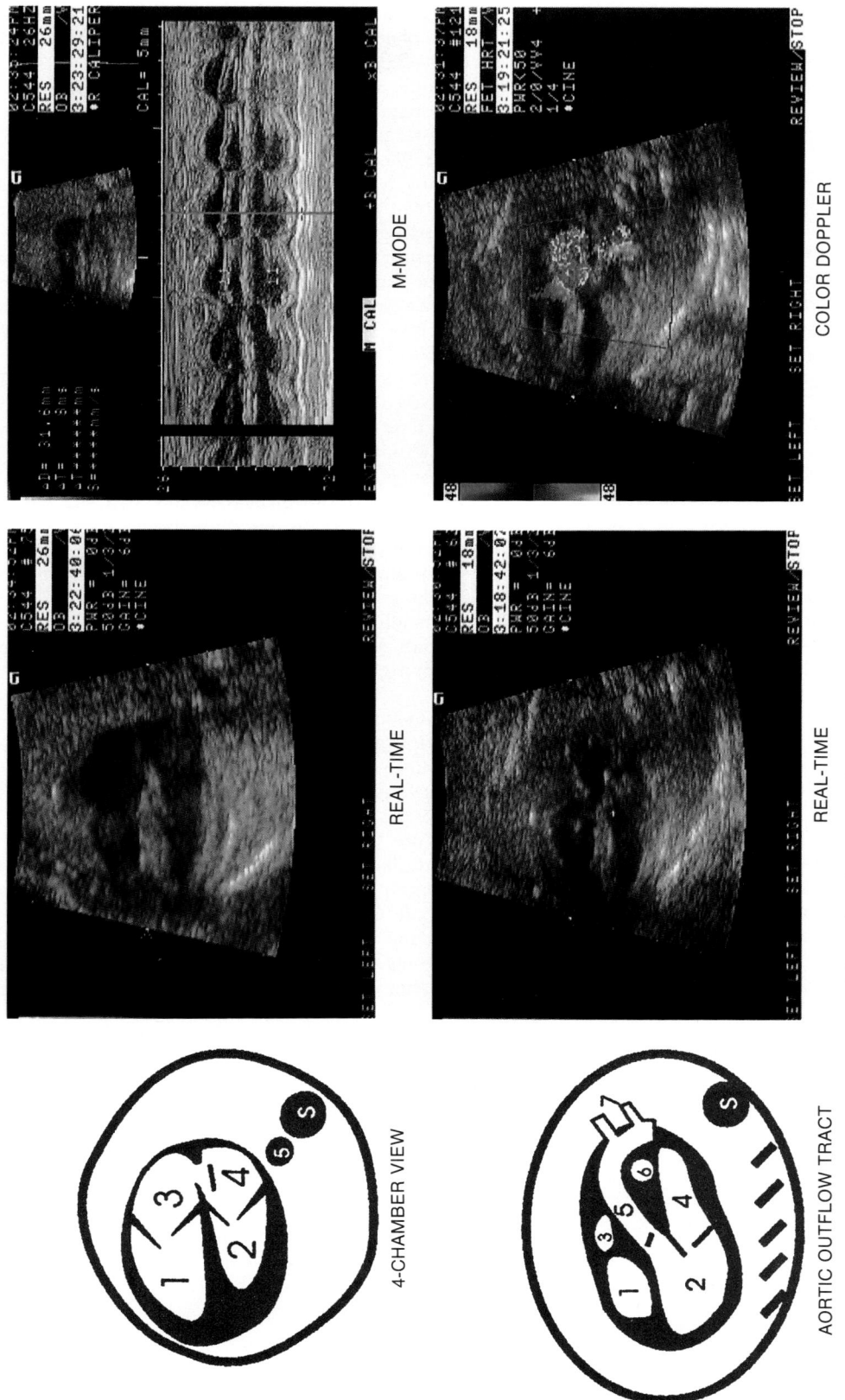

M-MODE

COLOR DOPPLER

REAL-TIME

REAL-TIME

4-CHAMBER VIEW

AORTIC OUTFLOW TRACT

FIGURE 13-15. Aortic stenosis with a normal four-chamber view. The upper panel illustrates the normal four-chamber view of the heart and the corresponding M-mode. The ventricles are of equal size (11 mm) and the walls are not hypertrophied. The aortic outflow tract does not appear abnormal except for minimal thickening of the aortic valve leaflets (*arrow*). Color Doppler, however, demonstrates aliasing and disturbed flow distal to the aortic valve. This fetus had moderate aortic stenosis. Note that the color bar is inverted. 1, right ventricle; 2, left ventricle; 3, right atrium; 4, left atrium; 5, aortic outflow tract; 6, right pulmonary artery; S, spine.

CONCLUSION

Evaluation of the four-chamber view and the outflow tracts with color Doppler adds information to the screening examination of the fetal heart. Although color Doppler devices may not be available in many clinical settings because of the cost of the equipment, it is my opinion that in the future this will not be the case. Because of the importance of color Doppler, physicians may wish to reconsider who performs the second-trimester ultrasound examination and request that patients be examined with color Doppler because of the added advantage of recognition of congenital heart disease, which has a high association with chromosomal aneuploidy.

REFERENCES

1. DeVore GR, Brar HS, Platt LD: Doppler ultrasound in the fetus: A review of current applications. JCU 1987; 15:687–703.
2. DeVore GR, Horenstein J, Siassi B, Platt LD: Fetal echocardiography. VII. Doppler color flow mapping: A new technique for the diagnosis of congenital heart disease. Am J Obstet Gynecol 1987; 156:1054–1064.
3. Jacobson RL, Perez A, Meyer RA, et al: Prenatal diagnosis of fetal left ventricular aneurysm: A case report and review. Obstet Gynecol 1991; 78(3):525–528.
4. Gembruch U, Chatterjee MS, Bald R, et al: Color Doppler flow mapping of fetal heart. J Perinat Med 1991; 19:27–32.
5. Copel JA, Morotti R, Hobbins JC, Kleinman CS: The antenatal diagnosis of congenital heart disease using fetal echocardiography: Is color flow mapping necessary? Obstet Gynecol 1991; 78:1–8.
6. Gembruch U, Knopfle G, Chatterjee M, et al: Prenatal diagnosis of atrioventricular canal malformations with up-to-date echocardiographic technology: Report of 14 cases. Am Heart J 1991; 121:1489–1497.
7. Sharland GK, Chita SK, Allan LD: The use of colour Doppler in fetal echocardiography. Int J Cardiol 1990; 28:229–236.
8. Gentile R, Pearlman AS, Lagana B, Marsocci A: Development of echocardiographic diagnosis of congenital cardiopathies: From M-mode to color Doppler. Medicina (Firenze) 1989; 9:147–154.
9. Chiba Y, Kanzaki T, Kobayashi H, et al: Evaluation of fetal structural heart disease using color flow mapping. Ultrasound Med Biol 1990; 16:221–229.
10. Matsuura T: Study on intracardiac blood flow with color flow mapping in human fetus: The reverse flow at tricuspid valve in human fetus during labor. Nippon Sanka Fujinka Gakkai Zasshi 1989; 41:1373–1379.
11. Gembruch U, Hansmann M, Redel DA, Bald R: Fetal two-dimensional Doppler echocardiography (colour flow mapping) and its place in prenatal diagnosis. Prenat Diagn 1989; 9:535–547.
12. Huhta JC: Future directions in noninvasive Doppler evaluation of the fetal circulation. Cardiol Clin 1989; 7:239–253.
13. Gembruch U, Hansmann M, Redel DA, Bald R: Two-dimensional color-coded fetal Doppler echocardiography: Its value in prenatal diagnosis. Geburtshilfe Frauenheilkd 1988; 48:381–388.
14. Kurjak A, Breyer B, Jurkovic D, et al: Color flow mapping in obstetrics. J Perinat Med 1987; 15:271–281.
15. D'Amelio R, Giorlandino C, Masala L, et al: Fetal echocardiography using transvaginal and transabdominal probes during the first period of pregnancy: A comparative study. Prenat Diagn 1991; 11:69–75.
16. DeVore GR: The prenatal diagnosis of congenital heart disease: A practical approach for the fetal sonographer. J Clin Ultrasound 1985; 13:229–245.
17. DeVore GR: The use of color Doppler imaging to examine the fetal heart: Normal and pathologic anatomy. In Jaffe R, Warsof SL (eds): Color Doppler Imaging in Obstetrics and Gynecology. New York: McGraw-Hill, 1992: 121–154.
18. DeVore GR: The aortic and pulmonary outflow tract screening examination in the human fetus. J Ultrasound Med 1992; 11:345–348.

John P. McGahan and Manuel Porto:
DIAGNOSTIC OBSTETRICAL ULTRASOUND.
© 1994 J.B. Lippincott Company.

Kathryn L. Reed   Norman B. Duerbeck

Chapter *14*

Doppler Ultrasound in Obstetrics

The use of ultrasound has revolutionized the ability to detect congenital and growth abnormalities during the antenatal period, and the use of Doppler ultrasound has expanded the techniques available to assess the fetus. In this chapter, we describe the use of Doppler velocimetry in the evaluation of the fetus.

TECHNOLOGY AND DEFINITION OF TERMS

Originally, Doppler ultrasound instruments were used to detect velocities continuously and thus were termed *continuous wave* instruments. These instruments used two crystals or transducers, one that transmitted and another that received continuously. A disadvantage of continuous wave Doppler is that it is nonselective in that all signals along the ultrasound beam are recorded. In contrast, the *pulsed wave* Doppler device uses only one crystal that both transmits and receives. An important advantage of pulsed wave Doppler ultrasound is that it allows specification of the measurement site and its depth from the transducer. In addition, the in-

tegration of *real-time imaging* with pulsed wave Doppler not only allows the vessel of interest to be identified, but, because the diameter of the vessel and the angle of insonation can be measured, also allows for an estimation of velocity and volume of flow.

As sound waves hit a moving target (red blood cells in a vessel or chamber), the receiving frequency is altered from the transmitting frequency. This change in frequency is described as the Doppler shift and can be represented by the mathematical formula

$$f_d = (2f_0 \times V \times \cos\theta)/c$$

where f_d is the Doppler shift, f_0 is the transmitted frequency, V is the velocity of blood flow, $\cos\theta$ is the cosine of the angle of insonation, and c is the velocity of sound in tissue (assumed to be 1540 m/second).[1] Measurement of absolute blood velocity requires knowledge of the angle between the Doppler beam and the direction of blood flow (Fig. 14-1). Measurement of blood flow volume (Q) requires measurement of the cross-sectional area (A) through which blood is flowing, which is then multiplied by the average velocity (V), Q = VA.

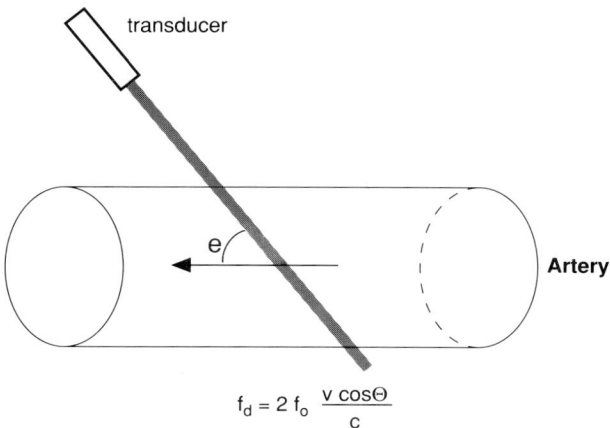

$$f_d = 2 f_o \frac{v \cos\Theta}{c}$$

FIGURE 14-1. Calculation of the Doppler shift. f_d, the Doppler shift; f_o, transmitted frequency; V, velocity of blood flow; $\cos \theta$, cosine of the angle of insonation; c, velocity of sound in tissue (assumed to be 1540 m/sec). (Modified from Techniques to evaluate fetal health. In Cunningham FG, MacDonald PC, Gant NF [eds]: Williams Obstetrics, 18th ed. Norwalk, CT: Appleton and Lange, 1989: 277–305.)

UMBILICAL ARTERY

The most extensively studied vessel in the evaluation of the fetus with Doppler ultrasound has been the umbilical artery. Because the fetus is completely dependent on the supply of oxygen and nutrients from the placenta, examination of the blood flow through the umbilical circulation would appear to have great potential for the assessment of fetal health.

Absolute umbilical blood flow increases up to 35 weeks' gestational age; blood flow relative to fetal weight is constant at about 120 ml/kg/minute.[2] There appears to be a slight drop-off at 40 weeks down to 90 ml/kg/minute.[2] Volume blood flow (Q) is equal to the average velocity multiplied by the cross-sectional area. Several errors can be made when using Doppler ultrasound to assess umbilical arterial flow (Table 14-1).

TABLE 14-1.   Pitfalls in the Use of Doppler Ultrasound to Assess Umbilical Flow

Umbilical artery diameter measurements are small (2.4 mm at term).[3]

Angles of insonation may be estimated incorrectly.[4]

Indexes have high false-negative rate for detection of intrauterine growth retardation.

Fetal breathing alters waveforms.

Diastolic velocities vary with fetal heart rate.

Indexes are higher at fetal site and lower at placental site.

The normal diameter of the umbilical artery at term is 2.4 mm.[3] It was demonstrated in a study by Gill that a difference as small as 0.5 mm could produce a 25% calculation error in volume flow estimates in a 4-mm vessel.[4] This error is further compounded by errors of estimation of the angle of insonation. Therefore, waveform analysis is used instead of direct blood velocity measurements because it is more easily reproducible and is essentially independent of these potential sources of error.

Under normal circumstances in the umbilical artery, there are relatively high forward velocities during diastole, consistent with blood flow into a low-impedance vascular bed, the placenta. With advancing gestation, there is an increase in end-diastolic flow velocity relative to peak systolic velocity (Figs. 14-2 and 14-3). This is attributed to

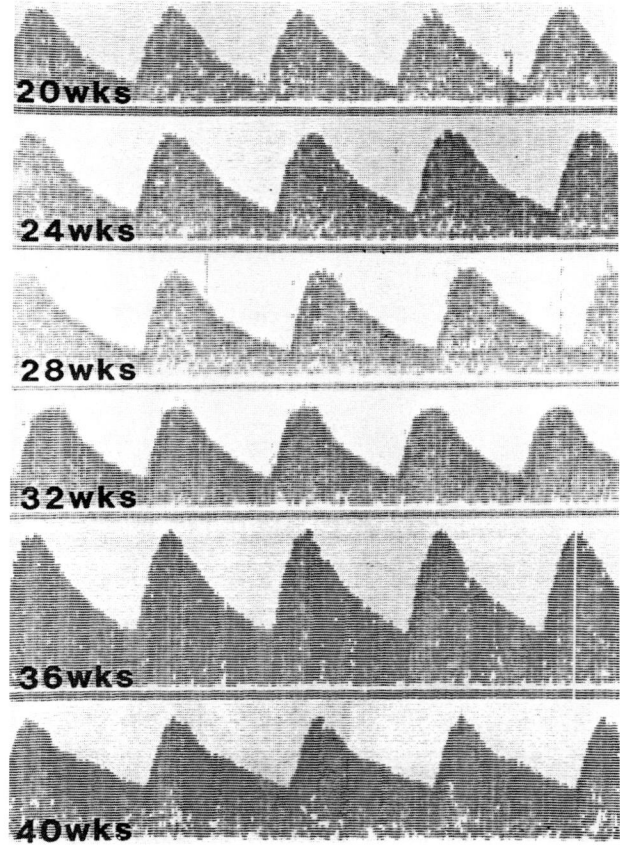

FIGURE 14-2. Gradual increase in the diastolic velocities relative to systolic velocities in the umbilical artery with gestational age from 20 menstrual weeks through 40 menstrual weeks. (Trudinger B: Doppler ultrasonography and fetal well-being. In Reece EA, Hobbins JC, Mahoney MJ, Petrie RH [eds]: Medicine of the Fetus and Mother. Philadelphia: JB Lippincott, 1992: 105.)

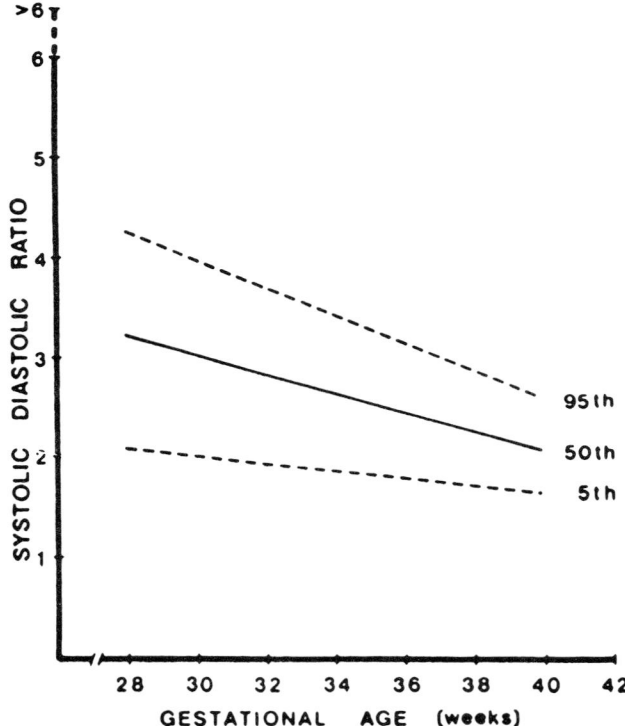

FIGURE 14-3. Changes in the systolic diastolic ratio (S/D) as a function of advancing gestational age. (Trudinger B: Doppler ultrasound assessment of blood flow. In Creasy RK, Resnik R [eds]: Maternal and Fetal Medicine Principles and Practice. Philadelphia: WB Saunders, 1989: 254–287.)

decreased resistance in the placental circulation with advancing gestation.[5] This change in the waveform can be quantified by the pulsatility index (PI), the Pourcelot index or resistance index (RI), or the systolic-to-diastolic ratio (S/D ratio; Fig. 14-4). In pregnancies in which the S/D ratio is elevated, there is an increase in intrauterine growth retardation and adverse perinatal outcome.[6] This may be due to a placental circulation that has diminished in volume owing to placental vascular occlusion.

DIFFERENT INDICES

Investigators have differing opinions about which Doppler index (ie, PI or RI, S/D ratio) provides the best predictor of fetal outcome.

Maulik and colleagues compared the predictive power of S/D ratio, PI, and diastolic/average ratio with abnormal neonatal outcome in 350 pregnant patients who underwent Doppler flow studies at 34 to 36 weeks.[7] In their study, abnormal fetal out-

come was defined by a small-for-gestational-age fetus (less than the 10th percentile), an Apgar score of less than 7 at 5 minutes, fetal distress, a fetal scalp pH of less than 7.2, thick meconium, or admission to the neonatal intensive care unit for longer than 48 hours. The authors concluded that, of the various Doppler indices, the RI offers the best diagnostic efficacy in predicting perinatal compromise.

Another opinion regarding the best index was derived from an analysis of 133 studies comparing the correlation coefficient for the three different indices.[8] In this review, Thompson and colleagues were unable to demonstrate any significant differences between indices. Therefore, none of the indices was demonstrated to be superior to the other in terms of the information provided. Of the three, the S/D ratio of the umbilical artery is the simplest to calculate. Not surprisingly, it is the most widely used and described in the literature.

INTRAUTERINE GROWTH RETARDATION

The fetus with growth retardation is at increased risk for intrauterine or neonatal mortality or morbidity.[9] Early identification of the fetus with abnor-

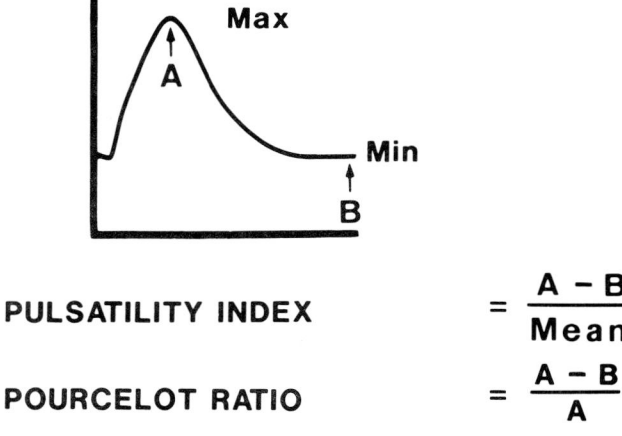

$$\text{PULSATILITY INDEX} = \frac{A - B}{\text{Mean}}$$

$$\text{POURCELOT RATIO} = \frac{A - B}{A}$$

SYSTOLIC/DIASTOLIC RATIO = A/B

FIGURE 14-4. Methods of quantification of the umbilical artery waveform using the pulsatility index, Pourcelot or resistance index, or the systolic/diastolic ratio. A, systolic velocity; B, diastolic velocity; mean, mean velocity. (Trudinger B: Doppler ultrasonography and fetal well-being. In Reece EA, Hobbins JC, Mahoney MJ, Petrie RH [eds]: Medicine of the Fetus and Mother. Philadelphia: JB Lippincott, 1992: 704.)

TABLE 14-2. Sensitivity of Umbilical Arterial Doppler S/D Ratios for the Detection of Fetuses With Abnormal Outcomes and IUGR

Investigation	S/D Ratio #/# (High Risk)	Criteria	Cutoff	SN	SP	PPV	NPV
Maulik et al. (1989)[17]	350/350	IUGR 5 min Apgar < 7 Thick meconium Fetal distress → NICU	3	79	93	83	91
Fleischer et al. (1985)[14]	189/mixed	IUGR	≥3	78	83	49	95
Schulman et al. (1989).[19]	255/195	IUGR	≥3	65	91	43	96
Trudinger et al. (1985)[20]	172/172	IUGR 5 min Apgar < 7 Neonatal death	95%	64 62	77 79	55 63	83 78
Marsal (1987)[16]	142/142	IUGR	±2 SD	57	85	80	64
Arduini et al. (1987)[11]	75/75	IUGR	±1 SD	61	73	50	81
Gaziano et al. (1988)[15]	256/256	IUGR	≥4	79	66	79	96
Divon et al. (1988)[13]	127/127	IUGR	>3	49	94	81	77
Berkowitz et al. (1988)[12]	168/168	IUGR	≥3	45	89	58	86
Al-Ghazali et al. (1988)[10]	300 + 71	IUGR	95%	72	87	82	79

IUGR, intrauterine growth retardation; S/D; systolic/diastolic; SN, sensitivity; SP, specificity; PPV, positive predictive value; NPV, negative predictive value; NICU, neonatal intensive care unit.

(Reed KL: Comment. In Maulik D, Yarlagadda P, Youngblood JP, Ciston P: The diagnostic efficacy of the umbilical arterial systolic/diastolic ratio as a screening tool: A prospective blinded study. Am J Obstet Gynecol 1990; 162:1518–1525.)

mal growth allows increased surveillance and early delivery if distress is present. Some fetuses identified as small by ultrasound are relatively normal and benefit from prolonging pregnancy, thereby allowing the lungs and other organ systems the needed time to mature. In other fetuses, however, the intrauterine environment is so marginally supportive that the risk of intrauterine death or serious damage outweighs the risk of preterm birth. A noninvasive test that could distinguish the stable fetus from the fetus developing irreversible morbidity would be of use in obstetrical management. It was hoped that Doppler velocimetry of the umbilical artery might be such a test. Doppler studies of the umbilical artery comparing S/D ratios for a number of different populations are listed in Table 14-2.[10–20]

When evaluating the umbilical arterial flow, absence of end-diastolic velocity in the umbilical artery is thought to represent an extreme abnormality of fetoplacental hemodynamics (Fig. 14-5). A perinatal mortality rate of 50% to 90% has been associated with this Doppler flow pattern.[21,22] Most investigators advocate intensive fetal surveillance if absent umbilical arterial velocities are documented.[23,24]

Possible mechanisms to explain the clinical finding of the absence of end-diastolic flow are an obliteration of the arterial lumen by a thickened intima or a reduction in the number of small muscular arteries in the tertiary villi.[25–27]

TWINS

The high morbidity and mortality rates among twins justify intense surveillance; this is another potential area for use of Doppler velocimetry. In twins with appropriate-for-gestational-age fetal weight, S/D ratios are comparable to normal singleton pregnancies. Detection of an S/D ratio of greater than 3 after 30 weeks of gestation using Doppler velocimetry could identify small-for-gestational-age twins. In addition, Giles and col-

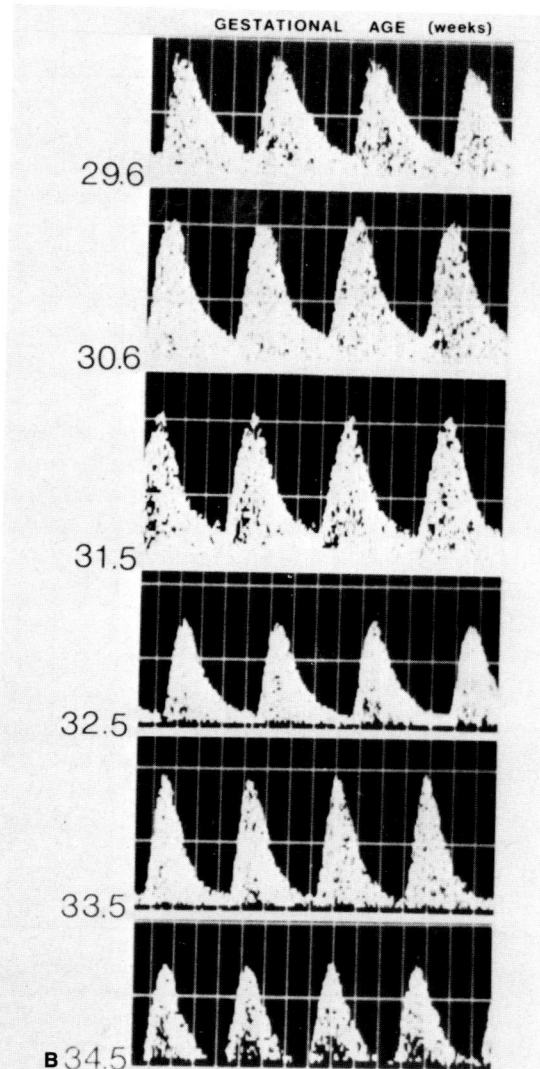

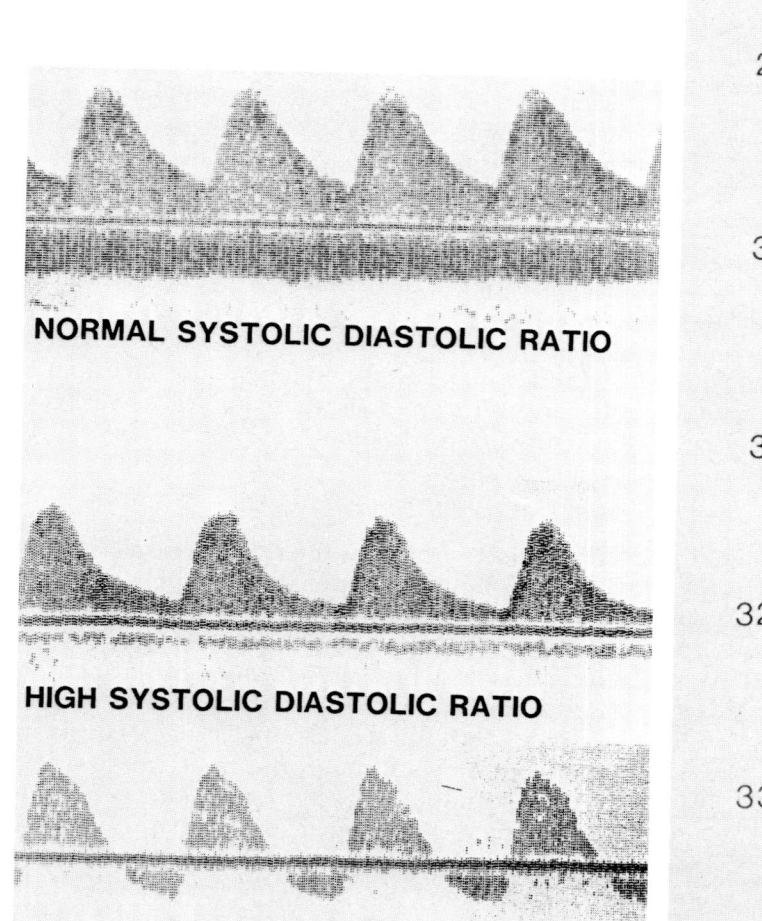

FIGURE 14-5. **(A)** Normal systolic to diastolic ratio compared to abnormal ratio with decrease and eventual reversal of diastolic component. **(B)** High systolic/diastolic ratio in the umbilical artery from 29.6 weeks to 34.5 weeks of menstrual age is seen in some fetuses with growth retardation. There is absent diastolic flow at 34 weeks. (Trudinger B: Doppler ultrasonography and fetal well-being. In Reece EA, Hobbins JC, Mahoney MJ, Petrie RH [eds]: Medicine of the Fetus and Mother. Philadelphia: JB Lippincott, 1992: 710, 713.)

leagues demonstrated that when there is discordant growth, nearly 80% of the S/D ratios are abnormal for at least one fetus.[28] Other investigators found that a difference in the S/D ratio of more than 0.4 had a positive predictive value of nearly 70% for a difference of fetal weights of more than 350 g.[29]

Based on these results, it was hoped that abnormal Doppler flow studies could aid in the diagnosis of twin transfusion, which is a common complication of monochorionic twin pregnancies and is one of the major causes of growth discrepancy in this group.[30]

Initial reports were encouraging. Investigations by Farmakides and colleagues[29] and Pretorius and colleagues[31] indicated that a difference in the umbilical artery S/D ratio of more than 0.4 was associated with twin transfusion syndrome.[29,31] These studies were criticized, however, because of the lack of fetal hematologic data to substantiate the diagnosis of twin transfusion syndrome.

In a series of 456 twin pregnancies, of which 11 had documented transfusion syndrome, Giles and colleagues demonstrated that, in all 11 cases, the umbilical artery S/D ratios were concordant even in the presence of discordancy in fetal size[32] (Table

TABLE 14-3. Umbilical Artery Doppler Studies in Twin Pregnancies

Abnormal S/D ratio in one fetus: 80% of twins are discordant[28]
S/D ratio difference of 0.4: 70% have 350 g weight difference[29]
S/D ratio difference of 0.4: possible twin-to-twin transfusion syndrome[31]
No difference in S/D ratio: 11 with documented twin-to-twin transfusion syndrome[32]

S/D, systolic/diastolic umbilical arterial velocity ratio.

14-3). This was explained by the theoretical possibility that a similarity in waveforms would point to the absence of an underlying placental vascular resistance lesion as a contributing factor to fetal growth discordancy under these circumstances.

OTHER USES OF UMBILICAL DOPPLER

Other proposed uses of umbilical arterial Doppler are listed in Table 14-4.[33–56]

TABLE 14-4. Other Uses of Umbilical Artery Doppler

Anemia[33–37]	Descending aortic and umbilical venous velocities are increased.
	Intracardiac velocities are increased.
	Umbilical artery velocities may be normal.
	Umbilical venous pulsations may be seen.
	Hematocrit cannot be reliably predicted.
Syphilis[38]	S/D ratios are statistically increased.
	Not useful to confirm infection
	Not useful to confirm response to treatment
Postdates[39–41]	Worse fetal outcome if abnormal Doppler
	Not a good predictor of postmaturity
Medications[42,43]	Pseudoephedrine—no effect
	Nifedipine—no effect
Preeclampsia[44–46]	Doppler is not useful as a screening test.
Diabetes[47,48]	Doppler is independent of glucose control.
	Doppler is abnormal if vascular disease is present.
Screening[49–54]	Not useful in low-risk populations
Acidosis[55–56]	Variable results

OTHER VESSELS FOR DOPPLER EXAMINATION

Umbilical Vein

Umbilical venous blood flow velocities were initially studied with Doppler to provide information about the volume of blood flow in the umbilical vessels.[2] Subsequently, variations in umbilical venous velocities coincident with heart rate were seen in fetuses with increased perinatal morbidity.[57] These venous pulsations are seen in some fetuses with abnormal cardiac function.[58] The pulsations appear to correlate with increases in reverse flow velocities in the inferior vena cava with atrial contraction. Variations in umbilical venous velocities are also seen in fetuses during intrauterine breathing episodes; these are not usually coincident with heart rate.

Inferior Vena Cava

Blood flows from the inferior vena cava into the right atrium in three phases. The highest velocity occurs during ventricular systole as the atrium relaxes and the atrioventricular valve ring descends, creating lower pressures in the right atrium. The next velocity peak occurs during early diastole, during which the atrioventricular valves open and the blood flows through the right atrium as if it were a conduit. The third velocity peak occurs with atrial contraction. During atrial contraction, blood usually flows in a reverse direction into the inferior vena cava (Fig. 14-6). The velocity of this reverse flow is determined by a number of factors, including the rate of ventricular relaxation, ventricular compliance, end-diastolic pressure, and venous pressure.[58] Increases in the velocity of blood flow in the reverse direction in the inferior vena cava with atrial contraction have been associated with increases in fetal morbidity and mortality.[58]

Other Arteries

As described previously, most assessments of the fetus with Doppler velocimetry described in the literature are of umbilical artery waveforms. In addition, however, other arteries have been examined, including the descending aorta, the renal arteries, the internal iliac arteries, and the internal carotid, middle cerebral, and posterior cerebral arteries.

In normal gestation, the relative amount of flow during diastole in the umbilical artery increases as the pregnancy advances. The same is true of the

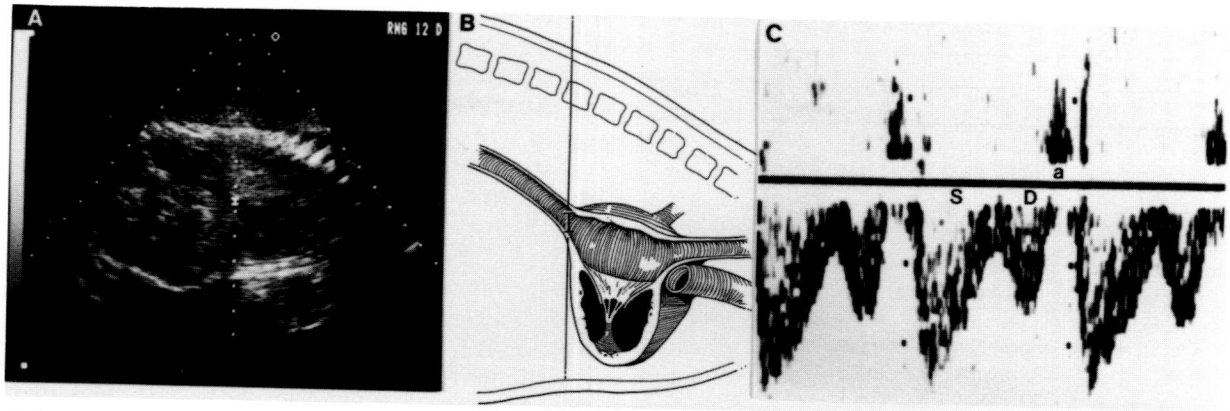

FIGURE 14-6.   Inferior vena caval blood flow velocities. **(A)** Two-dimensional ultrasound with Doppler gate placement. **(B)** Schematic of **A,** showing gate in inferior vena cava. **(C)** Doppler flow velocity tracing. S, systole; D, early diastole; a, atrial kick. (Reed KL, Appleton CP, Anderson CF, et al: Doppler studies of vena cava flows in human fetuses: Insights into normal and abnormal cardiac physiology. Circulation 1990; 81:498–505.)

intraabdominal and intracerebral arteries. The S/D ratios are usually higher in the nonumbilical and intracerebral arteries. Abnormally low ratios in the intracerebral vessels or abnormally high ratios in the renal arteries are associated with an increase in intrauterine growth failure.[59]

Although these multiple other vessels have been investigated by Doppler waveform analysis to identify fetuses at risk for poor perinatal outcome, they offer little additional information when used with umbilical artery Doppler studies.

FETAL INTRACARDIAC DOPPLER

Fetal intracardiac Doppler examinations may be used in normal fetuses and in fetuses with complications of pregnancy (Table 14-5). The Doppler examination of the fetal heart begins with a four-

TABLE 14-5.   Applications of Fetal Doppler Echocardiography

Normal fetuses
Congenital heart disease
Intrauterine growth retardation
Hydrops
   Isoimmunization
   Twins
   Unexplained
Arrhythmia
Prostaglandin synthetase inhibition

chamber view of the heart. Blood velocity in the *tricuspid* and *mitral* valves is examined by placing the sample volume immediately distal to the valve leaflets in the right or left ventricle. The most accurate measurements are obtained if the Doppler beam is less than 30 degrees from the estimated direction of blood flow. If the angle between the beam and the blood flow is greater than 30 degrees, the values must be angle-corrected, and small errors in the estimation of the angle may result in unacceptably large errors in velocity measurement. By moving the Doppler sample volume retrograde through the respective valve, the presence of valvular insufficiency may be detected. This is noted as reversal of the Doppler flow. Valvular stenosis is associated with increased velocity through the affected valve.[59] We do not grade stenosis in utero but simply measure peak velocities and compare these with normal values. Normal values for Doppler velocities are listed in Tables 14-6 and 14-7.

The *aortic* blood flow velocity is sampled in a view in which the aorta is imaged as it exits the left ventricle. Similar to sampling the atrioventricular valves, the most accurate measurement is obtained when the Doppler beam is parallel to the long axis of the aorta. The sample volume is placed immediately distal to the valve leaflets, with as little difference as possible between the Doppler beam and the estimated direction of blood flow. *Pulmonary* Doppler flow velocity waveforms are often obtained from the short axis view as the pulmonary artery exits the right ventricle. These views are presented in Chapter 12. Again, the Doppler sam-

TABLE 14-6. Doppler Measurements

Measurement*	Method	Units
Peak or maximal velocity	Zeroline to peak	cm/sec
Mean velocity	Time velocity integral/time of cardiac cycle	cm/sec
Volume flow	Mean velocity × area† × 60	ml/min
Acceleration time	Time from onset to peak	msec
Deceleration time	Time from peak to zeroline along slope of descent	msec
A/E ratio	Peak velocity with atrial contraction (A)/peak velocity during early diastole (E)	—

* Velocities should be measured within 30 degrees of estimated direction of flow or be angle-corrected.

† Area obtained from diameters measured with two-dimensional ultrasound

(Reed KL: Fetal Doppler echocardiography. Clin Obstet Gynecol 1989; 32:728–737.)

ple is ideally parallel to the long axis of the pulmonary artery or less than 30 degrees. The normal pulse Doppler tracing of the tricuspid valve, mitral valve, pulmonary artery, and aorta are presented in Figure 14-7.

From the waveforms generated by Doppler interrogation, various measurements may be obtained (see Table 14-6). Peak, or maximal, velocities are obtained by measuring the highest velocity of the time–velocity integral. Mean velocities are obtained by digitizing the area of the time–velocity integral and dividing by the time of the cardiac cycle. Cardiac output may be calculated by multiplying the mean temporal velocity by the area through which the blood is flowing (Figs. 14-8 and 14-9). The valve area is calculated from the diameter measurements of the valve annulus, obtained using two-dimensional ultrasound. Two velocity peaks are seen in atrioventricular flow velocity waveforms, the first during early diastole or passive filling (E) and the second with atrial contraction (A). A ratio between A and E can be calculated, and varies with gestational age, heart rate, and ventricular compliance. Deceleration time is measured from the early diastolic peak to the zeroline as the blood flow decelerates and varies with ventricular relaxation properties. Acceleration time is measured from the beginning of flow to peak velocity (see Figs. 14-8 and 14-9).

Intrauterine Growth Retardation and Intracardiac Doppler

Normally in the fetal heart, both ventricles eject blood into the systemic circulation simultaneously. Blood flow through the fetal heart is in parallel rather than in series, as is normal in extrauterine life. Using two-dimensional pulsed Doppler studies in the human fetal heart, it was demonstrated that the ratio of right ventricular blood flow to left ventricular blood flow is 1.33:1.[60,61] In addition, tricuspid valve velocities and diameters are greater than mitral valve velocities and valve diameters. Previous investigation has demonstrated that in fetuses with intrauterine growth retardation and no diastolic flow in the umbilical artery, the right-sided/left-sided volume flow ratio in the heart was increased to 2.15:1.[21]

TABLE 14-7. Normal Doppler Echocardiography in the Fetus

Valve	Tricuspid	Mitral	Pulmonary	Aorta
Maximal velocity (cm/sec)	51 ± 4	47 ± 4	60 ± 4	70 ± 3
Mean velocity (cm/sec)	12 ± 1	11 ± 1	16 ± 2	18 ± 2
Valve diameter (mm)*	8 ± 0.5	6.6 ± 0.4	7.6 ± 0.3	6.7 ± 0.2
Cardiac output (ml/kg/min)*	307 ± 30	232 ± 25	312 ± 11	250 ± 9
A/E ratio*	1.29 ± 0.04	1.35 ± 0.01	—	—
Deceleration time (msec)*	97 ± 29	110 ± 31	—	—
Acceleration time (msec)*	—	—	50.6 ± 12.0	46.7 ± 9.1

Note: See Table 14-6 for explanation of Doppler measurements and the method used for obtaining these measurements.

* Varies with gestational age.

A/E, atrial contraction/early diastole.

(Reed KL: Fetal Doppler echocardiography. Clin Obstet Gynecol 1989; 32:728–737.)

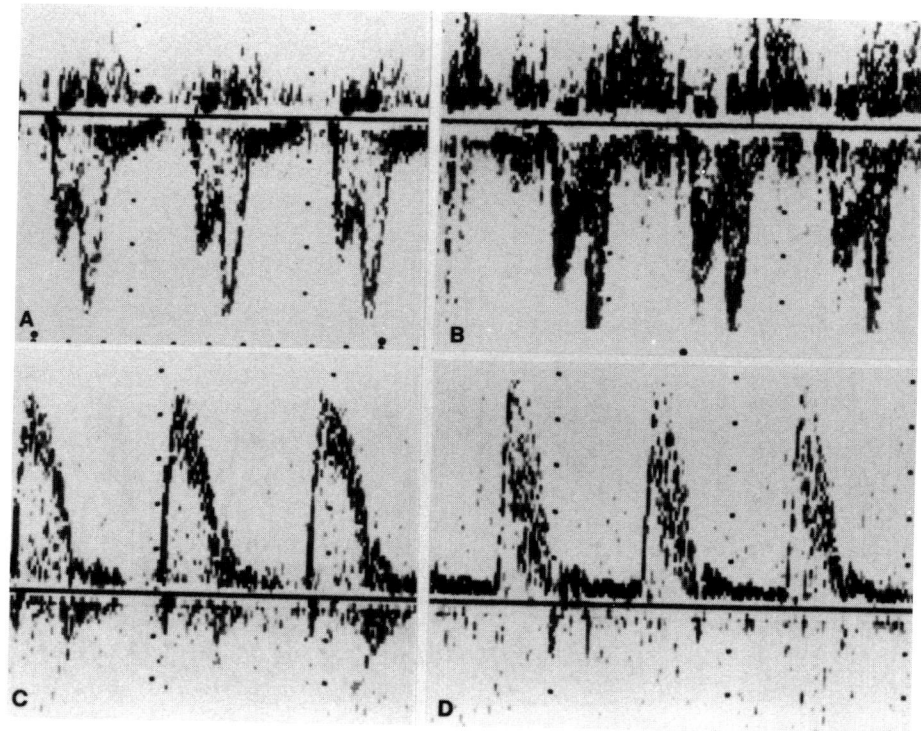

FIGURE 14-7. Pulsed Doppler ultrasound tracings through normal pregnancy in the **(A)** tricuspid valve and **(B)** mitral valve. Note the two peaks that always occur in the atrioventricular Doppler tracings (see Figure 14-8). Doppler tracings through **(C)** pulmonary artery and **(D)** aortic valve. Note single peak of the semilunar valve tracings (see Figure 14-9). Dots are 0.5 seconds apart on the horizontal axis; velocities are listed in Table 14-7. Direction of peak corresponds with direction of blood flow, with flow above the line representing flow toward the transducer and flow below the line representing flow away from the transducer. Direction of the peak varies with position of the fetus and depends on the orientation of the valves in relation to the transducer. (Shenker L, Reed KL, Marx GR, et al: Fetal cardiac Doppler flow studies in prenatal diagnosis of heart disease. Am J Obstet Gynecol 1988; 158:1267–1273.)

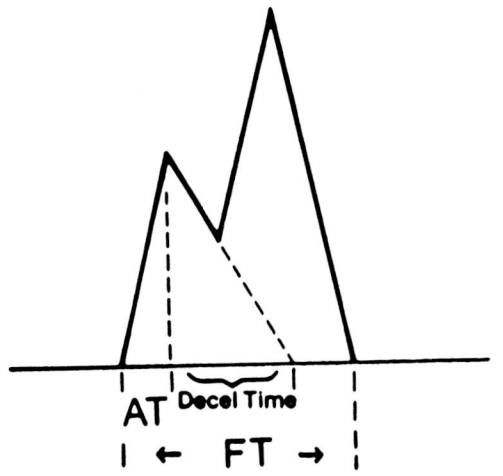

FIGURE 14-8. Schematized atrioventricular Doppler tracing (tricuspid and mitral valve). Two peaks are demonstrated: the first occurs during early diastole, the second during atrial contraction. Mean velocity may be calculated by digitizing the area under the curve and dividing by the time of the cardiac cycle. AT, acceleration time, which is the time from the onset of flow to peak velocity; FT, filling time, which is the total time of the blood flowing into the ventricle from the atrium. (Reed KL: Fetal Doppler echocardiography. Clin Obstet Gynecol 1989; 32:728–737.)

A possible explanation for these intracardiac changes is that developing hypoxia results in dilation of the cerebral vasculature and constriction of the peripheral pulmonary vasculature with enlargement of the ductus. To increase volume blood flow to the brain from the left ventricle, in the face of a dilated ductus supplied by the right ventricle, the volume flow must increase across both ventricles. Because the fetal heart operates in parallel, the net effect of increased volume flow through the right side of the heart is an increased combined ventricular output.

Intracardiac Studies in Fetuses With Cardiac Abnormalities

Although two-dimensional real-time ultrasound remains the primary method of diagnosing fetal cardiac disease, Doppler blood flow velocity estimates can provide pathophysiologic information to support the diagnosis. As described by Shenker and colleagues, if Doppler flow velocities are not consistent with the observed morphologic changes, further observations are indicated.[62] Changes of Doppler flow velocities result from cardiac defects are listed in Table 14-8. Several examples of cardiac defects with Doppler values obtained in the tricuspid, mitral, pulmonary, and aortic valves are listed in Table 14-9.

Tetralogy of Fallot

A schematic of the four-chamber view of the heart revealed a ventricular septal defect and an overriding aorta. On Doppler interrogation, increased aortic velocities with no pulmonary artery velocities were identified (Fig. 14-10). In this case, velocities were essentially normal through the mitral and tricuspid valves (see Table 14-9).

Right Ventricular Hypoplasia

Typical ultrasound findings were schematically illustrated and included a small right ventricle accompanied by tricuspid atresia. A ventricular septal defect also might be present. Doppler flow velocity studies in this case demonstrated decreased tricuspid velocities due to nearly complete tricuspid atresia. Blood flow through the left heart was increased, and therefore mitral velocities were increased. Aortic flow velocity was slightly increased, with normal pulmonary artery flow (Fig. 14-11; see Table 14-9).

(*text continues on page 311*)

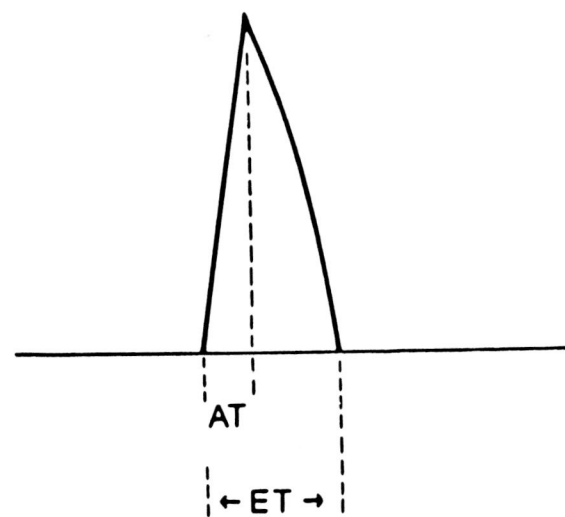

FIGURE 14-9. Schematized semilunar valve Doppler tracing (aortic and pulmonary artery). A single peak is present. Mean velocity may be calculated by digitizing the area under the curve and dividing by the time of the cardiac cycle. AT, acceleration time, which is the time from the onset of flow to the peak velocity; ET, ejection time, which is from the time from beginning to end of flow. (Reed KL: Fetal Doppler echocardiography. Clin Obstet Gynecol 1989; 32:728–737.)

**TABLE 14-8.   Changes in Doppler Flow Velocities
With Cardiac Anomalies**

Anomaly	TV	MV	PA	AO
Hypoplastic right ventricle	Decreased	Increased	Decreased	Increased
Hypoplastic left ventricle	Increased*	Absent	Increased	Absent
Tricuspid atresia	Absent	Increased	Decreased	Increased
Ebstein's anomaly	Increased*	Increased	Decreased	Increased
Pulmonary atresia	Increased*	Increased	Absent	Increased
Tetralogy of Fallot	Unchanged	Unchanged	Decreased	Increased
Transposition of the great vessels	Unchanged	Unchanged	Decreased	Increased
Double-outlet right ventricle	Unchanged	Unchanged	Unchanged	Unchanged
Atrioventricular canal defect	Increased	Decreased	Varies	Varies
	Increased*	Increased*	Varies	Varies

* Regurgitant flow may be present.
TV, tricuspid valve; MV, mitral valve; PA, pulmonary artery; AO, aorta.
(Reed KL: Fetal Doppler echocardiography. Clin Obstet Gynecol 1989; 32:728–737.)

TABLE 14-9.   Doppler Flow Velocities (cm/sec)

Anomaly	Tricuspid	Mitral	Pulmonary	Aorta
Normal				
Maximum	51 ± 4	47 ± 4	60 ± 4	70 ± 3
Mean	12 ± 1	11 ± 1	16 ± 2	18 ± 2
Tetralogy of Fallot				
Maximum	44	33	ND	113
Mean	16	12	ND	29
Hypoplastic right ventricle				
Maximum	ND	54	60	80
Mean	ND	15	20	22
Hypoplastic left ventricle				
Maximum	60	ND	86	ND
Mean	23*	ND	30	ND
Pulmonic atresia				
Maximum	65	36	ND	120
Mean	23*	15	ND	36

* Insufficient valve.
ND, Not detected.
(Shenker L, Reed KL, Marx GR, et al: Fetal cardiac Doppler flow studies in prenatal diagnosis of heart
disease. Am J Obstet Gynecol 1988; 158:1267–1273.)

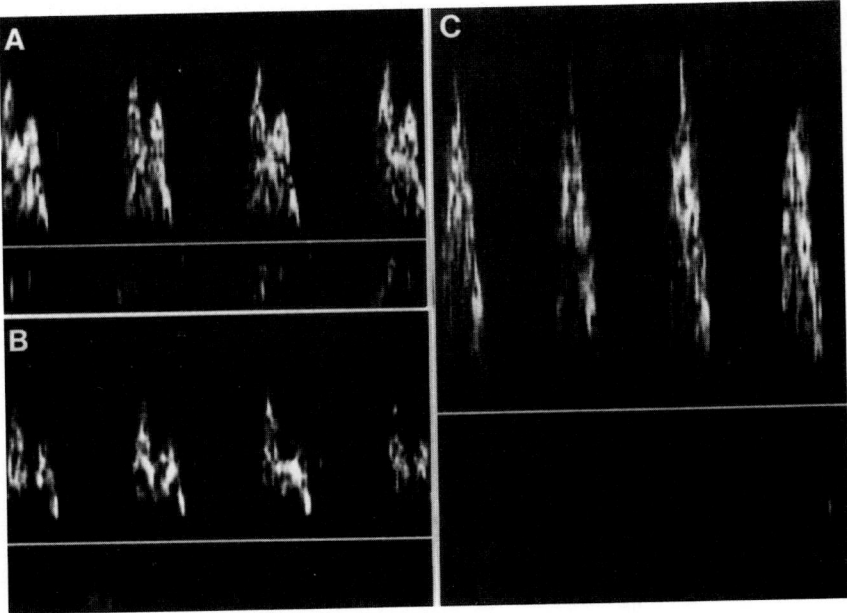

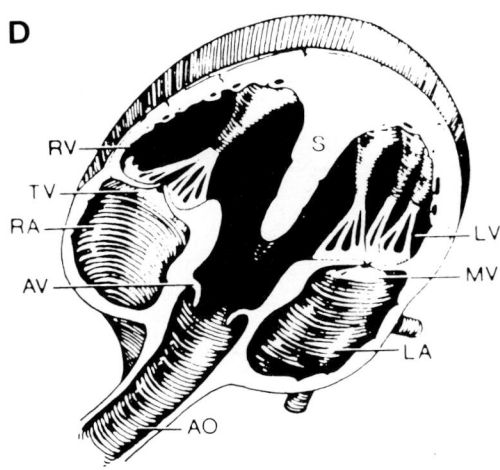

FIGURE 14-10. Pulsed Doppler ultrasound in a 26-week fetus with tetralogy of Fallot. Doppler through (A) tricuspid valve and (B) mitral valve shows the velocity in the normal range, both with flows toward the transducer. (C) Aortic valve velocity, which is obtained with a change in the fetal position to obtain flow toward the transducer, shows velocities increased over normal because the combined ventricular output must exit primarily through the aorta. Velocities are listed in Table 14-9. (Shenker L, Reed KL, Marx GR, et al: Fetal cardiac Doppler flow studies in prenatal diagnosis of heart disease. Am J Obstet Gynecol 1988; 158:1267–1273.) (D) Corresponding illustration shows aorta (AO) overriding ventricular septal defect. LA, left atrium; RA, right atrium; MV, mitral valve; LV, left ventricle; S, septum; TV, tricuspid valve; AV, aortic valve; MV, mitral valve. (Reed KL: The abnormal fetal heart. In Reed KL, Anderson CF, Shenker L [eds]: Fetal Echocardiography: An Atlas. New York: Wiley/Liss, 1988: 47–109.)

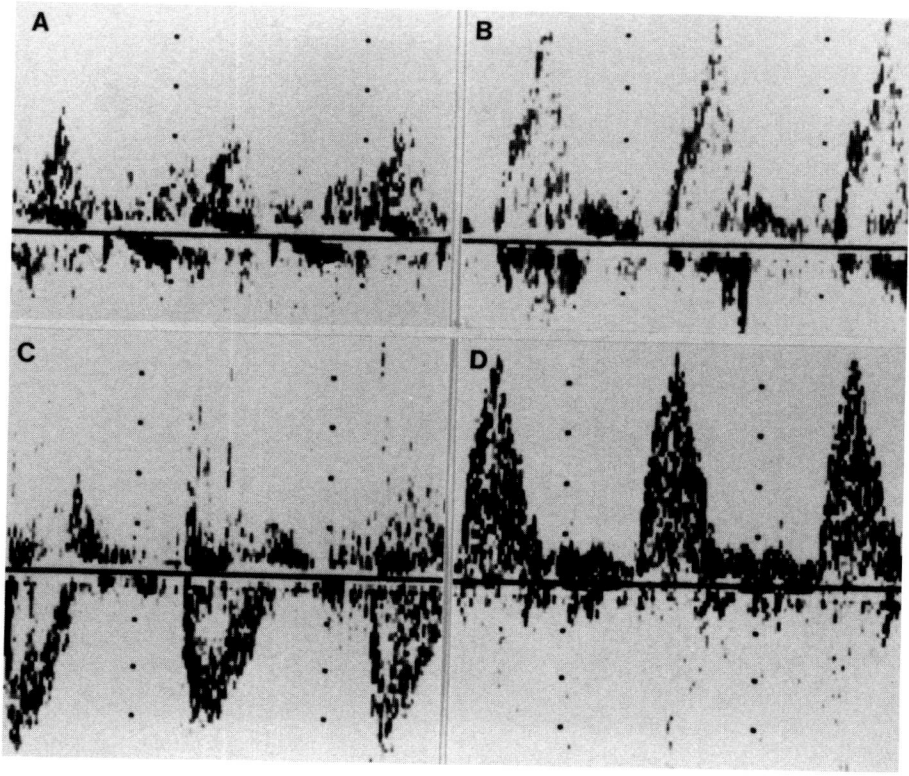

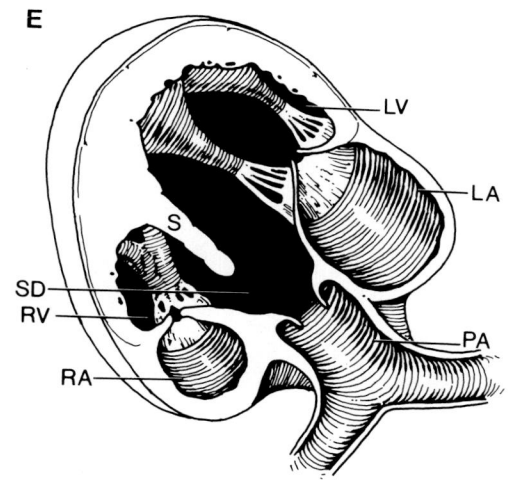

FIGURE 14-11.   Pulsed Doppler ultrasound velocity tracings across four valves in a 33-week fetus with hypoplastic right heart. **(A)** Tricuspid valve velocities are decreased. **(B)** Mitral valve velocities are increased. **(C)** Pulmonary valve velocities are normal. **(D)** Aortic valve velocities are increased. Velocities are listed in Table 14-9. Again, direction of peak velocities depend on orientation of flow either to or away from the transducer. (Shenker L, Reed KL, Marx GR, et al: Fetal cardiac Doppler flow studies in prenatal diagnosis of heart disease. Am J Obstet Gynecol 1988; 158:1267–1273.) **(E)** Corresponding illustration shows that left ventricle (LV) is greater than the right ventricle (RV). No tricuspid valve leaflets were identified. PA, pulmonary artery; LA, left atrium; RA, right atrium; SD, septal defect; S, septum. (Reed KL: The abnormal fetal heart. In Reed KL, Anderson CF, Shenker L [eds]: Fetal Echocardiography: An Atlas. New York: Wiley/Liss, 1988: 47–109.)

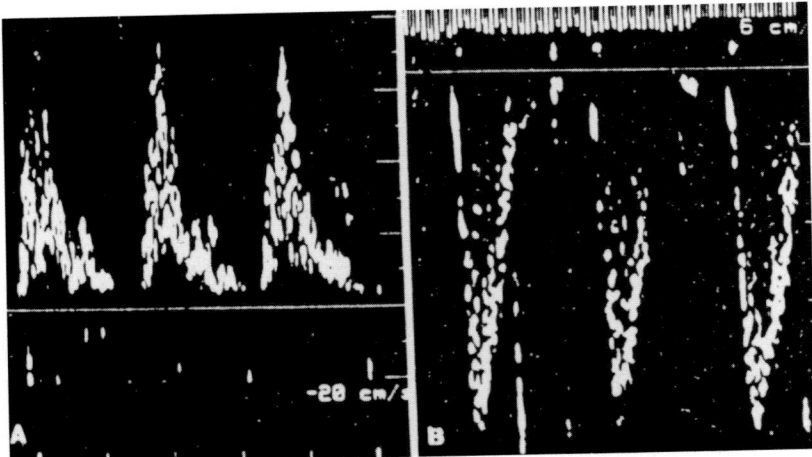

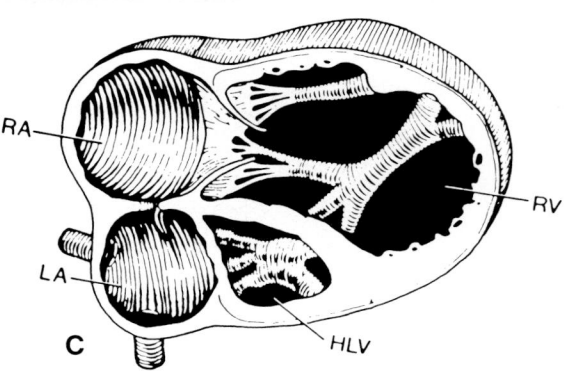

FIGURE 14-12. Pulsed Doppler tracings from a fetus with a hypoplastic left ventricle at 25 weeks. **(A)** Tricuspid valve and **(B)** pulmonary artery velocities are increased. However, no flow could be demonstrated through the mitral and aortic valves, consistent with both mitral atresia and aortic atresia and confirming the diagnosis of hypoplastic left ventricle. Velocities are listed in Table 14-9. (Shenker L, Reed KL, Marx GR, et al: Fetal cardiac Doppler flow studies in prenatal diagnosis of heart disease. Am J Obstet Gynecol 1988; 158:1267–1273.) **(C)** Corresponding illustration shows hypoplastic left ventricle (HLV). RV, right ventricle; RA, right atrium; LA, left atrium. (Reed KL: The abnormal fetal heart. In Reed KL, Anderson CF, Shenker L [eds]: Fetal Echocardiography: An Atlas. New York: Wiley/Liss, 1988: 47–109.)

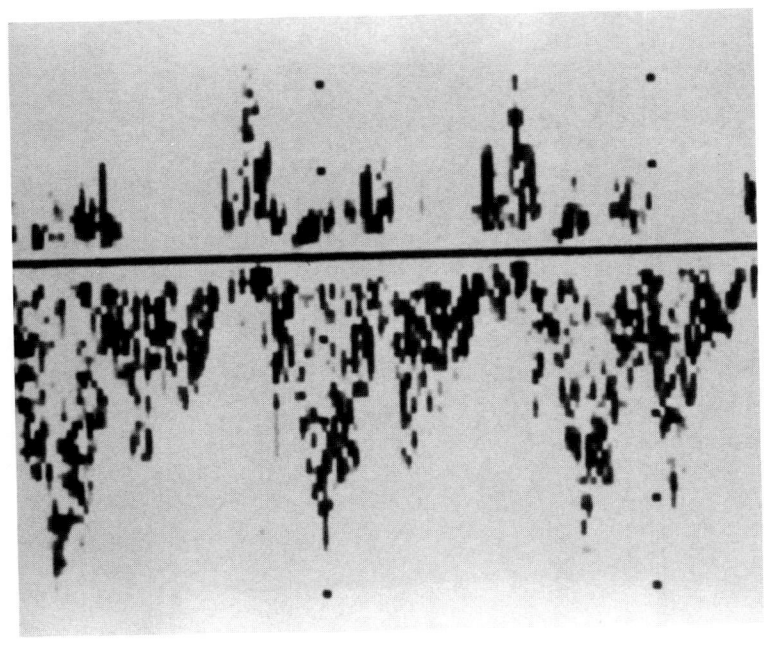

FIGURE 14-13. Pulsed Doppler ultrasound tracing from a fetus with a double-outlet right ventricle and a ventricular septal defect. Pulsed Doppler was placed over the ventricular septal defect, illustrating flow through the ventricular septal defect from left to right. Pulsed Doppler may thus be used to confirm the real-time ultrasound findings of a ventricular septal defect. Color Doppler may also be used to detect the defect. (Shenker L, Reed KL, Marx GR, et al: Fetal cardiac Doppler flow studies in prenatal diagnosis of heart disease. Am J Obstet Gynecol 1988; 158:1267–1273.)

Left Ventricular Hypoplasia

Doppler flow velocities were increased in the tricuspid valve and pulmonary artery. Antegrade flow velocities were not obtained through the ascending aorta or mitral valve because, in this case, both valves were completely atretic (Fig. 14-12; see Table 14-9). Echocardiography performed after birth confirmed left ventricular hypoplasia with both mitral and aortic atresia.

Ventricular Septal Defect

This was a case with complex heart disease and double-outlet right ventricle. Doppler was helpful to evaluate the findings, including flow through a ventricular septal defect, which was from left to right. Doppler may be used to confirm the possible findings of ventricular septal defect identified on real-time ultrasound. Color Doppler may also be used to document the defect (Fig. 14-13; see also Chapter 13).

Pulmonary Atresia

Ultrasound findings included pulmonary stenosis or atresia and an enlarged right atrium (Fig. 14-14). Doppler studies showed markedly increased tricuspid flow, with tricuspid insufficiency as noted by bidirectional flow. Aortic flow velocity was increased, but pulmonary velocities were not mea-

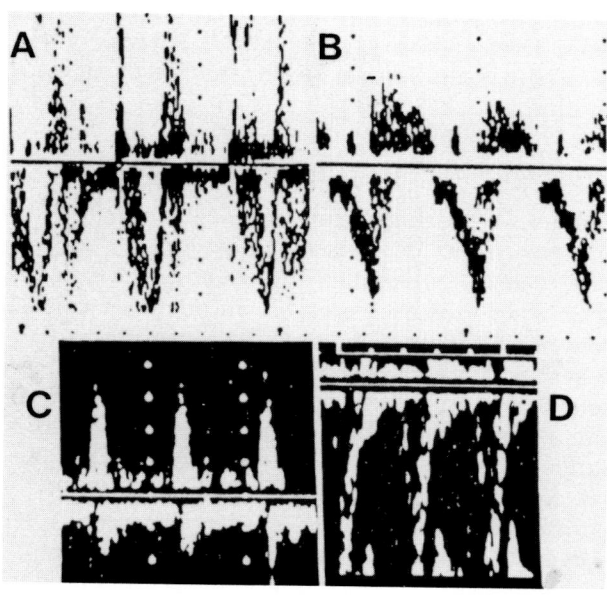

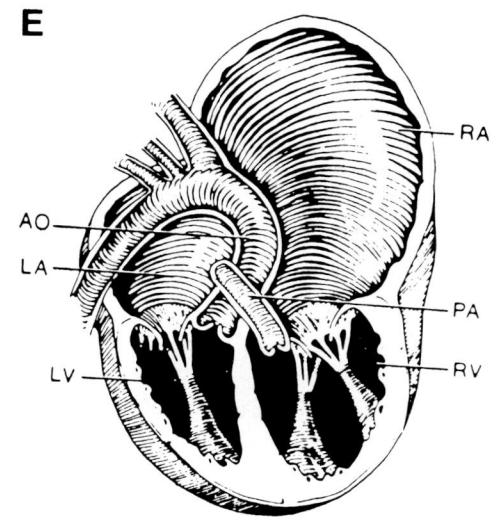

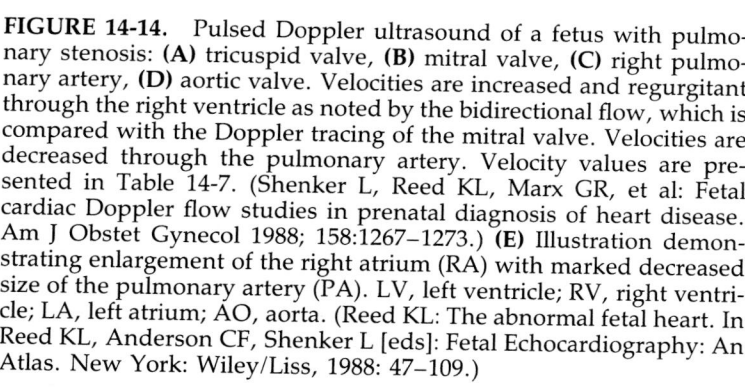

FIGURE 14-14. Pulsed Doppler ultrasound of a fetus with pulmonary stenosis: **(A)** tricuspid valve, **(B)** mitral valve, **(C)** right pulmonary artery, **(D)** aortic valve. Velocities are increased and regurgitant through the right ventricle as noted by the bidirectional flow, which is compared with the Doppler tracing of the mitral valve. Velocities are decreased through the pulmonary artery. Velocity values are presented in Table 14-7. (Shenker L, Reed KL, Marx GR, et al: Fetal cardiac Doppler flow studies in prenatal diagnosis of heart disease. Am J Obstet Gynecol 1988; 158:1267–1273.) **(E)** Illustration demonstrating enlargement of the right atrium (RA) with marked decreased size of the pulmonary artery (PA). LV, left ventricle; RV, right ventricle; LA, left atrium; AO, aorta. (Reed KL: The abnormal fetal heart. In Reed KL, Anderson CF, Shenker L [eds]: Fetal Echocardiography: An Atlas. New York: Wiley/Liss, 1988: 47–109.)

surable due to pulmonary atresia (see Fig. 14-14). Cardiac catheterization after birth confirmed the prenatal diagnosis of pulmonary atresia.

Doppler Flow With Arrhythmias

With premature atrial or ventricular contractions, there is typically diminished or no flow with the premature beat, with compensatory increased flow during the beat that follows the pause after the premature beat. This finding of an increase in the time velocity integral after a diastolic pause has been used to confirm the operation of a Frank-Starling mechanism in the fetus.[63]

With supraventricular tachycardia, mean velocities decrease as a result of the rapid heart rate.[62] In addition, during the atrial contraction, there is more reverse flow in the inferior vena cava.[57] These two factors contribute to a decrease in forward flow and explain in part the development of hydrops in fetuses with sustained tachyarrhythmias.

Prostaglandin Synthetase Inhibition

The use of prostaglandin synthetase inhibitors for preterm labor tocolysis has triggered a series of observations of Doppler flow velocity through the ductus arteriosus. Increased ductal flows consistent with constriction have been reported in fetuses of mothers receiving indomethacin.[64] Systolic ductus arteriosus velocities in normal fetuses range from 91 to 135 cm/second; diastolic velocities range from 14 to 25 cm/second. Fetuses with ductal constrictions have elevated systolic (141–235 cm/second) and diastolic (37–168 cm/second) velocities.[63] In addition, in animal models, the transplacental cardiovascular effects of acetaminophen, aspirin, ibuprofen, and indomethacin have been examined. In all instances, intrauterine ductal constriction and tricuspid regurgitation were seen after maternal treatment. Fetal ductal constriction and persistent pulmonary hypertension in the newborn were observed clinically after maternal treatment with nonsteroidal antiinflammatory drugs. Ibuprofen was the most potent in constriction of the fetal ductus arteriosus.[65]

CONCLUSION

The initial enthusiasm about the use of Doppler ultrasound of the umbilical artery to identify the fetus experiencing intrauterine difficulties has been tempered by results from prospective studies. This may be an inevitable consequence of asking too much of a single test. The positive predictive value of abnormal umbilical artery S/D ratios for adverse neonatal outcome is highest in those pregnancies already at risk for intrauterine growth retardation. Initial reports were hampered by population selection biases.

The interpretation of umbilical artery Doppler velocimetry also suffers from our incomplete understanding of fetal circulatory physiology. In its simplest interpretation, Doppler flow measures the velocity of blood flow through the umbilical and fetal vessels. This velocity, in turn, is theoretically inversely related to vascular resistance. In adults, the velocity is also directly related to blood pressure. Because acute blood pressure changes are small in the fetus, however, most of the effect on S/D ratios is thought to be due to placental resistance.[52] Such a view may be too simplistic.

Because of the complex nature of fetal physiology and growth, it is therefore likely that testing of flow will be of better diagnostic value when used in conjunction with other forms of antenatal testing, such as growth measurement, heart rate testing, and amniotic fluid indices.

For the specialist, however, there does appear to be a role for Doppler ultrasound as an aid in the diagnosis of fetal cardiac anomalies noted on two-dimensional ultrasound. The assessment of blood flow changes that occur in hearts with anomalies or in normally formed hearts complicated by heart or growth failure allows the identification of physiologic changes that provide confirmatory evidence of observed morphologic changes.

The advantages of fetal cardiac diagnosis as opposed to neonatal assessment lie in the fact that because the ductus remains open after birth, some cardiac lesions are not identified before discharge of the neonate. When the ductus does finally close, the infant may become cyanotic. This delay in diagnosis ultimately results in the development of acidosis. When this occurs, the assessment and repair of lesions becomes more difficult. Intracardiac Doppler flow velocimetry in those fetuses at risk can be a valuable adjunctive tool to two-dimensional ultrasound in the management of fetuses with cardiac disease.

REFERENCES

1. Schulman H: Doppler ultrasound. In Eden RD, Boehm FH (eds): Assessment and Care of the Fetus. Norwalk, CT: Appleton and Lange, 1990: 397–407.
2. Gill RW, Warren PS: Doppler measurement of umbilical blood flow. In Sanders RC, James AE Jr (eds): The Principles and Practice of Ultrasonography in

Obstetrics and Gynecology, 3rd ed. Norwalk, CT: Appleton-Century-Crofts, 1985: 87–97.

3. Moinan M, Meyer WW, Lind J: Diameters of umbilical cord vessels and weight of the cord in relation to clamping time. Am J Obstet Gynecol 1969; 105:604–606.

4. Gill RW: Pulsed Doppler with B-mode imaging for quantitative blood flow measurement. Ultrasound Med Biol 1979; 5:223–235.

5. Schulman H, Fleischer A, Stern W: Umbilical velocity waveforms in human pregnancy. Am J Obstet Gynecol 1984; 148:985–990.

6. Schulman H: The clinical implications of Doppler ultrasound analysis of the uterine and umbilical arteries. Am J Obstet Gynecol 1987; 156:889–893.

7. Maulik D, Yarlagadda D, Youngblood JD: Comparative efficacy of umbilical arterial Doppler indices for predicting adverse fetal outcome. Am J Obstet Gynecol 1991; 164:1434–1440.

8. Thompson RS, Trudinger BJ, Cook CM: A comparison of Doppler ultrasound waveforms in the umbilical artery: Indices derived from mean velocity. Ultrasound Med Biol 1986; 12:845–850.

9. Seeds JW: Impaired fetal growth: Definition and clinical diagnosis. Obstet Gynecol 1984; 64:303–310.

10. Al-Ghazali W, Chapman MG, Allan LD: Doppler assessment of the cardiac and uteroplacental circulation in normal and complicated pregnancies. Br J Obstet Gynaecol 1988; 95:575–580.

11. Arduini D, Rizzo G, Romanini C, Mancuso S: Fetal blood flow velocity waveforms as predictors of growth retardation. Obstet Gynecol 1987; 70:7–10.

12. Berkowitz GS, Chitkara U, Rosenberg J, et al: Sonographic estimation of fetal weight and Doppler analysis of umbilical artery velocimetry in the prediction of intrauterine growth retardation: A prospective study. Am J Obstet Gynecol 1988; 158:1149–1153.

13. Divon MY, Guidetti DA, Braverman JJ, et al: Intrauterine growth retardation: A prospective study of the diagnostic value of real-time sonography combined with umbilical artery flow velocimetry. Obstet Gynecol 1988; 72:611–614.

14. Fleischer A, Schulman H, Farmakides G, et al: Umbilical artery velocity waveforms and intrauterine growth retardation. Am J Obstet Gynecol 1985; 151:502–505.

15. Gaziano E, Knox GE, Wager GP, et al: The predictability of the small-for-gestational age infant by real-time ultrasound-derived measurements combined with pulsed Doppler umbilical artery velocimetry. Am J Obstet Gynecol 1988; 158:1431–1439.

16. Marsal K: Ultrasound assessment of fetal circulation as a diagnostic test: A review. In Lipshitz J, Maloney J, Nimrod, Carson G (eds): Perinatal Development of the Heart and Lung. Ithaca, NY: Perinatology Press, 1987: 127–142.

17. Maulik D, Yarlagadda AP, Youngblood JP, Willoughby L: Components of variability of umbilical arterial Doppler velocimetry: A prospective analysis. Am J Obstet Gynecol 1989; 160:1406–1412.

18. Reed KL: Comment on Maulik D, Yarlagadda P, Youngblood JP, Ciston P: The diagnostic efficacy of the umbilical arterial systolic/diastolic ratio as a screening tool: A prospective blinded study. Am J Obstet Gynecol 1990; 162:1518–1525.

19. Schulman H, Winter D, Farmakides G, et al: Pregnancy surveillance with Doppler velocimetry of uterine and umbilical arteries. Am J Obstet Gynecol 1989; 1760:192–196.

20. Trudinger BJ, Giles WB, Cook CM: Flow velocity waveforms in the maternal uteroplacental and fetal umbilical placental circulations. Am J Obstet Gynecol 1985; 152:155–163.

21. Reed KL, Anderson CF, Shenker L: Changes in intracardiac Doppler blood flow velocities in fetuses with absent umbilical artery diastolic flow. Am J Obstet Gynecol 1987; 157:774–779.

22. Brar HS, Platt LD: Reverse end-diastolic flow velocity on umbilical artery velocimetry in high risk pregnancies: An ominous finding with adverse pregnancy outcome. Am J Obstet Gynecol 1988; 159:559–562.

23. Divon MY, Lieblich R, Langer O: Clinical management of the fetus with markedly diminished umbilical artery end-diastolic flow. Obstet Gynecol 1989; 161:1523–1527.

24. Karsdorp VHM, Ujgt JM, Dekker GA, Geijn P: Reappearance of end-diastolic velocities in the umbilical artery following maternal volume expansion: A preliminary study. Obstet Gynecol 1992; 80:679–683.

25. Fox RY, Pailova Z, Bernirscheke K, et al: The correlation of arterial lesions with umbilical artery Doppler velocimetry in placentas of small for dates pregnancies. Obstet Gynecol 1990; 75:578–583.

26. Giles WB, Trudinger BJ, Baird PJ: Fetal umbilical artery flow velocity waveforms and placental resistance: Pathologic correlation. Br J Obstet Gynaecol 1985; 92:31–38.

27. McCowan LM, Mullen BM, Ritchie K: Umbilical artery flow velocity waveforms and the placental vascular bed. Am J Obstet Gynecol 1987; 157:900–902.

28. Giles WB, Trudinger BJ, Cook CM: Fetal umbilical artery velocity wave forms in twin pregnancies. Br J Obstet Gynaecol 1985; 92:490.

29. Farmakides G, Schulman L, Saldana L, Bracero L: Surveillance of twin pregnancy with umbilical arterial velocimetry. Am J Obstet Gynecol 1985; 153:789–792.

30. Naeye RL: The fetal and neonatal development of twins. Pediatrics 1964; 33:546–553.

31. Pretorius DH, Manchester D, Barkin S: Doppler ultrasound of twin transfusion syndrome. J Ultrasound Medicine 1988; 7:117–119.

32. Giles WB, Trudinger BJ, Cook CM: Doppler umbilical artery studies in the twin twin transfusion syndrome. Obstet Gynecol 1990; 76:1097–1100.

33. Rightmire DA, Nicolaides KH, Rodeck CH: Fetal blood velocities in Rh isoimmunization: Relation-

ship to gestational age and to fetal hematocrit. Obstet Gynecol 1986; 68:233–236.

34. Moise KJ, Mari G, Fisher DJ, Carpenter RJ: Acute fetal hemodynamic alterations after intrauterine transfusion for treatment of severe red blood cell alloimmunization. Am J Obstet Gynecol 1990; 163:776–784.

35. Copel JA, Grannum PA, Green JJ, et al: Pulsed Doppler flow velocity waveforms in the prediction of fetal hematocrit of the severely isoimmunized pregnancy. Obstet Gynecol 1989; 161:341–344.

36. Mari G, Moise K, Deter R, Carpenter RJ: Flow velocity waveforms of the vascular system in the anemic fetus before and after intravascular transfusion for severe red blood cell alloimmunization. Am J Obstet Gynecol 1990; 162:1060–1064.

37. Weiner CP, Anderson TL: The acute effect of cordocentesis with or without fetal curarization and of intravascular transfusion upon umbilical artery waveform indices. Obstet Gynecol 1989; 73:219–224.

38. Lucas M, Theriot S, Wendel GD: Doppler systolic diastolic ratios in pregnancies complicated by syphilis. Obstet Gynecol 1991; 77:217–222.

39. Rightmire DA, Campbell S: Fetal and maternal Doppler flow parameters in post term pregnancies. Obstet Gynecol 1987; 69:891–894.

40. Guidetti DA, Divon MY, Cavalieri O, Larger L: Fetal umbilical artery flow velocimetry in post date pregnancies. Am J Obstet Gynecol 1987; 157:1521–1523.

41. Pearce JM, McParland PJ: A comparison of Doppler flow velocity waveforms, amniotic fluid columns, and the non-stress test as a means of monitoring post-dates pregnancies. Obstet Gynecol 1991; 77:204–208.

42. Smith CV, Rayburn WF, Anderson JC, et al: Effect of single dose oral pseudoephedrine on uterine and fetal Doppler blood flow. Obstet Gynecol 1990; 76:803–806.

43. Pirhonen JP, Ekblad VV, Nysman L: Single dose nifedipine in normotensive pregnancy: Nifedipine concentrations, hemodynamic responses, and uterine and fetal flow velocity waveforms. Obstet Gynecol 1990; 76:807–811.

44. Sorenson TK, Hendricks S, Carlson KL, Benedetti JJ: Effect of orthostatic stress on umbilical Doppler waveforms in normal and hypertensive pregnancies. Am J Obstet Gynecol 1992; 167:643–647.

45. Hanretty KP, Whittle MJ, Rubin PC: Reappearance of end-diastolic velocity in pregnancy complicated by severe pregnancy-induced hypertension. Am J Obstet Gynecol 1988; 158:1123–1124.

46. Hume RF, Hertzberg BS, McCoy C, Killam AP: Fetal umbilical artery Doppler response to graded maternal aerobic exercise and subsequent maternal mean arterial blood pressure: Predictive value for pregnancy-induced hypertension. Am J Obstet Gynecol 1990; 163:826–829.

47. Landon MB, Gabbe SG, Bruner JP, Ludmir J: Doppler umbilical artery velocimetry in pregnancy complicated by insulin dependent diabetes mellitus. Obstet Gynecol 1989; 73:961–965.

48. Bracero L, Schulman H, Fleischer A, et al: Umbilical artery velocimetry in diabetes and pregnancy. Obstet Gynecol 1986; 68:654–658.

49. Trudinger BJ, Cook CM, Jones L, Giles WB: A comparison of fetal heart rate monitoring and umbilical artery waveforms in the recognition of fetal compromise. Br J Obstet Gynaecol 1986; 93:171–176.

50. Ogunyem D, Stanley R, Lynch C, Fukushima T: Umbilical artery velocimetry in predicting perinatal outcome with intrapartum fetal distress. Obstet Gynecol 1992; 80:377–380.

51. Ratnam SS: Umbilical artery Doppler velocimetry as a labor admission test. Obstet Gynecol 1991; 77:10–14.

52. McParland P, Pearce JM: Review article: Doppler blood flow in pregnancy. Placenta 1988; 9:427–450.

53. Newnham JP, Patterson LL, James IR, Reid E: An evaluation of the efficacy of Doppler flow velocity waveform analysis as a screening test in pregnancy. Am J Obstet Gynecol 1990; 162:403–410.

54. Newnham JP, Dea MR, Reid KP, Diepeveen DA: Doppler flow velocimetry waveforms analysis in high risk pregnancies: A randomized controlled trial. Br J Obstet Gynaecol 1991; 98:956–963.

55. Morrow RJ, Adamson SL, Shelley B, Ritchie K: Hypoxic acidemia, hyperviscosity, and maternal hypertension do not affect the umbilical arterial velocity waveform in fetal sheep. Am J Obstet Gynecol 1990; 163:1313–1320.

56. Copel JA, Schafer D, Belanger K, et al: Does umbilical artery systolic diastolic ratio reflect flow or acidosis? Am J Obstet Gynecol 1990; 163:751–756.

57. Indik JH, Chen V, Reed KL: Association of umbilical venous with inferior vena cava blood flow velocities. Obstet Gynecol 1991; 77:551–557.

58. Reed KL, Appleton CP, Anderson CF, et al: Doppler studies of vena cava flows in human fetuses: Insights into normal and abnormal cardiac physiology. Circulation 1990; 81:498–505.

59. Reed KL: Fetal Doppler echocardiography. Clin Obstet Gynecol 1989; 32:728–737.

60. Reed KL, Meijboom EJ, Scagnelli SA, et al: Cardiac Doppler flow velocities in human fetuses. Circulation 1986; 73:41–46.

61. Reed KL, Anderson CF, Shenker L: Fetal pulmonary artery and aorta: Two-dimensional Doppler echocardiography. Obstet Gynecol 1987; 69:175–178.

62. Shenker L, Reed KL, Marx GR, et al: Fetal cardiac Doppler flow studies in prenatal diagnosis of heart disease. Am J Obstet Gynecol 1988; 158:1267–1273.

63. Reed KL, Sahn DJ, Marx GR: Cardiac Doppler flow during fetal arrhythmias: Physiologic consequences. Obstet Gynecol 1987; 70:1–5.

64. Moise KJ, Huhta JG, Sharif DS: Indomethacin in the treatment of premature labor. N Engl J Med 1988; 319:327–330.

65. Momma K, Takao A: Transplacental cardiovascular effects of four popular analgesics in rats. Am J Obstet Gynecol 1990; 162:1304–1306.

John P. McGahan and Manuel Porto:
DIAGNOSTIC OBSTETRICAL ULTRASOUND.
© 1994 J.B. Lippincott Company.

Richard A. Humes

Chapter *15*

Diagnosis of Fetal Cardiac Arrhythmias

PERSPECTIVE

Fetal cardiac arrhythmias are an interesting and important antenatal problem. It is estimated that 2% of fetuses exhibit a fetal arrhythmia.[1] In a select population, different authors have reported that fetal arrhythmias represent about 20% of referrals for fetal echocardiography at large centers.[2,3] The consequences of the arrhythmia to the fetus depends largely on the type of rhythm, the underlying ventricular rate, and the duration of the rhythm disorder. Fetal cardiac tachyarrhythmia and bradyarrhythmia may lead to congestive heart failure, hydrops fetalis, or intrauterine death. Echocardiographic techniques have been employed for over 10 years to detect and define fetal arrhythmias.

This chapter defines the different types of fetal arrhythmias and describes the echocardiographic techniques used to diagnose the rhythm disorder. It also provides a systematic approach to the diagnosis of fetal cardiac arrhythmias.

DEFINITIONS AND INCIDENCE

All cardiac rhythm disorders must be defined by regularity and rate. The normal fetal heart rates are shown in Table 15-1. The types of rhythms commonly seen in a referral population are shown in Table 15-2.

DIAGNOSTIC METHODS

The echocardiographic modalities typically used for defining fetal arrhythmias are M-mode tracings and Doppler.[2,3,5,6] There is no consensus about the relative methodologic superiority of one ultrasound technique over another. Factors such as fetal position, maternal obesity, and fetal activity may have an overwhelming influence on the success of any echocardiographic technique in the individual patient. A combination of techniques may be employed and individualized with each patient to achieve the best overall results. The goal is to

315

TABLE 15-1.   Definitions of Fetal Heart Rate

	Rate (beats/min)	R–R Interval (s)
Normal		
20 weeks	120–160	0.5–0.375
36 weeks	110–150	0.55–0.4
Tachycardia	>180	<0.33
Bradycardia	<100	>0.6

make inferences about the electrical activity of the heart based on the mechanical activity of the walls and valves.

M-Mode Techniques

M-mode echocardiography traces a linear drawing of cardiac motion along a timeline. When used for a postnatal transthoracic echocardiogram, an electrocardiogram (ECG) is superimposed on the image to aid in timing cardiac events. The electrical activity of the P-wave on the ECG produces atrial contraction. This is seen on the M-mode as atrial inward motion (when the atrial wall is drawn) or the A-wave tracing of either atrioventricular (mitral or tricuspid) valve as it opens. The R-wave on the ECG produces ventricular contraction or semilunar valve (aortic or pulmonary) opening. These phenomena are shown in Figures 15-1 and 15-2.

Advantages

M-mode is a sensitive, high-fidelity recording of motion. The M-mode cursor records events along a line and can sometimes be positioned through atrial and ventricular chambers simultaneously.

TABLE 15-2.   Fetal Arrythmias: Abnormal Rhythms Seen at Three Centers

Arrhythmia	No.
Premature atrial contractions	242
Premature ventricular contractions	31
Complete heart block	25
Supraventricular tachycardia	23
Sinus bradycardia	14
Atrial flutter	5
Atrial fibrillation	2
Ventricular tachycardia	2
TOTAL	344

When this can be done with high fidelity, it may be the best technique for recording simultaneous atrial and ventricular events.

Disadvantages

Atrial wall contractions in the small fetus are often difficult to see. The ability to record *simultaneous* atrial and ventricular contractions depends on the clarity of image and fetal position.

Doppler Techniques

The use of Doppler flow to record atrial and ventricular events is a relatively newer technique that may be employed to assess heart rhythm. The goal is similar to that of M-mode recordings: to use Doppler to establish the timing of atrial and ventricular contractions to make inferences about the electrical activity of the heart. Pulsed Doppler is used to ensure sampling at precise locations. Widening the pulsed Doppler sample volume or "gate" can allow sampling in regions of flow where both systolic and diastolic events occur.

Atrial events (corresponding to the P-wave of the electrocardiogram) may be recorded by Doppler in several areas. Recording of inflow into either ventricle across the atrioventricular valves (mitral or tricuspid) during normal sinus rhythm produces a characteristic biphasic waveform of early filling (E-wave) and late filling (A-wave).[2,3] This later filling corresponds to atrial contraction (Fig. 15-3). The atrial activity may also be recorded by positioning the sample volume near the foramen ovale on the left atrial side[2] (Fig. 15-4). Chan and colleagues described a technique of sampling in the inferior vena cava to analyze atrial activity.[7]

Recording of the ventricular activity (R-wave on ECG) is performed by sampling in the ventricular outflow tracts or great arteries (aorta and pulmonary). Simultaneous recording of inflow and outflow may be achieved by expanding the pulsed Doppler sample volume in the area of the left ventricular inflow (Fig. 15-5) or in the abdomen to include inferior vena caval flow as well as aortic flow.

Advantages

Because the quantitative aspects of the Doppler in this instance are less important than the timing, the Doppler sampling may be carried out from a variety of angles, making this technique somewhat less dependent on fetal position than M-mode. Doppler flow is often more sensitive than the two-dimensional image in cases of poor image quality,

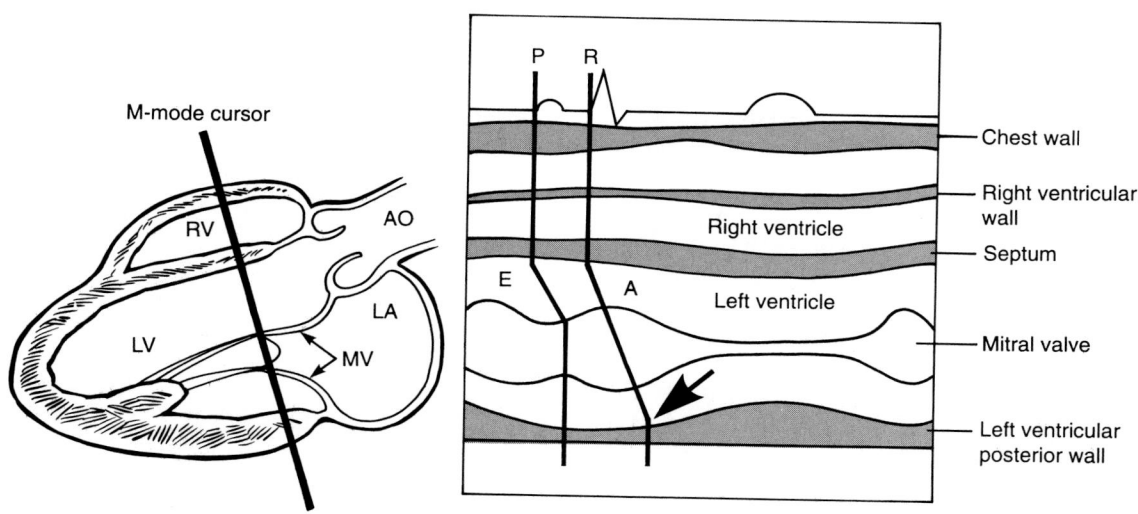

FIGURE 15-1. M-mode echocardiogram with the cursor through the mid-portion of the left ventricle demonstrates how atrial and ventricular events may be displayed. The P-wave (P) on the surface electrocardiogram produces an atrial "kick," and after a short time, delay between electrical and mechanical events reopens the mitral valve, producing an A-wave (A). The R-wave on the electrocardiogram initiates ventricular contraction, which is displayed as thickening and inward movement of the left ventricular posterior wall (*arrow*). AO, aorta; LA, left atrium; MV, mitral valve; LV, left ventricle; RV, right ventricle.

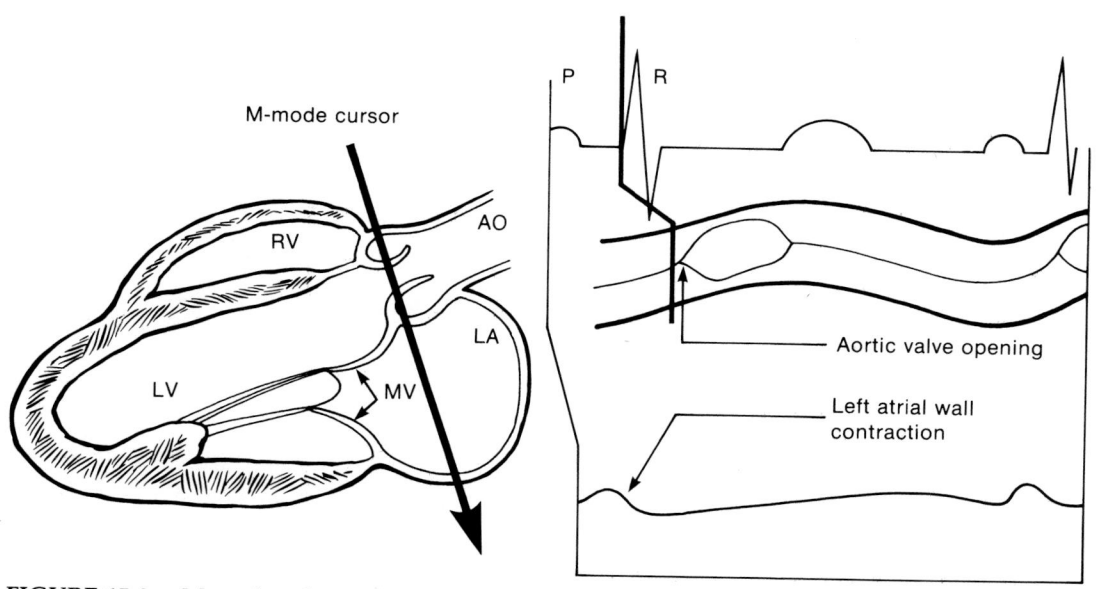

FIGURE 15-2. M-mode echocardiogram with cursor through the aortic valve and left atrium (LA) demonstrates left atrial wall contraction corresponding to the P-wave (P) of the electrocardiogram and aortic valve opening afterward, with R-wave (R) on the electrocardiogram. AO, aorta; RV, right ventricle; LV, left ventricle; MV, mitral valve.

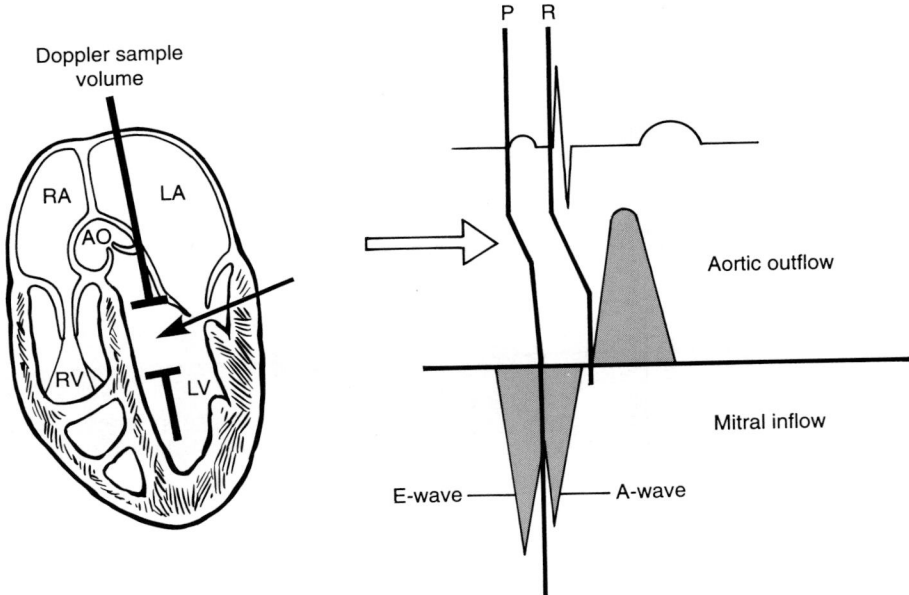

FIGURE 15-3. The Doppler sample volume is placed in the mid-portion of the body of the left ventricle (LV) with the sample gate opened widely (*solid arrow*). After a short time delay (*open arrow*), the electrical events of the P-wave (P) produce the second phase of ventricular filling (A-wave). The R-wave initiates ventricular contraction, and flow is directed out through the aortic valve in an opposite direction to ventricular inflow. AO, aorta; LA, left atrium; RA, right atrium; RV, right ventricle.

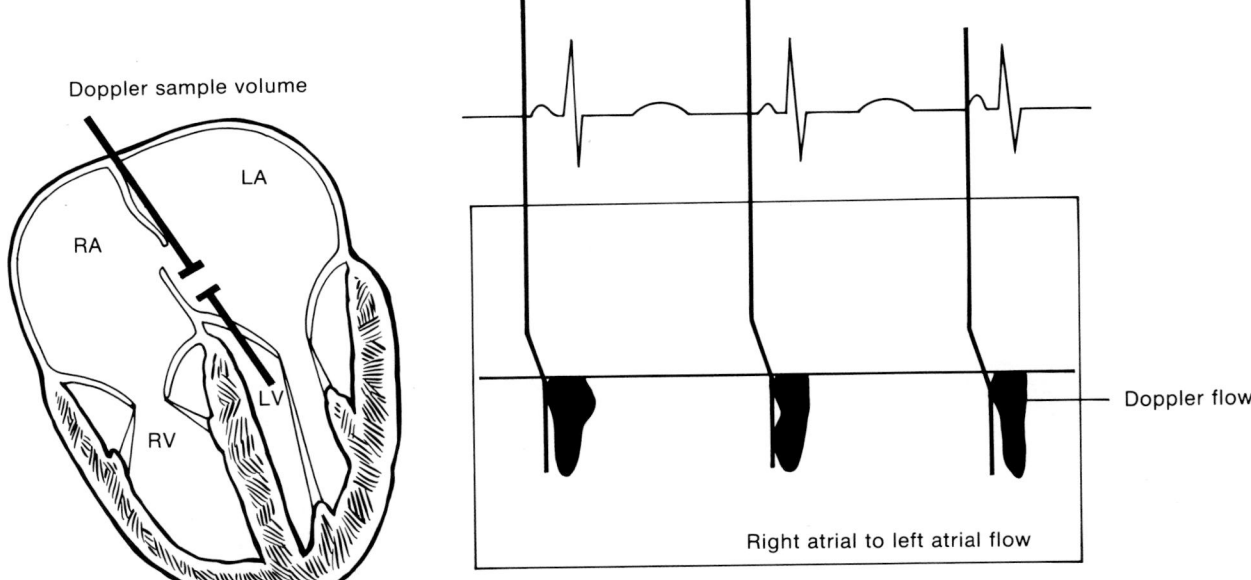

FIGURE 15-4. To detect atrial events, Doppler sample volume may be placed on the left atrial side of the atria, and right atrial to left atrial flow may be detected corresponding to atrial contractions. RA, right atrium; LA, left atrium; RV, right ventricle; LV, left ventricle.

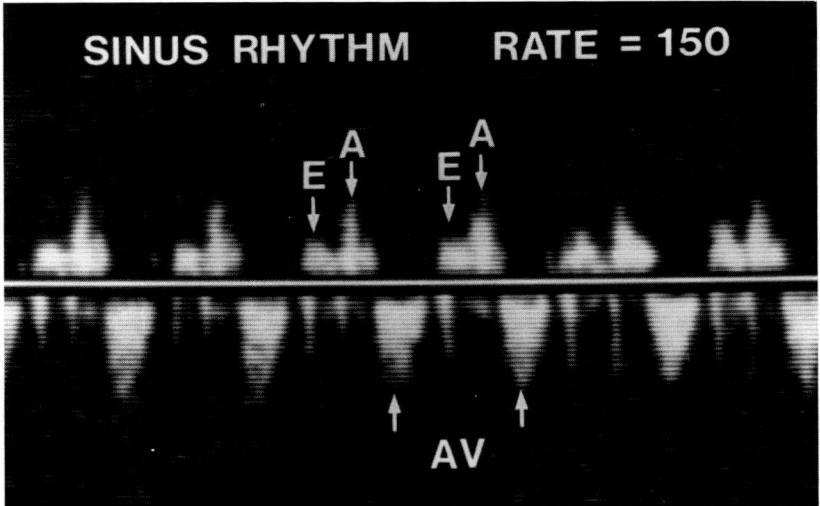

FIGURE 15-5. An example of a Doppler tracing in a normal sinus rhythm with a rate of 150 beats/min. The sample volume is placed in the mid-left ventricle so that mitral inflow, as shown with characteristic E- and A-waves, is seen. The A-wave corresponds to atrial contraction and is usually the dominant wave in the fetus. Ventricular contraction and aortic valve (AV) flow is seen immediately afterward (*arrows*).

which would hamper M-mode quality. Additionally, the Doppler flow may provide insight into the hemodynamic effects of the rhythm on the fetus.

Disadvantages

Electrical events, particularly atrial events, do not always produce mechanical opening of the atrioventricular valves. In addition, some premature beats occur at a time that impedes flow, such as a premature ventricular beat producing early closure of the atrioventricular valves. Thus, flow may not be present in some areas, which can lead to interpretive errors. At very fast heart rates such seen in rapid tachycardia, the early and late ventricular filling signals across the atrioventricular valves blend into one another, impeding the ability to distinguish ventricular relaxation (E-wave) from atrial activity (A-wave).

SYSTEMATIC APPROACH TO ARRHYTHMIA ANALYSIS

Analysis of echocardiographic events to reconstruct electrical events can follow various schema that have been described to interpret electrocardiograms for rhythm disorders.[8–15] The algorithm for those diagnostic pathways is shown in Figure 15-6. The highly variable nature of some rhythms and the presence of varying degrees of atrioventricular block make this diagram imperfect for every possible rhythm. Rhythms are seen in the categories in which they are *most often* encountered in clinical practice. The major branching points of this sche-

matic diagram represent clinical decision points and are discussed briefly next.

The first part of the decision process includes making an assessment of ventricular rhythm *regularity* (Fig. 15-7). Regular rhythms may then be characterized by their rate. Irregular rhythms are described as continuously (or regularly) irregular or intermittently (or irregularly) irregular.

Regular Arrhythmias

Regular arrhythmias are defined by their rates (Fig. 15-8).

1. An increased rate with a 1:1 atrioventricular relation produces a regular tachycardia. The type of tachycardia may be further defined by the rate itself. Sinus tachycardia is rarely over 210 beats/minute, whereas supraventricular tachycardia is faster, usually occurring at 250 to 260 beats/minute. Atrial ectopic tachycardia is seen postnatally and usually exists as an intermittent, unsustained rhythm. This confusing rhythm, however, may occur for some sustained time periods (minutes or hours) at a variety of rates.
2. Bradycardias are defined by their ventricular rate, but the type of bradycardia is determined by the atrioventricular relation (Fig. 15-9). If there is a 1:1 atrioventricular relation, then sinus or ectopic atrial bradycardia may be considered. If the P–P interval (time between atrial activity) is less than the R–R interval (time between

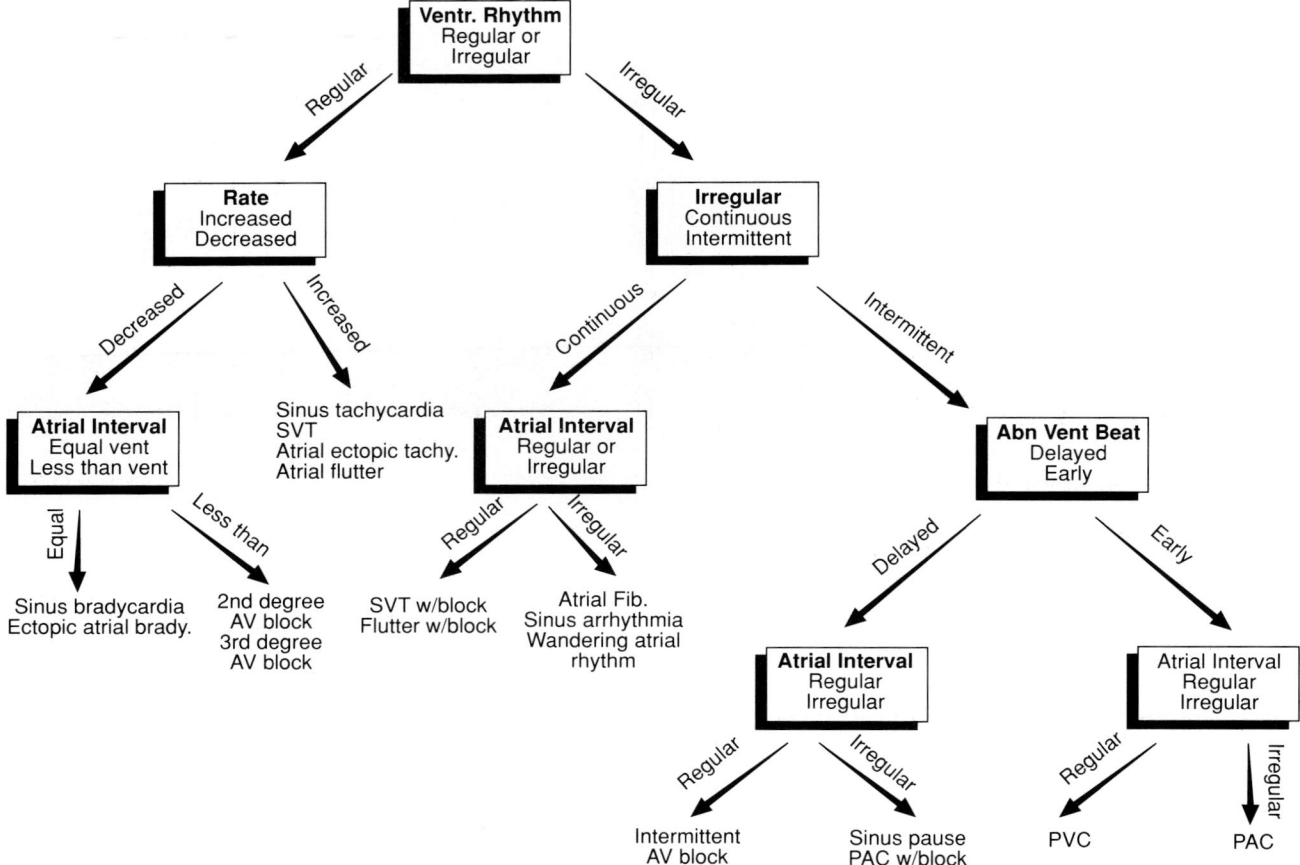

FIGURE 15-6. Algorithm of a systematic approach to rhythm analysis. AV, atrioventricular; PAC, premature atrial contractions; PVC, premature ventricular contractions; SVT, supraventricular tachycardia.

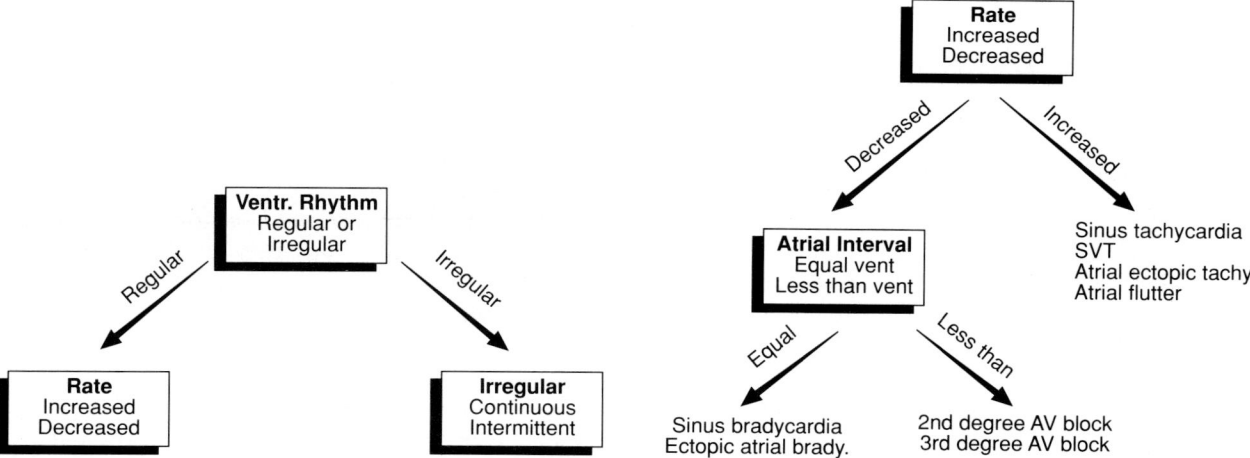

FIGURE 15-7. The top of the arrhythmia algorithm involves a decision about the regularity of ventricular activity. If the ventricular rhythm is regular, the rate is then examined. If the ventricular rhythm is irregular, the pattern of irregularity is then examined.

FIGURE 15-8. For regular arrhythmia with increased rate, the diagnosis can often be made by simply measuring the rate (see text). If the rate is decreased, the atrial and ventricular intervals need to be compared. AV, atrioventricular; SVT, supraventricular tachycardia.

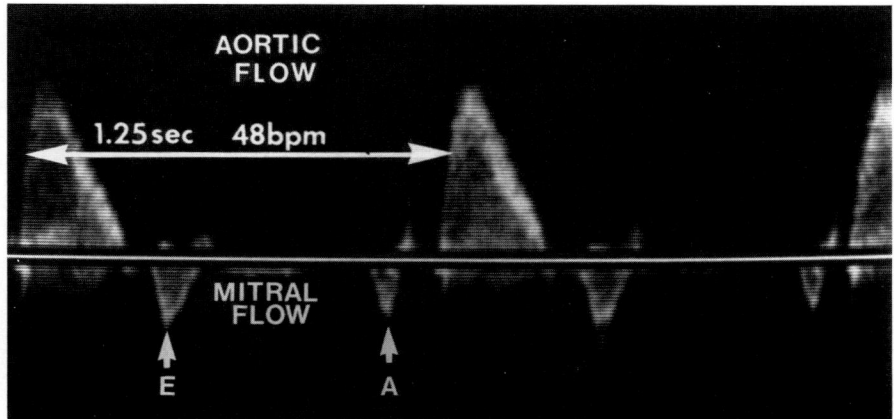

FIGURE 15-9. An example of severe sinus bradycardia that was initially thought to be heart block because of the slow ventricular rate (48 beats/min). The regular relation between the atrial activity E-wave (E) and A-wave (A) is shown on subsequent beats.

ventricular activity), then a regular, second- or third-degree heart block may be considered. If some (usually a 2 : 1 relation) atrial beats appear to conduct to the ventricle, then second-degree atrioventricular block is present. If there is no relation between the atrial and ventricular rates, then third-degree block is present.

Continuously Irregular Rhythms

Irregular heart rhythms may or may not have a regular pattern (Fig. 15-10). When irregular

rhythms exhibit a regular pattern, the atrial P–P interval is examined. If it is regular (and smaller than the R–R interval), then supraventricular tachycardia (SVT) or atrial flutter with a regular block is present. Classifying these rhythms as irregular may be somewhat confusing. SVT or atrial flutter with a regular block can be regular (Fig. 15-11) and last for extended periods. Similarly, SVT or flutter without block may come and go as the fetus goes into and out of the rhythm, thus producing irregularity. Irregular atrial activity or P–P interval is seen in atrial fibrillation, sinus arrhythmia, and wandering atrial rhythm. Atrial fibrillation usually

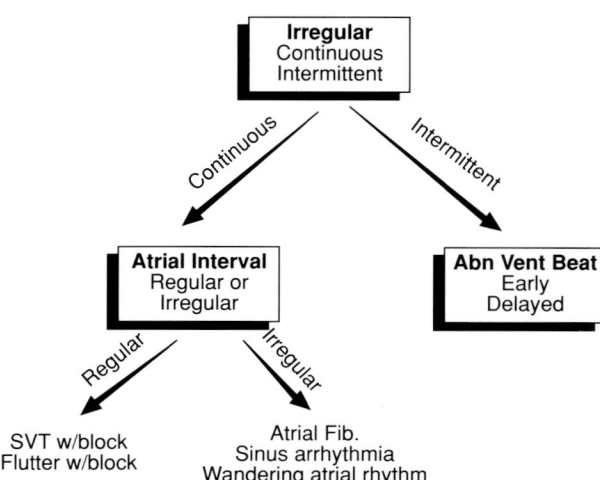

FIGURE 15-10. When the ventricular rhythm is continuously irregular, the atrial interval is then examined. Regular atrial intervals occur with supraventricular tachycardia (SVT) and atrial flutter with variable block. Irregular atrial intervals usually indicate atrial fibrillation. Intermittently irregular ventricular rate is further examined in Figure 15-12.

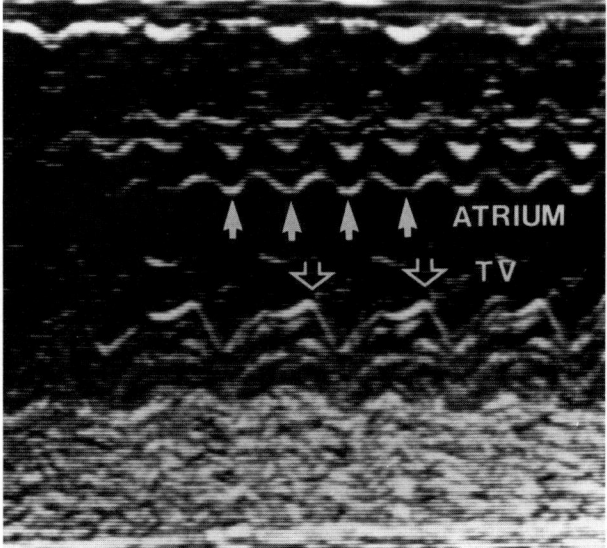

FIGURE 15-11. M-mode tracing of atrial flutter with 2 : 1 atrioventricular block. Rapid atrial contractions at a rate of 400 beats/min are shown (*solid arrows*). The tricuspid valve (TV) is shown opening only with every other atrial contraction (*open arrows*), establishing the 2 : 1 atrioventricular relation.

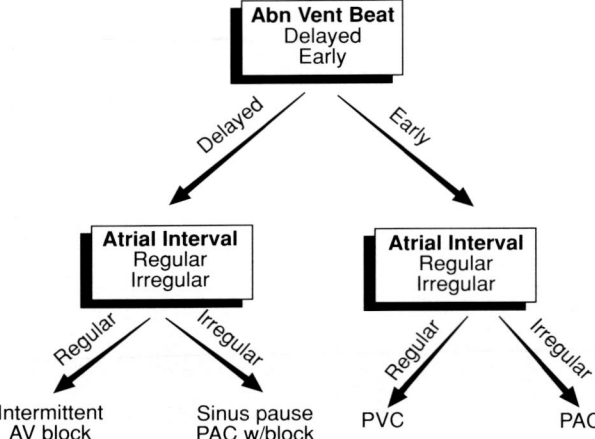

FIGURE 15-12. With irregular ventricular rhythms, a determination must be made about whether the abnormal ventricular beat is delayed or early with respect to normal (see text). AV, atrioventricular; PAC, premature atrial contractions; PVC, premature ventricular contractions.

produces a rapid and chaotic atrial rate. Sinus arrhythmia and wandering atrial rhythm are difficult, if not impossible, diagnoses to make in the fetus without actually seeing the fetal electrocardiogram.

Intermittently Irregular Rhythms

Intermittently irregular rhythms are the most common fetal arrhythmias seen, making this portion of the diagram (Fig. 15-12) the most often used. Examination of the ventricular rate should reveal that the irregular beats are occurring either early or late.

Early ventricular activity should represent either premature atrial (PAC) or ventricular (PVC) contractions. If the atrial activity is irregular, then PAC should be suspected (Figs. 15-13 and 15-14). If the atrial activity remains regular, the most likely cause is PVC (Figs. 15-15 and 15-16). Occasionally, a PVC is timed such that it is conducted in a retrograde fashion to the atria and resets the sinus node. This produces a PVC with an *irregular* atrial rate, in contradistinction to the diagram.

Delayed ventricular beats with regular atrial activity are found in intermittent atrioventricular block. This rhythm is the intermittent version of a regular, second-degree atrioventricular block (see Fig. 15-8). Irregular atrial activity produces a delayed ventricular beat in cases of sinus pause or premature atrial contraction with block.

TREATMENT

Treatment of fetal arrhythmias must be undertaken with a firm concept of the mother and fetus as a single entity (the "maternal–fetal unit"), since medical therapy is often given to the mother in hopes of achieving a therapeutic effect in the fetus. The decision for therapy involves an initial two-part decision: (1) should therapy be given? and (2) what therapy to give?

The correct rhythm diagnosis is essential to beginning the therapeutic decision process. Once this has been established, decision making can proceed in a logical fashion, as seen in Figure 15-17. This scheme is meant to be a general guideline for deciding about therapy and does not represent an established standard of care.

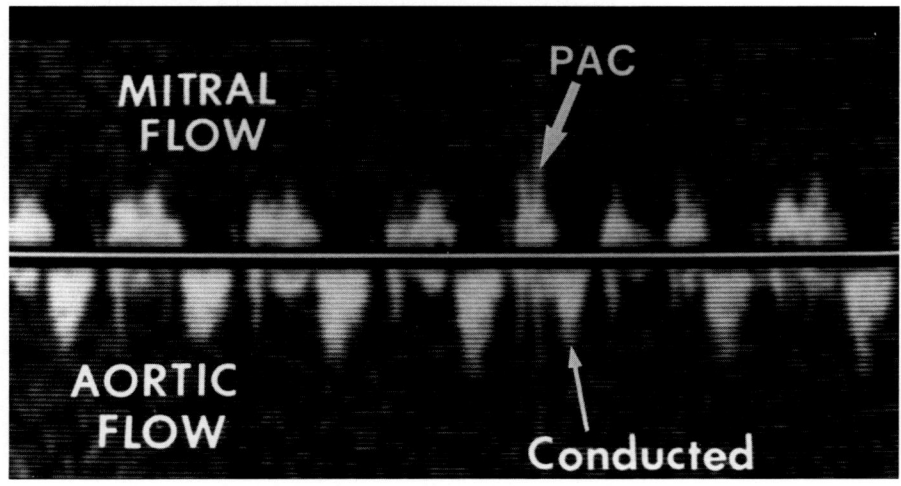

FIGURE 15-13. Doppler flow in the left ventricle during a premature atrial contraction. Four normal beats with biphasic mitral flow are followed by four normal aortic flow beats. An early beat (PAC) produces an early conducted aortic flow beat (*thin arrow*). After a compensatory pause, the regular rhythm resumes.

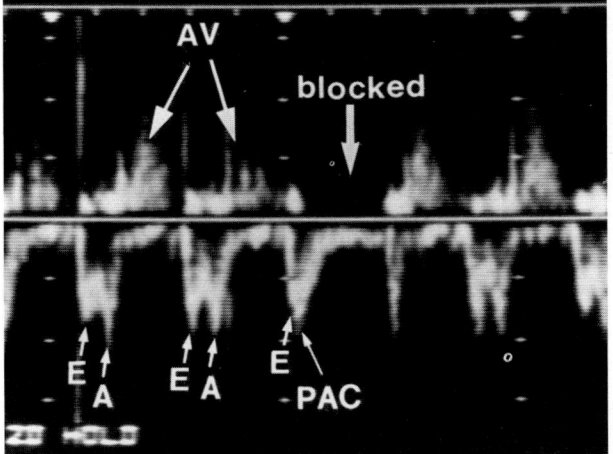

FIGURE 15-14. Doppler interrogation of a blocked, premature atrial contraction. The Doppler sample volume is in the mid-left ventricle and once again demonstrates three regular beats with normal E- and A-waves. The aortic valve (AV) flow is less distinct but follows the atrial contraction. An early atrial beat (PAC) is shown fused with the early ventricular filling (E). No aortic flow follows (blocked). A single atrial beat followed by a ventricular beat and then resumption of normal rhythm is seen after the blocked beat.

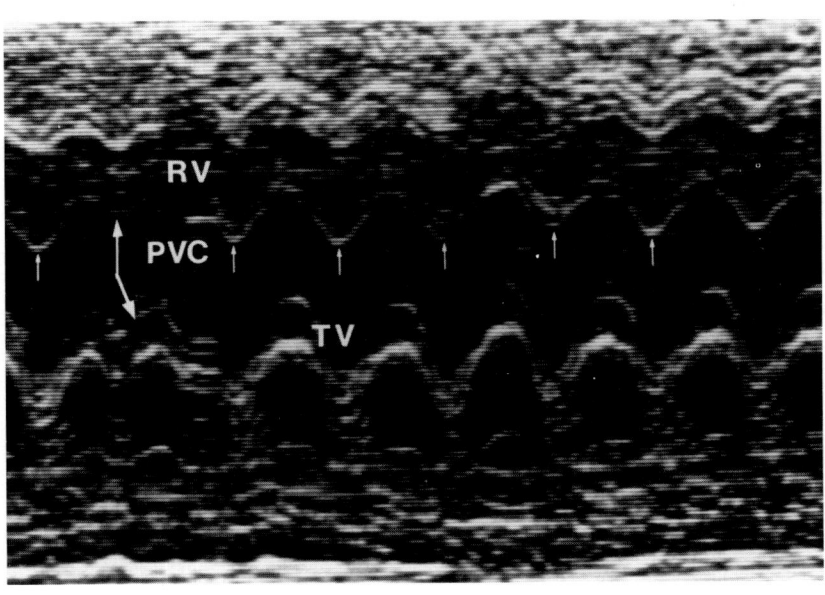

FIGURE 15-15. M-mode tracing through the right ventricle (RV) and tricuspid valve (TV). Regular ventricular contractions are seen (*small arrows*). An early and somewhat less forceful contraction (PVC) produces early closure of the tricuspid valve (*connected arrows*).

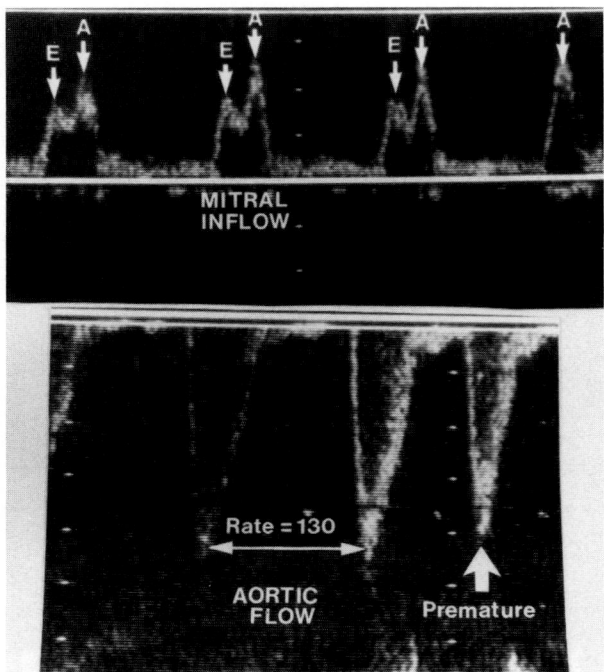

FIGURE 15-16. Nonsimultaneous Doppler tracings in the same patient from the mitral inflow position show characteristic E- and A-waves. The final beat has a solitary A-wave, which is normally timed. The E-wave is missing, presumably because of impaired mitral opening due to the premature ventricular contraction. In the lower panel, the premature ventricular beat creating a less intense and early aortic flow is shown (*thick arrow*).

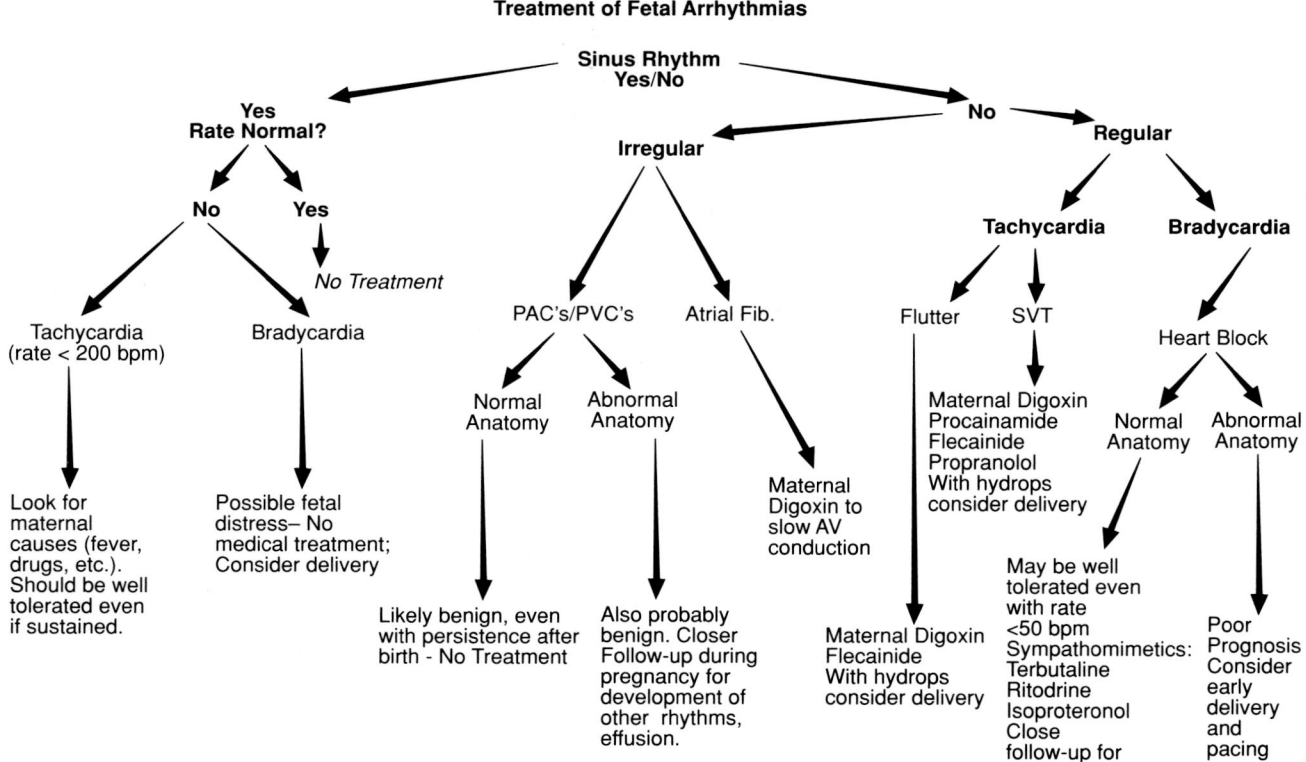

FIGURE 15-17. Schematic treatment approach to some of the more commonly encountered fetal arrhythmias. PAC, premature atrial contraction; PVC, premature ventricular contraction; SVT, supraventricular tachycardia.

The use of different types of medical therapy, the delivery route (eg, to the mother or directly to the fetus), and the relative efficacy are not firmly established in the literature.[16-22] Different groups have developed different practices and experience over time that do not result in a consensus. A thorough knowledge of the dosing, side effects, and mode of action of each of the drugs is required before clinical use.

REFERENCES

1. Elkayham U, Gleicher N: Cardiac problems in pregnancy. In Diagnosis and Management of Maternal and Fetal Disease. New York: Alan R Liss, 1990: 723–748.
2. Steinfeld L, Rappaport HL, Rossbach HC, Martinez E: Diagnosis of fetal arrhythmias using echocardiographic and Doppler techniques. J Am Coll Cardiol 1985; 8(6):1425–1432.
3. Strasburger JF, Huhta JC, Carpenter RJ, et al: Doppler echocardiography in the diagnosis and management of persistent fetal arrhythmias. J Am Coll Cardiol 1985; 7(6):1386–1391.
4. Southall DP, Richerdo J, Hardwick RA, et al: Prospective study of fetal heart rate and rhythm patterns. Arch Dis Child 1980; 55:506–511.
5. Kleinman CS, Donnerstein RL, Jaffe CC, et al: Fetal echocardiography: A tool for evaluation of in utero cardiac arrhythmias and monitoring of in utero therapy. Analysis of 71 patients. Am J Cardiol 1983; 51:237–243.
6. DeVore GR, Siassi B, Platt LD: Fetal echocardiography III. The diagnosis of cardiac arrhythmias using real-time–directed M-mode ultrasound. Am J Obstet Gynecol 1983; 146:792–799.
7. Chan FY, Woo SK, Ghosh A, et al: Prenatal diagnosis of congenital fetal arrhythmias by simultaneous pulsed Doppler velocimetry of the fetal abdominal aorta and inferior vena cava. Obstet Gynecol 1990; 76(2):200–205.
8. Garson A: Standard electrocardiograph diagnosis of dysrhythmias: The first step. In Gillette PC, Farson A (eds): Pediatric Cardiac Dysrhythmias. New York: Grune and Stratton, 1981.
9. Crowley DC, Dick M, Raybum WF, Rosenthal A: Two-dimensional and M-mode echocardiographic evaluation of fetal arrhythmia. Clin Cardiol 1985; 8:1–10.
10. D'Cruz IA, Prabhu R, Cohen HC, Glick G: Echocardiographic features of second degree atrioventricular block. Chest 1977; 72:459–464.
11. Fujii J, Foster JR, Mills PG, et al: Dual echocardiographic determination of atrial contraction sequence in atrial flutter and other related arrhythmias. Circulation 1978; 58:314–319.
12. Petsas AA, Pinto R, Mower MM: Mitral valve motion in atrial tachycardia with block. Chest 1974; 66:182–185.
13. Prabhu R, D'Cruz IA, Cohen HC, Glick G: Echocardiographic correlates of atrial contraction in normal and abnormal rhythm. Prog Cardiovasc Dis 1978; 20:436–440.
14. Procacci PM, Levites R, Kotter MN, Anderson GJ: Dissimilar atrial rhythms diagnosed by echocardiography. Chest 1978; 73:429–431.
15. Zoneraich S, Zoneraich O, Rhel JJ: Echocardiographic findings in atrial flutter. Circulation 1975; 52:455–458.
16. Kleinman CS: Prenatal diagnosis and management of intrauterine arrhythmias. Fetal Ther 1986; 1:92–95.
17. Martin GS, Ruckman RN: Fetal echocardiography: A large clinical experience and follow-up. J Am Soc Echocardiogr 1990; 3:4–8.
18. Silverman NS, Enderlein MA, Stanger P, et al: Recognition of fetal arrhythmias by echocardiography. J Clin Ultrasound 1985; 13:255–263.
19. Allan LD, Crawford DC, Anderson RH, Tyran M: Evaluation and treatment of fetal arrhythmias. Clin Cardiol 1984; 7:467–473.
20. Wiggins JW, Bowes W, Clewell W, et al: Echocardiographic diagnosis and intravenous digoxin management of fetal tachyarrhythmias and congestive heart failure. Am J Dis Child 1986; 140:202–204.
21. Azancot-Benisty A, Jacqz-Aigrain E, Guirgis NM, et al: Clinical and pharmacologic study of fetal supraventricular tachyarrhythmias. J Pediatr 1992; 121:608–613.
22. Schmidt KG, Ulmer HE, Silverman NH, et al: Perinatal outcome of fetal complete atrioventricular block: A multicenter experience. J Am Coll Cardiol 1991; 17:1360–1366.

John P. McGahan and Manuel Porto:
DIAGNOSTIC OBSTETRICAL ULTRASOUND.
© 1994 J.B. Lippincott Company.

Ralph M. Steiger   Manuel Porto

Chapter *16*

The Anterior Abdominal Wall

The focus of this chapter is the group of anomalies that result from defective closure of the ventral abdominal wall. These anomalies include omphalocele, gastroschisis, and rare defects such as body stalk anomaly and exstrophy of the bladder and cloaca. Patients with cloacal exstrophy usually have an omphalocele. The incidence of these disorders (Table 16-1) increases significantly when the sonographer participates in a selective screening program, such as α-fetoprotein screening, in which case ventral wall defects are the second most common lesion after neural tube defects.[7] Some cystic lesions of the proximal umbilical cord and anterior abdominal wall that may be confused with omphalocele also are discussed; these include persistent urachus, allantoic cysts, and omphalomesenteric cysts.

The fetal abdomen is bounded superiorly by the diaphragm, posteriorly by the back and retroperitoneum, inferiorly by the pelvic bones and pelvic diaphragm, and anteriorly by the ventral abdominal wall. Open defects of these boundaries are unique to the diaphragm and ventral wall. A diaphragmatic hernia may coexist with an omphalocele. Diaphragmatic hernias are covered in Chapter 11. Abnormalities of the pelvic floor are extremely uncommon, although it is feasible to see the separation of the pubic bones with absence of the pubic symphysis in bladder and cloacal exstrophy.[8]

It is difficult to approach this subject without a brief discussion of the abnormal development involved. *Body stalk anomaly* can arise from failed closure of the lateral body folds in embryogenesis[9] (Fig. 16-1). Alternate hypotheses for the development of the body stalk anomaly include early rupture of the amnion at 4 to 5 weeks of gestation, possibly leading to mechanical compression of the body against the placenta before closure of the lateral folds.[10] A third theory is that body stalk anomaly is a severe form of amniotic band syndrome.

Incomplete closure of the lateral body folds may also be partially responsible for *omphalocele*, but more typically failure of the bowel to return to the abdomen after the normal herniation into the cord at 8 weeks of gestation is held to be responsible[11] (Fig. 16-2). *Gastroschisis* is thought to arise from the occlusion of the right omphalomesenteric artery early in embryonic life, leading to infarction of the right anterior abdominal wall.[12] *Exstrophy of the*

TABLE 16-1.   Abdominal Wall Defects and Associated Rate of Occurrence

Defect	Frequency	Reference
Omphalocele	1/5000	1, 2
Gastroschisis	1/12,000	1, 2, 3
Body stalk anomaly	1/15,000	4
Exstrophy of bladder	1/30,000	5
Exstrophy of cloaca	1/200,000	6

bladder and *cloaca* is thought to result from persistence of the cloacal membrane, inhibiting normal development of the lower anterior abdominal wall, symphysis pubis, and perineum (Fig. 16-3). If the urorectal septum fails to develop completely as well, the bladder and hindgut continue to communicate with each other in a common chamber (the cloaca), and the anus remains imperforate (Fig. 16-4). Cloacal and bladder exstrophy or eversion results when the cloacal membrane finally breaks down.[13]

NORMAL ANATOMY

Standards

The American Institute of Ultrasound has issued recommended guidelines for ultrasound in pregnancy, which include the following statement. During the second and third trimester of pregnancy, "the study should include, but not necessarily be limited to, the following fetal anatomy: . . . stomach, urinary bladder, umbilical cord insertion site on the anterior abdominal wall. . . ."[14] This statement essentially delineates the minimal standard views of the abdomen that are necessary to visualize the defects discussed in this chapter. The stomach, bladder, and umbilicus must be seen. The contour of the abdomen should also be studied. The normal approach is as follows:

The fetal abdomen is generally viewed in serial transverse planes. The smooth contour of the abdominal wall should be noted as one scans from one end of the abdomen to the other. On the inner aspect of the abdominal wall is a thin, 1- to 3-mm anechoic zone that is the muscle tissue of the abdominal wall. This should not be confused with

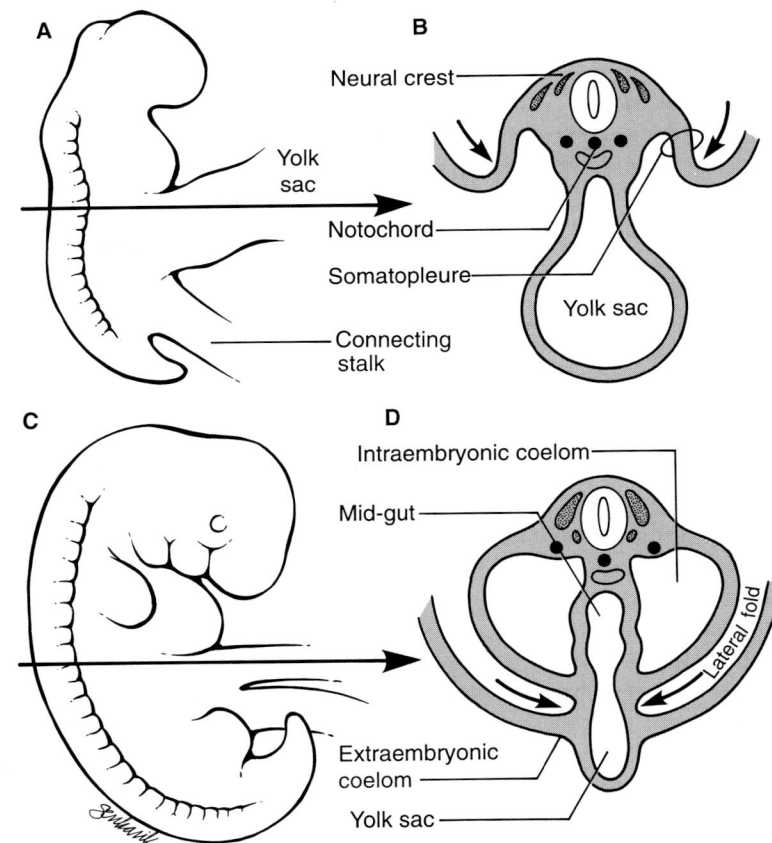

FIGURE 16-1. Normal closure of the lateral body folds. Failure to close may result in the body stalk anomaly without an umbilical cord (body stalk) between the abdominal wall and the placenta. (Modified from Moore KL [ed]: The embryonic period. In The Developing Human, 3rd ed. Philadelphia: WB Saunders, 1982: 71)

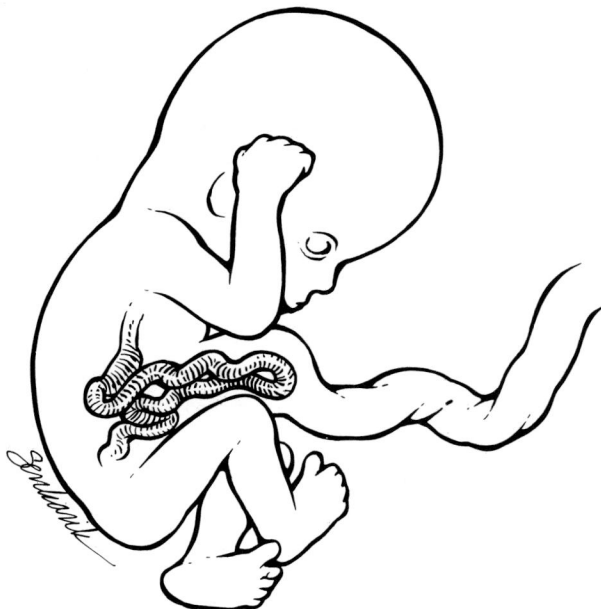

FIGURE 16-2. Normal gut migration. The bowel normally herniates into the base of the umbilical cord between 8 and 12 menstrual weeks and returns to the abdominal cavity by 12 weeks. This early herniation should not be confused with an omphalocele. (Modified from Cyr DR, Bach LA, Schoeneker SA, et al: Bowel migration in the normal fetus: US detection. Radiology 1986; 1961:119.)

ascites because it is smooth and not crescent-shaped, as is ascites when bounded by bowel. This anechoic zone can also be noted to be continuous with the ribs. After identifying the fetal stomach and bladder, the umbilicus should be identified. This can be difficult in situations in which the extremities are close to the abdominal wall. The level of difficulty is increased when the fetus is prone and in the third trimester, when there is relatively less amniotic fluid. The location of the umbilicus can be inferred in these situations by identifying the umbilical vein in the upper abdomen and following it caudally until it approaches the abdominal wall and finally disappears from the abdomen. This point of disappearance should be at or just below the umbilicus. Sagittal views can also be helpful in following the umbilical vein and studying the contour of the abdominal wall. When possible, visualization of the proximal umbilical cord with enumeration of the vessels is ideal to rule out cystic lesions of the umbilical cord, such as a patent urachus. The umbilicus can be a good place to count the vessels, with the two umbilical arteries coming in from the lower abdomen and the vein entering from the upper abdomen. Cloacal ex-

strophy is usually associated with a single umbilical artery.[13] As a word of caution, some of the omphaloceles associated with chromosomal defects can be small[15] (Fig. 16-5).

Artifacts

Common artifacts that can be mistaken for abdominal wall defects are listed in Table 16-2.

1. The bowel normally herniates into the proximal umbilical cord in the 8th menstrual week but returns to the abdomen during the 12th week.[10] The diagnosis of omphalocele or gastroschisis can be made at or after 13 weeks of gestation[16–18] (see Fig. 16-2).
2. Oblique views of the fetus can give the false impression of an omphalocele. This is especially true in the flexed fetus with decreased amniotic fluid (Fig. 16-6). Viewing the abdomen in the proper plane when the fetus is at rest with the spine relatively straight, and also noting subcutaneous fat covering the anterior abdominal wall, usually resolves this problem.
3. Normal umbilical cord can be confused with gastroschisis in the fetus when the umbilical cord is bunched and compressed against the abdomen. This confusion may be worsened if the cord is large or has large umbilical veins. The use of color Doppler studies quickly resolves this if flow cannot be otherwise appreciated.
4. Localized deposition of Wharton's jelly at the umbilicus can lead to the impression of a small omphalocele,[19] but the mass is hyperechoic, not anechoic, as with bowel in an omphalocele, and the vessels run through it, not around it. Omphaloceles with predominately liver contents are also hyperechoic, but these defects are larger.
5. Focal masses of the umbilical cord, such as omphalomesenteric cysts or allantoic cysts, may be confused with abdominal wall defects. These cysts can occur in conjunction with abdominal wall defects and are reviewed in more detail in Chapter 7.

THE ABNORMAL VENTRAL WALL

The two levels of approach to the diagnosis of ventral wall defects are detection and diagnosis. The first level is the outcome of a careful and thorough

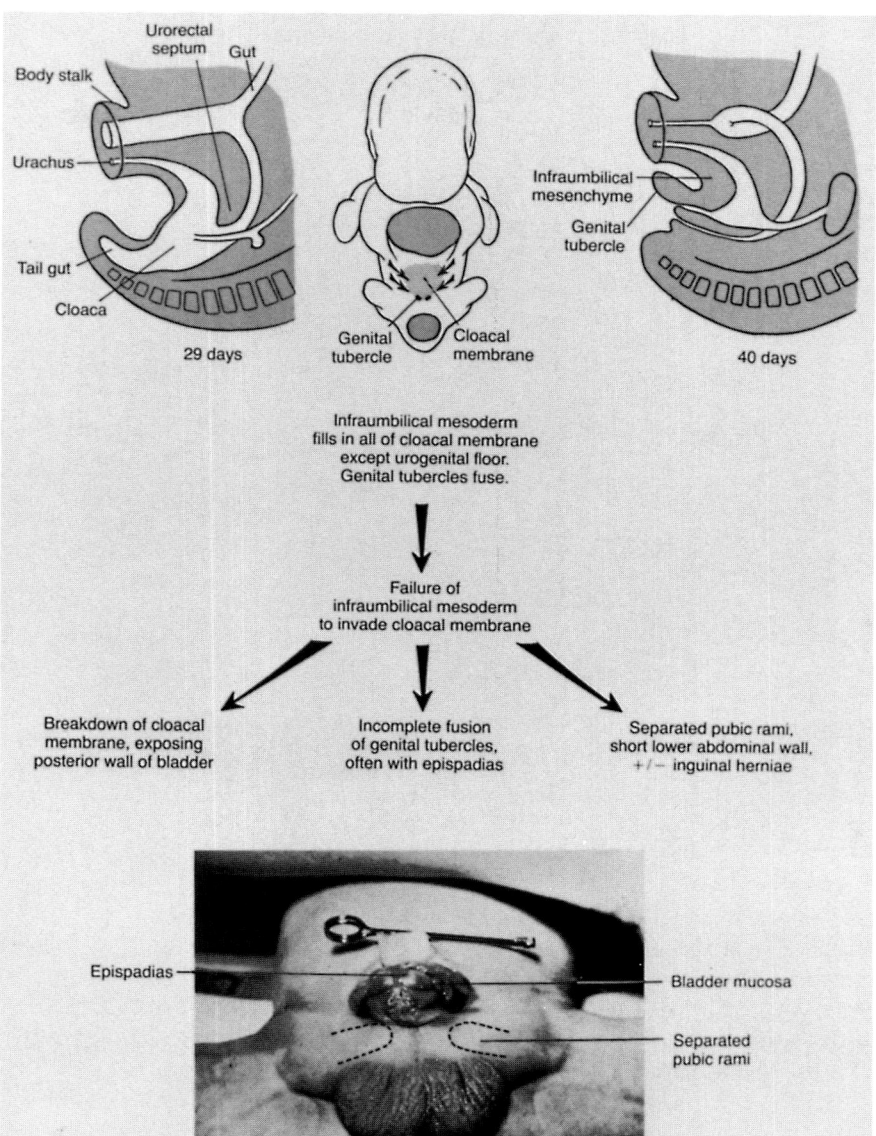

FIGURE 16-3. Exstrophy of the bladder sequence. Normally, the infraumbilical mesenchyme migrates to give rise to the abdominal wall, genital tubercle, and pubic rami. Failure of migration leads to exposed bladder wall, incomplete fusion of the genital tubercle, and separation of the pubic rami. (Jones KL [ed]: Smith's Recognizable Pattern of Human Malformations, 4th ed. Philadelphia: WB Saunders, 1988: 567)

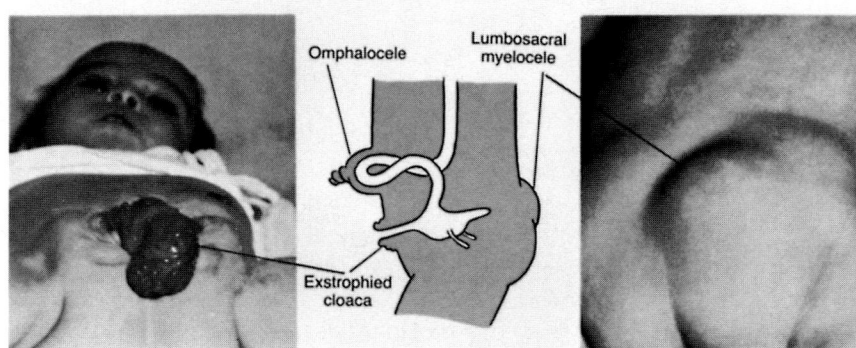

FIGURE 16-4. Developmental sequence of cloacal exstrophy. Normally, the mesoderm contributes to the (1) infraumbilical mesenchyme, (2) cloacal septum, and (3) caudal vertebra. Defective development of the early mesoderm leads to exstrophy of the cloacae with omphalocele and lumbosacral myelocele, as outlined above. (Jones KL [ed]: Smith's Recognizable Pattern of Human Malformations, 4th ed. Philadelphia: WB Saunders, 1988: 569.)

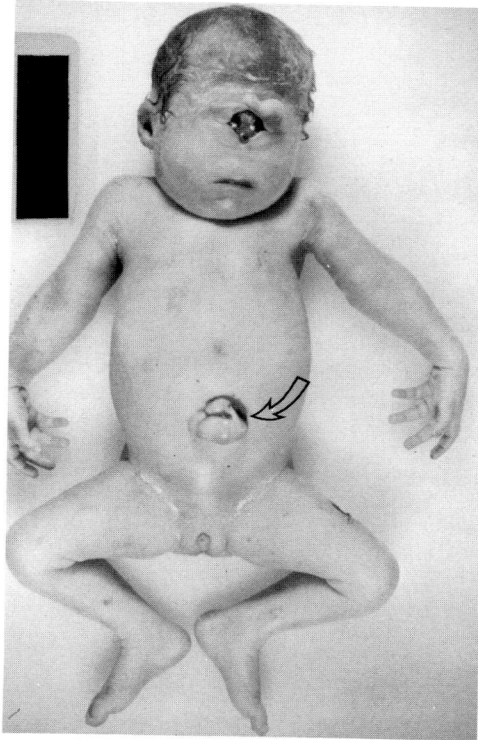

FIGURE 16-5. Typical facial features of trisomy 13 with cyclopia, proboscis, and very small bowel containing omphalocele (*arrow*). (Courtesy of John P. McGahan, MD, Sacramento, CA.)

survey of fetal anatomy as outlined previously. Detection can be greatly aided by an organized α-fetoprotein screening program; this is discussed separately. Once a lesion is detected, the examination is focused to determine the exact nature and extent of the lesion as well as the presence of associated anomalies. This is critical in predicting the

TABLE 16-2. Artifacts Commonly Confused With Ventral Wall Defects

Artifact	Comment
Bowel herniation into umbilical cord	Normally present at 8–12 menstrual weeks
Oblique fetal abdomen (pseudoomphalocele)	Note elongated rather than oval shape of abdomen
Normal umbilical cord	Doppler or color to check for flow
Localized Wharton's jelly	Hyperechoic appearance with vessels transversing
Cord cysts or masses	Focal lesions of cord (see Chapter 7)

prognosis of the fetus and the relative need for karyotype determination.

An outline to the approach of ventral wall defects is given in Table 16-3 and is presented in more detail here. First, it is important to localize the site of the defect in relation to the umbilicus. If a break in the contour of the abdominal wall or herniation of abdominal contents is detected, then the approximate site of the defect must be determined. When it is at the level of the umbilicus, it is either a gastroschisis or omphalocele. Lesions that extend below the umbilicus suggest exstrophy of the bladder or cloaca. *Cantrell's pentalogy* is an omphalocele with a defect extending upward toward the thorax, which includes a herniated heart (ectopia cordis).[20] This defect is presented in Chapter 12. When the ventral wall defect is so large that it is hard to tell where it begins or ends, then a body stalk anomaly should be suspected (Fig. 16-7).

When the herniated abdominal contents include bowel, the lesion is either a gastroschisis, omphalocele, or body stalk anomaly (Table 16-4). Omphaloceles and gastroschisis are the most common abnormalities and have distinguishing features and important differential points (Table 16-5). *Omphaloceles* can contain only liver on occasion but more typically also include portions of bowel (Figs. 16-8 through 16-10). Omphaloceles may contain liver that appears solid with hepatic vessels, small bowel that appears echogenic, or other intraabdominal contents, such as the stomach or gallbladder (see Fig. 16-9). Omphaloceles that contain only bowel and no liver are more often associated with karyotypic abnormalities (see Fig. 16-5). Ascites may be seen with omphaloceles (see Fig. 16-9). An omphalocele herniates through the umbilicus into the cord, creating a sac that is bounded by a thin membrane consisting of peritoneum and amnion. The presence of this sac is the easiest way to differentiate between omphalocele and gastroschisis (see Fig. 16-9). Unfortunately, this sac ruptures about 15% of the time.[21] Localization of the umbilicus and its vessels in relation to the defect is then important. The ventral wall defect is on the right side of the umbilical vessels in *gastroschisis* (Figs. 16-11 through 16-13). The umbilical vessels come off the top of an omphalocele. Herniated liver in a gastroschisis has only been reported infrequently.[22] The presence of a herniated liver in a ventral wall defect without a limiting membrane is more suggestive of a *ruptured omphalocele*. Extraabdominal and intraabdominal bowel obstruction is more common to gastroschisis, so that dilated bowel loops suggest gastroschisis (Fig. 16-14). Dis-

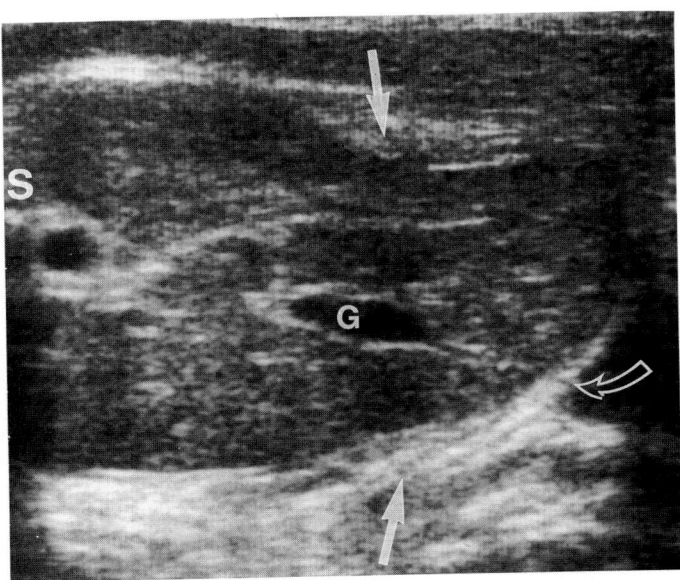

FIGURE 16-6. Pseudoomphalocele. Oblique scan through the compressed abdomen demonstrates an apparent omphalocele in the anterior abdominal wall, which was not in fact an omphalocele but compression of the anterior abdominal wall (*arrows*). Note echogenic subcutaneous fat (*curved arrow*), which is noted to cover the anterior abdominal wall in this defect. Also, anechoic muscle layer is noted just below this. Neither layer would be present in true omphalocele. (Courtesy of John P. McGahan, MD, Sacramento, CA.)

tinguishing features that separate gastroschisis from omphalocele are listed in Table 16-5.

The diagnostic features of the *body stalk anomaly* are the large ventral wall defect, absence of the umbilical cord (the body stalk), and presence of fetal scoliosis from immobilization of the mid-trunk (see Fig. 16-7). The absence of the umbilical cord can be difficult to confirm because the umbilical vessels usually travel together along the edge of the membranes. The vessels, however, are amazingly straight because torsion of the cord is not possible.[23] (This is covered in Chapter 7.) The high incidence of amputation defects of extremities from amniotic bands in body stalk anomaly has led to the synonym *limb–body–wall complex* (see Fig. 16-7).

When there is a defect below the umbilicus, consider *exstrophy of the bladder*. The presence of this defect and a persistently absent fetal bladder are diagnostic of this condition (see Fig. 16-3). The diagnosis should also be actively pursued when a normal bladder is persistently absent and the kidneys appear normal. Although bladder exstrophy is several times more common than cloacal exstrophy, it appears to have been diagnosed antenatally only once.[24] In this one case a solid 5-cm mass was seen protruding from the anterior abdominal wall below the umbilicus in the absence of a fetal bladder. This finding was not observed until 36 weeks of gestation despite a prior scan at 15 weeks. It may be that eversion of the bladder is not evident early in pregnancy. The ability to see the everted bladder is not possible if there has not been a breakdown of the cloacal membrane, but if the outflow of urine is still possible, then the lesion appears as a normal bladder. Once there is eversion of the bladder, the typical anechoic internal fetal bladder should not be seen. There is separation of the pubic bones with absence of the symphysis in both cloacal and bladder exstrophy, but this has only occasionally been noted antenatally.

The presentation of *cloacal exstrophy* is much more complex. Cloacal exstrophy, in addition to being the rarest of ventral wall defects, is also the most complex and varied in its sonographic appearance. There are about 17 fetuses with cloacal exstrophy who had ultrasound examinations before birth, and among these, there are only about 14 with adequate description of ultrasound findings.[8,25–34] Only 30% of the cases were noted to have a ventral wall defect, and these were almost all thought to be omphaloceles, which are frequently seen in the disorder. A lower abdominal

TABLE 16-3.   Site of Ventral Wall Defects in Relation to Umbilicus

1. Above umbilicus: consider pentalogy of Cantrell
2. At umbilicus: consider gastroschisis or omphalocele
3. Below umbilicus: Consider exstrophy of bladder or cloaca
4. Difficult to tell because of size: consider body stalk anomaly

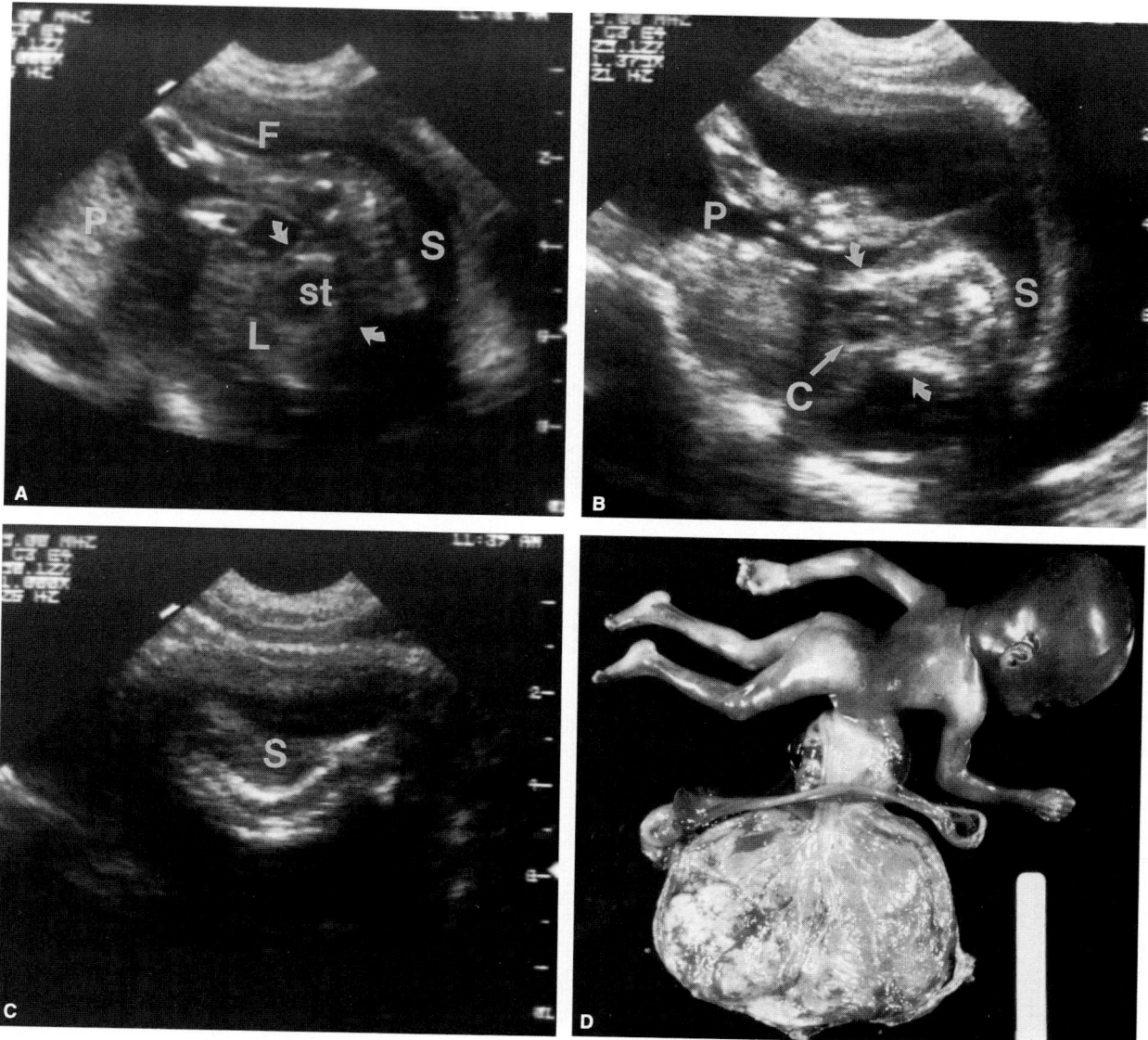

FIGURE 16-7. Body stalk anomaly. **(A)** Oblique sagittal view through the leg and spine shows the waste of the ventral wall defect (*arrows*), with the defect containing stomach (st) and liver (L). **(B)** Transverse view through the thorax demonstrates the waste of the defect (*arrows*). The cardiac silhouette (C) noted in defect is contiguous with the placenta (P). S, spine. **(C)** Coronal view through the fetal spine (S) demonstrates typical scoliosis. **(D)** Postmortem specimen demonstrates defect in the anterior abdominal wall, which is contiguous with the placenta.

TABLE 16-4. Initial Approach to Ventral Wall Defect

I. Bowel involved
    A. Contained in sac → Omphalocele, unless
       1. Large defect, no separate cord, → Body stalk anomaly
         fetal scoliosis
       2. Bladder persistently not seen, → Cloacal exstrophy
         neural tube defect present
    B. Not contained in sac—cord to left → Gastroschisis, unless
       side
       1. Liver involved → Probable ruptured omphalocele
       2. Malformations other than bowel → Probable ruptured omphalocele
      (Dilated bowel loops are consistent with obstruction and imply gastroschisis.)
II. Solid mass
    A. Smooth border
       1. Large → Probably omphalocele with liver
       2. Relatively small with umbilical → Umbilical cord
        vessels, no bowel
    B. Irregular border, below umbilicus → Bladder exstrophy
III. Large septate cystic mass in lower → Cloacal exstrophy
    abdomen or pelvis; neural tube defect
    present

wall defect consistent with exstrophy of the cloaca was thought to be seen on only three occasions in the literature[8,34] and once at our institution (Fig. 16-15). The most common finding (54%) was that of a large cystic mass in the pelvis or abdomen, frequently noted to be septate and not usually protruding from the anterior abdominal wall. This cyst may be accompanied by hydronephrosis and oligohydramnios in most cases and is not infrequently misinterpreted as an obstructed bladder outflow tract. These cystic structures technically are more likely to represent a persistent cloaca

TABLE 16-5. Important Distinguishing Factors Between Gastroschisis and Omphalocele

Gastroschisis	Omphalocele
Right-sided, paraumbilical	Umbilical
Free-floating bowel	Defect covered by peritoneum and amnion
Liver in defect—extremely rare	Liver in defect—common
Bowel obstruction (intra- or extraabdominal)—common	Bowel obstruction—rare
Associated anomalies—extremely rare	Associated anomalies—common, especially cardiac
Chromosomes—aneuploidy not increased	Chromosomes—frequently abnormal
Associated syndromes—rare	Associated syndromes—common (see Table 16-6)

than cloacal exstrophy, but the diagnosis is based on the findings at the time of birth. Ascites was noted 38% of the time, as were neural tube defects. Neural tube defects are thought to be uniformly present in cloacal exstrophy. The presence of a lumbar sacral neural tube defect in the presence of an omphalocele or in the absence of a bladder should lead to suspicion of cloacal exstrophy. In at least one case, ascites was noted to predate the development of the abdominal cyst.[32]

A sequence of events may be used to attempt to explain the varied sonographic presentations of cloacal exstrophy. In cases of cloacal exstrophy, the cloacal membrane initially remains intact. The cloaca may leak as urine fills it and cause ascites, possibly through the fallopian tubes attached to the cloaca, as proposed by Petrikovsky and colleagues.[32] If there is no leak, or after the leak seals, the cloaca becomes distended and, in turn, the kidneys show changes consistent with hydronephrosis. The incomplete urorectal septum causes the cyst to appear septate. The cloacal membrane may then rupture, leading to the classic findings of cloacal exstrophy. When the membrane does not rupture, it is preferable to refer to the abdominal cyst as a persistent cloaca or cloacal cyst. There is documentation by serial ultrasound of rupture of the persistent cloacal membrane.[8] Omphaloceles have not been seen in the presence of the cloacal cysts. A normal fetal bladder was seen only once, and it

(text continues on page 338)

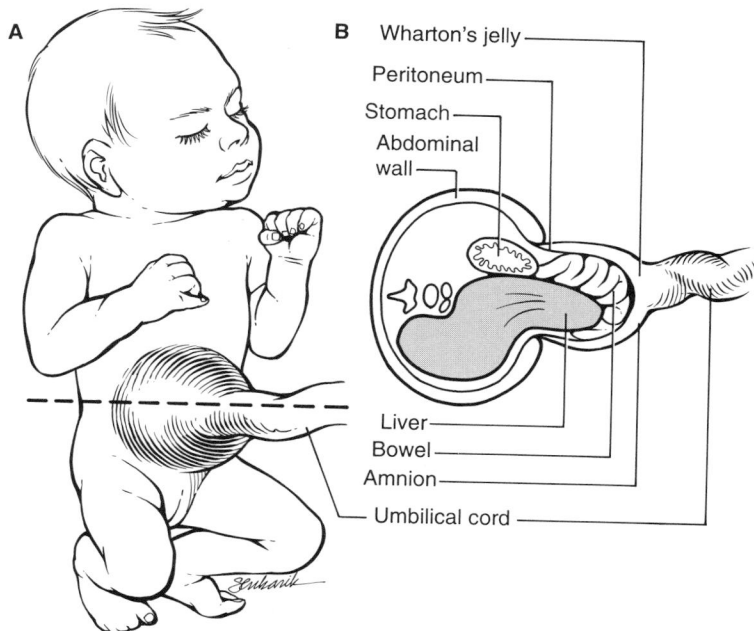

FIGURE 16-8. Typical features of omphalocele containing liver and bowel on external examination **(A)** and cross-sectional **(B)** view. This defect, unlike gastroschisis, is covered by both the amnion and peritoneum and can contain a number of structures, including the liver, bowel, and fetal stomach. (Modified from Callen PW [ed]: Ultrasonography in Obstetrics and Gynecology, 2nd ed. Philadelphia: WB Saunders, 1988: 245.)

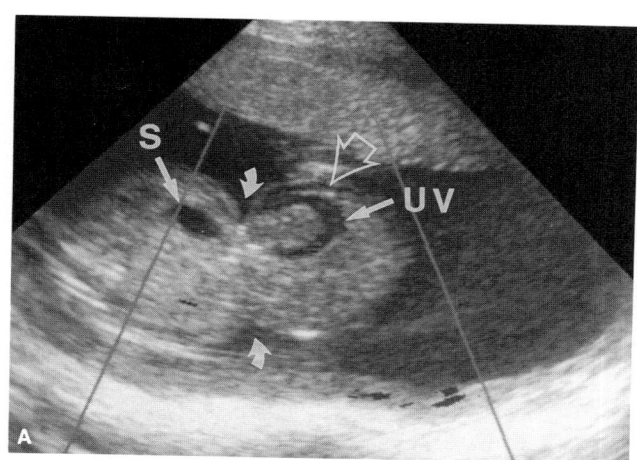

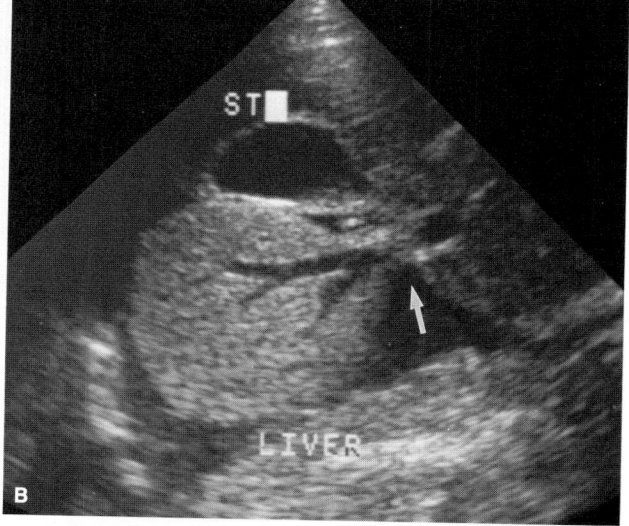

FIGURE 16-9. Variable appearance of omphalocele. **(A)** Typical appearance of liver containing omphalocele with a figure-eight appearance of the omphalocele, as noted on transverse scan of the abdomen. Note the acute angle of the omphalocele with the anterior abdominal wall (*curved arrows*). Also note the small amount of abdominal ascites (*open arrow*) between the liver and the peritoneal or amniotic membrane covering the omphalocele. UV, umbilical vein, S, stomach. **(B)** Both stomach (ST) and liver are herniated in this large abdominal defect. Note the acute angle of the defect with the anterior abdominal wall (*arrow*). **(C)** Typical omphalocele with peritoneal or amniotic membrane noted (*arrows*) covering the herniated liver (L) and gallbladder (G). Note the small amount of ascites between the liver and the covering membranes. Note the acute angle of the defect with anterior abdominal wall (*curved arrow*). (Courtesy of John P. McGahan, MD, Sacramento, CA.)

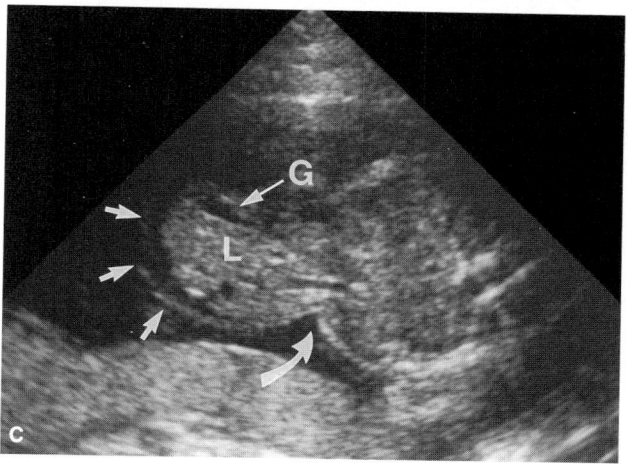

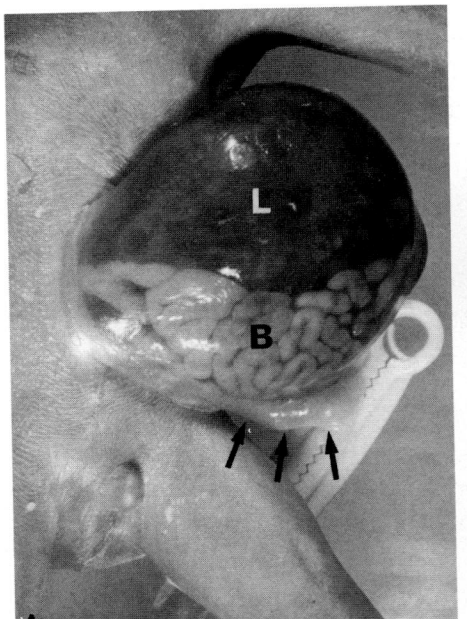
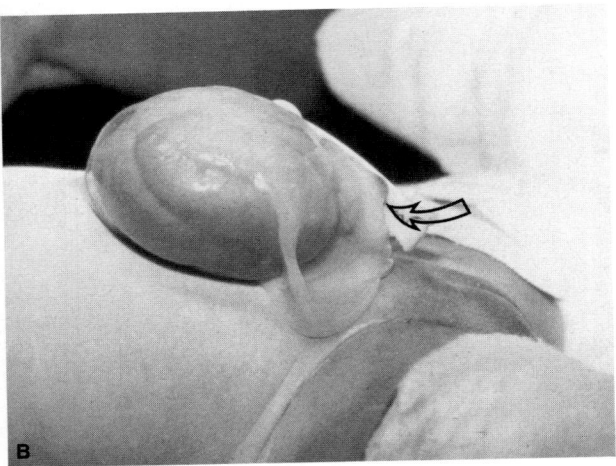

FIGURE 16-10.   (A) Omphalocele containing both liver (L) and bowel (B). Umbilical cord is marked with arrows. **(B)** Small bowel containing omphalocele. Umbilical cord is marked with curved arrow. (Courtesy of Marshall Z. Schwartz, MD, Children's Hospital, Pittsburgh, PA.)

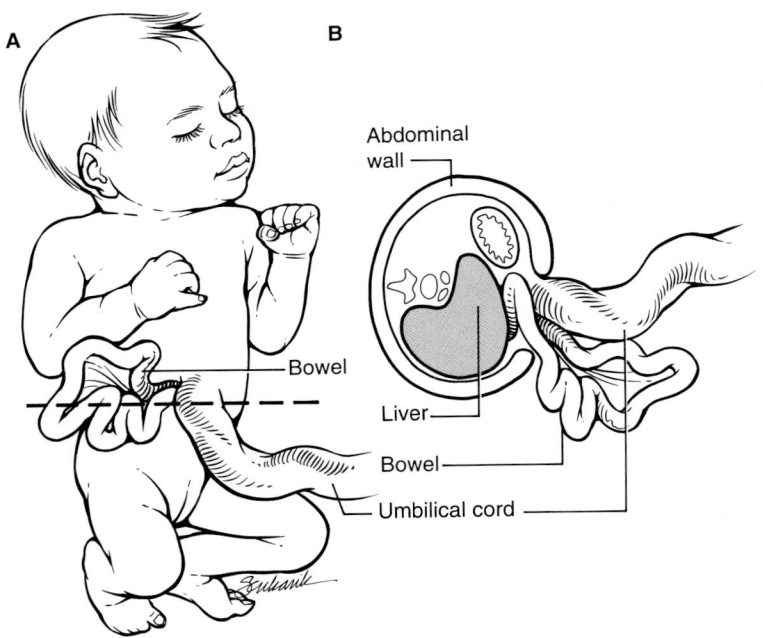

FIGURE 16-11. Typical features of gastroschisis demonstrated on both external examination **(A)** and cross-sectional **(B)** view. The ventral wall defect is right paraumbilical, with bowel loops floating free in the amniotic fluid. (Modified from Callen PW [ed]: Ultrasonography in Obstetrics and Gynecology, 2nd ed. Philadelphia: WB Saunders, 1988: 241.)

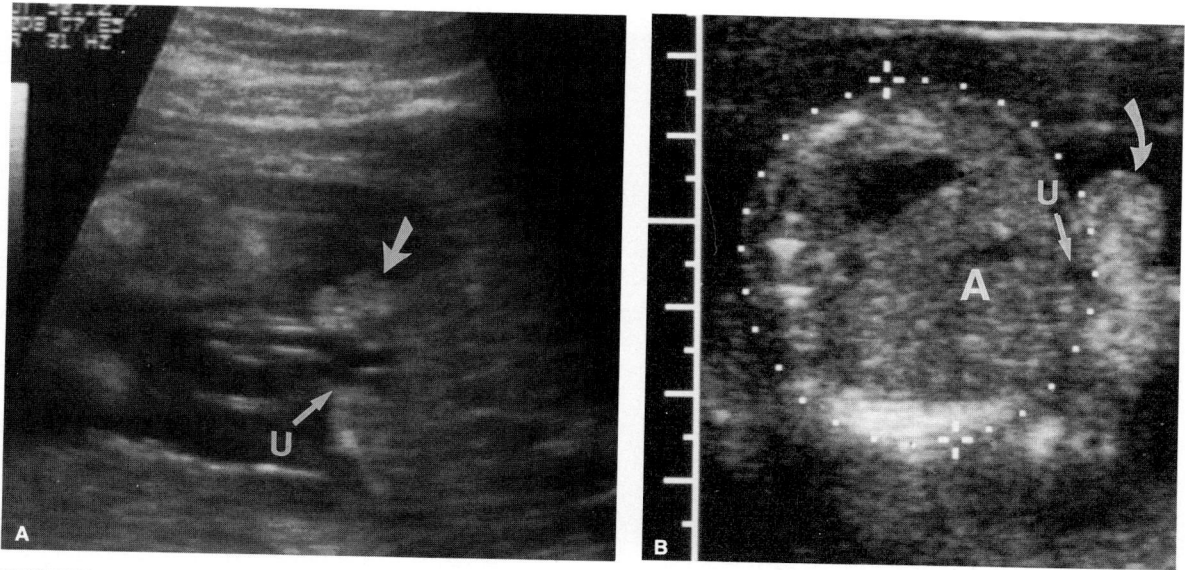

FIGURE 16-12.   Gastroschisis. **(A)** Scan through the anterior abdominal wall demonstrates a small amount of echogenic bowel (*arrow*) herniated to the right of the umbilical insertion site (U). **(B)** Transverse scan through the abdomen (A) demonstrates echogenic, free-floating loops of bowel (*curved arrow*) that have herniated to the right of the umbilical vein (U), representing gastroschisis. (Courtesy of John P. McGahan, MD, Sacramento, CA.)

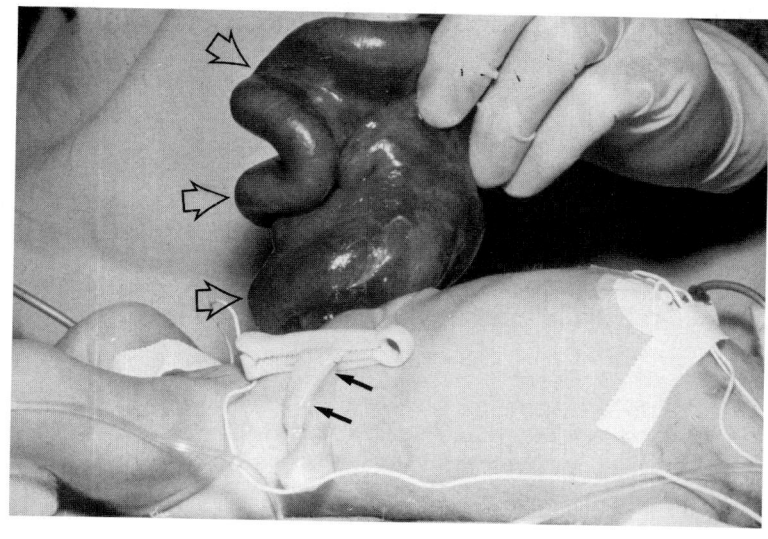

FIGURE 16-13.   Gross examination of gastroschisis at the time of delivery demonstrates right paraumbilical defect with loops of bowel (*open arrows*). Closed arrows point to umbilical cord. (Courtesy of Marshall Z. Schwartz, MD, Children's Hospital, Pittsburgh, PA.)

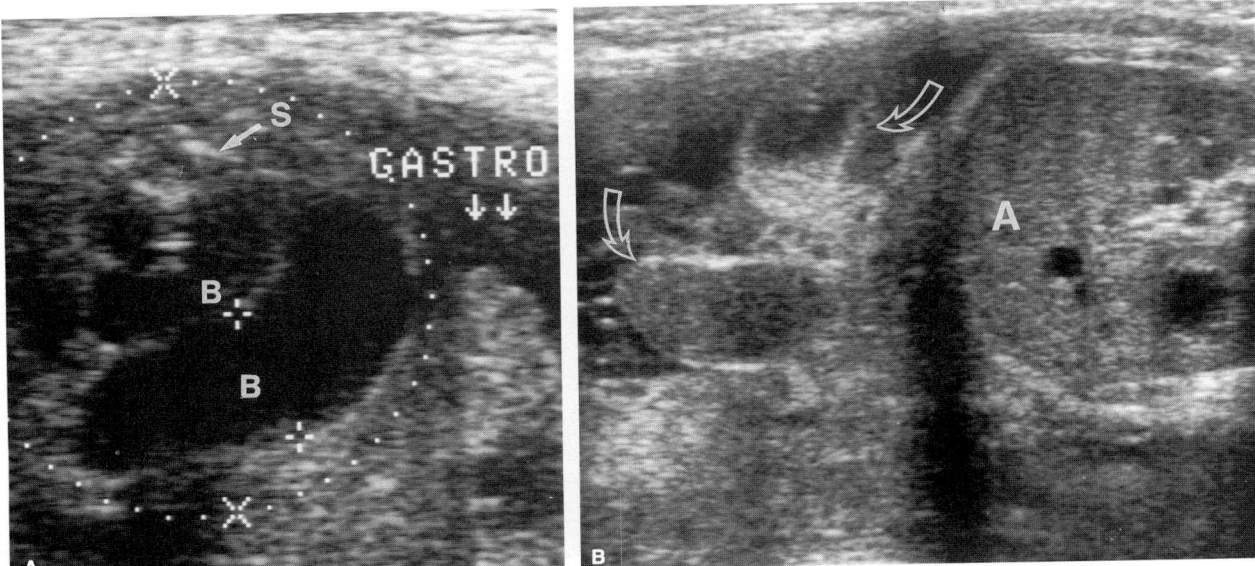

FIGURE 16-14. Gastroschisis with bowel obstruction. **(A)** Third-trimester intraabdominal bowel obstruction as noted by dilated loops of bowel (B) is associated with fetal gastroschisis (Gastro). S, spine. **(B)** Transverse scan through the fetal abdomen (A) demonstrates free-floating loops of bowel that became distended (*curved arrows*) and were associated with bowel ischemia at the time of delivery. (Courtesy of John P. McGahan, MD, Sacramento, CA.)

was subsequently replaced by a large septate cystic structure.[32] Other than this one case, a normal bladder has never been seen—it is either absent or thought to be very large. The large cloacal cyst is not infrequently mistaken for megacystis secondary to posterior urethral valves. The spinal lesions seen with cloacal exstrophy are discussed in the sections below.

Maternal Serum α-Fetoprotein and Ventral Wall Defects

Maternal serum α-fetoprotein (MSAFP) levels are higher in *gastroschisis* than *omphalocele*, possibly because the defect is covered by a membrane, albeit thin.[35] The other possibility is the association of trisomies with omphalocele. Trisomic fetuses, especially trisomy 18, are known to result in lower MSAFP levels.[36] The combined effects of these two trends may result in normalization of the MSAFP values. This has been specifically addressed in trisomy 18 fetuses.[37] The authors of this study compared multiples of the median (MoM) in trisomy 18 fetuses without ventral wall defects and neural tube defects to those in fetuses with omphalocele and to a small group of three fetuses with both defects. The median MoM with uncomplicated tri-

somy 18 was 0.6, but with an omphalocele it was 1.1 MoM, and the trisomy 18 fetuses with both omphalocele and neural tube defects had a median MoM of 4.5. The fetus with trisomy 18 and omphalocele may not be picked up with a screening MSAFP, and as previously stated the omphalocele in the aneuploid fetus may be small.

Body stalk anomalies are associated with high MSAFP levels, as would be expected from the size of the defect. In the one reported case in which an MSAFP value was reported, the value was 10.1 MoM.[38] The last three body stalk anomalies from our facility yielded an average MSAFP of 9.9 MoM, with a range of 6.8 to 11.6 MoM. None of our cases had an open neural tube defect.

Cloacal exstrophy is generally thought to be associated with an elevated MSAFP, based on a series of six patients reported to have exstrophy of the cloaca.[30] The description of five of the six cases is more consistent with body stalk anomaly. This leaves only one reported case of cloacal exstrophy with an elevated MSAFP from Gosden and Brock's series[30] and two from Kutzner and colleagues' series.[34] The MSAFP levels in the latter report are high (30.4 and 23.7 MoM). There is no mention of MSAFP in the other reported cases of cloacal exstrophy noted previously. In a case of cloacal ex-

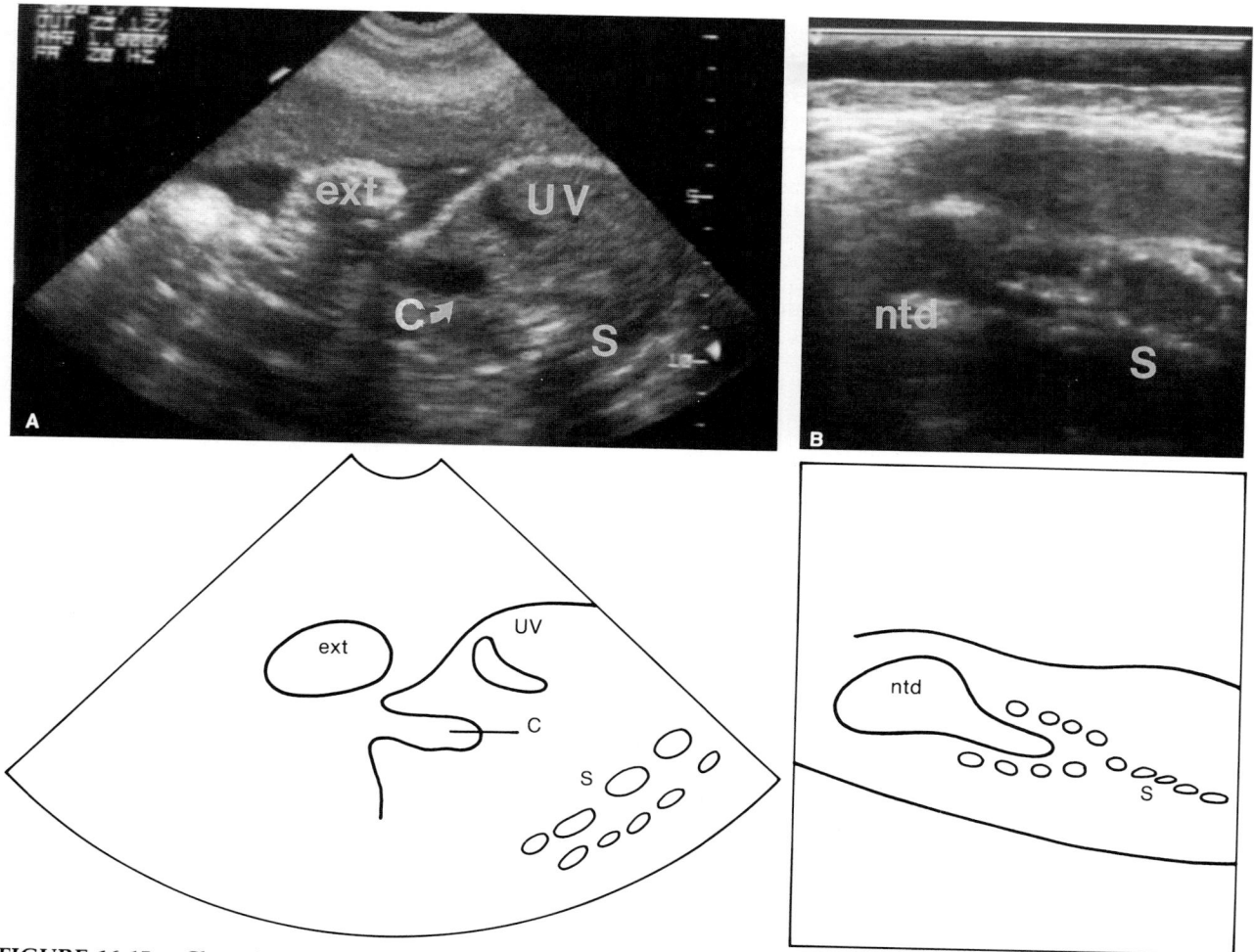

FIGURE 16-15.   Cloacal exstrophy. **(A)** Sagittal ultrasound through the abdomen and corresponding drawing demonstrate the cloacal defect (C) identified to the left of the abdominal portion of the umbilical vein (UV). The cloacal defect is open anteriorly into the amniotic fluid. S, spine; ext, extremity. **(B)** Coronal view through the spine (S) shows a large neural tube defect (NTD) of the lower lumbosacral spine.

strophy seen at our facility, the 32-week fetus previously had a normal MSAFP of 0.78 MoM. There are three reported cases in which only an amniotic fluid α-fetoprotein level was obtained with cloacal exstrophy, and all were reported to be normal.[25,27,32] An elevated MSAFP would be expected in this disorder, which is associated with omphalocele and neural tube defects. The neural tube defect, however, may be a hydromyelia, which is not an open defect and is skin covered.[13] The cloacal and bladder exstrophy themselves do not cause contact between the peritoneal cavity and the amniotic fluid. The omphalocele may be small, as it was in the case from our facility. There are no publications in our survey that report MSAFP levels in bladder exstrophy.

Associated Conditions

Omphalocele

In addition to being the most frequent ventral wall defect, omphalocele is the most complex in terms of its causes. Some of the syndromes in which one of the manifestations is omphalocele are listed in Table 16-6, along with other sonographically detectable features seen in the particular syndrome. Most of these syndromes are covered in greater detail in other chapters throughout this book.

The large number of karyotypic abnormalities linked to this disorder is of special importance. The incidence of abnormal karyotypes reported in fetuses with omphalocele ranges from 18% to 54%.[15,39–41] This risk has been shown to increase to

TABLE 16-6.   Syndromes Associated With Omphalocele

Syndrome	Sonographically Detectable Features
Beckwith-Wiedemann	Macrosomia (increased kidneys, liver), enlarged protuberant tongue (macroglossia)
Cloacal exstrophy	Absent bladder, lumbar sacral neural tube defect, single umbilical artery
Pentalogy of Cantrell	Omphalocele, ectopia cordis, diaphragmatic hernia, pericardial defect, intrinsic cardiac abnormality
Meckel-Gruber	Encephalocele, enlarged echogenic kidneys, polydactyly, cleft lip, Dandy-Walker malformation
Trisomy 13	Multiple cardiac defects, midline facial defects, microcephaly, holoprosencephaly, polydactyly, rocker-bottom feet, single umbilical artery
Trisomy 18	Multiple cardiac defects, intrauterine growth retardation, cleft lip, single umbilical artery, cystic hygroma, hydrocephaly, overlapping fingers, rocker-bottom feet
Trisomy 21	Multiple cardiac defects, duodenal atresia, cystic hygroma
Polyploidy	Severe early onset, asymmetric intrauterine growth retardation, molar degeneration of the placenta, multiple defects of the heart and central nervous system, oligohydramnios

53% to 100% if the omphalocele contains only bowel as opposed to liver[15,40–42] (see Figs. 16-5 and 16-9). The incidence of chromosomal abnormalities, although it is much less when the liver is involved in the omphalocele, is not zero and should not preclude an amniocentesis. The presence of other malformations also increases the risk of chromosomal abnormalities.[15,40,42]

Omphalocele is the only type of ventral wall defect that has been proved to be associated with increased risk of chromosomal anomalies (see Fig. 16-5). Unfortunately, the number of reported cases of bladder and cloacal exstrophy is too small for us to be comfortable with the lack of an association. Cloacal exstrophy is also of concern because omphalocele is a feature of the disorder. Gastroschisis, therefore, is the only lesion with which we can be comfortable that there is a lack of associated risk of chromosomal abnormalities. There is always that lingering doubt, however, that one is dealing with a ruptured omphalocele.

One of the most important prognostic factors in omphalocele is the presence of congenital heart defects. As many as half of the neonatal deaths in babies born with omphalocele may be secondary to heart defects.[43] Although most cases of omphalocele with congenital heart defects are linked to aneuploidy, the incidence of congenital heart defects is more than expected even after the exclusion of fetuses with chromosomal abnormalities.[39,40]

A variety of other abnormalities have been linked to omphalocele, but it is difficult to determine whether these occur from common causes listed in Table 16-2. Ascites is frequently seen in association with omphalocele, but it does not appear to worsen the prognosis[40] (see Fig. 16-9).

Gastroschisis

The most common conditions associated with gastroschisis are the various types of bowel atresia, most commonly ileal atresia.[44] This is consistent with the theory that gastroschisis arises from early loss of the omphalomesenteric artery because this also develops into the superior mesenteric artery.[12] The atresia can lead to bowel obstruction, gangrene, and necrosis. This has led some authors to recommend early delivery if the findings of marked dilation of the bowel are present,[45] although it has not been proved that this improves the fetal outcome in any prospective clinical trials (see Fig. 16-14).

Body Stalk Anomaly

Body stalk anomaly defect is frequently associated with several schisis-type defects of the neural tubes, such as exencephaly and encephalocele. A variety of defects of the limbs and heart are present. The ventral wall defect may involve the chest wall as well as the abdomen. The diaphragm is frequently also missing (74%).[46] The heart may be extracorporeal but is contained in the defect (see Fig. 16-7). The additional defects do not add substantially to the diagnosis because the defect is easily recognizable and the mortality is 100% regardless of associated defects. Chromosomal abnormalities were not noted in our review of the literature on body stalk anomaly.

Exstrophy of the Bladder

A variety of genital defects may be seen in both bladder and cloacal exstrophy, but these lesions are of minimal significance to the sonographer because they cannot be reliably seen with ultrasound. Separation of the symphysis is common to both exstrophies.

Exstrophy of the Cloaca

Disagreement can be found in the literature about whether omphalocele is a constant feature of cloacal exstrophy. *Smith's Recognizable Patterns of Human Malformations* states that there is "often omphalocele."[13] There is also confusion about whether the lumbosacral spinal defect always seen in association with cloacal exstrophy is a meningomyelocele. Smith's textbook also points out that a hydromyelia with incomplete development of the lumbosacral vertebra is part of cloacal exstrophy. Hydromyelia, however, is a closed spinal cord abnormality with a large dilated central canal. Whether this lesion should correctly be referred to as a *meningomyelocele* is unclear. The lesion is covered with skin and can be large. On antenatal sonograms, it is probably not feasible to separate hydromyelia from meningomyelocele. Of interest, the fetus in Figure 16-15 did not have a banana sign or lemon sign. To simplify matters in regard to what is included under the term *cloacal exstrophy*, one might use the term *OEIS syndrome* (omphalocele, exstrophy, imperforate anus, and spinal defects) instead.[47]

Cystic Lesions of the Anterior Abdominal Wall and Proximal Cord

Urachal cysts or a patent urachus are the most common cystic lesions of the anterior abdominal wall and proximal cord and should be considered in the differential diagnosis of common ventral wall defects. These anomalies are covered in more detail in Chapter 17. These are anechoic pockets that form in a line along the inner aspect of the anterior abdominal wall from the umbilical cord to the bladder. They are the remnants of the allantois, which is an embryonic precursor of the bladder and urachus. The cyst may be directly contiguous with or separate from the bladder. There can be more than one urachal cyst. The intervening urachus may be ligamentous or patent. Most ura-

chal cysts resolve by the time of delivery, but some newborns develop a patent urachus despite apparent resolution on the antenatal ultrasound.[48] The pediatrician should be made aware of this possibility.

Omphalomesenteric cysts have also been noted as anechoic cysts on antenatal ultrasound examinations.[49] They are embryologically different from urachal cysts. Other than the theoretical association with a Meckel's diverticulum, however, they are of no clinical significance.

Cystic structures of the umbilical cord can be separated from omphalocele in that there is usually only one anechoic area as opposed to the multiple anechoic areas seen in bowel loops. These are discussed in more detail in Chapter 7.

REFERENCES

1. Carpenter MW, Curci MR, Dobbins AW, Haddow JE: Perinatal management of ventral wall defects. Obstet Gynecol 1984; 64:646–651.
2. Lindham S: Omphalocele and gastroschisis in Sweden: 1965–1976. Acta Pediatr Scand 1981; 70:55–60.
3. Baird PA, MacDonald EC: An epidemiologic study of congenital malformations in the anterior abdominal wall in more than a half million consecutive live births. Am J Hum Genet 1981; 33:470–478.
4. Mann L, Ferguson-Smith MA, Desai M, et al: Prenatal assessment of anterior wall defects and their prognosis. Prenat Diagn 1984; 4:427–435.
5. Engel RM: Exstrophy of the bladder and associated anomalies. Birth Defects 1974; 10:146–149.
6. Soper RT, Kilger K: Vesico-intestinal fissure. J Urol 1964; 92:490–501.
7. Brock JH, Barron L, Duncan P: Significance of elevated mid-trimester maternal plasma-alpha-fetoprotein values. Lancet 1979; 1:1281–1282.
8. Langer JC, Brennan B, Lappalainen RE, et al: Cloacal exstrophy: Prenatal diagnosis before rupture of the cloacal membrane. J Pediatr Surg 1992; 27:1352–1355.
9. Potter C: Diaphragmatic and abdominal hernias. In Pathology of the Fetus and the Infant, 3rd ed. Chicago: Year Book Medical Publishers, 1975: 384–392.
10. Higginbottom MC, Jones KL, Hall BD, DW Smith: The amniotic band disruption complex: Timing of amniotic rupture and variable spectra of consequent defects. J Pediatr 1979; 95:544–549.
11. Moore KL: The digestive system. In The Developing Human, 3rd ed. Philadelphia: WB Saunders, 1982: 227–254.
12. Hoyme HE, Higginbottom MC, Jones KL: The vascular pathogenesis of gastroschisis: Intrauterine interruption of the omphalomesenteric artery. J Pediatr 1981; 98:228–231.
13. Jones KL: Exstrophy of cloaca sequence. In Smith's

Recognizable Patterns of Human Malformation, 4th ed. Philadelphia: WB Saunders, 1988: 567–568.

14. AIUM guidelines. J Ultrasound Med 1991; 10:576.

15. Nyberg DA, Fitzsimmons J, Mack LA, et al: Chromosomal abnormalities in fetuses with omphalocele. J Ultrasound Med 1989; 8:299–308.

16. Scmidt W, Kubli F: Early diagnosis of severe congenital malformations by ultrasonography. J Perinat Med 1982; 10:233–241.

17. Kushnir O, Izquiero L, Vigil D, Curet LB: Early transvaginal sonographic diagnosis of gastroschisis. J Clin Ultrasound 1990; 18:194–197.

18. Gram DL, Martin CM, Crane JP: Differential diagnosis of first trimester ventral wall defect. J Ultrasound Med 1989; 8:255–258.

19. Ramanathan K, Epstein S, Yaghoobian J: Localized deposition of Wharton's jelly: Sonographic findings. J Ultrasound Med 1986; 5:339–340.

20. Cantrell JR, Haller JA, Ravitch MM: A syndrome of congenital defects involving the abdominal wall, sternum, diaphragm, pericardium, and heart. Surg Gynecol Obstet 1958; 107:602–614.

21. Schwaitzberg SD, Pokorny WJ, McGill CW, Harberg FJ: Gastroschisis and omphalocele. Am J Surg 1982; 144:650–654.

22. Argyle JC: Pulmonary hypoplasia in infants with giant abdominal wall defects. Pediatr Pathol 1989; 9:43–45.

23. Lockwood CL, Scioscia AL, Hobbins JC: Congenital absence of the umbilical cord resulting from maldevelopment of embryonic body folding. Am J Obstet Gynecol 1986; 155:1049–1051.

24. Mirk P, Calisti A, Fileni A: Prenatal sonographic diagnosis of bladder exstrophy. J Ultrasound Med 1986; 5:291–293.

25. King CR, Prescott GH: Amniotic fluid alpha-fetoprotein elevation with fetal omphalocele and a possible mechanism for its occurrence. Am J Obstet Gynecol 1978; 130:279–283.

26. Haygood VP, Wahbeh CJ: Prospects for the prenatal diagnosis and obstetric management of cloacal exstrophy: A report of two cases. J Reprod Med 1983; 28:807–810.

27. Hesser JW, Murata Y, Swalwell CI: Exstrophy of cloaca with omphalocele: Two cases. Am J Obstet Gynecol 1984; 150:1004–1006.

28. Lande IM, Hamilton EF: The antenatal sonographic visualization of cloacal dysgenesis. J Ultrasound Med 1986; 5:275–278.

29. McLaughlin JF, Marks W, Jones G: Prospective management of exstrophy of the cloaca and myelocystocele following prenatal ultrasound recognition of neural tube defects in identical twins. Am J Med Genet 1984; 19:721–727.

30. Gosden C, Brock DJ: Prenatal diagnosis of exstrophy of the cloaca. Am J Med Genet 1981; 8:95–109.

31. Meizner I, Bar-Ziv J: In utero prenatal ultrasonic diagnosis of a rare case of cloacal exstrophy. J Clin Ultrasound 1985; 13:500–502.

32. Petrikovsky BM, Walzak MP, D'Addario PF: Fetal cloacal anomalies: Prenatal sonographic findings and differential diagnosis. Obstet Gynecol 1988; 72:464–469.

33. Frenkel Y, Atlas M, Horowitz A, Mashiach S: Fetal common cloaca: A case report and review. Eur J Obstet Gynecol Reprod Biol 1980; 11:115–120.

34. Kutzner DK, Wilson WG, Hogge WA: OEIS complex (cloacal exstrophy): Prenatal diagnosis in the second trimester. Prenat Diagn 1988; 8:247–253.

35. Palomaki GE, Hill LE, Knight GJ, et al: Second-trimester maternal serum alpha-fetoprotein levels in pregnancies associated with gastroschisis and omphalocele. Obstet Gynecol 1988; 71:906–909.

36. Merkatz IR, Nitowshy HM, Macri JN, Johnson WE: An association between low maternal serum alpha-fetoprotein and fetal chromosomal abnormalities. Am J Obstet Gynecol 1984; 148:886–891.

37. Lindembaum RH, Ryynnen M, Holmes-Siedle M, et al: Trisomy 18 and maternal serum and amniotic fluid alpha-fetoprotein. Prenat Diagn 1987; 7:511–519.

38. Gorczyca DP, Lindfors KK, McGahan JP, Hanson FW: Limb-body-wall complex: Another cause for elevated maternal serum alpha fetoprotein. J Clin Ultrasound 1990; 18:198–201.

39. Gilbert WM, Nicolaides KH: Fetal omphalocele: Associated malformations and chromosomal defects. Obstet Gynecol 1987; 70:633–635.

40. Hughes MD, Nyberg DA, Mack LA, Pretorius DH: Fetal omphalocele: Prenatal detection of concurrent anomalies and other predictors of outcome. Radiology 1989; 173:371–376.

41. Benaceraff BR, Saltzman DH, Estroff JA, Frigoletto FD: Abnormal karyotype of fetuses with omphalocele: Prediction based on omphalocele contents. Obstet Gynecol 1990; 75:317–319.

42. De Veciana M, Major C, Porto M, Baucian M: Prediction of an abnormal karyotype in fetuses with omphalocele. Am J Obstet Gynecol 1993; 168:352.

43. Schwaitzberg SD, Pokorny WJ, McGill CW, Harberg FJ: Gastroschisis and omphalocele. Am J Surg 1982; 144:650–654.

44. Moore TC: Gastroschisis and omphalocele: Clinical differences. Surgery 1977; 82:561–568.

45. Bond SJ, Harrison MR, Filly RA, et al: Severity of intestinal damage in gastroschisis: Correlation with prenatal sonographic findings. J Pediatr Surg 1988; 23:520–525.

46. Van Allen MI, Curry C, Gallagher L: Limb body wall complex. I. Pathogenesis. Am J Med Genet 1987; 28:529–548.

47. Carey JC, Greenbaum B, Hall BD: The OEIS complex (omphalocele, exstrophy, imperforate anus, spinal defects). Birth Defects 1978; 14:253–263.

48. Persutte WH, Lenke RR, Knopp K, Ghareeb C: Antenatal diagnosis of fetal patent urachus. J Ultrasound Med 1988; 7:399–403.

49. Rosenberg JC, Chervenak FA, Walker BA, et al: Antenatal sonographic appearance of omphalomesenteric duct cyst. J Ultrasound Med 1986; 5:719–720.

John P. McGahan and Manuel Porto:
DIAGNOSTIC OBSTETRICAL ULTRASOUND.
© 1994 J.B. Lippincott Company.

Manuel Porto   John P. McGahan

Chapter *17*

The Fetal Abdomen and Pelvis

THE ABDOMINAL CONTENTS

The abdominal contents arise from several different organ systems; as a result, the sonographic diagnosis and identification of normal structures and anomalies is potentially difficult. This chapter focuses on a practical approach to the diagnosis of the major intraabdominal anomalies, using a differential diagnosis format based primarily on their sonographic appearance. It is divided into two major sections—the first primarily discussing the gastrointestinal tract and its anomalies, and the second detailing the urinary system and its anomalies—because the differential diagnosis of abdominal anomalies so often encompasses both. The abdominal wall and cord insertion are discussed in Chapter 16.

THE GASTROINTESTINAL SYSTEM

Embryology and Normal Sonographic Appearance

The embryonic gut has three major parts: the foregut (esophagus, stomach, proximal duodenum, liver, and pancreas), the midgut (distal duode-

num, jejunum, ileum and proximal colon), and hindgut (distal colon, rectum, anus, and parts of the vagina and bladder). Dilatation of the foregut during the 6th menstrual week leads to the formation of the stomach, which then descends into the abdominal cavity by the 8th to 9th week. The midgut typically returns to the abdominal cavity by the 10th to 11th week. Although intestinal peristalsis begins by week 11, it can rarely be visualized sonographically before the midtrimester.

Fetal swallowing is evident before the end of the first trimester, and beyond the 14th week, the *stomach* should be visualized in nearly all normal fetuses.[1] With a transvaginal probe, the stomach can be visualized as early as the 9th week of gestation. In contrast, the normal fetal esophagus is not generally visualized sonongraphically.

The *small* and *large bowel* can be imaged and distinguished from each other, particularly in the third trimester (Fig. 17-1). The more centrally located small bowel is often difficult to discern in normal fetuses, appearing as a relatively homogeneous, slightly echogenic mass. The small bowel remains more echogenic than the large bowel until near term, displaying active peristalsis during the third trimester. In the late third trimester, small bowel loops are commonly identified, generally

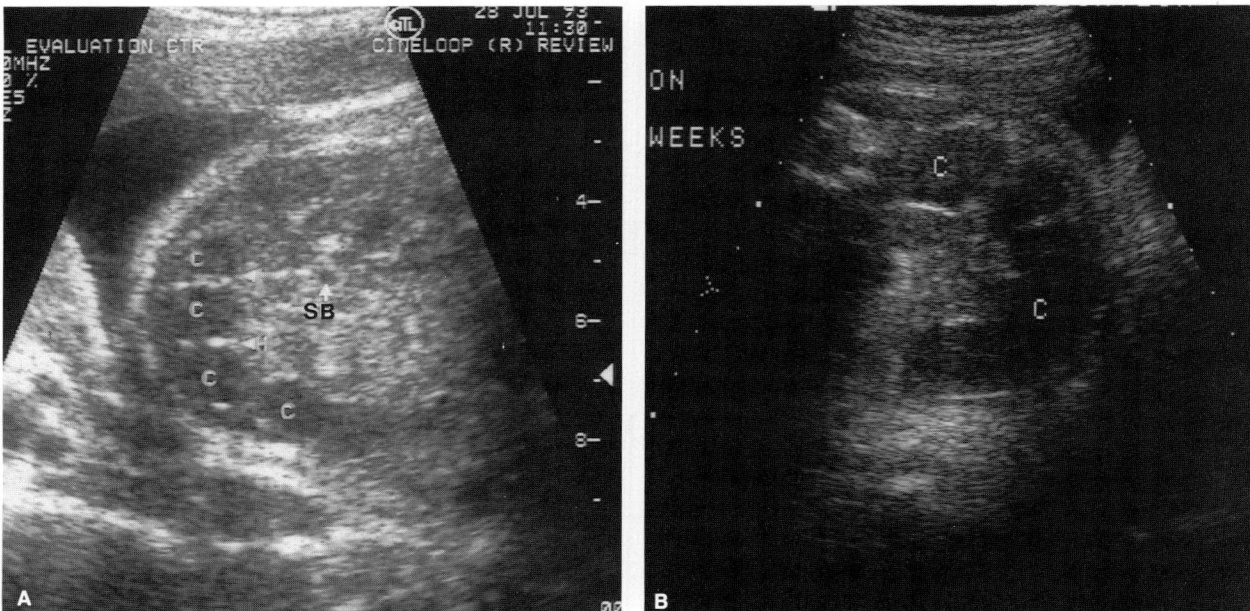

FIGURE 17-1.   Normal bowel. **(A)** Small bowel (SB) and colon (C) can be identified in this 36-week fetus. *Arrows* identify colonic haustra. **(B)** Colon (C) rims the perimeter of the fetal abdomen. The hypoechoic meconium in this near-term fetus allows easy identification of colonic haustra.

measuring less than 15 mm in length and rarely more than 5 mm in diameter.[2]

The *colon* frames the fetal abdomen, appearing as a continuous tube with a hypoechoic lumen (see Fig. 17-1). (Meconium creates this hypoechoic appearance, in contrast to the echogenic bowel wall.) In fact, normal colon with liquid meconium is often mistaken for pathology (dilated bowel, cysts). The colon exhibits far less peristalsis than the small intestine. By the middle of the third trimester, colonic haustra can be identified in nearly all fetuses. The diameter of the large bowel increases in linear fashion from 3 to 5 mm at 20 weeks to up to 20 mm at term. Although colonic grading has been attempted based on comparative echogenicity,[3] the clinical utility of this approach has not been demonstrated.

The *liver* is the dominant organ in the upper fetal abdomen, the area for standard abdominal circumference measurements (Fig. 17-2). The *gallbladder* is often overlooked or misrepresented sonographically (under the assumption that it represents an intrahepatic vein). Although it is a sonolucent structure, its ovoid/conical shape and lack of flow on Duplex or color Doppler, as well as its location inferior and to the right of the intrahepatic segment of the umbilical vein, should help distinguish it (see Fig. 17-2). The *spleen* is another upper

abdominal organ that is often overlooked or mistaken for an abnormal solid left-sided mass. Although not always easily visualized, it can usually be seen throughout the second half of gestation, posterior to the stomach and lateral and superior to the left kidney. It is homogeneous in appearance and slightly less echogenic than the liver, similar to the kidney.[4] The *pancreas* is sometimes visualized in the third trimester as well, especially with the fetus in a supine position.

Pitfalls and Artifacts

Absent Stomach

Inability to visualize the stomach in the second and third trimester of pregnancy requires further examination (Fig. 17-3). Repeated examination over time (several hours or days later) will confirm a normal fetal stomach in approximately 50% of cases. Esophageal atresia should always be considered when polyhydramnios is accompanied by failure to visualize the stomach bubble. The differential diagnosis for this problem is summarized in Table 17-1.

Gastric Pseudomass

A well-defined echogenic "focus" can be identified within the fluid-filled fetal stomach in approxi-

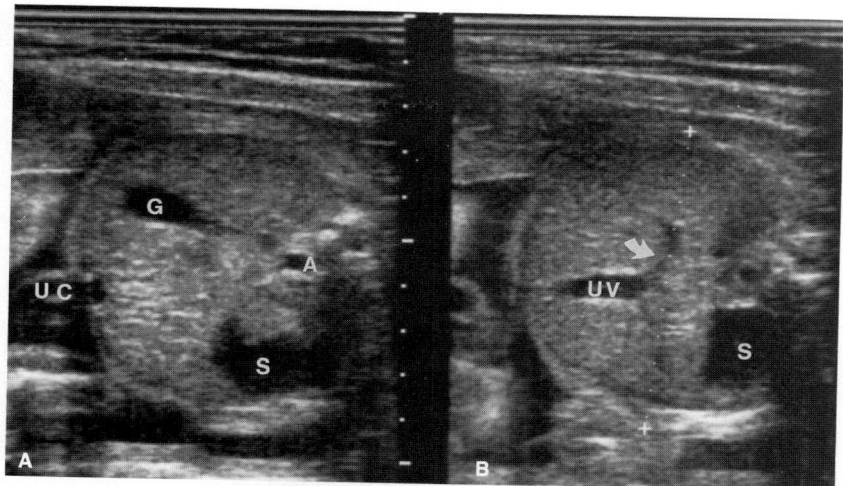

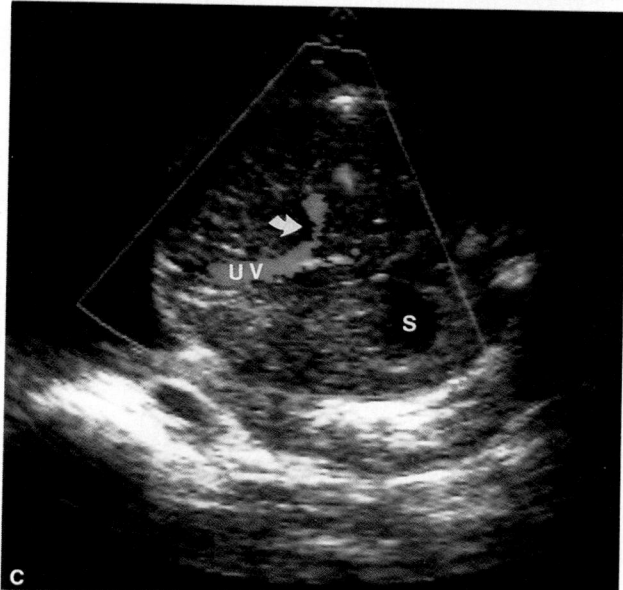

FIGURE 17-2. Normal abdomen. **(A,B)** Transverse scans of the abdomen of the fetus demonstrate umbilical cord insertion site (UC), fetal gallbladder (G), fetal stomach (S), and umbilical vein (V) draining into the portal vein (*arrow*). **(C)** Color flow demonstrating similar findings.

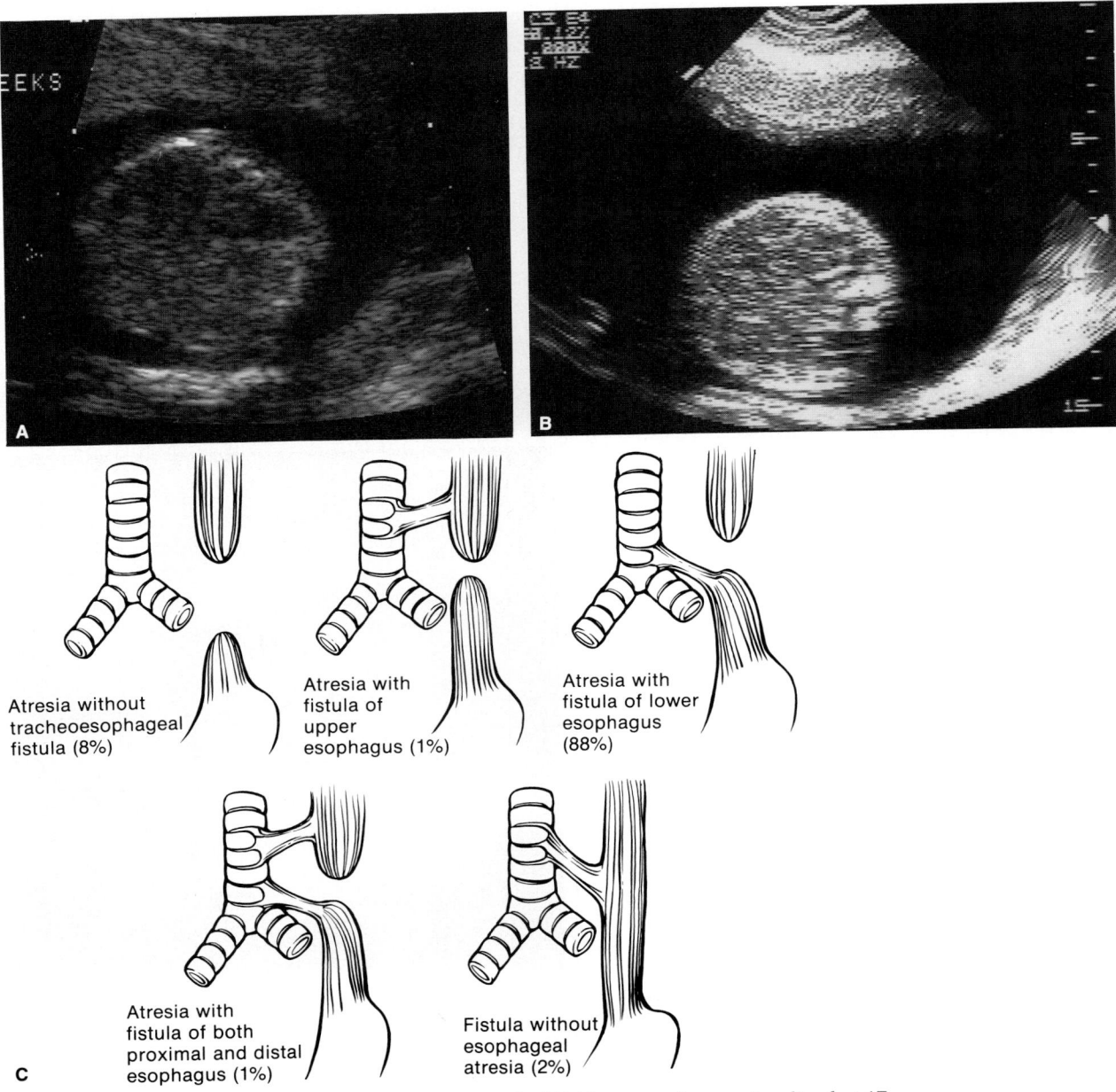

FIGURE 17-3. Nonvisualization of the fetal stomach. **(A)** No stomach was visualized at 17 weeks. Follow-up exam revealed a normal stomach. **(B)** No stomach was visualized in this case, and there was polyhydramnios indicative of esophageal atresia. **(C)** Diagram representing different types of tracheoesophageal fistulas occurring with esophageal atresia. Most commonly there is esophageal atresia with a tracheoesophageal fistula to the stomach. (Modified from Gwinn JL: Tracheoesophageal fistula with and without esophageal atresia—special aspects. In Kaufman HJ [ed]: Progress in Pediatric Radiology. Chicago: Year Book, 1969; and Singleton EB: X-Ray Diagnosis of the Alimentary Tract in Infants and Children. Chicago: Year Book, 1959.)

TABLE 17-1. Differential Diagnosis of Absent Stomach Bubble

Empty stomach (time)
Esophageal atresia ± tracheoesophageal fistula
Diaphragmatic hernia
Situs inversus
Oligohydramnios
Facial clefts
Central nervous system disorders

mately 1% of sonographic evaluations (Fig. 17-4). These echogenic pseudomasses are thought to represent swallowed cellular debris (although this has not been proved), and they generally resolve spontaneously. No association with clinical problems has been confirmed to date.[5]

Pseudoascites

A common pitfall in obstetrical ultrasound is the over-diagnosis of fetal ascites. This can occur even with a relatively experienced sonographer, especially when evaluating a patient at risk for hydrops (eg, Rh isoimmunized). Typically, a hypoechoic band that parallels the anterior abdominal wall is interpreted to represent free fluid (Fig. 17-5). This band is actually the abdominal wall musculature.[6,7] True ascites usually displays an irregular, hypoechoic area within the fetal abdomen, and even in its earliest stages allows visualization of both sides

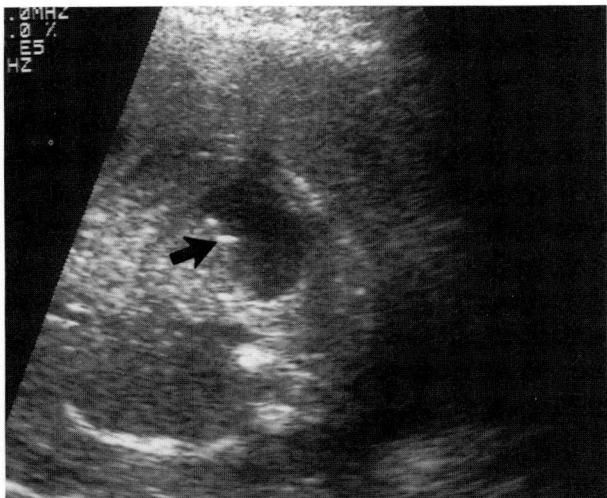

FIGURE 17-4. Gastric pseudomass. Echogenic foci along the wall of the stomach (*arrow*) are thought to represent swallowed echogenic debris. These are of no significance.

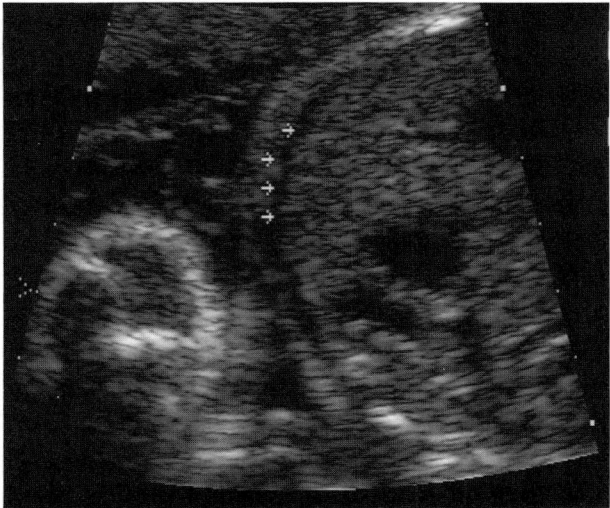

FIGURE 17-5. Pseudoascites. *Arrows* depict the hypoechoic abdominal wall musculature or "pseudoascites."

of the bowel wall.[8] Moreover, pseudoascites rarely exhibits some of the other signs of early hydrops fetalis (Table 17-2). However, it is important to avoid the pitfall of diagnosing early ascites when visualizing normal bowel in the late third trimester.

Anomalies

Situs Inversus

The diagnosis of situs inversus totalis requires a solid sense of orientation to fetal position, since the two key landmarks (stomach and heart) are on the same side of the body. By routine orientation, however, the fact that the stomach, heart axis, and aortic arch are on the right should be apparent. In

TABLE 17-2. Differentiating Ascites from Pseudoascites

	Pseudoascites	Ascites
Polyhydramnios	No	Often
Other hydropic signs (anasarca, effusions)	No	Often
Fluid between bowel loops	No	Yes
Fluid surrounding liver, omentum, or in the pelvis	No	Often
Symmetric hypoechoic rim of anterior abdominal wall	Yes	No
Outlines umbilical vein and falciform ligament	No	Often

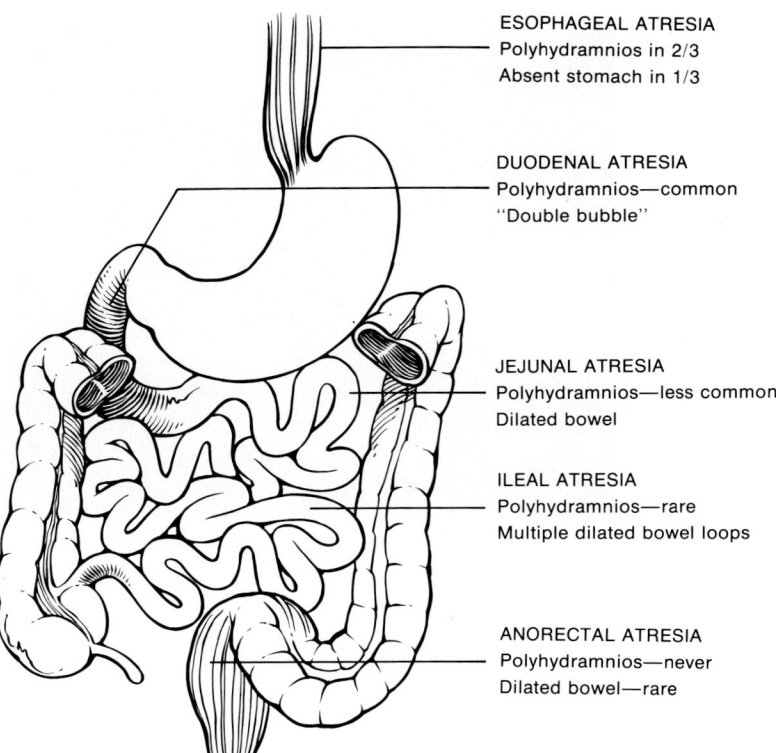

ESOPHAGEAL ATRESIA
Polyhydramnios in 2/3
Absent stomach in 1/3

DUODENAL ATRESIA
Polyhydramnios—common
"Double bubble"

JEJUNAL ATRESIA
Polyhydramnios—less common
Dilated bowel

ILEAL ATRESIA
Polyhydramnios—rare
Multiple dilated bowel loops

ANORECTAL ATRESIA
Polyhydramnios—never
Dilated bowel—rare

FIGURE 17-6. Sites of gastrointestinal obstruction and typical ultrasound findings.

addition, the liver and spleen are transposed, with the gallbladder on the left. This relatively rare disorder generally carries a good prognosis, with few associated anomalies, including Kartagener's syndrome. However, rare instances occur of situs inversus (thoracic and abdominal visceral situs are inverted) with the stomach on the right and the cardiac apex pointed to the left. This carries a high incidence of associated cardiac anomalies, which are explained in more detail in Chapter 12.

By way of contrast, situs ambiguous is associated with severe concurrent anomalies and a mortality rate of 80% to 90%. This disorder can best be divided into two types, asplenia and polysplenia, each with a distinct set of problems. The key sonographic feature of both subtypes is the presence of the stomach on the right side of the abdomen, discordant from the normally positioned heart. Complex cardiac anomalies are common, especially with the asplenia syndrome. Other sonographic clues to this anomaly include (1) an abnormal liver position (midline and horizontal), (2) midline gallbladder, (3) the aorta and inferior vena cava on the same side, and (4) as the name suggests, absence of the spleen.

In the polysplenia syndrome, the liver is on the left, the spleen is to the right, the gallbladder is absent, and the vena cava ends at the liver. The more common cardiac lesions seen with partial situs include endocardial cushion defect, outflow tract, and great vessel anomalies (see Chapter 12 for further details). Neural tube defects and genitourinary anomalies have also been reported with these conditions.

Esophageal Atresia

Esophageal atresia should always be considered when polyhydramnios is accompanied by failure to visualize the stomach bubble (see Fig. 17-3). Other sites of gastrointestinal atresia and associated ultrasound findings are presented in Figure 17-6. However, 90% of cases are associated with a communicating tracheoesophageal fistula, usually with a visible stomach. The gastric mucosa alone may produce enough fluid to allow visualization of the stomach in some cases of atresia without fistula.[9] Pretorius and colleagues reviewed 22 cases with tracheoesophageal fistula, noting polyhydramnios in two thirds and nonvisualization of the stomach in one third.[10] The blind pouch of the proximal esophageal segment has been seen infrequently, as has regurgitation after fetal swallowing

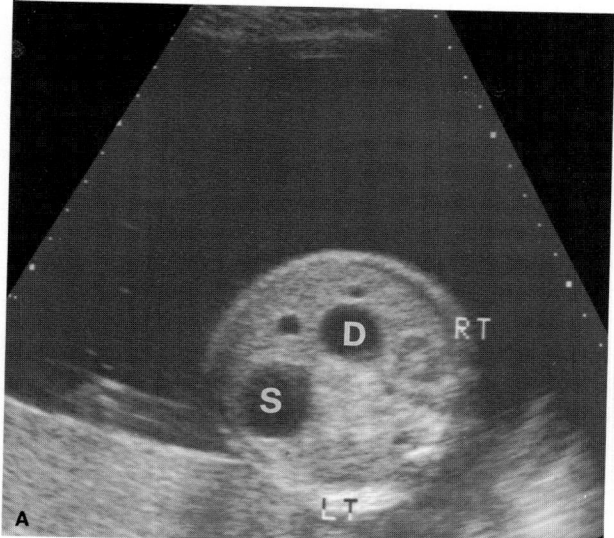 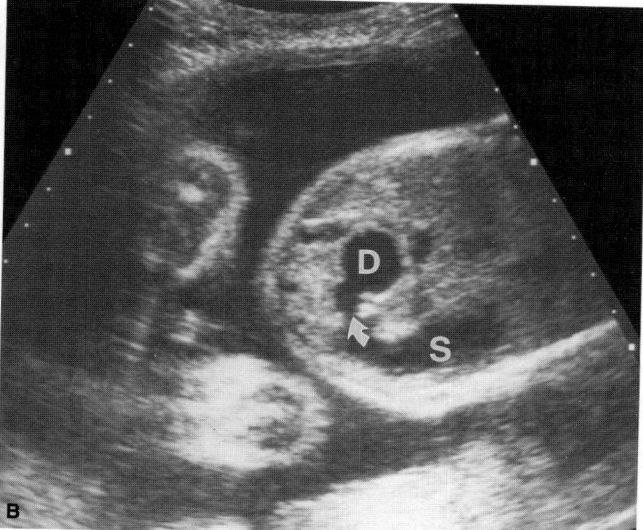

FIGURE 17-7. Duodenal atresia. **(A)** Classic "double bubble" of dilated stomach (S) and duodenum (D) associated with duodenal atresia. RT, right; LT, left. **(B)** Oblique scan showing continuity (*arrow*) between stomach (S) and duodenum (D).

during real-time observations. Associated anomalies are seen in nearly 60% of cases, with other gastrointestinal (28%), cardiac (24%), and chromosomal (19%) anomalies being the most common.[11] As with most intestinal atresias, esophageal atresia is rarely diagnosed before the third trimester. Although the survival rate is particularly poor overall (<50%), the prognosis is much improved with isolated esophageal atresia (85% survival).

Duodenal Atresia

Duodenal atresia, with an incidence of approximately 1 in 5000 births, is the most common intestinal obstruction encountered in the perinatal period. The lesion is most commonly caused by one or more membranes interrupting the duodenal lumen. The classic "double bubble" appearance (Fig. 17-7), almost invariably associated with polyhydramnios, makes the sonographic diagnosis relatively straightforward. However, it is extremely important to attempt to demonstrate the communication between the stomach and the first part of the duodenum (see Fig. 17-7).

Associated anomalies are the rule rather than the exception with this disorder, occurring in more than 50% of cases. In particular, 30% of fetuses with duodenal atresia have Down's syndrome; hence, prenatal diagnosis should be offered. By way of contrast, however, only 10% of Down's-syndrome fetuses have duodenal atresia. Other commonly associated anomalies with Down's syndrome include skeletal, cardiac, and other gastrointestinal malformations. Renal anomalies are seen in approximately 8%, and growth restriction is very common.

Although it is extremely uncommon to make the diagnosis of duodenal atresia before 24 weeks' gestation, it is important to reevaluate patients with a prominent stomach bubble during an early second-trimester sonogram. We recently diagnosed a case of duodenal atresia at 16 weeks after an ultrasound evaluation at 13 menstrual weeks revealed a prominent stomach.

A prominent stomach bubble may on occasion be mistaken for duodenal atresia if imaged in a coronal or oblique rather than a transverse plane. Another key to avoiding this pitfall is to note that the smaller duodenal bubble is generally located to the right of the midline. Pitfalls for duodenal atresia include a choledochal cyst, a hepatic cyst, or the gallbladder (Table 17-3). The lack of a communication between the two cystic structures, as well as the absence of polyhydramnios, should help clarify the diagnosis.[12]

Small Bowel Obstruction

The incidence of small bowel obstruction is approximately 1 in 5000 births. However, the prevalence of in utero or sonographic detection may be somewhat higher. It is often difficult, if not impossible, to differentiate jejunal from ileal atresia, although the extent of bowel dilatation is often a clue

TABLE 17-3. Common and Less Common Causes of Double Bubble Identified on Prenatal Ultrasound

Common
Duodenal atresia (associated with trisomy 21)

Less Common
Duodenal stenosis
Duodenal web
Ladd's bands
Annular pancreas
Proximal jejunal atresia
Bowel malrotation

(more loops are present with ileal abnormalities) (Fig. 17-8). A midgut volvulus is difficult, if not impossible, to differentiate from jejunoileal atresia; therefore, it is most accurate to refer to these disorders as small bowel obstructions rather than by the specific location (Fig. 17-9).

Polyhydramnios is often the initial clue to a small bowel obstruction and is present in the overwhelming majority of cases. Unfortunately, as with duodenal atresia, jejunal and ileal obstructive problems are invariably diagnosed late in preg-

nancy, specifically in the third trimester. Unlike duodenal atresia, however, non-gastrointestinal anomalies are rare in these cases. Other intestinal tract anomalies are common, with up to 45% exhibiting malrotations and/or enteric duplications, for example. Distal ileal obstructions seem to have the most favorable prognosis.

Multiple dilated loops of small bowel (>7 mm diameter) are the typical features in these cases, often with increased peristalsis (see Fig. 17-8). Differentiating small from large bowel obstruction is usually possible by the location of the loops, the absence of haustra in small bowel, and the presence of polyhydramnios. Colonic obstructions, however, are uncommonly diagnosed in utero, and Hirschsprung's disease (congenital aganglionic megacolon) is likely to present with dilated small bowel and polyhydramnios, making it difficult to differentiate from a jejunoileal lesion.[13]

Anorectal Atresia
The prenatal diagnosis of anorectal atresia has been reported, generally as part of a syndrome of multiple anomalies (eg, caudal regression syndrome, VACTERL syndrome, McKusick-Kaufman syndrome)[14] (Fig. 17-10). VACTERL syndrome may have a number of concurrent abnormalities,

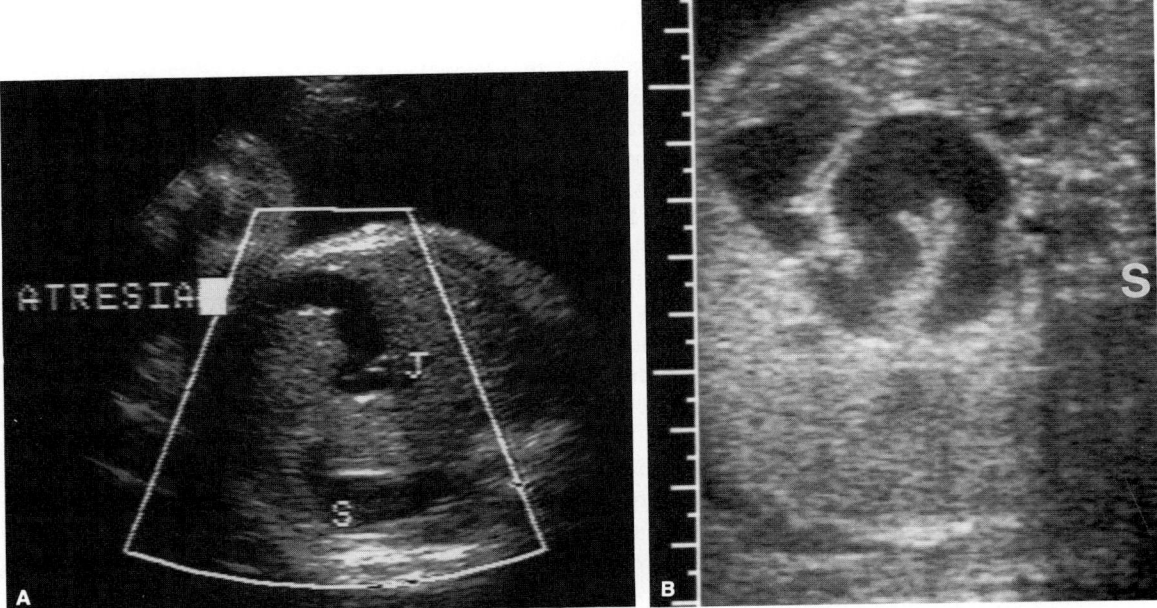

FIGURE 17-8. Jejunal atresia. **(A)** Dilated small bowel (J) and stomach (S) in this fetus with proximal jejunal atresia. **(B)** Transverse ultrasound showing dilatation of the stomach and the small bowel in this fetus with more distal jejunal atresia. S, spine.

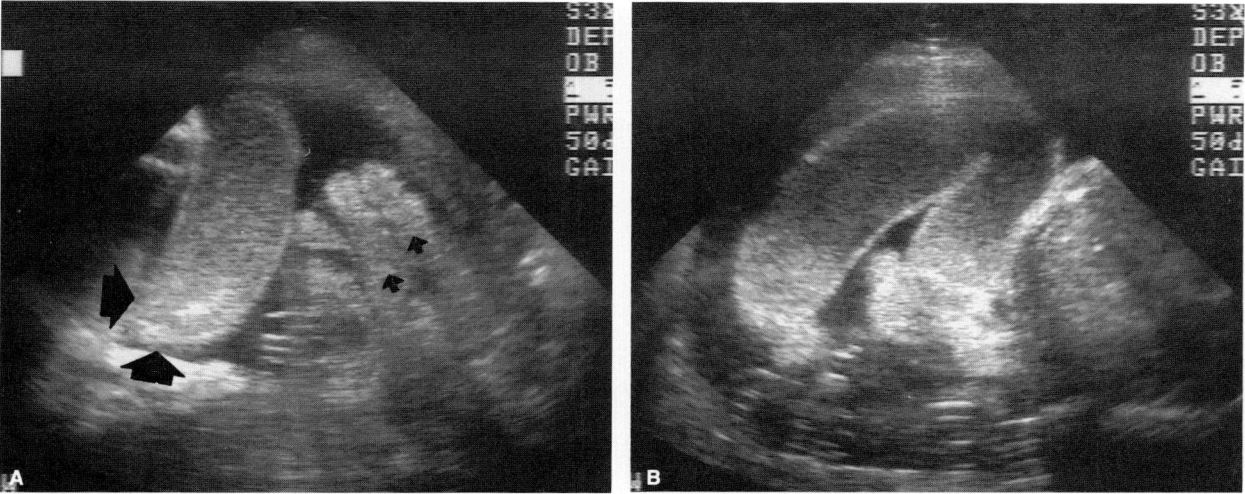

FIGURE 17-9.   Small bowel volvulus. **(A)** This loop of bowel (*large arrows*) measured nearly 3.0 cm in diameter in this fetus with gastroschisis. Adjacent normal small bowel loops are seen to the right (*small arrows*). **(B)** The same fetus depicting a more classic view of the small bowel volvulus.

including *v*ertebral abnormalities, *a*norectal atresia, *c*ardiac anomalies, *t*racheoesophageal fistulas, *e*sophageal atresia, *r*enal anomalies, and *l*imb abnormalities (Table 17-4). Harris and colleagues reported several cases with the salient features being dilated colon in the pelvis or lower abdominal cavity with normal amniotic fluid.[15] They stressed, however, that concomitant renal or upper gastrointestinal anomalies may lead to oligohydramnios or polyhydramnios, respectively.

Meconium Ileus

Meconium ileus results from a distal ileal obstruction with abnormally thick, viscous meconium. When this is present, the fetus is almost certain to have cystic fibrosis (CF), although only 10% to 15% of infants with CF have the condition.[16] The typical appearance of dilated ileum, with a normal jejunum, collapsed colon, and polyhydramnios, may be indistinguishable from other small bowel obstructions.[17] However, in some cases the bowel presents as an echogenic mass. Initially thought to be a highly specific finding for meconium ileus and CF, echogenic bowel has been associated with a number of other diagnoses, as discussed below (Table 17-5).

Meconium plug syndrome,[18,19] or an obstructed colon from intraluminal meconium, represents the large bowel equivalent of meconium ileus (Fig. 17-11). Although not as closely linked to CF (<25%), genetic counseling should be strongly advised for patients suspected of having a pregnancy with these findings.

Meconium Peritonitis

Meconium peritonitis is a condition resulting from a small bowel perforation. Although it is a relatively rare condition in neonates, this entity has been well described for over a century. The perforation generally leads to a chemical peritonitis, which results in intraabdominal calcifications that are the characteristic sonographic feature in this condition. The calcifications can occur anywhere within the peritoneal cavity but must be distinguished from intraluminal or intrahepatic calcifications. Typically the calcifications are linear in nature, sometimes rimming a hypoechoic mass or pseudocyst, and are usually associated with ascites and polyhydramnios. Meconium pseudocyst (Fig. 17-12) is usually the result of a contained bowel perforation, and nearly half of all cases of meconium peritonitis are the result of an underlying obstructive process.[20] Although ascites is a common feature of the condition, it is usually echogenic in appearance (intraperitoneal meconium). However, the ascites in conjunction with an inflamed abdominal wall can mimic the appearance of nonimmune hydrops.[21] The lack of generalized anasarca and the subsequent development of peritoneal calcifications are helpful clues in avoiding this pitfall. In male fetuses, scrotal calcifications also have been reported on occasion.[22]

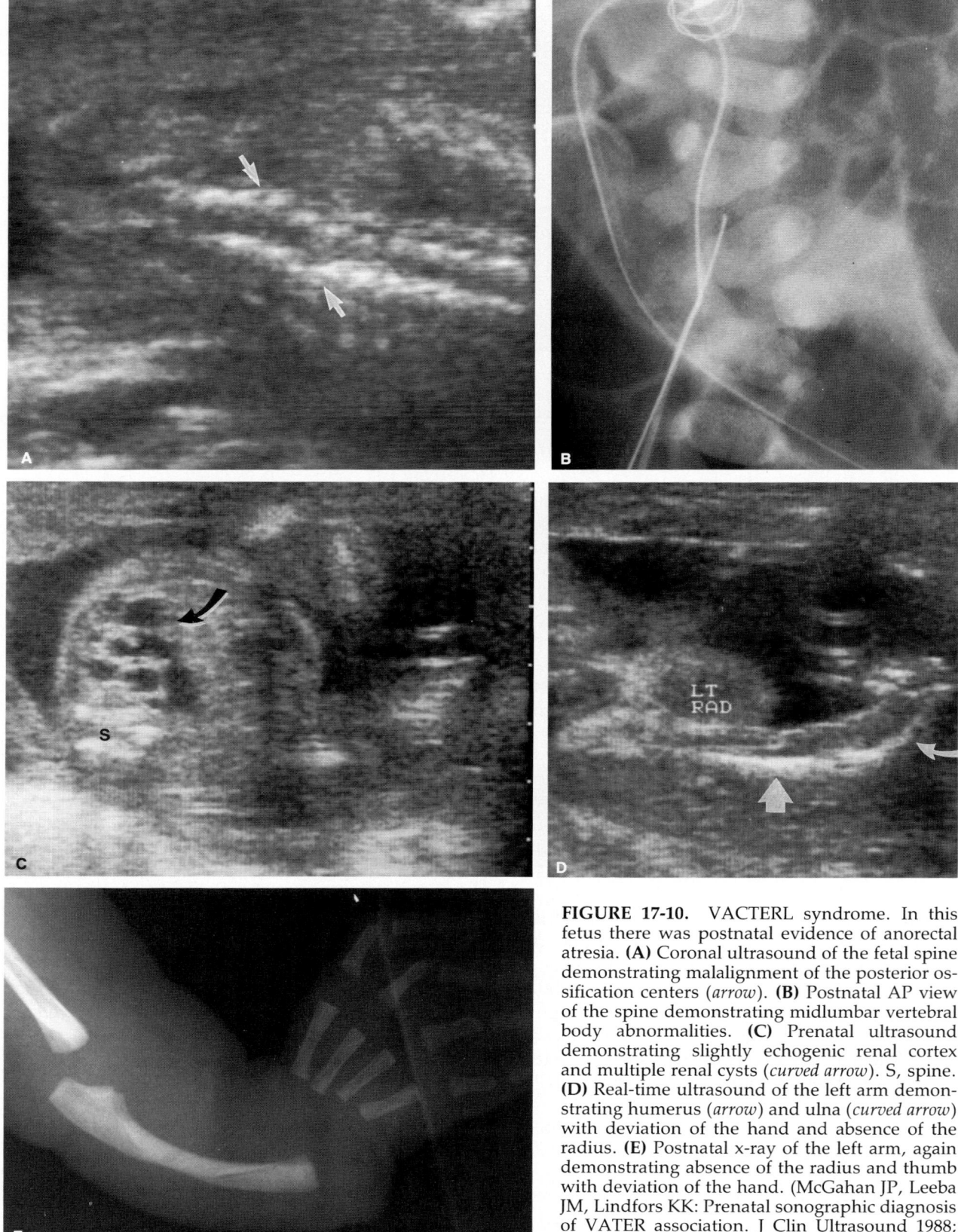

FIGURE 17-10. VACTERL syndrome. In this fetus there was postnatal evidence of anorectal atresia. **(A)** Coronal ultrasound of the fetal spine demonstrating malalignment of the posterior ossification centers (*arrow*). **(B)** Postnatal AP view of the spine demonstrating midlumbar vertebral body abnormalities. **(C)** Prenatal ultrasound demonstrating slightly echogenic renal cortex and multiple renal cysts (*curved arrow*). S, spine. **(D)** Real-time ultrasound of the left arm demonstrating humerus (*arrow*) and ulna (*curved arrow*) with deviation of the hand and absence of the radius. **(E)** Postnatal x-ray of the left arm, again demonstrating absence of the radius and thumb with deviation of the hand. (McGahan JP, Leeba JM, Lindfors KK: Prenatal sonographic diagnosis of VATER association. J Clin Ultrasound 1988; 16:588.)

TABLE 17-4. Malformations Associated With VACTERL Syndrome

Vertebral abnormalities
    Hemivertebra
    Sacral agenesis
    Syringomyelia
Anorectal atresia
Cardiovascular malformation
    Central nervous system anomalies
    Chromosomal abnormalities
Tracheoesophageal fistula
Esophageal atresia
Renal abnormalities
    Renal agenesis
    Renal dysplasia
    Horseshoe kidney
Limb abnormality
    Radial ray malformations

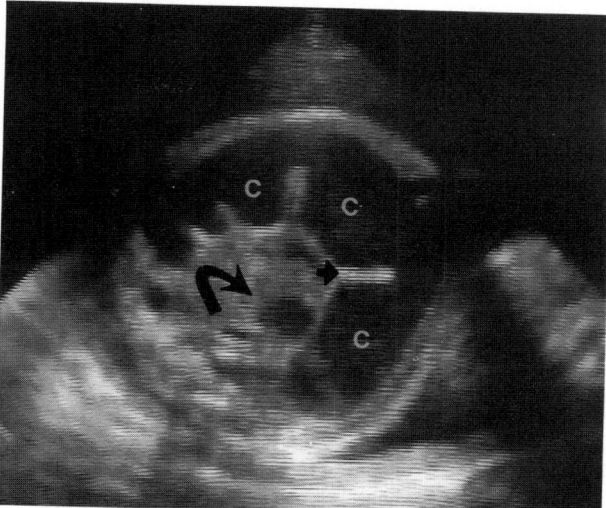

FIGURE 17-11. Meconium plug syndrome. Transverse abdominal scan showing dilated large bowel (C) with colonic haustra (*arrow*) and central echogenic small bowel (*curved arrow*).

Meconium peritonitis is sometimes confused with meconium ileus, a problem that is fostered by the fact that up to 40% of infants with the condition may also have cystic fibrosis (meconium ileus).[23] However, in utero series suggest that this association is far less common.[24] Therefore, despite a 10% to 15% risk of cystic fibrosis, most cases of meconium peritonitis have a good prognosis, sometimes without postnatal detection of the primary perforation. As with many of the anomalies discussed in this section, the diagnosis of meconium peritonitis is typically made in the third trimester.

Echogenic Bowel

A wide range of associated fetal conditions have been suggested when the bowel displays a hyperechoic appearance (Fig. 17-13). These range from artifacts to devastating abnormalities (see Table 17-5). How to approach the differential diagnosis of this not infrequent finding has remained a controversy for the better part of the past decade. One of

TABLE 17-5. Differential Diagnosis of Echogenic Bowel

Normal second-trimester variant
High gain and/or low dynamic range settings
Bloody amniotic fluid (intraluminal red blood cells)
Meconium ileus (cystic fibrosis)
Down's syndrome

the biggest problems is the somewhat subjective nature of the finding. The bowel will commonly display some relative echogenicity; hence, how echogenic must it be to be classified as abnormal? At times certain ultrasound units will routinely present the bowel with a somewhat echogenic appearance. Some settings with high gain and low dynamic range can simulate a hyperechoic appearance as well. Perhaps the best criterion is to describe the bowel as echogenic only when it achieves a brightness equivalent to that of the surrounding pelvic bones. Despite this, several authors have described echogenic bowel as a normal variant in the second trimester.[25] As mentioned above, meconium ileus (cystic fibrosis) and meconium peritonitis can be described as displaying an echogenic bowel appearance. Although this finding typically ocurs in the third trimester,[26] a few second-trimester cases of cystic fibrosis have been diagnosed prenatally with hyperechoic bowel as the only sonographic finding.[27]

Most recently, Scioscia and colleagues reported a series of 22 fetuses with echogenic bowel, suggesting a strong association with Down's syndrome.[28] Although the frequency of this association remains in question, when the bowel exhibits the same echogenicity as the pelvic bones, a detailed search for other anomalies associated with trisomy 21 should be undertaken and prenatal diagnosis considered (for a more detailed discussion of this issue see Chapter 21).

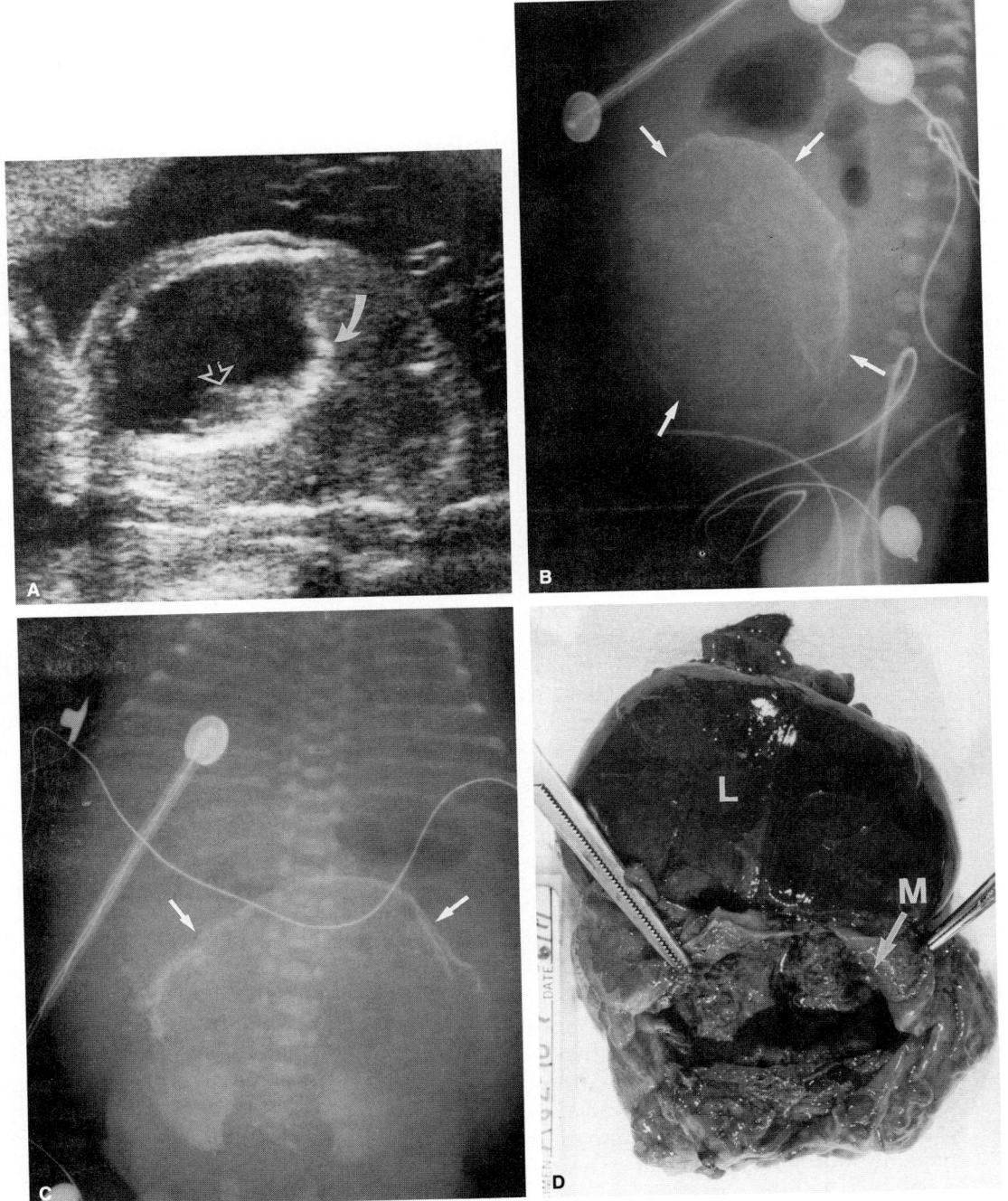

FIGURE 17-12.   Meconium pseudocyst. **(A)** Oblique scan of the fetal abdomen demonstrates a large midabdominal anechoic mass with thick echogenic walls (*curved arrows*). *Open arrows* depict echogenic material layered in the dependent portion of the cyst. **(B,C)** Lateral and anterior-posterior radiographs of the neonate shortly after birth with *arrows* demonstrating a well-calcified mass. **(D)** Gross specimen demonstrates an opened, thick-walled meconium pseudocyst (M) adherent to the surrounding bowel, bladder, and liver (L). (McGahan JP, Hanson F: Meconium peritonitis with accompanying pseudocyst: Prenatal sonographic diagnosis. Radiology 1983; 148:125.)

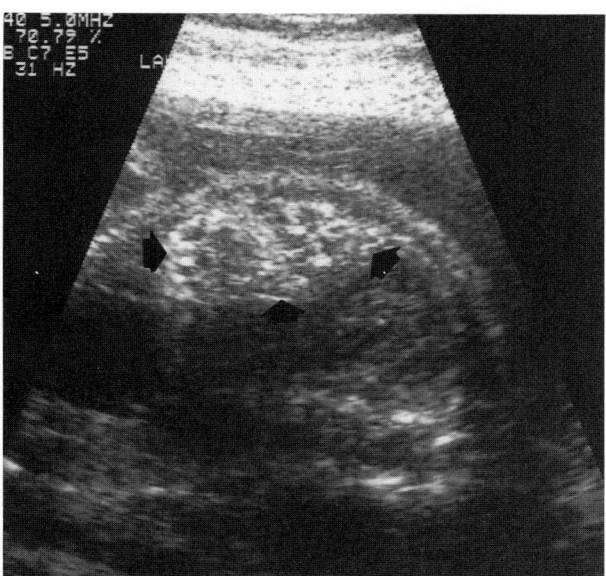

FIGURE 17-13. Echogenic bowel (*arrows*) in a patient with high maternal serum alpha-fetoprotein (MSAFP) and evidence for in utero bleeding (brown fluid at amniocentesis). The echogenic appearance may represent intraluminal red blood cells.

In our experience, red blood cells in the intestinal tract can produce this appearance as well. We have occasionally observed echogenic bowel at amniocentesis when discolored (old blood) amniotic fluid is noted, as with high maternal serum alpha-fetoprotein (MSAFP) or during follow-up examinations after an invasive procedure such as fetal blood sampling and intravascular transfusion.

Abdominal Cyst: Differential Diagnosis

When faced with the dilemma of an anechoic, presumably cystic mass in the fetal abdomen, a systematic approach is critical to making an appropriate diagnosis (Tables 17-6 and 17-7). Preliminary assessments to make include:

1. Location and orientation of the mass
2. Relationship to other abdominal organs
3. Size and shape of the lesion
4. Fetal gender
5. The wall and contents of the cyst

In addition, the change in appearance over time may be extremely helpful in difficult cases. (Many of these cystic-appearing abnormalities are covered in the preceding section on bowel obstruction and/or meconium pseudocyst.)

Ovarian cyst is among the more common anechoic abdominal anomalies seen in a female fetus in the third trimester. They are usually, though not exclusively, located within the lower fetal abdomen. They may have changed in position in the abdomen or pelvis and may undergo torsion since they are on a pedicle (Fig. 17-14). Although most fetal ovarian cysts are simple in nature, it is important to look for septae in these typically benign lesions. It is thought that these cysts arise as a result of hormonal stimulation from the mother and placenta. Given the minimal contribution of placental hormones in early pregnancy, a cystic abdominal mass in the first or second trimester of pregnancy is most unlikely to be an ovarian neoplasm; indeed, none has been reported to date.

More commonly, cystic lesions in the abdomen are related to bowel or urinary tract pathology, making it critical to examine the apparent cyst in multiple planes, addressing its relationship to adjoining structures—particularly the kidneys, bladder, and stomach (Figs. 17-15 to 17-19). For example, a unilateral or bilateral cystic structure in the dorsal, paraspinal region of the midabdomen most likely represents some form of *obstructive uropathy* (eg, hydronephrosis, hydroureter). In many cases, involvement with the renal fossa can be demonstrated and the diagnosis clarified. Other cystic masses localized to the kidney, such as *multicystic dysplastic kidneys*, are discussed below.

The urachus represents the communication from the embryonic allantois (umbilical cord) to the urogenital sinus (urinary bladder), a structure that usually fibroses to form the umbilical ligament. Although often confused with an abdominal wall defect (see Chapter 16), a *urachal cyst* or diverticulum can be located within the anterior abdomen (Fig. 17-20). The key to the diagnosis is the cyst's communication with the bladder and often with the umbilicus as well. Obviously, it can occur in males or females and is unilocular and singular in nature.

A urachal cyst should not be confused with a *persistent right umbilical vein*. A urachal cyst is located caudal to the umbilical cord insertion, whereas a persistent right umbilical vein is located cephalad to the umbilical cord insertion. The umbilical veins are paired between 2 and 4 weeks' gestation, usually with the right umbilical regressing and the left umbilical vein persisting. The left umbilical vein then drains into the portal venous system. However, if the reverse occurs, the persistent right umbilical vein will not drain directly into the portal vein but will instead drain into vari-

TABLE 17-6. Differential Diagnosis of Abdominal Cyst

Anomaly	Location	Appearance	Other Anomalies	Gender
Choledochal	Right upper	Single cyst near gallbladder, dilated adjacent hepatic ducts	Rare	Usually female
Hepatic	In liver	Usually single	None	Usually female
Multicystic renal disease	Dorsal, left, and/or right	Cysts of variable size, which are noncommunicating	Various syndromes	Either
Hydronephrosis	Dorsal, left, and/or right	Often multiple communicating cysts within renal fossa	Other GU anomalies	Usually male
Hydroureter	Lateral	Often tubular, communicates with kidney or bladder	Other GU anomalies; associated obstructed, enlarged bladder	Usually male
Ureterocele	In bladder	Single cyst or "septated" bladder	Hydronephrosis, hydroureter, MCDK	Usually male
Megacystis–microcolon–intestinal hypoperistalsis syndrome	Mid-abdomen	Increased bladder, hydronephrosis, hydroureter	± Dilated bowel	Either
Meconium pseudocyst	In mid-abdomen	Thick or calcified wall; echogenic debris	Associated bowel obstruction	Either
Bowel atresia	Dependent on site of obstruction	"Double bubble" to dilated bowel	Common; trisomy 21	Either
Mesenteric/omental	Mobile, middle	Variable: small–large, unilocular–septated	None	Either
Ovarian	Pelvis, lower	Unilocular, round, occasional septae; bilateral uncommon	None	Female
Umbilical vein varix	Cord insertion	Single "cyst," Doppler venous flow	High MSAFP, stillbirth	Either
Urachal	Ventral	Smooth cyst, communicates with bladder	None	Either
Sacrococcygeal teratoma	Off coccyx with both internal and external extension	Usually solid but may be cystic	None	Either
Anterior meningocele	Sacral	Cystic to complex	CNS malformations	Either
Hydrometrocolpos	Pelvis, retrovesical anomalies	Cyst or solid	Frequent GU	Female

MCDK, multicystic dysplastic kidney; MSAFP, maternal serum alpha-fetoprotein.

TABLE 17-7. Cystic Abdominal Masses by Location*

Right Upper Quadrant

Hepatic cyst
Choledochal cyst

Left Upper Quadrant

Splenic cyst

Posterior (Renal)

Renal cyst (see Tables 17-21 for types)
Hydronephrosis
Urinoma/urine ascites (secondary to rupture of calyx in utero with hydronephrosis)

Throughout Abdomen

Bowel atresia (see Fig. 17-6)
Megacystis–microcolon–intestinal hypoperistalsis syndrome

Anterior or Mid-Abdomen

Mesenteric cyst
Omental cyst
Meconium pseudocyst
Umbilical vein varix

Lower Abdomen

Ovarian cyst (but may migrate to mid-abdomen)
Ureterocele
Urachal cyst
Hydrometrocolpos
Sacrococcygeal teratoma (most commonly solid but may be cystic)
Anterior meningocele

* Many cystic abdominal masses may be in variable locations other than those listed.

able locations, including the right atrium, the inferior vena cava, or the iliac vein (Fig. 17-21). The importance of this finding lies in the fact that persistent right umbilical vein is associated with a number of different anomalies.[29]

Mesenteric or *omental cysts* are usually located in the midabdomen and are frequently mobile. Enteric duplication cysts are generally tubular in appearance, do not communicate with the bowel, and are more common in male fetuses. These anomalies are extremely difficult, if not impossible, to differentiate from an ovarian cyst or from each other. *Hydrometrocolpos* is a rare anomaly characterized by a retrovesical cystic mass in a female fetus (Fig. 17-22). This represents hormonal secretions filling the vagina as a result of a hymenal obstruction or a vaginal anomaly (atresia or septum). Other genitourinary anomalies such as renal atresia and intestinal atresias may be seen in

association with hydrometrocolpos. McKusick-Kaufman syndrome is an autosomal recessive triad of hydrometrocolpos, congenital heart disease, and polydactyly.

Another relatively uncommon lesion is the *umbilical vein varix* (Fig. 17-23). Although not truly a cyst, it may be confused with one located in the anterior mid-abdomen at the cord insertion site.[30] The key to the diagnosis is the communication with the umbilical and portal vasculature; in difficult cases, pulsed and/or color flow Doppler should clarify the vascular nature of this "cystic"-appearing lesion. Although little is known about the frequency of umbilical vein varices, a recent series points out a strong association with elevated MSAFP and sudden intrauterine fetal demise in 4 of 10 cases.[31]

Outside Japan, prenatal detection of *choledochal cysts* is quite rare (Fig. 17-24). These cysts of the biliary tree are usually single and, as expected, are found in the right upper quadrant near the gallbladder. The keys to differentiating this cyst from a gastrointestinal anomaly are documenting the hepatic communication, the absence of peristalsis, the lack of polyhydramnios, or any communication with the stomach or small bowel.[32] A *hepatic cyst* is another rare lesion of the right upper quadrant.[33] Like choledochal cysts, these lesions are far more common in female fetuses.

Sacrococcygeal teratomas are discussed in more detail in Chapter 9. Usually they are solid masses, but they may have cystic components. They originally arise from the deep pelvis coccyx and may have both intrapelvic and extrapelvic components.

(*text continues on page 360*)

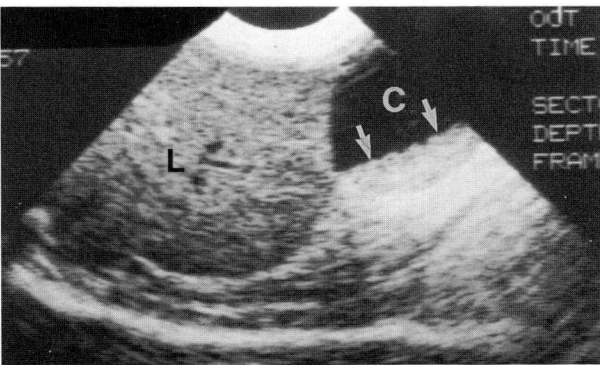

FIGURE 17-14.   Ovarian cyst. Longitudinal scan of the right upper quadrant of the abdomen shows a cyst (C) with debris (*arrows*) adjacent to the liver (L). This corresponds to a pedunculated ovarian cyst. The cyst was on a pedicle and changed in position throughout the abdomen and pelvis in utero.

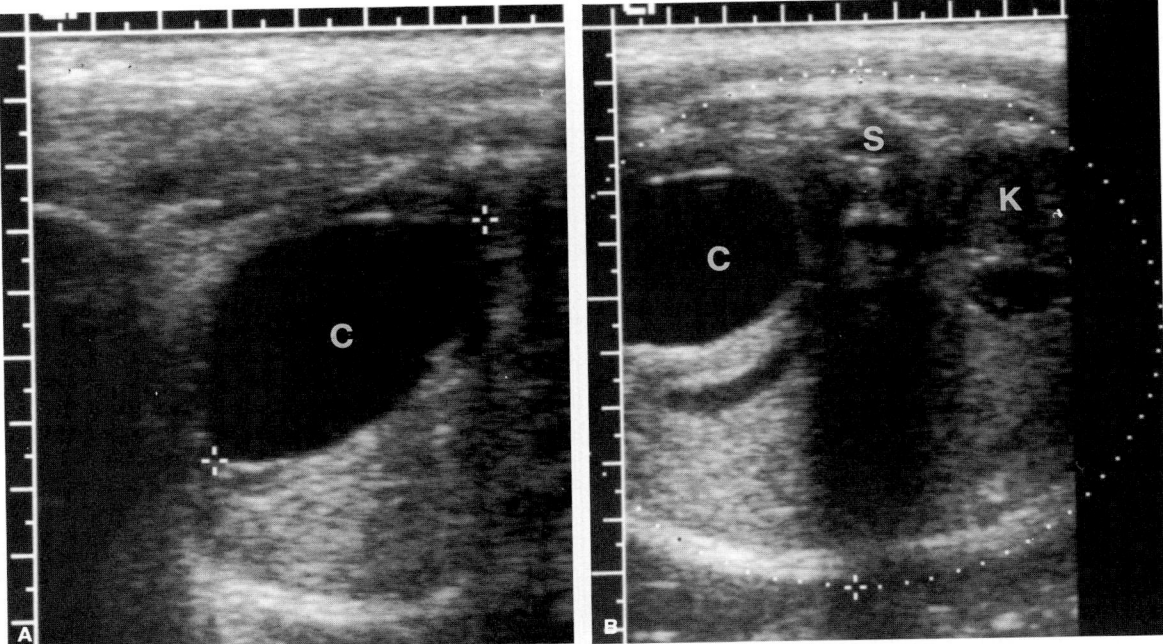

FIGURE 17-15.   Fetal cystic mass—ureteropelvic junction obstruction. **(A)** Longitudinal scan through the fetal abdomen demonstrating a cystic mass (C) in the renal fossa. Careful scanning demonstrates renal cortex surrounding this cyst. **(B)** Transverse scan demonstrates the cyst (C) to be in a paraspinal (S) location and corresponds to a ureteropelvic junction obstruction (K marks opposite kidney).

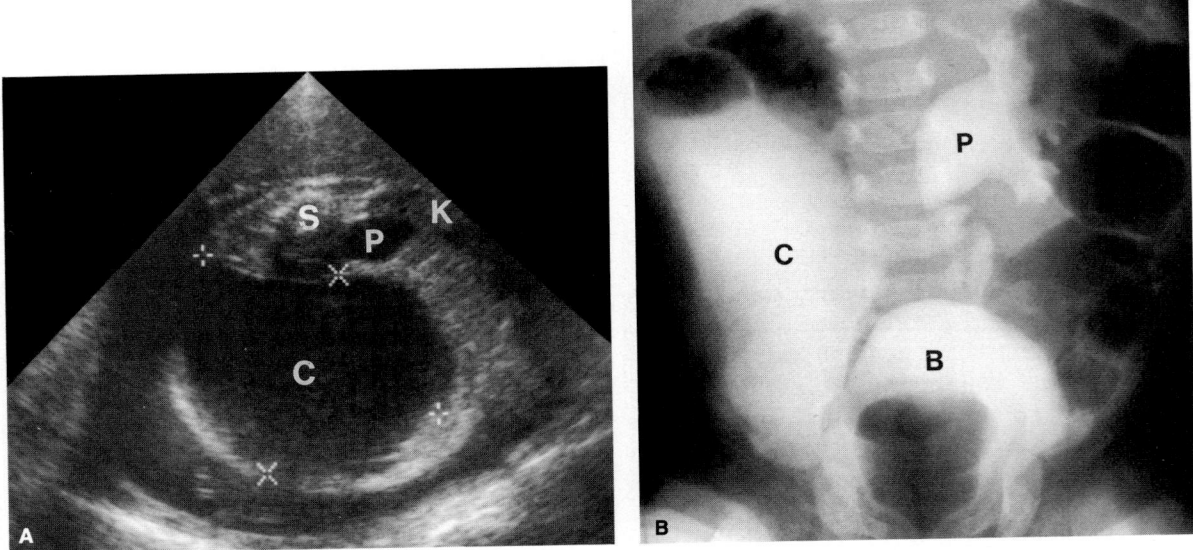

FIGURE 17-16.   Giant fetal cystic mass—ureteropelvic junction obstruction. **(A)** Transverse ultrasound demonstrating the left kidney (K) with dilatation of the renal pelvis (P). The right kidney was difficult to visualize; however, there was a very large cystic mass (C) noted extending from the paraspinal location (S) to the midabdomen. **(B)** Postnatal delayed intravenous pyelogram demonstrating mild UPJ obstruction of the left kidney (P), a normal bladder (B), and a large cyst (C) corresponding to massive UPJ obstruction on the right side.

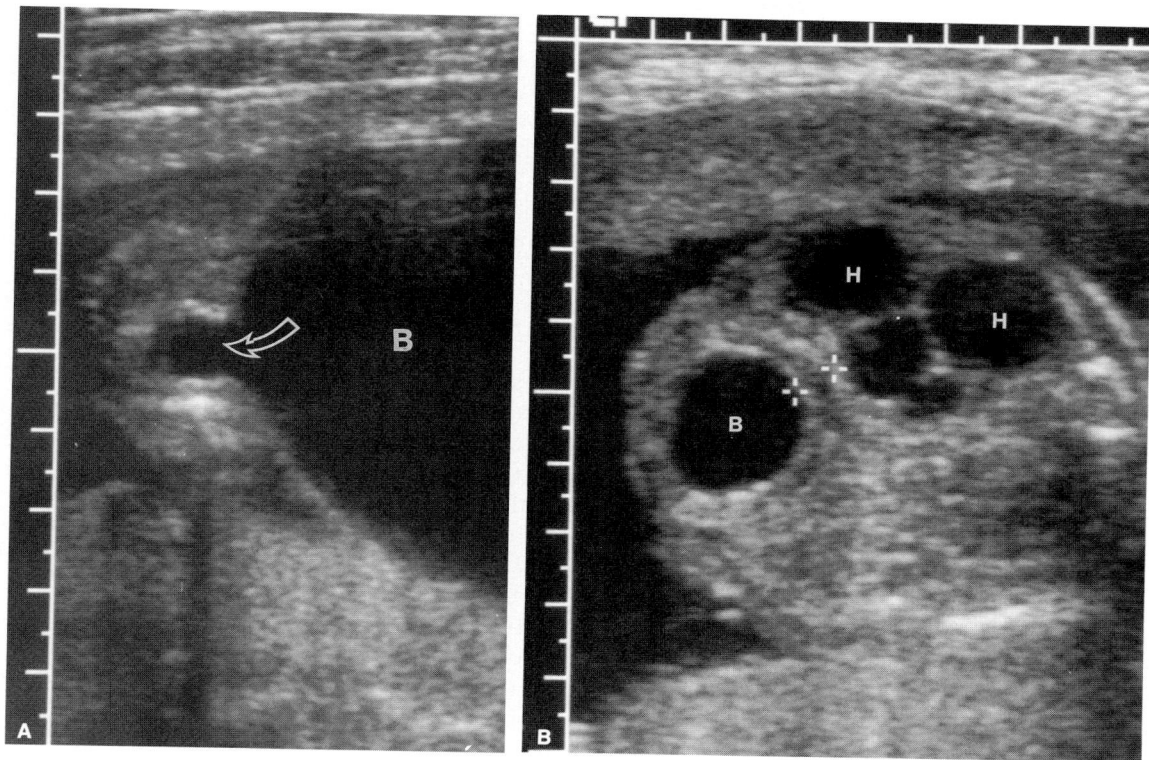

FIGURE 17-17.   Posterior urethral valves with decompression. **(A)** Coronal ultrasound show-ing typical key-hole appearance of dilated urethra (*open arrow*) with massive dilatation of the bladder (B). **(B)** Later there was decompression of the bladder (B), and now there is marked bladder wall thickening (to greater than 6 mm [*calipers*]). There is persistent bilateral hydrone-phrosis (H) and hydroureter.

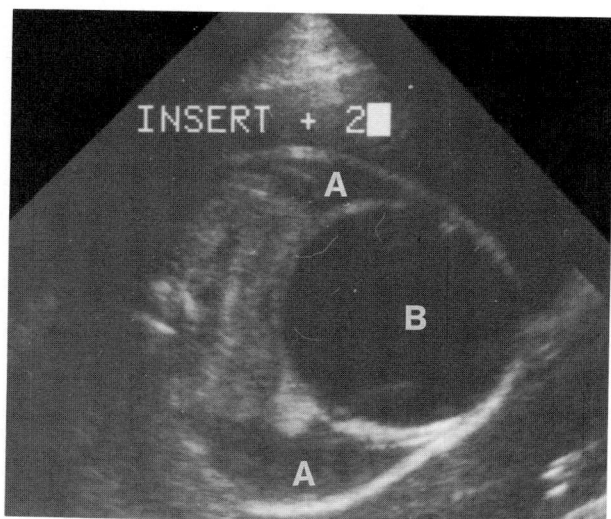

FIGURE 17-18.   Transverse ultrasound of the fetal ab-domen demonstrating massive dilatation of the bladder (B) with urine ascites (A) in this fetus with posterior urethral valves.

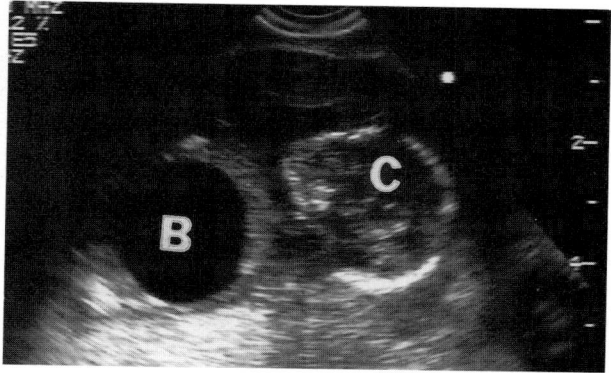

FIGURE 17-19.   Urethral atresia. Massive bladder (B) dilatation in a 16-week fetus with oligohydramnios. C, fetal head.

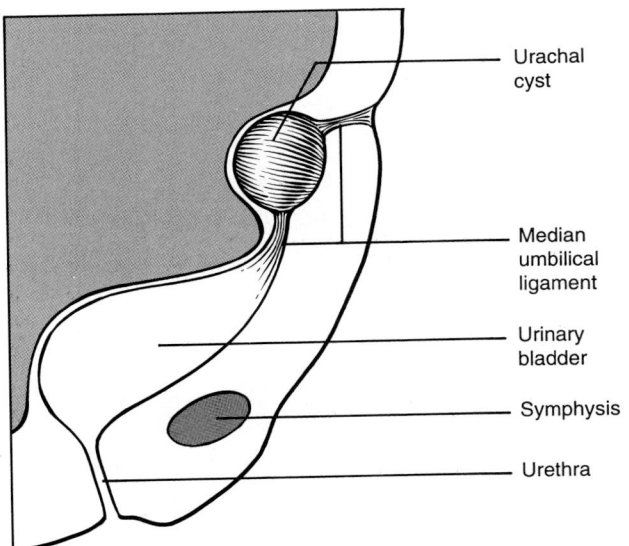

FIGURE 17-20. Sagittal diagram of a urachal cyst lying cephalad to the bladder in the median umbilical ligament, which is somewhere along its course between the umbilicus and the most cephalad portion of the bladder.

One pitfall in the differential diagnosis is mistaking the gallbladder for an abdominal cyst. This structure is usually visible throughout the second half of pregnancy, and the sonographer should become comfortable with its location and appearance.

Ascites

The presence of fluid within the fetal abdomen, or ascites, is always abnormal. As discussed above, however, the over-diagnosis (pseudoascites) is quite common (see Fig. 17-5). Although often seen as an isolated finding, it frequently represents an early stage of hydrops fetalis, immune or non-immune (see Chapter 18); as such, an accurate, early diagnosis is of critical importance in patients at risk.

Truly isolated ascites may be caused by a myriad of conditions, including infections and a large number of "idiopathic" causes. However, it is important to perform a detailed search for anomalies, not only to discover those associated with hydrops but also to rule out bowel obstructions or urinary ascites associated with obstructive uropathy.

The early diagnosis of ascites is aided by awareness of the more common sites for its detection: surrounding the liver, in the flanks, surrounding

the bowel, and in the pelvis (see Figs. 17-18 and 17-23). As stated earlier, the earliest sign of ascites may be the appearance of prominent fetal bowel loops, particularly in the second and early third trimester.[8] In its more advanced stages, one can see the liver and spleen completely outlined by fluid, as well as the falciform ligament, umbilical vein, mesentery, and omentum.

Abdominal Calcifications

Abdominal calcifications are relatively common sonographic findings in pregnancy; it is also quite common to misrepresent a bright echogenic area as an abnormality. To avoid this pitfall it is important to document the acoustic shadow cast by the reflecting mass (Fig. 17-25). Meconium peritonitis is the most common cause for calcific lesions in the subhepatic peritoneal cavity (Table 17-8).

Intrahepatic calcifications are seen with relative frequency, often as a result of a viral or other congenital infection such as toxoplasmosis, cytomegalovirus (CMV), rubella, and varicella. Many of these TORCH infections will also manifest with periventricular calcifications in the brain and intrauterine growth restriction. Vascular lesions such as hemangiomas,[34] hepatoblastomas, and ischemic hepatic infarcts may be seen as well.

Intraabdominal tumors must be considered in the differential diagnosis (see Table 17-8), particularly when the calcification is associated with a mass; neuroblastomas and teratomas should be high on the differential list because they can occur in a variety of sites within the abdomen.

Intraluminal calcifications in the right upper quadrant may represent fetal gallstones. Although quite uncommon, these lesions usually resolve postnatally without any symptoms or treatment.

Although it is important to rule out the potentially significant diagnoses mentioned above, it is also notable that small intrahepatic calcifications are commonly seen during the second and third trimesters of pregnancy without any etiology or sequelae.

Hepatosplenomegaly

Enlargement of the liver or spleen may occur secondary to an isolated finding such as a liver tumor (hemangioendothelioma) or systemic abnormalities such as fetal hydrops (Table 17-9). Fetal hydrops is explained in more detail in Chapter 18.

(text continues on page 364)

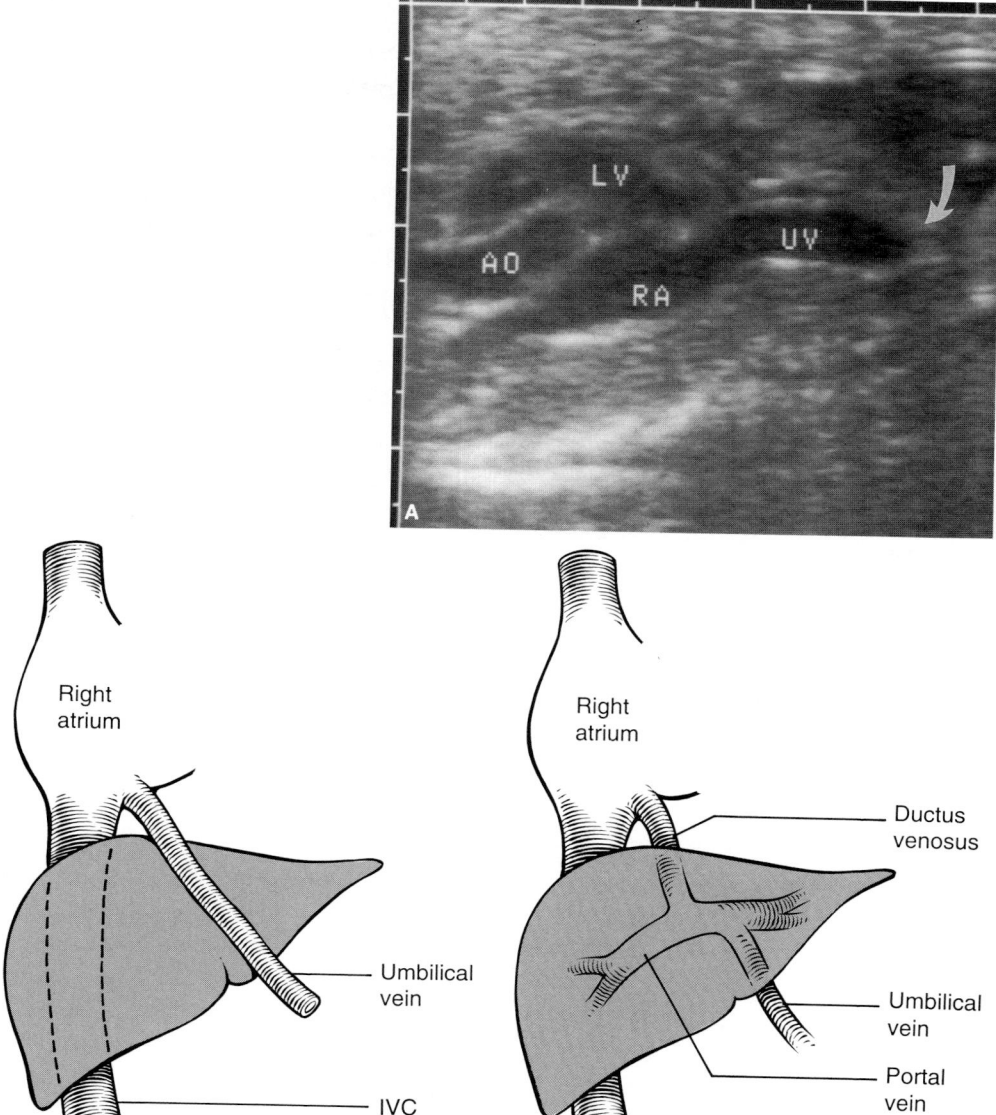

FIGURE 17-21.   Persistent right umbilical vein. **(A)** Oblique transverse image showing the course of the umbilical vein as it enters the anterior abdomen (*arrow*). The umbilical vein drains directly into the right atrium in this case instead of into the portal vein. AO, aorta; LV, left ventricle; RA, right atrium; UV, umbilical vein. **(B)** Abberrant right umbilical vein with direct communication of the right atrium bypassing the portal venous system. **(C)** Normal course of the umbilical vein entering the portal vein with connection to the right atrium via the ductus venosis. (Modified from Greiss HB, McGahan JP: Umbilical vein entering the right atrium: Significance of in utero diagnosis. J Ultrasound Med 1992; 11:111.)

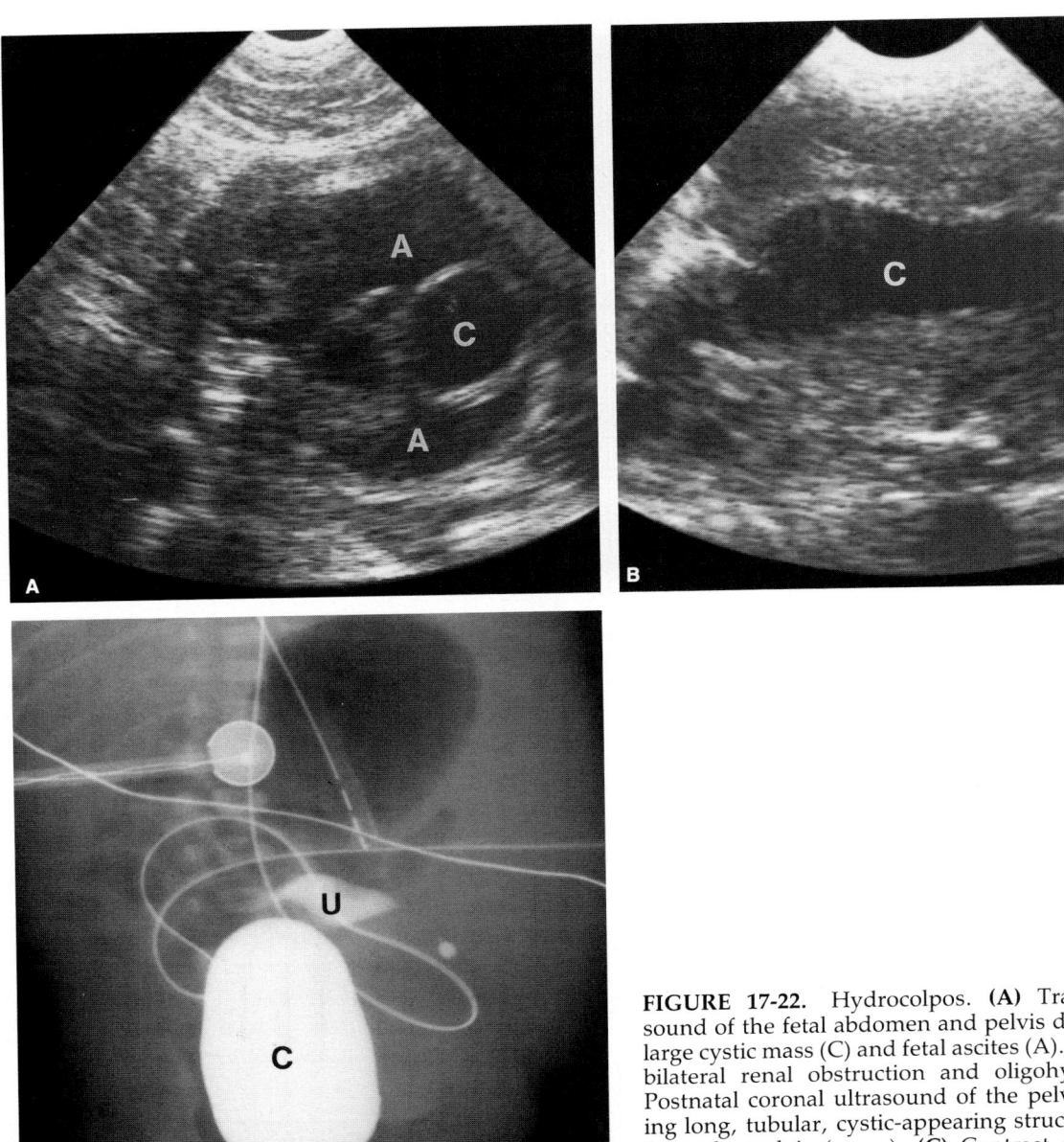

FIGURE 17-22. Hydrocolpos. **(A)** Transverse ultrasound of the fetal abdomen and pelvis demonstrating a large cystic mass (C) and fetal ascites (A). There was also bilateral renal obstruction and oligohydramnios. **(B)** Postnatal coronal ultrasound of the pelvis demonstrating long, tubular, cystic-appearing structure (C) arising from the pelvis (*arrow*). **(C)** Contrast study with the catheter in the distal vagina demonstrating a cyst (C), which corresponds to dilatation of the vagina and contrast flowing into the uterus (U).

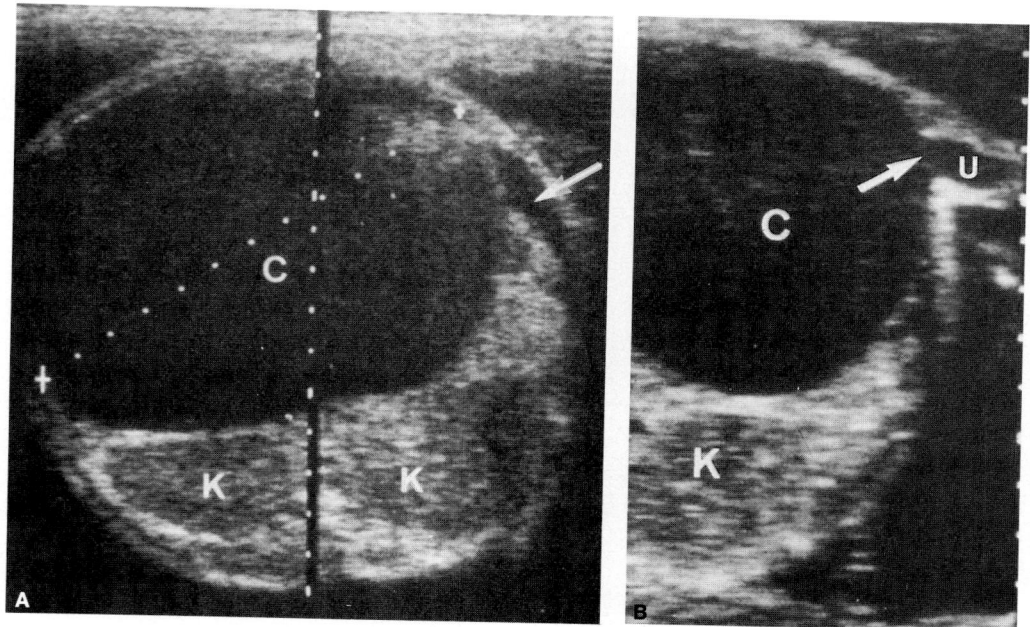

FIGURE 17-23. Giant umbilical vein varix/ascites. **(A)** Ultrasound of the fetal abdomen demonstrates large intraabdominal cyst (C). Arrow indicates ascites. K, kidney. **(B)** Transverse scan at the level of the umbilicus demonstrates a cyst (C), which communicates with the umbilical vein (U) and was noted to be a varix of the umbilical vein. Fetal demise occurred later in pregnancy. (Fuster JS, et al: Giant dilatation of the umbilical vein. J Clin Ultrasound 1985; 13:363.)

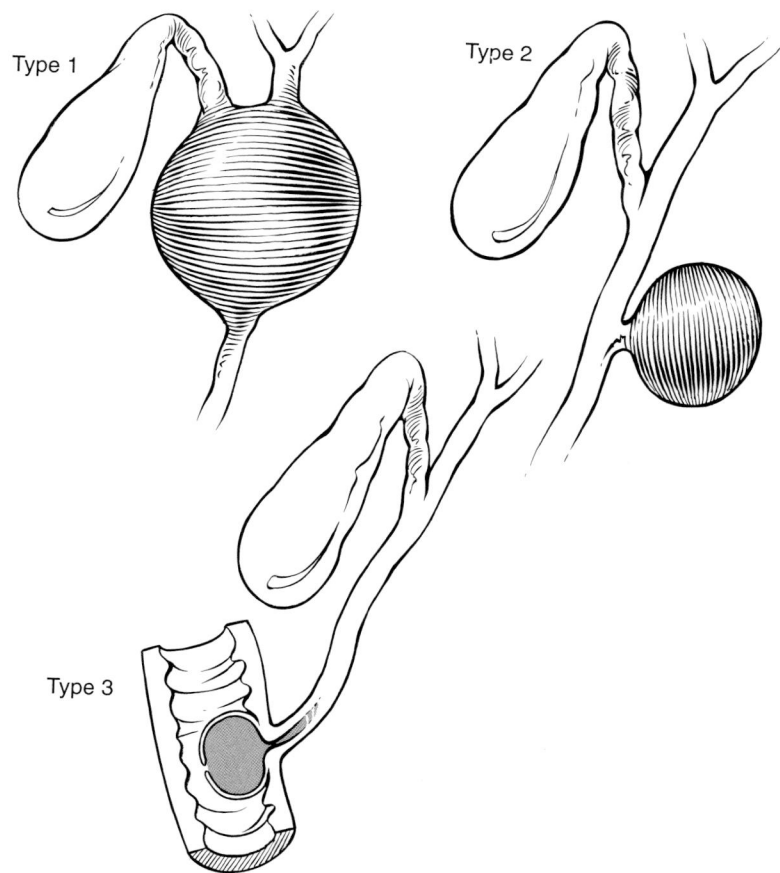

FIGURE 17-24. Different types of choledochal cyst. Type 1 is the most common and represents dilatation of the common duct, which may extend into the common hepatic duct and the proximal cystic duct. Type 2 is a focal diverticula of the common bile duct. Type 3 is a smaller diverticula of the common bile duct as it enters the duodenum. (Modified from Gray SW, Skandalakis JF: Embryology for Surgeons. Philadelphia: WB Saunders, 1972.)

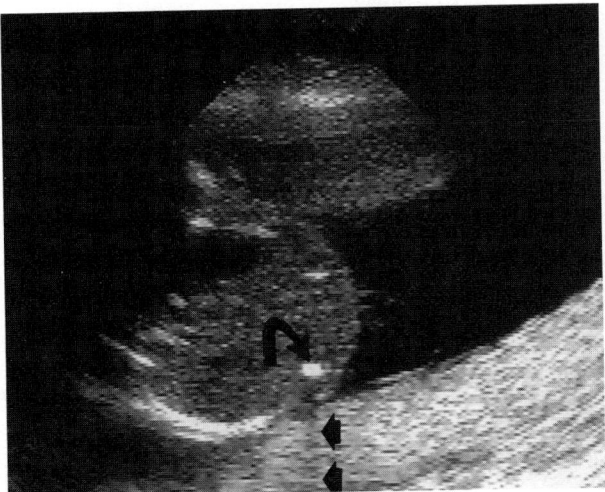

FIGURE 17-25. Intrahepatic calcifications. Curved arrow depicts a densely echogenic calcification in the right upper quadrant of this 20-week fetus. *Short arrows* point out the acoustic shadow cast by the lesion. (A work-up for infection, etc., proved negative, and upon serial examination the echogenic areas resolved.)

TABLE 17-8. Differential Diagnosis of Intraabdominal Calcifications

Meconium (Extraluminal)
Focal or diffuse (meconium peritonitis)
Associated cyst (meconium pseudocyst)

Meconium (Intraluminal)
Anorectal atresia
Small bowel atresia
Meconium ileus

Idiopathic (Focal)
No etiology determined

Infection
Cytomegalovirus, toxoplasmosis

Tumors
Neuroblastoma
Teratoma
Hemangioma
Hepatoblastoma

Parenchymal
Liver
Spleen

Cholelithiasis (Gallbladder)
Usually regress postnatally

TABLE 17-9. Fetal Hepatosplenomegaly

Common
Hydrops
  Immune
  Nonimmune
Infection
  TORCH
  Hepatitis (liver)
Congestive heart failure
Congenital anemias

Uncommon
Errors of metabolism
  Tumors
    Infantile hemangioendothelioma (liver)
    Hepatoblastoma (liver)
Beckwith-Wiedemann syndrome
Systemic malignancy
  Metastatic neuroblastoma
  Leukemia

THE GENITOURINARY SYSTEM

Embryology and Normal Sonographic Appearance

The pronephros and mesonephros are the two primitive urinary systems of the human embryo. The pronephros regresses by week 6; at that time the mesonephros gives rise to the ureteral bud, preceding and inducing the development of the metanephros by the 8th to 10th week of gestation. The metanephros gives rise to the permanent kidney (nephron), whereas the ureteral bud is responsible for the formation of the renal collecting system (pelvis, calyces, etc.).

Although the kidneys and bladder can be imaged sonographically as early as 10 to 12 weeks' gestation, especially with newer equipment and transducers, the internal architecture of the kidneys cannot reliably be assessed before 16 weeks (Figs. 17-26 and 17-27). The kidneys appear as oval, hypoechoic, paraspinal structures in the dorsal area of the midabdomen. In the later half of pregnancy the renal capsule becomes more echogenic, and the kidneys are best viewed as circular, paraspinal structures in the transverse view of the mid to lower abdomen. The kidneys grow steadily throughout gestation, ranging from 2.0 cm in length at 20 weeks to nearly 4.0 cm at term (Table 17-10). Anterior-to-posterior dimension is approximately 1.0 to 1.1 cm at 20 weeks, increasing to 2.5

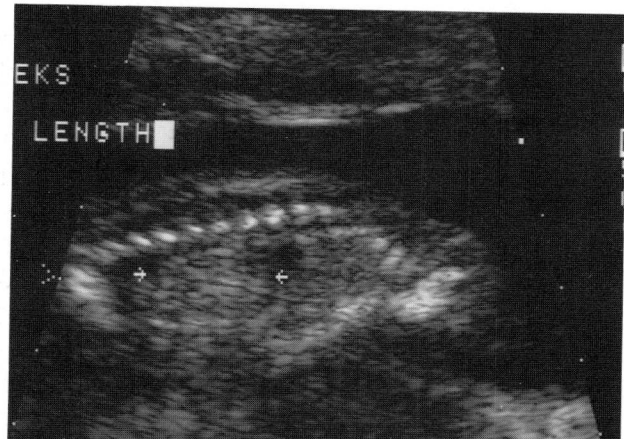

FIGURE 17-26. Sagittal view of renal length at 16 weeks. Note the close relationship to the spine and the difficulty in distinguishing the kidney from other surrounding structures.

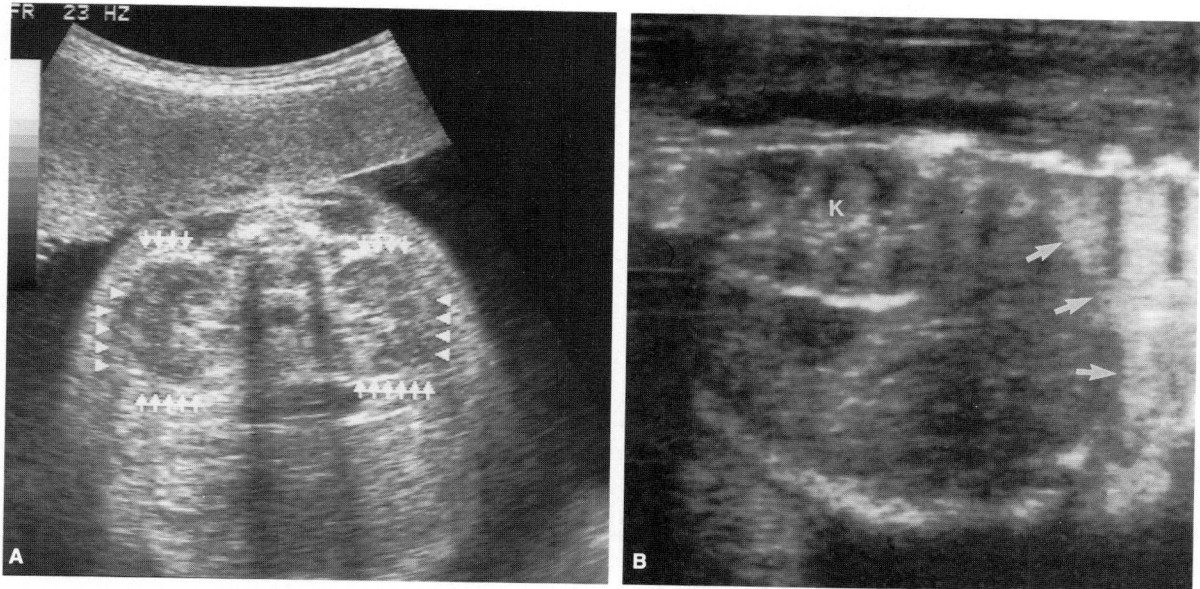

FIGURE 17-27. Normal kidneys, 30 weeks. **(A)** Transverse views of both kidneys. *Arrows* depict the echogenic renal capsule. **(B)** Longitudinal ultrasound in another case demonstrates the kidney (K) with good cortical medullary distinction. *Arrows* indicate the diaphragm.

TABLE 17-10. Normal Length of Fetal Kidneys at Different Gestational Ages

Menstrual Age (wk)	−2 SD* (mm)	Predicted Value† (mm)	+2 SD* (mm)
24	22.0	24.5	27.0
25	22.6	25.1	27.7
26	23.3	25.8	28.3
27	24.0	26.5	29.0
28	24.7	27.2	29.8
29	25.5	28.0	30.5
30	26.3	28.8	31.3
31	27.1	29.6	32.1
32	27.9	30.4	32.9
33	28.8	31.3	33.8
34	29.6	32.2	34.7
35	30.5	33.1	35.6
36	31.5	34.0	36.5
37	32.4	35.0	37.5
38	33.4	36.0	38.5
39	34.5	37.0	39.5
40	35.5	38.0	40.5
41	36.6	39.1	41.6
42	37.7	40.2	42.7

* Standard deviation = 1.259 mm.

† Length = 16.8933 + 0.0132 (menstrual age)^2.

(Bertagnoli L, Lalatta F, Gallicchio R, et al: Quantitative characterization of growth of the fetal kidney. J Clin Ultrasound 1983; 11:349–356. Used by permission.)

cm at 40 weeks (Table 17-11). A good rule of thumb is that in the second and third trimesters the kidneys increase in length at approximately 1 mm per week and increase in diameter at approximately 0.5 mm per week. Grannum and colleagues reported the ratio of kidney circumference to abdominal circumference in normal gestation, a useful ratio that remains relatively constant throughout the later half of pregnancy at approximately 28% to 30%[35] (Table 17-12). The normal ureter is not seen sonographically. The normal adrenal gland can often be visualized at the superior border of the kidney (Fig. 17-28).

Although the fetal kidneys are functionally immature throughout fetal life, urine production in the fetus begins by 10 weeks' gestation. However, fetal urine does not become the primary source of amniotic fluid volume until 16 to 18 weeks' gestation. This point is critical in the evaluation of possible urinary tract anomalies because amniotic fluid volume, particularly in the latter half of pregnancy, is a reliable indicator of fetal urine output.

Oligohydramnios

A detailed discussion of amniotic fluid volume is beyond the scope of this chapter; however, some sense of oligohydramnios is critical to the evaluation of urinary tract malformations. Although the subjective impression of oligohydramnios by experienced sonologists and sonographers is generally quite accurate, a semiquantitative estimate of amniotic fluid can be accomplished using a four-quadrant measurement technique, the *amniotic fluid index*.[36] With this technique, the sum of the largest vertical pocket in each quadrant is added together to form the index. A value below 5.0 cm is consistent with severe oligohydramnios beyond 16 weeks' gestation; before 32 to 34 weeks, a value below 8.0 cm raises concern of decreased amniotic fluid volume as well. The index is a very useful tool for serial examination and management of patients by multiple examiners of varying experience using different equipment. The test is very repro-

TABLE 17-11. Normal Anteroposterior Diameter of Kidneys at Different Gestational Ages

Menstrual Age (wk)	−2 SD* (mm)	Predicted Value† (mm)	+2 SD* (mm)
22	8.9	11.3	13.7
23	9.3	11.7	14.1
24	9.7	12.1	14.5
25	10.2	12.6	15.0
26	10.7	13.1	15.5
27	11.3	13.7	16.1
28	11.9	14.3	16.7
29	12.5	15.0	17.4
30	13.2	15.6	18.0
31	14.0	16.4	18.8
32	14.8	17.2	19.6
33	15.6	18.0	20.4
34	16.5	18.9	21.3
35	17.5	19.9	22.3
36	18.5	20.9	23.3
37	19.5	21.9	24.4
38	20.7	23.1	25.5
39	21.8	24.3	26.7
40	23.1	25.5	27.9

* Standard deviation (SD) = 1.209.

† Predicted value = 8.457278951 + .00026630314 (menstrual age)^3.

(Bertagnoli L, Lalatta F, Gallicchio R, et al: Quantitative characterization of growth of the fetal kidney. J Clin Ultrasound 1983; 11:349–356. Used by permission.)

TABLE 17-12.   Fetal Kidney and Abdominal Parameters by Gestational Age Group in Normal Fetuses

	Gestational Age (wk)					
Variable	<16 (n = 9)	17–20 (n = 18)	21–25 (n = 7)	26–30 (n = 11)	31–35 (n = 19)	>36 (n = 25)
Fetal Kidney						
Anteroposterior (cm)						
Mean	0.84	1.16	1.49	1.93	2.20	2.32
SD	0.24	0.24	0.37	0.19	0.32	0.32
Transverse (cm)						
Mean	0.86	1.13	1.64	2.00	2.34	2.63
SD	0.14	0.25	0.40	0.28	0.42	0.50
Circumference (cm)						
Mean	2.79	3.80	5.40	6.58	7.86	8.42
SD	0.64	0.72	0.68	0.67	0.86	1.39
Fetal Abdomen						
Anteroposterior (cm)						
Mean	2.92	3.73	5.12	6.74	8.50	8.88
SD	0.62	0.72	0.80	0.58	0.82	0.94
Transverse (cm)						
Mean	2.93	3.68	5.12	7.09	8.76	9.68
SD	0.59	0.56	0.49	0.61	0.89	1.44
Circumference (cm)						
Mean	9.66	12.37	17.36	22.03	28.11	30.45
SD	1.88	2.28	1.77	1.77	2.31	3.45
KC/AC* Ratio						
Mean	0.28	0.30	0.30	0.29	0.28	0.27
SD	0.02	0.03	0.02	0.02	0.03	0.04

Calculations of ratio used variables measured to eight decimal places.

* KC, kidney circumference; AC, abdominal circumference.

(Reprinted with permission from Grannum P, Bracken M, Silverman R, et al: Assessment of fetal kidney size in normal gestation by comparison of ratio of kidney circumference to abdominal circumference. Am J Obstet Gynecol 1980; 136:253.)

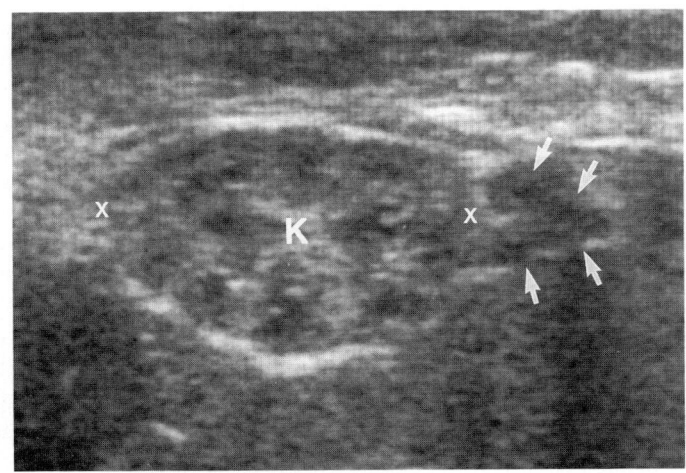

FIGURE 17-28. Normal kidney—adrenal. Longitudinal scan of the kidney (K) demonstrates cortical medullary distinction. At the most cephalad border of the kidney is the Y- or V-shaped adrenal gland (*arrows*).

ducible as well, with inter- and intra-observer error of less than 7%.[37]

Anomalies

It is important to realize that urinary tract anomalies represent some of the most common anomalies seen in fetal and neonatal life. In our practical scheme, the basic questions to ask include:

1. Are the bladder and both kidneys documented in their normal location?
2. Are the renal pelvises, ureters, and/or bladder dilated?
3. Are renal cysts present? If so, do they communicate?
4. Are the kidneys abnormal in size or echogenicity?
5. Are the abnormalities bilateral or unilateral?
6. Is the amniotic fluid volume normal?

Are the Bladder and Both Kidneys Documented in Their Normal Location?

Renal Agenesis: Bilateral. The incidence of complete bilateral renal agenesis (Potter syndrome) is approximately 1 in 4000 births.[38] The malformation is more common in males (as are most urinary tract anomalies) and is invariably accompanied by oligohydramnios beyond 18 to 20 weeks' gestation. In earlier gestation, amniotic fluid volume is not dependent on urine production and may be normal despite absent renal function. The diagnosis of bilateral renal agenesis should be suspected when severe oligohydramnios is seen and the kidneys and bladder cannot be visualized. The differential diagnosis includes symmetric intrauterine growth retardation with oligohydramnios as well as early preterm premature rupture of membranes.

Potential pitfalls in the diagnosis include:

1. Assuming that amniotic fluid volume is normal despite nonvisualization of kidneys and bladder
2. Inability to image the kidneys and bladder due to the poor image quality associated with severe oligohydramnios (especially with an anterior placenta and/or a thick maternal abdominal wall)
3. Adrenal hypertrophy associated with renal agenesis (Fig. 17-29). Because the kidneys and adrenals are embryologically different, the adrenal glands are almost always present with renal agenesis. The adrenals appear larger and assume a discoid shape, have a distinct cortex

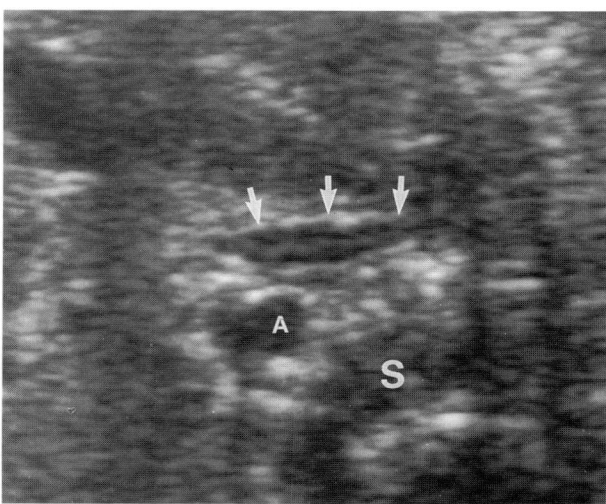

FIGURE 17-29. Adrenal gland with renal agenesis. Transverse ultrasound of the fetal abdomen demonstrating the spine (S) posteriorly, the aorta (A), and the "pancake"-shaped adrenal gland (*arrows*). The adrenal gland is nearly 2 cm in length with very distinct hypoechoic adrenal cortex and echogenic adrenal medulla.

and medulla, and thus may be mistaken for renal tissue when there is renal agenesis. Methods to help avoid this pitfall are listed below.

Until recently, a *furosemide challenge test*[39] was suggested as a diagnostic aid in the diagnosis, to accelerate the prolonged scanning time often required to visualize the bladder. Normal fetal bladder filling and emptying cycles every 20 to 45 minutes. Failure to demonstrate the bladder after intravenous furosemide administration to the mother, despite frequent observations over more than 2 hours, was reported to be a reliable indicator of Potter syndrome. More recently the reliability of this technique has been questioned.[40] In one series, among six fetuses with oligohydramnios and failure of furosemide to demonstrate the bladder, two growth-retarded fetuses with normal urinary tracts were reported.[41] However, a negative test may still be useful, for if the fetal bladder is identified to fill and empty, bilateral renal agenesis can be ruled out. The other potential etiologies for absent bladder are listed in Table 17-13.

Many experienced sonologists have begun to utilize the transvaginal transducer, particularly in the second trimester and with breech presentations, to aid in visualizing the kidneys and bladder.[42] A transabdominal infusion of saline via amniocentesis has been employed with great success

TABLE 17-13.   Nonvisualization of the Fetal Bladder

Renal Abnormality

Bilateral renal agenesis
Bilateral ureteral pelvic junction obstruction
Bilateral multicystic dysplastic kidney
Bilateral combinations of any of the above
Infantile polycystic kidney disease

Bladder Abnormality

Cloacal (or bladder) exstrophy
Persistent cloaca

Systemic

Severe intrauterine growth retardation

to enhance the image quality in these difficult cases.[43]

When the adrenal glands are enlarged with Potter sequence, *color flow Doppler* is now sensitive enough to depict the renal vasculature with some reliability[44] (Fig. 17-30). Inability to visualize renal arterial blood flow supports the diagnosis of renal agenesis, but perhaps more importantly, color flow mapping can often help delineate the kidneys in difficult cases of oligohydramnios, thereby avoiding confusion.

Associated anomalies with bilateral renal agenesis are quite common, although many of these represent deformations rather than malformations, the consequences of oligohydramnios. The abnormal facies so typical of "Potter's sequence," the limb deformities and pulmonary hypoplasia invariably seen, are all a direct result of the prolonged lack of amniotic fluid volume for the fetus[45] (Fig. 17-31). The small chest circumference and an abnormal chest-to-abdominal circumference ratio[46] support the diagnosis of pulmonary hypoplasia. In addition, musculoskeletal anomalies are reported in 40% of cases, cardiac anomalies are seen in nearly 15%, and central nervous system and gastrointestinal anomalies have been reported as well.

If the diagnosis is certain, pregnancy termination should be offered owinge to the uniform lethality of the condition. Although severe oligohydramnios alone carries a dismal prognosis, it is critical, particularly in later gestation, to be certain of the diagnosis of bilateral renal agenesis before offering nonintervention for the fetus in these cases. With this in mind, it is important to avoid the pitfalls noted above and certainly appropriate to use vaginal transducers, color flow Doppler, and amnioinfusion if necessary to confirm the diagnosis.

Unilateral renal agenesis is a much more common disorder, although the diagnosis may be far more difficult (Table 17-14). The presence of a normal-appearing bladder and amniotic fluid volume, coupled with the hyperplastic adrenal gland occu-

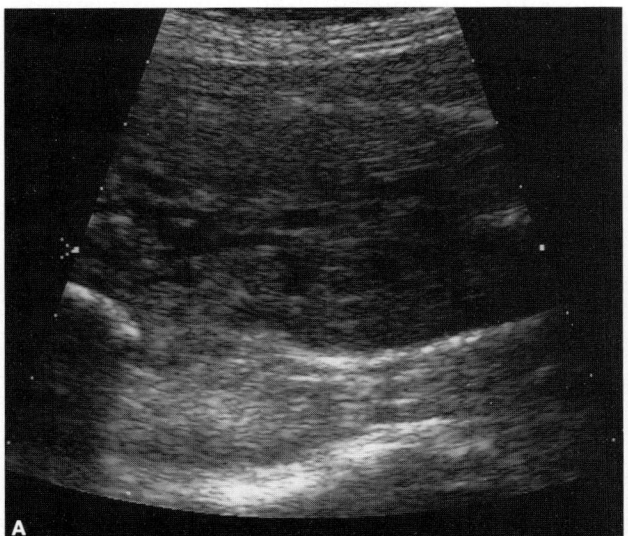
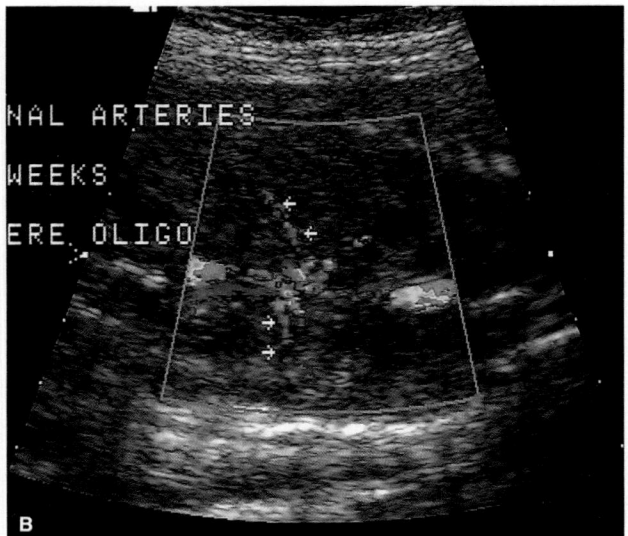

FIGURE 17-30.   Nonvisualization of kidney—color flow. **(A)** A sagittal view of the abdomen in this 21-week fetus referred for oligohydramnios to rule out Potter syndrome. Kidneys are not clearly identified. **(B)** Color flow Doppler maps out the renal arteries bilaterally (*arrows*) and demonstrates the kidneys clearly.

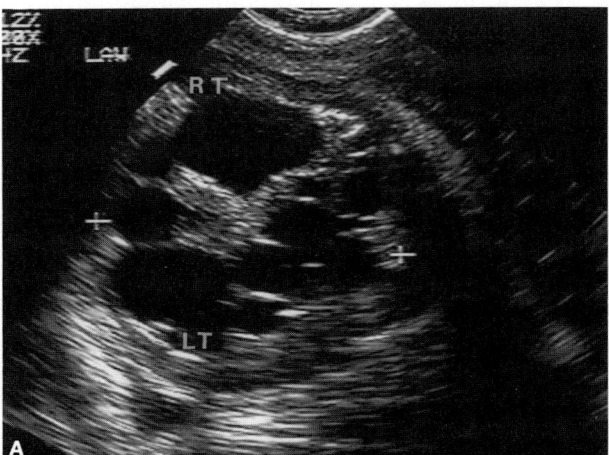
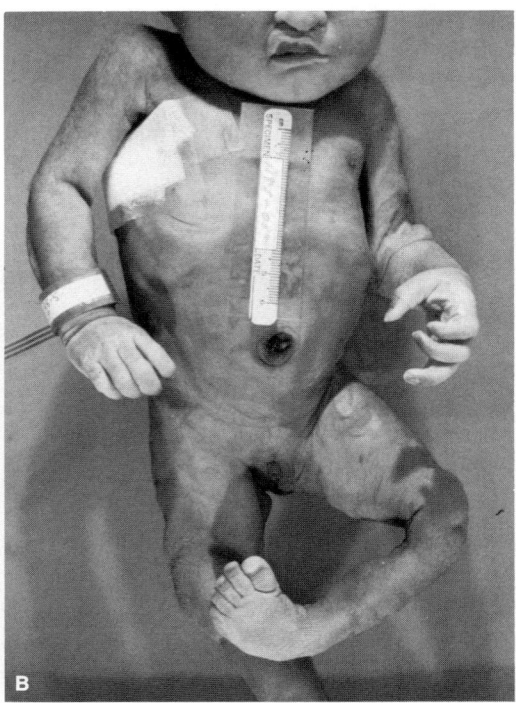

FIGURE 17-31. Multicystic dysplastic kidneys (MCDK)—bilateral. **(A)** Right (RT) and left (LT) kidneys demonstrating multiple cysts of varying sizes corresponding to MCDK or Potter type II. There was associated severe fetal oligohydramnios. **(B)** Fetal specimen demonstrating limb deformities and abnormal facies due to oligohydramnios with Potter's syndrome.

pying the renal fossa on the affected side, makes it easy to see why this diagnosis is often overlooked (see Fig. 17-29). In many cases other anomalies are present. A common pitfall in this diagnosis results from failure to image one kidney in a transverse plane owing to acoustic shadowing from the spine (see Table 17-14). Rotating the transducer to image both renal fossa is critical (Fig. 17-32).

Ectopic Kidney. Pelvic kidney is a relatively frequent occurrence (approximately 1 in 1000 births) and a common pitfall in the diagnosis of unilateral

renal agenesis.[47] When both kidneys are not clearly identified in their usual paraspinous location, a high index of suspicion is required to make the diagnosis (Fig. 17-33). Ectopic kidneys can also be found in the thorax and other areas within the abdomen.

Less commonly, crossed renal ectopia[48] may be confused with unilateral renal agenesis. In this condition the kidney is located on the opposite side from its ureter. Typically the kidney is bilobed, enlarged, and S- or L-shaped, often with findings of obstructive uropathy.

Horseshoe Kidney. Horseshoe kidney is a relatively common renal anomaly, with an incidence of approximately 1 in 400 births. The kidneys are usually joined at the lower pole by an isthmus adjacent to the third or fourth lumbar vertebra. Associated anomalies—including cardiac, central nervous system, and chromosomal anomalies such as Turner syndrome (45, XO) and trisomy 18—are quite common with this disorder. In the absence of other anomalies, horseshoe kidney is a relatively benign disorder that often goes undetected.

TABLE 17-14.   Differential Diagnosis of Absent Fetal Kidney (Unilateral)

Shadowing from the fetal spine
Pelvic kidney
Unilateral renal agenesis
Crossed renal ectopia

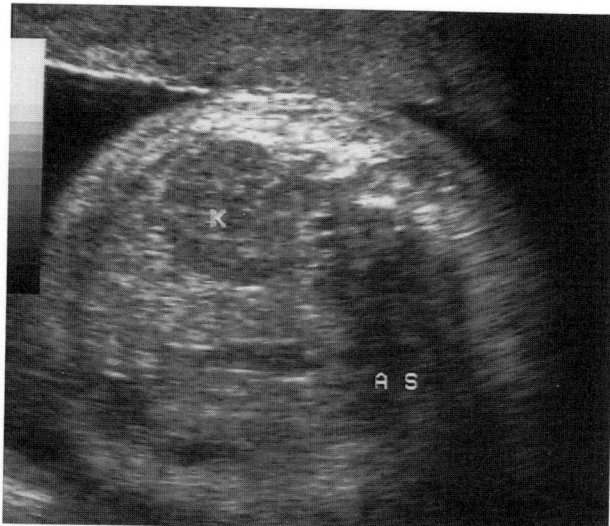

FIGURE 17-32.   Kidney visualization—pitfall. Acoustic shadowing (AS) from the spine obliterates the view of one kidney in this transverse view of a 32-week fetus. K, kidney.

Are the Renal Pelvises, Ureters, and/or Bladder Dilated?

Obstructive lesions of the genitourinary system are among the most common sonographic findings in obstetrics. In a study of 142 neonates with obstructive uropathy, over 75% were initially diagnosed

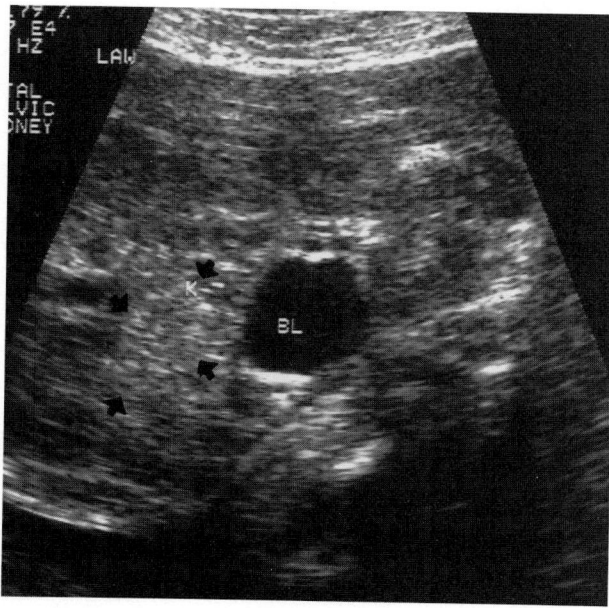

FIGURE 17-33.   Pelvic kidney (K), noted by *arrows*, is located immediately superior to the bladder (BL) and not in the usual paraspinal location.

prenatally.[49] Fifty percent of the cases involved a ureteropelvic junction obstruction, 25% exhibited ureterovesical junction obstruction, 15% had a duplicate collecting system, and 5% had a bladder obstruction (posterior urethral valve). It seems appropriate to discuss these anomalies in their order of frequency.

Ureteropelvic Junction Obstruction.   Ureteropelvic junction obstruction (UPJ) is by far the most common form of obstructive uropathy, representing fully two thirds of fetal hydronephrosis cases (Fig. 17-34 and 17-35; see also Figs. 17-15 and 17-16). It is also important because congenital hydronephrosis often has a subtle clinical presentation for neonates; in some series less than 25% of cases are diagnosed by 1 year of age, and only 55% of cases are diagnosed by age 5. Given the fact that diagnostic delay may increase the risk of permanent renal impairment, it is crucial to make an early and accurate diagnosis whenever possible.

Although an early diagnosis of fetal UPJ obstruction is clearly important for optimal outcome, minimal or mild renal collecting system dilation, or pyelectasis (see Fig. 17-34), generally resolves without clinical sequelae.[50] Frequent rescanning of these individuals increases health care costs and patients' anxieties, all without any benefit to the fetus. Currently there is no consensus of management for patients with minimal pyelectasis. However, until very recently many had followed the guidelines of Grignon and colleagues.[51] Specifically, they found that a pelvic diameter (measured in the AP direction) (see Fig. 17-34) in a transverse plane of less than 1 cm and a ratio of pelvic-to-kidney diameter of less than 50% were rarely associated with a kidney requiring postnatal therapy (Table 17-15).

A more recent study by Corteville and co-workers challenged this dictum.[52] They reported a 41% incidence of congenital hydronephrosis in fetuses who had AP measurements of the renal pelvis in the 4- to 6-mm range before 24 weeks' gestation (Table 17-16). They recommended a repeat scan in 3 to 4 weeks if the AP diameter of the renal pelvis is 4 mm before 33 weeks and 7 mm after 33 weeks (Table 17-17). This approach may yield a high sensitivity for the detection of hydronephrosis, although, clearly, many false positive diagnoses would result. In fact, using a pelvis-to-kidney ratio of greater than 28% as a threshold (as Corteville suggests) led to a greater than 90% sensitivity but at the expense of a false positive rate of 20% to 50% for the diagnosis of congenital hydronephro-

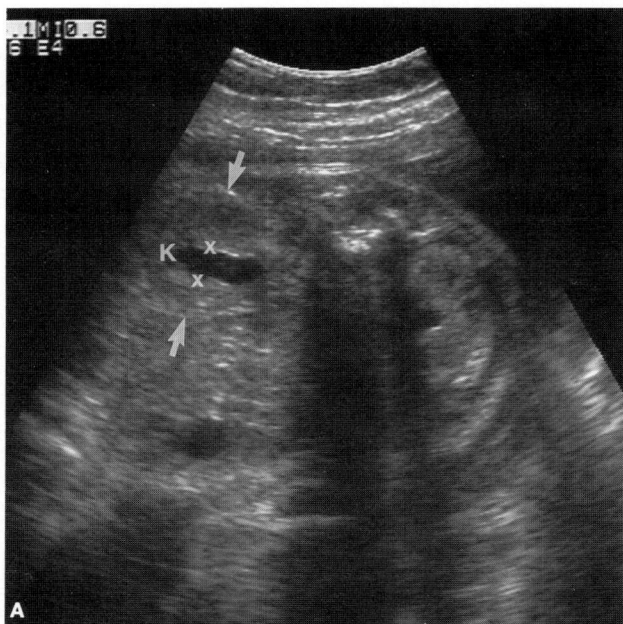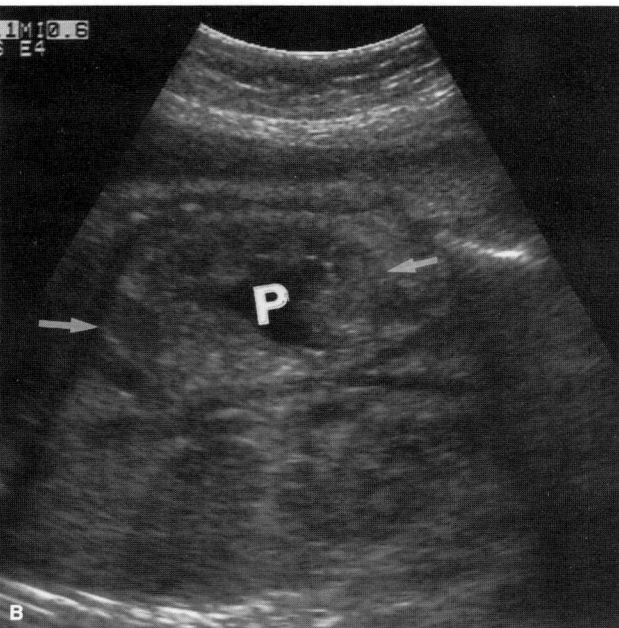

FIGURE 17-34.   Pyelectasis. **(A)** Transverse view of the abdomen in this fetus returning for re-exam at 21 weeks to follow prominent renal pelvis. The AP measurement of the renal pelvis (calipers) was 7 mm. AP dimension of the kidney (K) is marked by *arrows*. **(B)** Sagittal view of the same fetus reveals a dilated renal pelvis (P). The patient developed moderate hydronephrosis due to a ureteropelvic junction (UPJ) obstruction but did well postnatally.

sis (Table 17-18). One potential pitfall in accurately determining the false positive rate in these studies is the fact that postnatal dehydration in the first 48 hours can lead to a falsely normal report.[53] Reevaluation of cases at risk should be considered at 5 to 7 days after birth when initial postnatal sonograms appear normal.

Mandell and colleagues[54] suggest a slightly different approach, which in our center has helped maintain a high sensitivity for the diagnosis of significant hydronephrosis while minimizing the false positive rate. Their thresholds for follow-up pre- and postnatal scanning are based on the renal pelvic diameter in the AP plane:

>4 mm between 15 and 20 weeks
>8 mm between 20 and 30 weeks

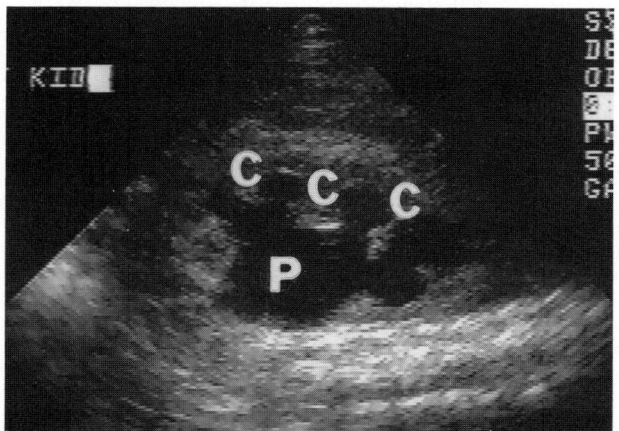

FIGURE 17-35.   Moderate hydronephrosis. Note the renal pelvis (P) and calyceal (C) dilatation in this fetus near term.

TABLE 17-15.   Grading of Degrees of Fetal Hydronephrosis After 20 Menstrual Weeks

Grade	Size of Renal Pelvis	Calyceal Dilatation
I	<10 mm	Physiologic
II	10–15 mm	Normal calyces
III	>15 mm	Slight dilatation
IV	>15 mm	Moderate dilatation
V	>15 mm	Severe dilatation

(Modified from Grignon A, Filion R, Filiatrault D, et al: Urinary tract dilatation in utero: Classification and clinical applications. Radiology 1986; 160:645.)

TABLE 17-16. Anteroposterior Diameter of Fetal Renal Pelvis at Different Stages of Gestation Correlated With Subsequent Congenital Hydronephrosis Confirmed Postnatally and With Postnatal Urinary Tract Corrective Surgery or Renal Compromise

Anteroposterior Pelvic Diameter (mm)	14–23 Wk		24–32 Wk		33–42 Wk	
	CH (%)	S/C (%)	CH (%)	S/C (%)	CH (%)	S/C (%)
<3	0	0	0	0	0	0
4–6	41	19	38	13	0	0
7–9	53	40	33	6	67	50
>10	82	73	86	72	82	59

CH, congenital hydronephrosis confirmed postnatally; S/C, postnatal surgery and/or evidence of renal compromise.

(Corteville JE, Gray DL, Crane JP: Congenital hydronephrosis: Correlation of fetal ultrasonographic findings with infant outcome. Am J Obstet Gynecol 1991; 165:384.)

>10 mm beyond 30 weeks. Patients with less renal pelvic dilatation appear to have minimal risk of progressive obstructive uropathy.

Recently, second-trimester renal pyelectasis has been associated with Down's syndrome.[55] Benacerraf and coworkers, using similar criteria for pyelectasis as shown above, noted retrospectively that 25% of 44 Down's syndrome fetuses exhibited mild pyelectasis. These authors do not suggest prenatal diagnosis unless pyelectasis is accompanied by other sonographic signs of Down's syndrome.[56] (For an in-depth discussion of Down's syndrome see Chapter 21.)

Despite the controversy surrounding second-trimester pyelectasis, few would argue that at any gestational age, a renal pelvic diameter greater than 10 mm is associated with a need for intervention in the majority of cases. In Corteville's series such patients had a greater than 80% incidence of confirmed neonatal hydronephrosis, and the majority required surgical intervention and/or had evidence for compromise (see Tables 17-16 to 17-18 and Figs. 17-34 and 17-35). Another approach to grading severity has been suggested by Harrison and colleagues.[57] Specifically, they suggest reserving the severe designation for patients with large unilocular dilatation, while mild to moderate would describe dilated renal pelvis and dilated calyces, respectively (see Figs. 17-35 and 17-36).

Most commonly the obstruction is unilateral, maintaining normal or sometimes compensatory polyhydramnios, and requires no prenatal inter-

TABLE 17-17. Anteroposterior Diameter of Fetal Renal Pelvis at Different Stages of Gestation Correlated With Risk of Postnatal Congenital Hydronephrosis

Anteroposterior Pelvic Diameter	14–23 Wk		24–32 Wk		33–42 Wk	
	Sensitivity (%)	False-Positive Rate (%)	Sensitivity (%)	False-Positive Rate (%)	Sensitivity (%)	False-Positive Rate (%)
≥4	100	55	100	42	100	24
≥7	61	35	91	34	100	21
≥10	32	18	74	14	82	18

(Corteville JE, Gray DL, Crane JP: Congenital hydronephrosis: Correlation of fetal ultrasonographic findings with infant outcome. Am J Obstet Gynecol 1991; 165:384.)

TABLE 17-18.   Ratio of Anteroposterior Diameter of Fetal Renal Pelvis to Kidney at Different Stages of Pregnancy Correlated With Risk of Postnatal Congenital Hydronephrosis

Anteroposterior Diameter Pelvis/Kidney Ratio	14–23 Wk		24–32 Wk		33–42 Wk	
	Sensitivity (%)	False-Positive Rate (%)	Sensitivity (%)	False-Positive Rate (%)	Sensitivity (%)	False-Positive Rate (%)
>0.28	100	50	90	37	91	20
>0.30	92	48	88	33	84	20
>0.40	64	47	69	15	68	21
>0.50	40	47	52	8	50	15

(Corteville JE, Gray DL, Crane JP: Congenital hydronephrosis: Correlation of fetal ultrasonographic findings with infant outcome. Am J Obstet Gynecol 1991; 165:384.)

vention. When unilateral hydronephrosis is accompanied by oligohydramnios, a search for contralateral pathology must be made (eg, agenesis, dysplasia, etc.). With bilateral hydronephrosis, serial ultrasound evaluations are necessary in the third trimester to address amniotic fluid volume and progression of renal pelvic dilatation.

Severe oligohydramnios in the second trimester carries an extremely poor prognosis, and termination of pregnancy is a definite option. In the third trimester, decisions regarding delivery versus conservative management must be made based on the overall clinical circumstances and the patient's wishes. When bilateral UPJ obstruction is associated with normal or increased amniotic fluid, a targeted search for a concomitant gastrointestinal anomaly is warranted. Of course, the obstetrical ultrasound axiom cannot be overstated: *whenever one anomaly is encountered another should be expected.* The presence of ascites in conjunction with severe UPJ obstruction strongly suggests urinary ascites and generally carries a poor prognosis for the kidney with a presumed ruptured collecting system (see Fig. 17-18). Open surgical intervention for severe bilateral hydronephrosis, using a hysterotomy approach to perform open cutaneous ureterostomies, has been tried only a few times.[58] This procedure clearly remains experimental.

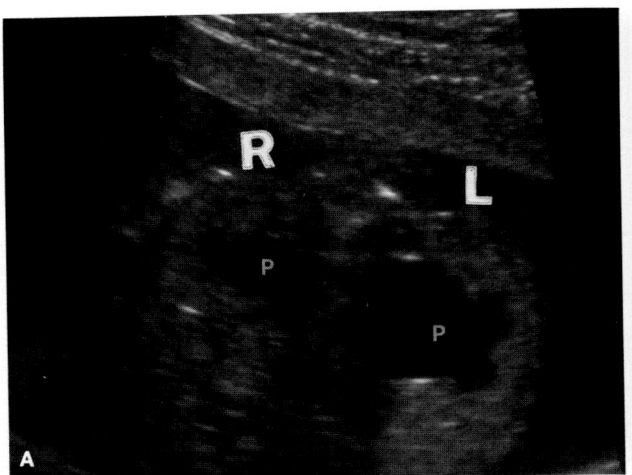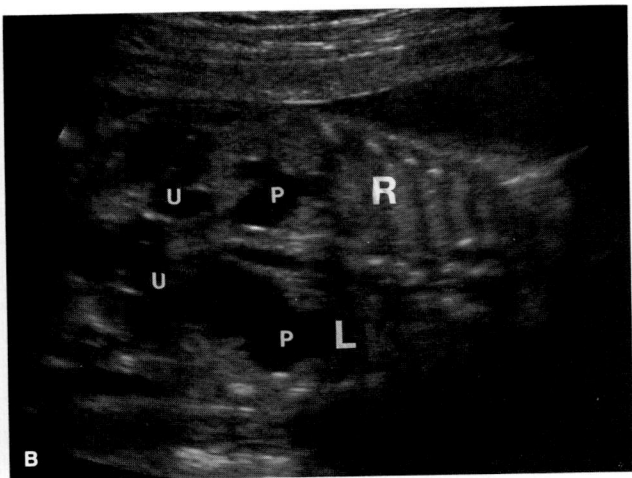

FIGURE 17-36.   Bilateral hydroureter. **(A)** Transverse scan revealing right-sided (R) pyelectasis (P), with 8-mm AP dilatation, and moderate hydronephrosis (P) on the left (L) with 1.6-cm dilatation. **(B)** Coronal ultrasound demonstrating bilateral pyelectasis (P) and hydroureters (U). R, right; L, left.

Hydroureter and Ureterovesical Junction Obstruction. Ureteral dilatation is typically the result of urinary obstruction or reflux, often beginning at the ureterovesical junction (UVJ). This disorder is several times more common in males and is more frequently encountered on the left side. As mentioned previously, the normal fetal ureter is generally 1 to 2 mm in diameter and is not readily visualized sonographically. Primary megaureter refers to a defect in the ureter, as in ureteral valve stenosis and ureterocele. Secondary megaureter refers to an anomaly elsewhere resulting in megaureter, such as in the classic posterior urethral valve syndrome. Hydronephrosis and hydroureter are concomitant findings in typical UVJ cases, although the ureter tends to be more dilated than the renal pelvis (Fig. 17-36). The diagnosis of UVJ is fairly secure when one encounters dilated ureters in the absence of megacystis.

The sonographic appearance of hydroureter may be difficult to distinguish from that of bowel. It should also be pointed out that the presence of active peristalsis of a sonolucent tubular structure on real-time sonography does not confirm bowel; it is often seen with hydroureter as well. The snakelike sonolucent segments must be meticulously tracked to demonstrate their communication with the kidney and/or bladder[59] (see Fig. 17-36). In addition, the ureter generally comes into close contact with the spine, which the small bowel does not. These structures can be several centimeters in width, so that size alone does not preclude megaureter as a possible diagnosis (Table 17-19).

Ureterocele. Ureterocele is a dilated ureter that has prolapsed into the bladder either at the normal ureteral orifice (simple) or at an atypical orifice location at the bladder neck or urethra (ectopic) (Fig.

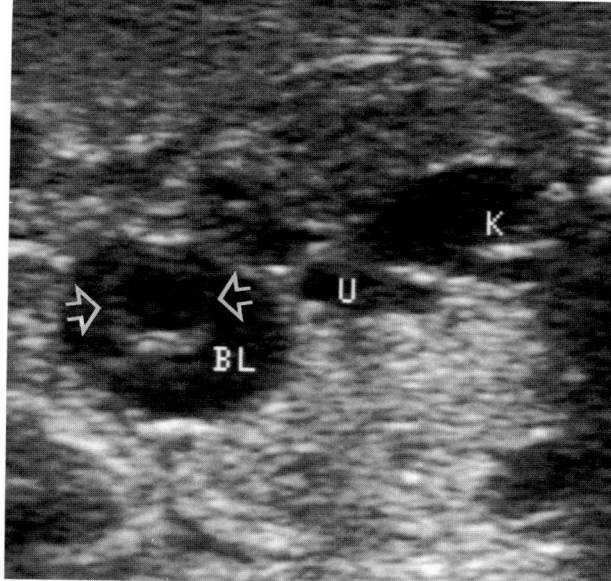

FIGURE 17-37. Simple ureterocele. Prenatal coronal ultrasound of the fetal abdomen demonstrating dilatation of the pelvis of the kidney (K), hydroureter (U), and bladder (BL) with ureterocele (*arrows*).

17-37). Unlike most urinary tract disorders, ureterocele is nearly four times more common in females and is generally left sided.[60] A duplicate renal collecting system is a commonly associated anomaly, typically with the upper pole obstructed in an ectopic ureterocele.[61] Therefore, if focal hydronephrosis is detected, a careful search of the urinary bladder is necessary to exclude a ureterocele. The kidney on the side of the ureterocele tends to be significantly affected, often with dysplastic and/or cystic changes.

The sonographic diagnosis is fairly straightforward when the bladder is at least partially full. Under these circumstances, a cystlike structure can be readily detected within the bladder. If the bladder is empty or only minimally distended, the diagnosis can often be overlooked. Therefore, it is important to evaluate the bladder over a prolonged period of time when upper urinary tract pathology is detected, to avoid missing a possible ureterocele.

Megacystis. The most likely etiology for a persistently distended bladder is a urethral obstruction. Among the various causes, posterior urethral valve (PUV) is the most common, followed by a urethral membrane, urethral atresia, stricture, and persistent cloaca (Table 17-20). A nonobstructive

TABLE 17-19. Differentiating Hydroureter From Bowel

	Hydroureter	Bowel
Appearance	Anechoic, tubular	Anechoic, tubular
Kidneys and bladder	Often dilated	Usually normal
Location	Posterior	Anterior
Communication	Renal pelvis	Other loops
Peristalsis	Yes	Yes
Intraluminal particles	No	Yes
Gender	Usually male	Either

TABLE 17-20. Etiologies for Megacystis

Posterior urethral valves
Urethral diaphragmatic membrane
Urethral atresia (agenesis)
Urethral stricture
Persistent cloaca
Megacystis–microcolon–intestinal hypoperistalsis syndrome

cause for megacystis (megacystis–microcolon–intestinal hypoperistalsis syndrome) will be discussed separately. Because of its bilateral destructive effects, urethral obstruction, if complete, is potentially one of the most devastating fetal anomalies.

Classically, the diagnosis of PUV consists of a distended fetal bladder with a dilated proximal urethra ("keyhole appearance") in a male fetus, often with oligohydramnios (see Figs. 17-17 and 17-18). If the bladder does not completely obscure more detailed abdominal examination, the kidneys and ureters will display evidence of bilateral obstruction as well, in the form of hydroureter and hydronephrosis. If the obstruction is longstanding, the kidneys may actually be small and echogenic, consistent with dysplasia (Fig. 17-38), an extremely poor prognostic sign. Once decompressed, either by spontaneous rupture or percutaneous aspiration (cystocentesis), the bladder usually displays a thickened muscular wall (>2 mm) (see Fig. 17-17).

Whereas PUV and urethral membrane often cause an intermittent obstruction, urethral atresia

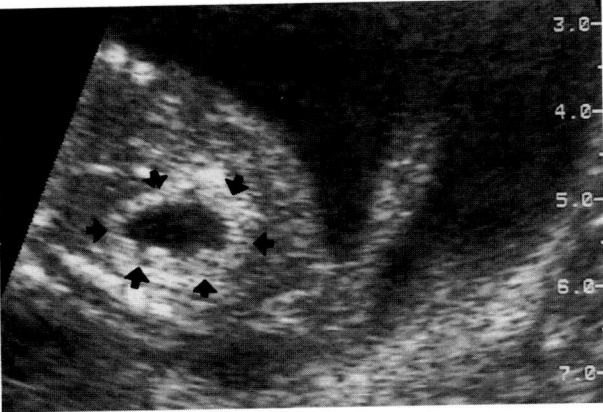

FIGURE 17-38. Echogenic kidney (*arrows*) with collecting system dilatation in a patient with posterior urethral valve. This represents a poor prognostic sign for renal function, suggesting renal dysplasia.

can be detected in the first trimester.[62] Bulie and coworkers noted a 2-cm sonolucent mass in the fetal pelvis as early as 11 weeks' gestation, providing strong support for early fetal urine production. More disturbing, however, was the fact that both cases showed serious renal lesions at pathologic examination despite delivery at 14 and 15 weeks. Such data raise serious questions regarding the feasibility of fetal therapy in this disorder.

Management. Fetal therapy for urethral obstruction has been a controversial subject of intense interest for more than a decade. Although much has been learned over that time, major questions remain as to patient selection criteria, timing of intervention, and surgical technique. On the surface it would appear straightforward to conclude that if urethral obstruction leads to renal dysplasia and pulmonary hypoplasia over time, then diverting the urine to the amniotic cavity via a timely vesicoamniotic shunt should prevent further renal damage and pulmonary hypoplasia. Data from the International Fetal Surgery Registry noted that nearly all neonatal deaths after vesicoamniotic shunt were secondary to pulmonary hypoplasia.[63] As with most urinary tract anomalies, the presence or absence and duration of oligohydramnios are critical factors in the fetal prognosis. Mahoney and colleagues evaluated 40 bladder outlet obstructions to determine the important prognostic prenatal ultrasound features.[64] Over 50% of survivors had a normal amniotic fluid volume, whereas only 7% survived with oligohydramnios. By way of contrast, 80% of those suffering a subsequent demise had decreased amniotic fluid, whereas only 12% had a normal volume. The only other predictor in their series appeared to be the degree of caliectasis. Over 70% of survivors had moderate to marked collecting system dilatation, whereas 80% of demises had little or no caliectasis. Other authors have found the presence of renal cortical cysts to have a 100% specificity for renal dysplasia but less than 60% sensitivity.[82,83] The presence of increased renal echogenicity has had similar predictability.

Recently, fetal urine analysis obtained by percutaneous aspiration has been utilized extensively to help predict renal function in utero.[65] Normally, fetal urine is very hypotonic; measuring urine electrolytes has produced some useful cutoff values for prognosis. The thresholds for good function include: sodium less than 100, chloride less than 90, osmolality less than 210, calcium less than 1.5, and urine output greater than 2 ml/hour. Urine electrolytes above these values suggest that the prognosis for normal kidney function is small. Other investi-

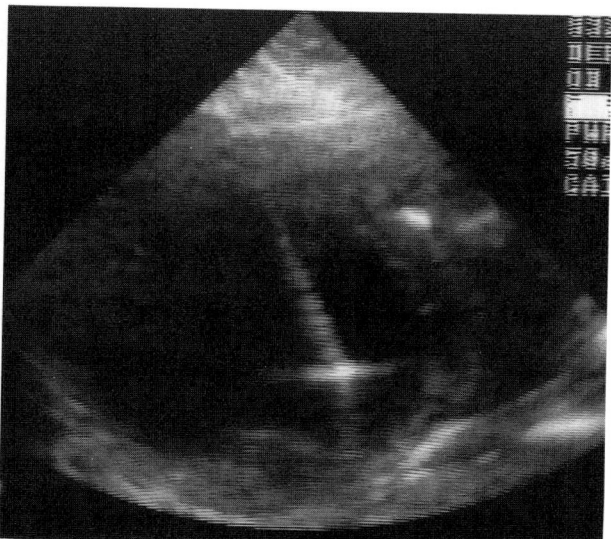

FIGURE 17-39. Huge megacystic bladder undergoing cystocentesis for decompression and diagnosis.

gators have challenged the efficacy of these thresholds,[66,67] but to date no more reliable predictor of successful outcome or candidacy for intervention has been proposed. At our center the fresh fetal urine analysis, obtained via cystocentesis (Fig. 17-39), is combined with the ultrasound appearance of the kidneys and amniotic fluid volume to counsel the patient regarding the prognosis and options. The need for a *fresh* urine sample from the fetal bladder cannot be emphasized enough. In our experience, fetal urine that may have resided in the fetal bladder for many days may not accurately depict the current status of renal function.

Once the patient is determined to be a good candidate for intervention, one fetal surgical choice is the percutaneous placement (under ultrasound guidance) of a "pig-tailed" catheter (Fig. 17-40) into the bladder with the distal end on the anterior abdominal wall draining into the amniotic cavity. Crombleholme and colleagues reviewed an uncontrolled experience of 40 cases, many of whom underwent a shunt procedure.[68] In the group with normal-appearing kidneys and normal amniotic fluid, there was an 89% survival rate among the group treated surgically; however, the nonintervention group had a 70% survival rate with the same favorable criteria. In those with dysplasia and/or hypertonic urine, there were no survivors without intervention and a 30% survival rate with shunting. Among the vesicoamniotic shunt cases reported to the International Registry for Fetal Surgery, nearly 80% survival has been noted when candidates exhibited normal urinary electrolytes and ultrasound findings preoperatively.[69]

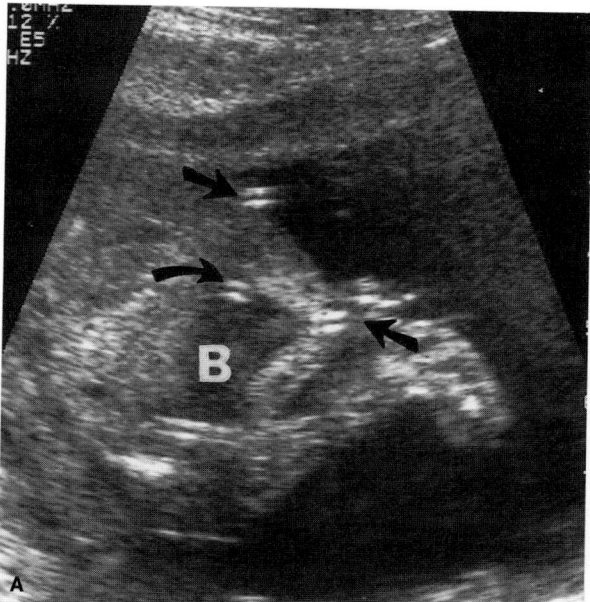
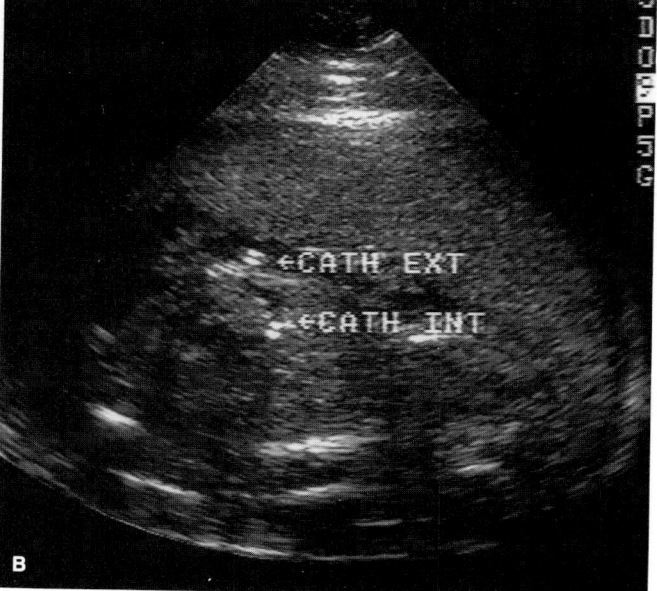

FIGURE 17-40. **(A)** Vesicoamniotic shunt 72 hours after placement at 14 weeks' gestation for a fetus with urethral atresia. Note the irregular bladder shape (B). (*Arrows* indicate catheter.) **(B)** Another vesicoamniotic shunt placed at 18 weeks' gestation. Echogenic catheter tips aid in placement and subsequent follow-up.

The problem with catheter placement is the potential for complications such as preterm labor, ruptured membranes, fetal trauma, infection, and, above all, shunt migration or occlusion. As a result of some of these concerns, Harrison and coworkers have performed several open vesicostomies through a hysterotomy incision in the late second trimester.[70] This procedure carries the risks of major surgery and anesthesia, as well as those associated with an open uterine cavity (preterm delivery infection, fetal hypoxia, hypothermia, and premature rupture of the membranes). Much more work is needed to evaluate the relative efficacy of these approaches.

Megacystis–Microcolon–Intestinal Hypoperistalsis Syndrome. Megacystis–microcolon–intestinal hypoperistalsis syndrome (MMIH) is another cause for an enlarged bladder. Although MMIH is far less common than PUV, differentiating between these two very distinct lesions is critical, especially if fetal therapy is being considered. MMIH carries a dismal prognosis, with the overwhelming majority of neonates dying soon after birth. The syndrome involves not only an unobstructed distended bladder but also a dilated small bowel and distal microcolon. The key features differentiating megacystis from urethral obstruction are the following:

1. Amniotic fluid is normal or increased in MMIH.

2. In MMIH the fetus is usually female; in PUV the fetus is almost always male.
3. A dilated small bowel is present with MMIH.

Although fetal surgery is of no benefit to the fetus with MMIH, the overdistended bladder may cause a soft tissue dystocia, which cystocentesis before delivery may prevent.

Are Renal Cysts Present?

Among neonatal renal anomalies, cystic lesions of the kidney are second only to hydronephrosis and hydroureter in frequency of diagnosis.[71] The various conditions are often confused, given the similarity of the names involved: polycystic, multicystic dysplastic, cystic dysplasia, and Potter types I, II, III, and IV. This section attempts to clarify these anomalies (Table 17-21).

Multicystic Dysplastic Kidney (Potter Type II). Multicystic dysplastic kidney (MCDK), or Potter type II, usually represents the end result of an early, severe urinary obstruction. This embryonic insult leaves a functionless kidney replaced by multiple cysts, both grossly and sonographically (Figs. 17-31 and 17-41). The lesion is unilateral in 70% to 80% of patients, although 20% to 30% have a renal anomaly of the contralateral kidney[72] (see Fig. 17-31). Bilateral processes such as bilateral MCDK or unilateral MCDK with renal agenesis are usually fatal to the fetus. However, unilateral MCDK most commonly occurs with some form of contralateral hydronephrosis as the associated

TABLE 17-21.   Classification of Major Renal Cystic Diseases

	Potter Type I	Potter Type II	Potter Type III	Potter Type IV
Nomenclature	Infantile polycystic kidney disease	Multicystic dysplastic kidney disease (MCDK)	Adult polycystic kidney disease	Renal cystic disease associated with hydronephrosis
Location	Bilateral	Unilateral 30% with contralateral renal disease including hydronephrosis, renal agenesis, or MCDK	Bilateral	Dependent upon etiology of hydronephrosis
Ultrasound appearance	Enlarged, echogenic	Cysts of variable size; noncommunicating	Rare in utero, enlarged, echogenic	Hydronephrosis + cortical cysts may change in appearance during pregnancy
Amniotic fluid	Often oligohydramnios	Normal to oligohydramnios (if bilateral)	Usually normal	Normal to oligohydramnios dependent on underlying etiology
Prognosis	Poor	Good—dependent on contralateral kidney and associated malformations	Adult onset	Dependent on underlying etiology
Risk of subsequent pregnancies	25%	Probably <5%	50%	Dependent on underlying etiology

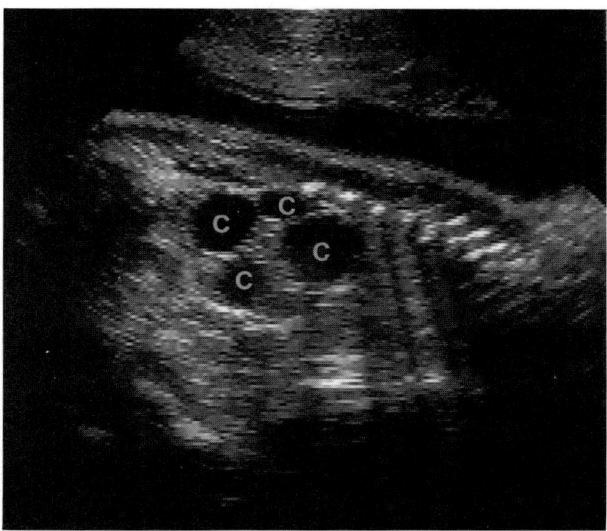

FIGURE 17-41. Unilateral multicystic dysplastic kidney (MCDK). Sagittal scan of the kidney demonstrating multiple cysts (C) of variable size noted within this MCDK or Potter type II. Note that the cysts are haphazardly arranged in this kidney and are of variable size, which helps to distinguish this from hydronephrosis.

anomaly, which carries with it a much better prognosis. Given the lack of function of MCDK, the presence of oligohydramnios strongly suggests a serious contralateral renal anomaly. Unilateral renal agenesis occurs in 10% of cases, and a similar percentage will develop hydronephrosis. The corollary to this statement is also true in that bilateral cystic disease of the kidneys in the presence of a normal amniotic fluid volume essentially precludes the diagnosis of bilateral MCDK.

Differentiating severe hydronephrosis from MCDK is sometimes less than straightforward.[73] The key to the differential diagnosis (Table 17-22) is the cysts themselves;[74] if they communicate and are of similar size, they most likely represent calyceal dilatation of hydronephrosis. In MCDK the cysts tend to be round and of varying size, often giving the kidney the appearance of a cluster of grapes (see Figs. 17-31 and 17-41). Although the appearance and size of MCDK may change markedly over time,[75] the kidney generally loses its shape and is larger than normal, with no organizational pattern to the cysts or recognizable renal parenchyma.

Cystic Renal Dysplasia (Potter Type IV). Cystic renal dysplasia, or Potter type IV, is the consequence of an obstructive uropathy occurring in the second or third trimester of pregnancy. This contrasts with MCDK, which results from an early first-trimester insult. A posterior urethral valve obstruction frequently leads to this lesion, and given the lack of renal function of such dysplastic kidneys, it is critical to recognize them before considering in utero intervention. Less commonly, UPJ and UVJ obstructive uropathies can also lead to cystic renal dysplasia.

The sonographic appearance is that of parenchymal echogenicity and subcapsular cysts (Fig. 17-42). These cysts may change in size and appearance during pregnancy. However, the diagnosis is not always so straightforward, since the kidneys can be dysplastic without visible cysts and with normal-appearing parenchyma (see Table 17-21).

Renal Cyst. Renal cysts can be seen on occasion in the absence of other obvious genitourinary anoma-

TABLE 17-22.   Differential Diagnosis of Severe Ureteropelvic Junction Obstruction (UPJO) and Multicystic Dysplastic Kidney Disease (MCDK)

	UPJO	MCDK
Renal parenchyma visible	Usually	No
Cyst characteristics	Oval, irregular	Round,
	Communicating with each other and the renal pelvis peripheral	noncommunicating with each other or pelvis central
Ureteral dilatation	Often	No
Contralateral kidney	10%–40% with UPJO	40% abnormal
		20% bilateral
		10% agenesis
		10% UPJO

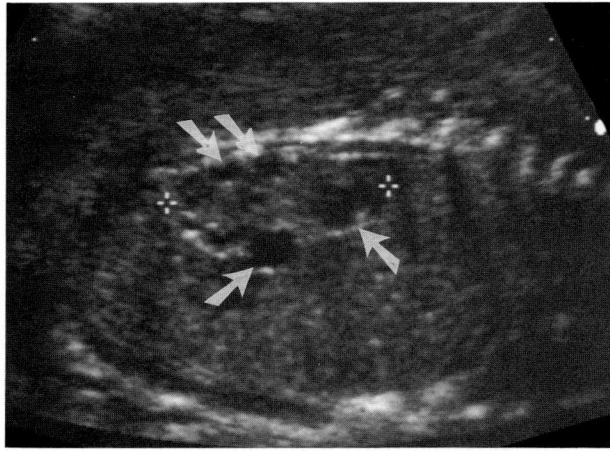

FIGURE 17-42.   Echogenic kidney with multiple renal cortical cysts (*arrows*) in this fetus in which unilateral hydronephrosis was earlier observed. The cysts changed in size and number throughout pregnancy.

lies (Fig. 17-43). Often they will be the result of an anomalous duplication of the collecting system with a nonfunctional pole. More often, however, the correct diagnosis will relate to an obstructive uropathy or cystic disease, as discussed above.

Are the Kidneys Abnormal in Size or Echogenicity?

Infantile Polycystic Kidney Disease (Potter Type I). Infantile polycystic kidney disease (IPKD), or Potter type I, is an autosomal recessive disorder with an incidence of 1 in 40,000 births. From the

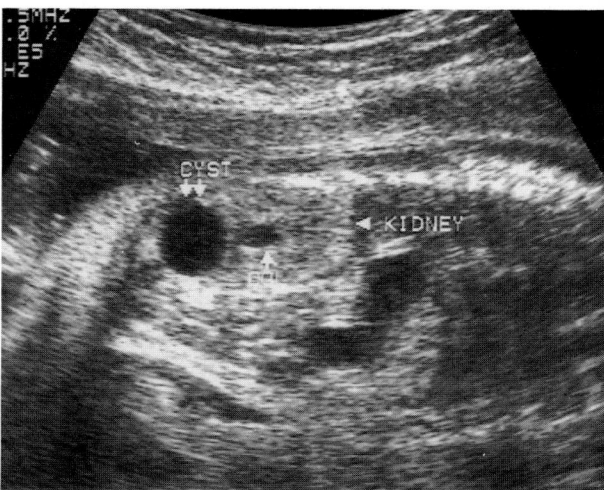

FIGURE 17-43.   Isolated renal cyst can be identified in the lower pole of this kidney.

sonologist's point of view, the name is a misnomer in that the kidneys generally do not appear cystic when imaged.[76] The disease is characterized by microscopic cysts, but sonographically the kidneys appear as bilaterally enlarged echogenic masses, in association with oligohydramnios and nonvisualization of the bladder (Fig. 17-44; see also Table 17-21). In patients at risk on the basis of family history, it is important to initiate sonographic evaluation by 16 weeks because the enlarged kidneys may be diagnosed early in some cases.

The disease carries a dismal prognosis owing to the poor renal function and pulmonary hypoplasia that can occur. However, several different subtypes of the disorder are now recognized, each with its own distinct presentation and prognosis. The foregoing discussion relates to the perinatal variety, which carries the worst prognosis and is unfortunately the most common. In the neonatal subtype, an in utero diagnosis can sometimes be suggested based on enlarged, echogenic kidneys; there often is hepatic fibrosis (probably not sonographically detectable), usually without pulmonary hypoplasia, and a relatively normal amniotic fluid volume. Renal failure may be delayed for several weeks after birth, and death typically occurs within the first year. The later subtypes have progressively more benign clinical courses from the renal standpoint, with increasingly severe hepatic involvement.

It is imperative that patients with IPCD have a detailed anatomic survey, with special scrutiny of the skull for an encephalocele and of the hands and feet for polydactyly and the triad of Meckel-Gruber syndrome, an autosomal recessive condition, as well (see Chapter 9).

Adult Polycystic Kidney Disease (Potter Type III). Adult polycystic kidney disease, or Potter type III, is an autosomal dominant condition, which as its name suggests is only rarely reported prenatally.[77] The vast majority of cases are diagnosed in early adult life. In families at risk, a fetus with symmetrically large, echogenic kidneys, similar in appearance to those of infantile polycystic kidney disease (see Fig. 17-44), should raise a suspicion of Potter type III. On occasion the kidneys may appear cystic (see Table 17-21).

Renal Fossa Mass. Fetal renal tumors usually present sonographically as a solid mass in the paraspinous area or renal fossa. The most common tumors are mesoblastic nephroma (or leiomyomatous hamartoma; Fig. 17-45) and, less frequently,

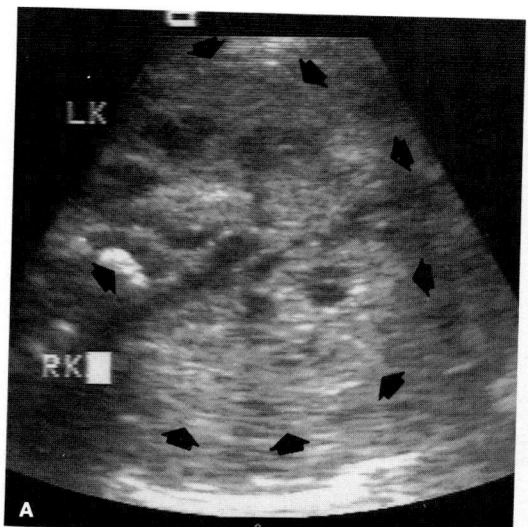
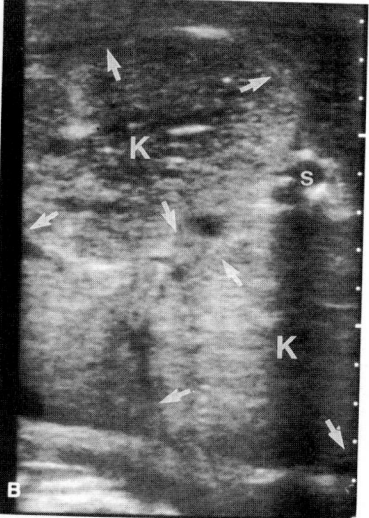
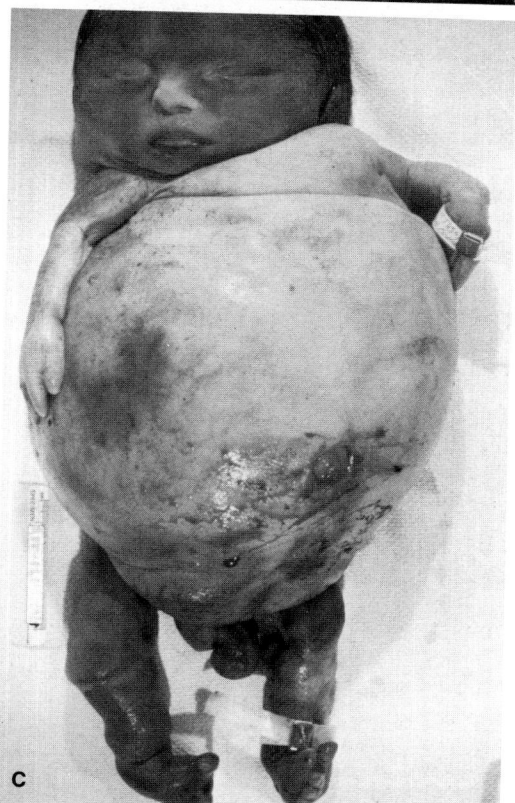

FIGURE 17-44. Infantile polycystic kidney disease. **(A)** Coronal ultrasound demonstrating echogenic, bilaterally enlarged kidneys (*arrows*). **(B)** In another fetus, bilaterally enlarged echogenic kidneys (K) are noted in the paraspinal (S) location. **(C)** In this fetus there is massive enlargement of the fetal abdomen owing to the enlarged kidneys.

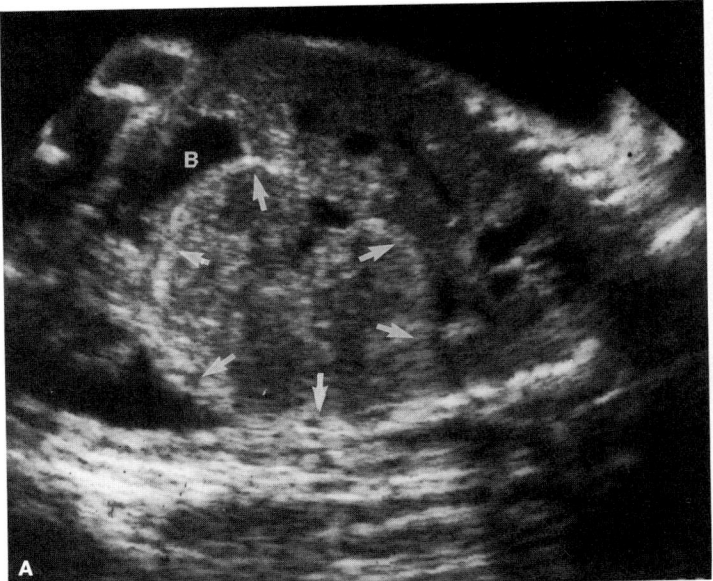

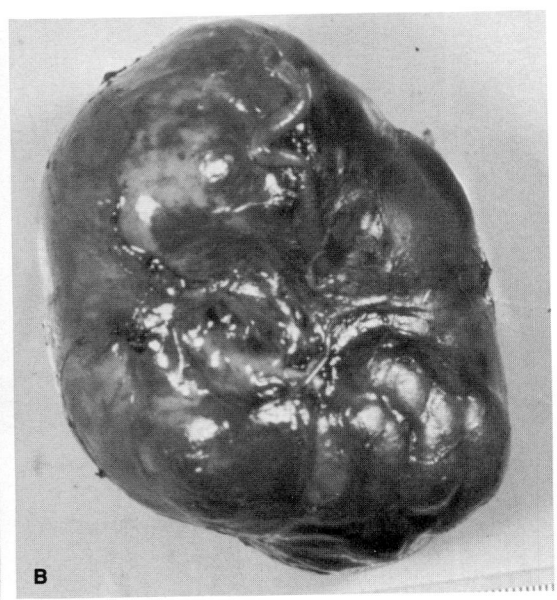

FIGURE 17-45.   Mesoblastic nephroma. **(A)** Sagittal ultrasound of the fetus showing echogenic mass (*arrows*) arising from the left renal fossa. B, bladder. **(B)** After delivery a well-encapsulated mass, which corresponded to a mesoblastic nephroma, was removed from the left perinephric space. (Walter JP, McGahan JP: Mesoblastic nephroma: Prenatal sonographic detection. J Clin Ultrasound 1985; 13:686.)

Wilms' tumor (or nephroblastoma). The two are indistinguishable by current sonographic techniques.[78] Although the sonographic distinction between the two lesions cannot be made, their prognoses are dramatically different. Mesoblastic nephroma is a benign entity, in contrast to Wilm's tumor, which is a malignant lesion. The prognosis for Wilm's tumor varies with the grade and extent of the lesion.

The differential diagnosis for a unilateral solid mass in the renal fossa includes the aforementioned renal lesions as well as an adrenal neuroblastoma and adrenal hemorrhage (Table 17-23). The mesoblastic nephromas reported to date have consistently been associated with polyhydramnios,[79,80] although the mechanism for this finding is not readily apparent.

TABLE 17-23.   Differential Diagnosis of Renal Fossa Mass

Mesoblastic nephroma
Adrenal neuroblastoma
Adrenal hemorrhage
Wilms' tumor
Retroperitoneal teratoma

Adrenal neuroblastoma is the most common adrenal lesion in prenatal and neonatal life. The usual sonographic appearance is of a mixed cystic and solid lesion (Fig. 17-46), occasionally with calcifications as well. Although adrenal neuroblasto-

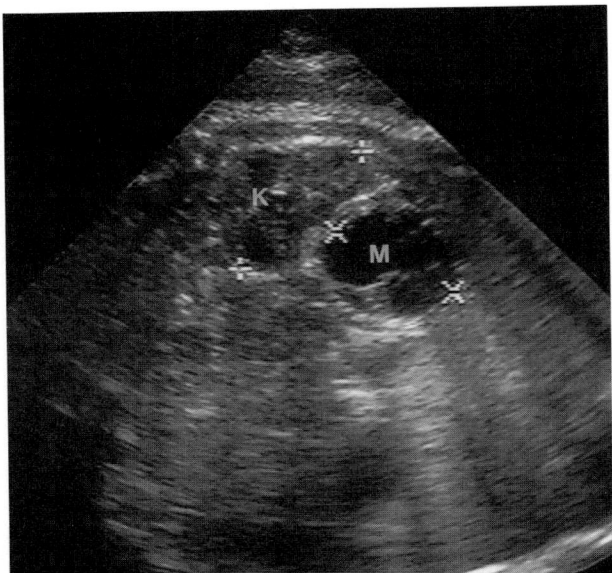

FIGURE 17-46.   Adrenal neuroblastoma. Mixed cystic/solid mass (M) at the superior pole of the right kidney (K) corresponding to a fetal neuroblastoma.

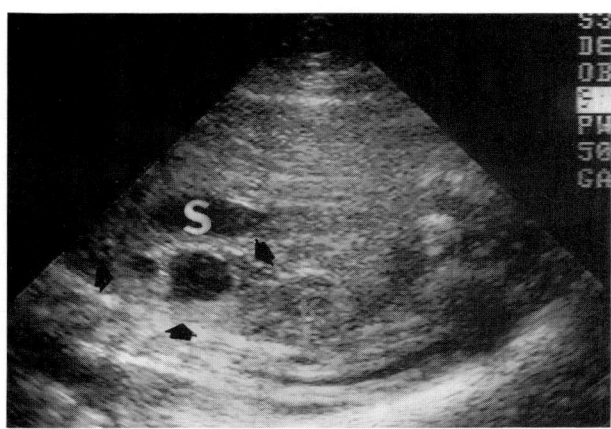

FIGURE 17-47. Adrenal hemorrhage. Mixed echogenic mass (*arrows*) with both cystic and solid components located superior to the left kidney (K). S, stomach.

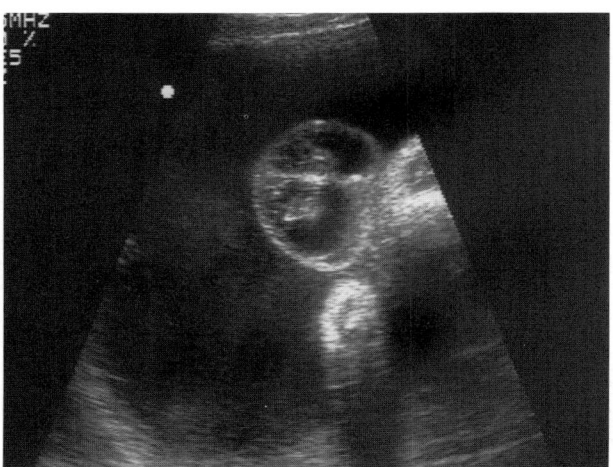

FIGURE 17-48. Scan of the scrotal sac demonstrating bilateral hydroceles.

mas are most commonly found in the superior renal fossa area, they can also be metastatic lesions in a variety of locations. Besides the usual location, the differential diagnosis can be aided by the endocrine nature of these lesions. Because they usually produce catecholamines, maternal symptoms may support the sonographic diagnosis. We have found amniotic fluid catecholamines to be markedly elevated in a recent case; thus, amniocentesis may also aid in the prenatal diagnosis.

Adrenal hemorrhage (Fig. 17-47) can have a sonographic appearance similar to that of an adrenal or renal neoplasm. The key to the diagnosis is the evolution of the lesion over time.

FETAL GENDER

Ultrasound can be used to assess fetal gender. In a study in the early 1980s approximately one third of all fetuses could not be sexed because of fetal position.[81] One third were correctly identified as male and one third correctly identified as female. In approximately 3% of cases fetal gender is incorrectly assigned. This inaccuracy often is due to the fact that the labial hypertrophy during pregnancy may be misinterpreted as the male scrotum.[81]

Hydroceles observed during pregnancy are common. Most of these have no significance; some may occur secondary to intraabdominal ascites that has tracked into the scrotum (Fig. 17-48). In either case there is usually little significance to the finding of a fetal hydrocele in a male fetus.

SUMMARY

The approach in this chapter has been to deal with the abdominal organs and anomalies in a practical and systematic manner. The key to the differential diagnosis of abnormal findings is to take time to evaluate the relationship of the abnormality to normal anatomic structures.

REFERENCES

1. Pretorius DH, Gosink BB, Clautice-Engle T, et al: Sonographic evaluation of the fetal stomach: Significance of nonvisualization. AJR 1988; 151:987.
2. Nyberg DA, Mack LA, Patten RM, et al: Fetal bowel: Normal sonographic findings. J Ultrasound Med 1987; 6:3.
3. Goldstein I, Lockwood C, Hobbins JC: Ultrasound assessment of fetal intestinal development in the evaluation of gestational age. Obstet Gynecol 1987; 70:682.
4. Schmidt W, Yarkoni S, Jeanty P, et al: Sonographic measurements of the fetal spleen: Clinical implications. J Ultrasound Med 1985; 4:667.
5. Fakhry J, Shapiro LR, Schecter A, et al: Fetal gastric pseudomasses. J Ultrasound Med 1987; 6:177.
6. Rosenthal SJ, Filly RA, Callen PW: Fetal pseudoascites. Radiology 1979; 131:195.
7. Hashimoto BE, Filly RA, Callen PW: Fetal pseudoascites: Further anatomic observations. J Ultrasound Med 1986; 5:151.
8. Benacerraf BR, Frigoletto FD Jr: Sonographic sign for the detection of early fetal ascites in the management of severe isoimmune disease without intrauterine transfusion. Am J Obstet Gynecol 1985; 152:1039 and 153:635.

9. Lacrampe M, Jeanty P: Polyhydramnios and small stomach: Clinical outcome and pathologic findings. Fetus 1991; 1:753.

10. Pretorius DH, Drose JA, Dennis MA, et al: Tracheoesophageal fistula in utero: 22 cases. J Ultrasound Med 1987; 6:509.

11. Holder TM, Cloud DT, Lewis JE Jr, et al: Esophageal atresia and tracheoesophageal fistula: A survey of its members by the surgical section of the American Academy of Pediatrics. Pediatrics 1964; 34:542.

12. Romero R, Jeanty P, Gianluigi P, et al: The prenatal diagnosis of duodenal atresia. Does it make any difference? Obstet Gynecol 1988; 71:739.

13. Vermesh M, Mayden KL, Confino E, et al: Prenatal sonographic diagnosis of Hirschsprung's disease. J Ultrasound Med 1986; 5:37.

14. Robinow M, Shaw A: The McKusick-Kaufman syndrome: Recessively inherited vaginal atresia, hydrometrocopos, uterovaginal duplications, anorectal anomalies, postaxial polydactyly and congenital heart disease. J Pediatr 1979; 94:776.

15. Harris RD, Nyberg DA, Mack LA, Weinberg E: Anorectal atresia: Prenatal sonographic diagnosis. AJR 1987; 149:395.

16. Caspi N, Elchalal U, Lancet U, et al: Prenatal diagnosis of cystic fibrosis: Ultrasonographic appearance of meconium ileus in the fetus. Prenat Diagn 1988; 8:379.

17. Goldstein RB, Filly RA, Callen PW: Sonographic diagnosis of meconium ileus in utero. J Ultrasound Med 1987; 6:663.

18. Park RW, Grand RJ: Gastrointestinal manifestations of cystic fibrosis. A review. Gastroenterology 1981; 81:1143.

19. Nyberg DA, Hastrup W, Watts H, et al: Dilated fetal bowel: A sonographic sign of cystic fibrosis. J Ultrasound Med 1987; 6:257.

20. McGahan JP, Hanson F: Meconium peritonitis with accompanying pseudocyst: Prenatal sonographic diagnosis. Radiology 1983; 148:125.

21. Dillard JP, Edwards DU, Leopold GR: Meconium peritonitis masquerading as fetal hydrops. J Utrasound Med 1987; 6:49.

22. Heydenrych JJ, Marcus PB: Meconium granuloma of the tunica vaginalis. Urology 1976; 115:596.

23. Finkel LI, Slovis TL: Meconium peritonitis, intraperitoneal calcifications, and cystic fibrosis. Pediatr Radiol 1982; 12:92.

24. Foster MA, Nyberg DA, Mahony BS, et al: Meconium peritonitis: Prenatal sonographic findings and clinical significance. Radiology 1987; 165:661.

25. Fakhry J, Reiser M, Shapiro LR, et al: Increased echogenicity in the lower fetal abdomen: A common normal variant in the second trimester. J Ultrasound Med 1986; 5:489.

26. Benacerraf B, Chaudhury AK: Echogenic fetal bowel in the third trimester associated with meconium ileus secondary to cystic fibrosis. J Reprod Med 1989; 34:299.

27. Dicke JM, Crane JP: Sonographically detected hyperechoic fetal bowel: Significance and implication for pregnancy management. Obstet Gynecol 1992; 80:778.

28. Scioscia AL, Pretorius DH, Budorick NE, et al: Second-trimester echogenic bowel and chromosomal abnormalities. Am J Obstet Gynecol 1992; 167:889.

29. Greiss HB, McGahan JP: Umbilical vein entering the right atrium: Significance of in utero diagnosis. J Ultrasound Med 1992; 11:111.

30. Fuster JS, Benasco C, Saa I: Giant dilation of the umbilical vein. J Clin Ultrasound 1985; 3:363.

31. Reisner DP, Mahony BS, McGahan JP, Nyberg DA: Adverse fetal outcome associated with varix of the fetal intraabdominal umbilical vein [SPO abstract #197]. Am J Obstet Gynecol 1992; 166:333.

32. Elrad H, Mayden KL, Ahart S, et al: Prenatal ultrasound diagnosis of choledochal cyst. J Ultrasound Med 1985; 4:553.

33. Chung WM: Antenatal detection of hepatic cyst. J Clin Ultrasound 1986; 14:217.

34. Hill LM: Sonographic detection of fetal gastrointestinal anomalies. Ultrasound Q 1988; 6:35.

35. Grannum P, Bracken M, Silverman R, et al: Assessment of kidney size in normal gestation by comparison of kidney circumference to abdominal circumference. Am J Obstet Gynecol 1980; 136:249.

36. Rutherford SE, Smith CV, Phelan JP, et al: Four-quadrant assessment of amniotic fluid volume. Interobserver and intraobserver variation. J Reprod Med 1987; 32:587.

37. Moore TR, Cayle JE: The amniotic fluid index in normal pregnancy. Am J Obstet Gynecol 1990; 162:1168.

38. Potter EL: Bilateral absence of ureters and kidneys. A report of 50 cases. Obstet Gynecol 1965; 25:3.

39. Keirse MJNC, Meerman RH: Antenatal diagnosis of Potter syndrome. Obstet Gynecol 1978; 52:64S.

40. Harman CR: Maternal furosemide may not provoke urine production in the compromised fetus. Am J Obstet Gynecol 1984; 150:322.

41. Raghavendra BN, Young BK, Greco MA, et al: Use of furosemide in pregnancies complicated by oligohydramnios. Radiology 1987; 165:455.

42. Benacerraf BR: Examination of the second trimester fetus with severe oligohydramnios using transvaginal scanning. Obstet Gynecol 1990; 175:491.

43. Nicolaides K, Rodeck C, Gosden C, et al: Rapid karyotyping in non-lethal fetal malformations. Lancet 1986; 1:283.

44. McGahan JP, Myracle MR: Adrenal hypertrophy: Potential pitfall in the sonographic diagnosis of renal agenesis. J Ultrasound Med 1986; 5:265.

45. Romero R, Cullen M, Grannum P, et al: Antenatal diagnosis of renal anomalies with ultrasound. III. Bilateral renal agenesis. Am J Obstet Gynecol 1985; 151:38.

46. Johnson A, Callan NA, Bhutani VK, et al: Ultrasonic ratio of fetal thoracic to abdominal circumference:

An association with fetal pulmonary hypoplasia. Am J Obstet Gynecol 1987; 157:764.

47. Hill LM, Peterson CM: Antenatal diagnosis of fetal pelvic kidneys. J Ultrasound Med 1987; 6:393.

48. Greenblatt AM, Beretsky I, Lankin DH, et al: In utero diagnosis of crossed renal ectopia using high resolution real-time ultrasound. J Ultrasound Med 1985; 4:105.

49. Brown T, Mandell J, Lebowitz RL: Neonatal hydronephrosis in the era of sonography. AJR 1987; 148:959.

50. Hoddick WK, Filly RA, Mahony BS, et al: Minimal fetal renal pyelectasis. J Ultrasound Med 1985; 4:51.

51. Grignon A, Filion R, Filiatrault D, et al: Urinary tract dilatation in utero: Classification and clinical applications. Radiology 1986; 160:645.

52. Corteville JE, Gray DL, Crane JP: Congenital hydronephrosis: Correlation of fetal ultrasonographic findings with infant outcome. Am J Obstet Gynecol 1991; 165:384.

53. Laing FC, Burke VD, Wing VW, et al: Postpartum evaluation of fetal hydronephrosis: Optimal timing for follow-up sonography. Radiology 1984; 152:423.

54. Mandell J, Blyth B, Peters CA, et al: Structural genitourinary defects detected in utero. Radiology 1991; 178:193.

55. Benacerraf BR, Mandell J, Estroff JA, et al: Fetal pyelectasis: A possible association with Down syndrome. Obstet Gynecol 1990; 76:58.

56. Benacerraf BR, Neuberg D, Bromley B, et al: Ultrasound scoring index for prenatal detection of chromosomal abnormalities. J Ultrasound Med 1992; 11:448.

57. Harrison MR, Golbus MS, Filly RA: The Unborn Patient. Prenatal Diagnosis and Treatment. Orlando, FL: Grune & Stratton, 1984.

58. Harrison MR, Golbus MS, Filly RA: The Unborn Patient, 2nd ed. Philadelphia: WB Saunders, 1991: 381.

59. Montana MA, Cyr DR, Lenke RR, et al: Sonographic detection of fetal ureteral obstruction. AJR 1985; 145:595.

60. Mandell J, Colodny AH, Lebowitz R, et al: Ureteroceles in infants and children. J Urol 1980; 123:921.

61. Nussbaum AR, Dorst JP, Jeffs RD, et al: Ectopic ureter and ureterocele: Their varied sonographic manifestations. Radiology 1986; 159:227.

62. Bulie M, Podobnik M, Korenie B, Bistricki J: First-trimester diagnosis of low obstructive uropathy: An indicator of initial renal function in the fetus. J Clin Ultrasound 1987; 15:537.

63. Manning FA, Harrison MR, Rodeck C, et al: Catheter shunts for fetal hydronephrosis and hydrocephalus—report of the International Fetal Surgery Registry. N Engl J Med 1986; 315:336.

64. Mahony BS, Callen PW, Filly RA: Fetal urethral obstruction: US evaluation. Radiology 1985; 157:221.

65. Nicolaides KH, Cheng HH, Snijders RJM, et al: Fetal urine biochemistry in the assessment of obstructive uropathy. Am J Obstet Gynecol 1992; 166:932.

66. Wilkins IA, Chitkara U, Lynch L, et al: The nonpredictive value of fetal urinary electrolytes: Preliminary report of outcomes and correlation with pathologic diagnosis. Am J Obstet Gynecol 1987; 157:694.

67. Elder JS, O'Grady JP, Ashmead G, et al: Evaluation of fetal renal function: Unreliability of fetal electrolytes. J Urol 1990; 144:574.

68. Crombleholme TM, Harrison MR, Golbus MS, et al: Fetal intervention in obstructive uropathy: Prognostic indicators and efficacy of intervention. Am J Obstet Gynecol 1990; 162:1239.

69. Manning FA: The International Fetal Surgery Registry. Winnipeg, Canada, personal communication, 1993.

70. Harrison MR, Golbus MS, Filly RA: The Unborn Patient, 2nd ed. Philadelphia: WB Saunders, 1991:383.

71. Helin I, Perrson PH: Prenatal diagnosis of urinary tract abnormalities by ultrasound. Pediatrics 1986; 78:879.

72. Kleiner B, Filly RA, Mack L, et al: Multicystic dysplastic kidney: Observations of contralateral disease in the fetal population. Radiology 1986; 161:27.

73. Rizzo N, Gabrielli S, Pilu G, et al: Prenatal diagnosis and obstetrical management of multicystic dysplastic kidney disease. Prenat Diagn 1987; 7:109.

74. Beretsky I, Labkin DH, Rusoff JH: Sonographic differentiation between the multicystic dysplastic kidney and ureteropelvic junction obstruction in utero using high resolution real-time scanners employing digital detection. J Clin Ultrasound 1984; 12:429.

75. Hashimoto BE, Filly RA, Callen PW: Multicystic dysplastic kidney: Changing appearance on ultrasound. Radiology 1986; 159:107.

76. Luthy DAM, Hirsch JH: Infantile polycystic kidney disease: Observations from attempts at prenatal diagnosis. Am J Med Genet 1985; 20:505.

77. Pretorius DH, Lee ME, Manco-Johnson ML: Diagnosis of autosomal dominant polycystic kidney disease in utero and in the young infant. J Ultrasound Med 1987; 6:249.

78. Walter JP, McGahan JP: Mesoblastic nephroma: Prenatal sonographic detection. J Clin Ultrasound 1985; 13:686.

79. Romano WL: Neonatal renal tumor with polyhydramnios. J Ultrasound Med 1984; 3:475.

80. Apuzzio JJ, Unwin W, Adhate A, Nichols R: Prenatal diagnosis of fetal renal mesoblastic nephroma. Am J Obstet Gynecol 1986; 154:636.

81. Elejalde BR, de Elejalde MM, Ketiman T: Visualization of the fetal genitalia by ultrasonography: A review of the literature and analysis of its accuracy and ethical implications. J Ultrasound Med 1985; 4:633.

82. Mahoney BS, Filly RA, Callen PW, et al: Fetal renal dysplasia: Sonographic evaluation. Radiology 1984; 152:143.

83. Sanders RC, Nussbaum AR, Solez K: Renal dysplasia: Sonographic findings. Radiology 1988; 167:623.

John P. McGahan and Manuel Porto:
DIAGNOSTIC OBSTETRICAL ULTRASOUND.
© 1994 J.B. Lippincott Company.

David C. Jones   Joshua A. Copel

Chapter *18*

Hydrops Fetalis

The term *hydrops fetalis* refers to a physical sign that may represent any of a number of causes. It is characterized by fetal fluid collections in at least two of several body compartments, including ascites, pleural or pericardial effusions, skin edema, placental edema, or polyhydramnios (Table 18-1). The incidence is about 1 in 2500 pregnancies. The causes of fetal edema are broadly divided into major categories (Table 18-2). Rh blood group immunization was once the leading cause of fetal hydrops, but since the availability of Rh immunoglobulin, the relative frequency of detection of nonimmune hydrops has increased. Through the careful application of history-taking and diagnostic testing, the cause hydrops fetalis can frequently be established (Table 18-3); however, a significant number of fetuses elude diagnosis even after autopsy.[1,2] Hydrops fetalis can thus be divided into *immune* and *nonimmune* (Tables 18-4 and 18-5).

ISOIMMUNE HYDROPS FETALIS

Until recently, the management of Rh and other red cell alloimmunized pregnancies was relatively straightforward. Since the early 1960s, assessment of amniotic fluid for bilirubin concentration, using spectrophotometric analysis of the change in optical density at 450 mμ (ΔOD450) plotted on a graph as a function of gestational age (Liley graph), has served as the gold standard for risk assessment and management of these high-risk pregnancies.[3-5] More recently, the use of ultrasound assessment and percutaneous umbilical cord blood sampling (PUBS, or cordocentesis) has challenged this standard.[5] In this section, we briefly explore these modalities, with particular emphasis on the ultrasound clues to the diagnosis of fetal anemia associated with hydrops fetalis.

Maternal Antibody Screening

Although sonography alone may make one diagnose hydrops fetalis, other modalities may be necessary to establish the cause (see Table 18-3). The maternal antibody screen differentiates between immune and nonimmune hydrops. Isoimmunization effects hydrops through fetal anemia. When the antibody screen is positive, the precise identity of the antibody must be made to establish the risk of fetal hydrops. To cause fetal anemia, the antibody must be an immunoglobulin G (IgG) di-

TABLE 18-1.   Definition of Hydrops

Fluid collection in two or more body cavities, including:
  Skin edema
  Pleural space
  Pericardial space
  Abdomen (ascites)
  Polyhydramnios
  Placental edema

rected against antigens present on the fetal red blood cells at the appropriate time in pregnancy. Some antibodies always present as IgG, but others, such as anti-M, may present as IgG or IgM. In these instances, further testing to determine the antibody type is necessary to establish risk. If it is determined that the antibodies present are a cause of hydrops fetalis, one can assume that they are probably the cause of the hydrops seen. Nonetheless, if the father of the fetus is available, it is appropriate to check his blood to establish the presence of the offending antigen.

ΔOD450

Through the late 1970s, patients positive for a significant (IgG) red cell antibody were managed by serial amniocentesis for ΔOD450, usually beginning at 22 to 28 weeks of gestation. The original data for the correlation between elevated ΔOD450

TABLE 18-2.   Major Etiologic Categories of Hydrops Fetalis

Fetal anemia due to isoimmunization, hemolysis, fetal infection, or hemorrhage
Cardiac failure due to structural heart defects or rhythm abnormalities
High-output failure due to arteriovenous malformation (ie, sacral coccygeal teratoma)
Cranial defects
Pulmonary defects, which probably act by decreasing venous return to the heart
Gastrointestinal and hepatic defects
Renal abnormalities, which often cause hypoalbuminemia
Fetal infection
Skeletal dysplasias
Inherited metabolic disorders
Genetic syndromes and chromosomal abnormalities
Placental abnormalities, which may act like arteriovenous malformations

and fetal anemia and hydrops, however, were obtained in pregnancies at 28 weeks of gestation and later[3] (Fig. 18-1). Since that time, numerous investigators and clinicians have extrapolated Liley graph back into the second trimester, particularly for the management of severely isoimmunized pregnancies in which hydrops fetalis can be seen as early as 18 weeks of gestation. Bowman reported perhaps the largest single-center experience with severe isoimmunization in North America.[6] His data support the utility of Liley graph determination and management. Nearly 95% of his amniotic fluid samples accurately predicted the severity of the isoimmunization in over 1000 tests, with only a 2% rate of serious inaccuracy. In particular, the slope (downward trend) of serial ΔOD450 measurements is reassuring in nearly all cases.

Nicolaides and colleagues challenged the validity of this approach in a series of 59 severely isoimmunized fetuses referred before 26 weeks of gestation.[5] They found a poor correlation between fetal hemoglobin and ΔOD450 in individual cases. Only 32% of the severely anemic fetuses (hemoglobin less than 6 g/dl) had Liley graph determinations in zone 3 (transfusion zone), and 4 of 11 (36%) severely affected fetuses with more than one amniocentesis revealed a downward (reassuring) trend in ΔOD450. More recently, Ananth and Queenan suggested that second-trimester ΔOD450 determinations below a threshold of 0.15 could be followed by serial amniocentesis.[7] They further suggested that levels below 0.9 indicated mild or no disease. Our own experience suggests that such a threshold may be falsely reassuring in high-risk cases (previous hydrops or high antibody titer), and thus cordocentesis may serve as the only reliable predictor of fetal anemia.

Ultrasound

Investigators have searched for more than a decade for ultrasound clues to the diagnosis of fetal anemia and isoimmunization. Although the classic sonographic findings of hydrops fetalis (ie, *pleural* and *pericardial effusions, ascites,* and *anasarca*) are relatively straightforward to detect, they are uniformly associated with severe fetal anemia[8] (fetal hematocrit less than 15%–20%; Figs. 18-2 through 18-4). Perinatal outcome and intrauterine treatment are severely compromised in many cases when diagnosis is delayed to this point. Moreover, not all isoimmunized fetuses manifest classic hydropic changes before fetal death.[6]

(*text continues on page 394*)

TABLE 18-3. Evaluation of Fetal Hydrops

History of previously affected infant; maternal medical conditions, such as anemia, diabetes, infections, or medications; familial history of metabolic or hereditary conditions

Maternal testing	Indirect Coombs' testing	Immune hydrops
	Mean corpuscular volume	
	Hemoglobin electrophoresis	α-Thalassemia
	Kleihauer-Betke syndrome	Fetomaternal bleed
	Syphilis, parvovirus, and TORCH titers	Congenital fetal infection
	Maternal blood chemistry	G6PD deficiency and pyruvate kinase deficiency
Ultrasound	Two-dimensional ultrasound	Congenital malformations
		Extent of fetal edema
Fetal echocardiography	Two-dimensional ultrasound Pulsed and color flow Doppler	Congenital heart malformations
	M-mode	Abnormalities in fetal rhythm
Amniocentesis	Fetal karyotype	Chromosomal abnormalities
	α-Fetoprotein	Congenital nephrosis, sacrococcygeal teratomas
	Metabolic testing	Tay-Sachs, Gaucher's, GM_1 gangliosidosis
	Restriction endonucleases	α-Thalassemia
	Amniotic fluid culture, antigen tests, PCR	CMV, toxoplasmosis
Fetal blood sampling	Fetal karyotype	Chromosomal abnormality
	Fetal complete blood count	Fetal anemia
	Hemoglobin electrophoresis	α-Thalassemia
	Fetal antigen-specific IgM, IgA, and PCR	Congenital infection
	Fetal albumin	Fetal hypoalbuminemia
	Metabolic testing	Tay-Sachs, Gaucher's, GM_1 gangliosidosis

TORCH, toxoplasmosis, rubella, cytomegalovirus, and herpes simplex; PCR, polymerase chain reaction; Ig, immunoglobulin; G6PD, glucose-6-phosphate dehydrogenase; CMV, cytomegalovirus

(Modified from Holzgreve W, Holzgreve B, Curry JR: Non-immune hydrops fetalis: Diagnosis and management. Semin Perinatol 1985; 95:52–67.)

TABLE 18-4. Conditions Associated With Fetal Hydrops (General Outline)

I. Immune hydrops
II. Nonimmune hydrops
   A. Fetal—focal abnormality
      1. Cranial
      2. Thorax
         a. Cardiac
         b. Pulmonary
      3. Gastrointestinal
      4. Hepatic
      5. Renal
      6. Vascular
   B. Fetal—generalized abnormality
      1. Infectious
      2. Skeletal
      3. Metabolic
      4. Syndromes
      5. Chromosomal
      6. Fetal anemia
      7. Twins
   C. Placental
   D. Maternal
      1. Medication
      2. Maternal disease
   E. Miscellaneous
   F. Unknown cause

TABLE 18-5.   Conditions Associated With Fetal Hydrops (Expanded Outline)

Condition	Features
I. Immune hydrops	Positive maternal antibody screen (Indirect Coombs test) Hepatosplenomegaly is a hallmark
II. Nonimmune hydrops	
A. Fetal—focal abnormality	
1. Cranial	
a. Encephalocele	Extracranial mass with underlying skull defect on ultrasound
b. Fetal intracranial hemorrhage	Lateral heterogeneous mass displacing normal structures
c. Porencephaly with absent corpus callosum	Cyctic structure in the brain
d. Vein of Galen aneurysm	May be visualized as intracranial mass; Doppler and color flow studies may be helpful
2. Thorax	
a. Cardiac (structural defect (ASD, VSD, hypoplastic left heart, subaortic stenosis, pulmonary valve insufficiency, Ebstein's anomaly)	Defects may be seen with fetal echocardiography; atrioventricular valve regurgitation
i. Rhabdomyoma	Tumors with two-dimensional ultrasound; half are associated with tuberous sclerosis
ii. Endocardial fibroelastosis	Endocardium > 30 μm thick with decreased contractility; endocardium often calcified
iii. Rhythm abnormality (supraventricular tachycardia, atrial flutter, heart block)	Arrhythmia defined by M-mode or Doppler echocardiography; may be secondary to a tumor; heart block may be associated with maternal anti-Ro or anti-La antibody
iv. Intrapericardial teratoma	Tumor mass adjacent to heart
v. Premature closure of the foramen ovale	Hypertrophic right heart, no flow across foramen on Doppler ultrasound
b. Pulmonary	
i. Congenital cystic adenomatoid malformation	Cysts of varying sizes (<1 cm to >2 cm) are seen in the chest, usually unilaterally. Polyhydramnios is usually present
ii. Congenital chylothorax	Initially unilateral or bilateral isolated pleural effusions that may progress to hydrops secondary to vena caval obstruction; pleural tap may reveal primary lymphocytes
iii. Diaphragmatic hernia	Stomach seen above the diaphragm at the level of the heart; heart often shifted into the right chest
iv. Extralobar pulmonary sequestration	Usually a well-defined homogeneous mass in the upper abdomen or lower thorax, often conical or triangular in shape
v. Mediastinal teratoma	Tumor seen on two-dimensional ultrasound
vi. Pulmonary lymphagectasia	May see cystic hygromas
3. Gastrointestinal	
a. Diaphragmatic hernia	May present as isolated ascites
b. Duodenal atresia	Mass effect with mediastinal shift; small lung; stomach present at the level of the heart in an axial view; double-bubble sign
c. Jejunoileal atresia	Multiple dilated loops of bowel
d. Imperforate anus	Dilated distal colon, may be a U-shaped mass
e. Meconium peritonitis	Echogenic peritoneal meconium plaques; associated with cystic fibrosis
f. Volvulus	Dilation of the proximal bowel
g. Duodenal diverticulum	
4. Hepatic	
a. Hepatic calcification	May be secondary to viral infection
b. Hepatic fibrosis	Hepatomegaly, polycystic kidneys as evidenced by increased echogenicity, pancreatic or splenic cysts may also be present
c. Polycystic disease of the liver	Multiple hepatic cysts and renal cysts
d. Cholestasis	
e. Cirrhosis with portal hypertension	
f. Congenital portal dysplasia	
g. Giant cell hepatitis	

(continued)

TABLE 18-5.   *(Continued)*

Condition	Features
5. Renal	
a. Congenital nephrosis (Finnish type)	Increased amniotic fluid α-fetoprotein, hypoproteinemia, and hypoalbuminemia; large placenta
b. Renal dysplasia secondary to urethral obstruction	Dilated renal pelvis; enlarged bladder; narrow renal cortex; may lead to ruptured bladder and urinary ascites
c. Pelvic kidney	Kidney visualized at the level of the bladder
d. Hypoplastic kidney	Small, poorly visualized kidney
e. Polycystic kidneys	Large, echogenic kidneys; cysts rarely seen
f. Renal vein thrombosis	
6. Vascular	
a. Arteriovenous malformation	High-output failure with increased contractility; echolucent mass may be seen with high end-diastolic flow by Doppler
b. Sacrococcygeal teratoma	Sacral mass may extend intra-abdominally or into pelvis
c. Vena caval thrombosis	Decreased flow in vena cava by Doppler
d. Hemangioendothelioma	Vascular mass may be visible intraabdominally
e. Arterial calcification	Echogenic masses along the aorta
B. Fetal—generalized abnormality	
1. Infectious causes	
a. Cytomegalovirus	Amniocentesis positive for cytomegalovirus antigen
b. Coxsackievirus	Myocardial calcifications
c. Syphilis	Placental edema; positive fetal IgM for *Treponema pallidum* wall antigen
d. Toxoplasmosis	Fetal IgM on PUBS after 21 weeks; fetal anemia, thrombocytopenia, leukocytosis, leukopenia; may diagnose by positive amniotic fluid or blood culture
e. Parvovirus B19	Positive maternal serology; positive fetal PCR; aplastic anemia of the fetus
f. Rubella	Positive maternal serology, fetal rubella-specific IgM
g. Herpes simplex	Microcephaly or microphthalmia may be present; extensive brain destruction may lead to hydranencephaly
h. Chagas' disease	Positive maternal serology for *Trypanosoma cruzi*
i. Leptospirosis	Positive maternal serology for *Leptospira*
j. Respiratory syncytial virus	
k. Varicella	Maternal chickenpox
2. Skeletal dysplasias	A family history is helpful
a. Achondroplasia	Disproportionately large head, frontal bossing, depressed nasal bridge; rhizomelic micromelia
b. Achondrogenesis types I and IA	Extreme limb shortening, barrel-shaped trunk, poorly ossified skull and pelvis; ribs are short, cupped, and flared
c. Achondrogenesis, Langer-Saldino	Short trunk and extremely short limbs; markedly enlarged skill with normal ossification; decreased ossification of vertebrae and absent ossification of the sacrum and pubis
d. Osteogenesis imperfecta type II	Intrauterine bone fractures, particularly femora and ribs
e. Lethal osteopetrosis	Dense bones with macrocephaly or hydrocephaly; hepatosplenomegaly
f. Asphyxiating thoracic dysplasia	Narrow thorax with short limbs
g. Thanatophoric dwarfism	Thorax is narrow in anteroposterior and transverse diameters with short cupped ribs; limbs are short
h. Koide's osteochondrodystrophy	Marked shortened extremities, dumbbell-shaped tibias; widened fibulas with proximal shortening; poor ossification of the feet and hands; markedly hypoplastic vertebral bodies
i. McGuire's osteochondrodysplasia	Severe rhizomelia, reduced skull mineralization, short, narrow ribs
j. Intrauterine dwarfism with thin bones and fractures (Kozlowski-Kan syndrome)	Short extremities with multiple fractures; mid-shaft tapering of the long bones of the lower extremity; extremely thin ribs; peculiar facies with frontal bossing; normally developed thorax and abdomen
k. Greenberg-Rimoin chondrodystrophy	Markedly short long bones, ectopic ossification centers, marked platyspondyly

(continued)

TABLE 18-5. *(Continued)*

Condition	Features
l. Lethal chondrodysplasia with Dandy-Walker cyst and multiple congenital anomalies (Moerman-Vandehberghe-Fryns syndrome)	Severe microcelia, bilateral talipes equinovarus, absent ribs, cleft palate, hydroureters; hypoplastic right ventricle, VSD, atresia of the pulmonary valve
m. Short-rib polydactyly syndromes	
i. Saldino-Noonan	Marked limb reduction, postaxial polysyndactyly, narrow constricted thorax, small iliac bones, vertebral abnormalities
ii. Majewski's	Marked limb reduction, preaxial and postaxial polysyndactyly, cleft lip, polycystic kidneys, ambiguous genitalia, low-set ears
iii. Verma-Naumoff	Marked limb reduction, postaxial polysyndactyly, narrow constricted thorax, vertebral abnormalities
iv. Beemer's	Hydrocephalus, cardiac defect, ambiguous external genitalia, thrombocytopenia, dense bones
n. Lethal Kniest-like dysplasia	Dumbbell-shaped long bones with shortened diaphyses and metaphyseal irregularities
o. Chondrodysplasia punctata, Conradi-Hünermann variant	Depressed nasal bridge, flattened nasal tip
p. Cumming's syndrome	Campomelia, cervical lymphocele, polycystic kidneys, cleft palate
q. Pyknoachondrogenesis	Similar to achondrogenesis with extreme sclerosis of bones as seen by increased density on radiograph
r. Wegmann-Jones-Smith syndrome	Short-limb dwarfism, edema and iris coloboma
s. Boomerang skeletal dysplasia	Shortened extremities with anterior bowing of lower limbs; boomerang-like, triangular or oval shaped long bones with absent radii and fibulas; equinovarus deformity of the feet; shortened trunk with a small chest
t. Lethal chondrodysplasia with advanced bone age (Blomstrand's syndrome)	Micromelia with normal-sized hands and feet; advanced ossification of metacarpal and tarsal bones; macroglossia; coarctation of the aorta
u. Herva-Leisti-Kirkinen syndrome (contractures, congenital lethal Finnish type)	Severe flexion contractures of the elbows, hips, wrists; severe hyperextension of the knees; micrognathia, hypertelorism, and hypoplastic heart
3. Metabolic disorders	Family history is essential to guide testing
a. Gaucher's disease	Increased glucocerebrosides in the plasma; deficiency of β-glucosidase, glucocerebrosidase, or both, on circulating white blood cells
b. GM$_1$ gangliosidosis	Decreased β-galactosidase activity in fetal leukocytes and possibly cultured amniotic fluid cells
c. Mucopolysaccharidosis IH (Hurler's syndrome)	Deficient α-L-iduronidase in leukocytes or fibroblasts
d. Mucolipidosis type I	Isolated deficiency of neuraminidase (sialidase) in amniocytes or chorionic villi
e. Mucolipidosis type II (I-cell disease)	Elevated serum levels of β-N-acetylhexosaminidase, arylsulfatase A, iduronate sulfatase, and glycosidases with a deficiency of these in cultured fibroblasts; β-galactosidase is absent from trophoblasts
f. Glucose phosphate isomerase (GPI) deficiency	Fetal anemia with reduced activity of erythrocyte GPI; fetal GPI may be thermolabile compared with normal enzyme
g. Pyruvate kinase deficiency	Decreased fetal pyruvate kinase activity (5–20% of normal); parents may exhibit 50% activity
h. Carnitine deficiency	Fetal cardiomyopathy, decreased plasma carnitine levels.
i. Mucopolysaccharidosis type IVb (Morquio's disease)	Dwarfism with short trunk; deficiency of N-acetyl-galactosamine-6-sulfate sulfatase in amniocytes or chorionic villi
j. Mucopolysaccharidosis type VII	Decreased β-glucuronidase activity in fetal plasma and cultured amniotic fluid cells
k. Niemann-Pick disease types A and C	Rarely, hepatomegaly
l. Sialic acid storage disorder	Fetal anemia, clear vacuoles in lymphocytes, and increased sialic acid in amniotic fluid and amniocytes
m. Galactosialidosis	Deficiency of both β-galactosidase and neuraminidase in fibroblasts and leukocytes

(continued)

TABLE 18-5. *(Continued)*

Condition	Features
4. Syndromes	
a. Autosomal dominant	
i. G. syndrome (Optiz-Frias syndrome)	Hypertelorism, micrognathia; cleft lip or palate in up to 25%
ii. Myotonic dystrophy (neonatal Steinert's disease)	Reduced fetal movements, joint contractures, and talipes equinus
iii. Cornelia de Lange's syndrome	Microcephaly, upper limb abnormalities of variable severity
iv. Noonan's syndrome	Hypertelorism, frequent congenital heart defects
v. Yellow nail syndrome	Maternal or paternal history of yellow nail dystrophy and chronic bronchitis
vi. Tuberous sclerosis	50% have cardiac rhabdomyoma
b. Autosomal recessive	
i. Orofaciodigital syndrome type II (Mohr's syndrome)	Cleft lip, duplication of the hallux, poly- and syndactyly; mild mesomelia may be present, especialy of the tibia
ii. Arthrogryposis multiplex congenita	Multiple joint contractures
iii. Polysplenia syndrome	Single cardiac ventricle; bradycardia, dextrocardia, and displaced intestinal loops may be present
iv. Pena-Shokeir syndrome	Multiple joint contractures, hypertelorism, micrognathia, intrauterine growth retardation
v. Lethal multiple pterygium syndrome	Limb contractures, intrauterine growth retardation, cystic hygroma, intracranial facial clefts, and abnormalities such as small choroid plexus or cerebellar cysts may be present
vi. Neu-Laxova syndrome	Intrauterine growth retardation, microcephaly; may have hypertelorism, micrognathia, limb contractures, hypoplastic cerebellum, or lissencephaly
vii. Idiopathic recurrent hydrops	
viii. Isolated recurrent cystic hygroma	Cystic mass seen on fetal neck, axilla, or groin
ix. Elejalde's syndrome	Multiple nuchal cysts extending into the fetal abdomen
x. McKusick-Kaufman syndrome	Polydactyly; hydrometrocolpos, which may be seen as a large mass extending into the fetal abdomen
xi. Hypophosphatasia	Decreased tissue; nonspecific alkaline phosphatase isozyme activity in amniotic fluid, amniocytes, and chorionic villi; may be craniosynostosis; severely affected fetuses show poor bone mineralization
xii. Prune belly syndrome	Enlarged bladder; kidneys may be cystic, hypoplastic or hydronephrotic; frequent clubfoot; females rarely are affected
xiii. Angioosteohypertrophy syndrome (Klippel-Feil-Trenaunay)	Hemihypertrophy of a limb, may see "port-wine" nevi on fetoscopy
xiv. Massive cystic hygroma	
xv. Fanconi's syndrome type III	
5. Chromosomal	Diagnosed by karyotype of amniocytes or chorionic villi
a. Trisomy 21	Associated with nuchal thickness >6 mm, dilated renal pelves, hypoplastic middle phalanx of the fifth digit, short humerus, actual/expected femur length ratio ≤ 0.91, congenital heart disease
b. Trisomy 18	Cardiac defect, choroid plexus cysts
c. Trisomy 13	Midline facial cleft, cardiac defect
d. 45,XO (Turner's syndrome)	Cystic hygroma, cardiac defect
e. Trisomy 15	
f. Trisomy 16	
g. Partial duplication of chromosome 11	

(continued)

TABLE 18-5.   *(Continued)*

Condition	Features
h. Partial duplication of chromosomes 15 and 17	
i. Partial duplication of chromosome 18	
j. Partial deletion of the short arm of chromosome 13	
k. Partial deletion of the short arm of chromosome 18	
l. Rearrangement of the long arm of chromosome 22	
m. 46,XX/XY mosaic	
n. Triploidy	
o. Tetraploidy	
6. Fetal anemia	Low fetal hematocrit on fetal blood sampling
a. α-Thalassemia	Low maternal MCV, abnormal maternal hemoglobin electrophoresis, abnormal restriction endonuclease testing; oligohydramnios may be present
b. Fetal closed-space hemorrhage	Ultrasound may show evidence of blood accumulation such as intracranial hemorrhage
c. Hemolysis	Fetal G6PD deficiency, fetal pyruvate kinase deficiency
d. Maternal–fetal hemorrhage	Positive Kleihauer-Betke
7. Twin-to-twin transfusion (including acardiac parasitic twin)	Monochorionic twin gestation with polyhydramnios in one sac and oligohydramnios in the other (hydrops may be seen in donor or receipt)
C. Placental and umbilical cord causes	
1. Chorioangioma	May see a placental mass on ultrasound
2. True knots of the cord	Rarely diagnosed on ultrasound
3. Angiomyxoma of the umbilical cord	Diagnosed histologically
4. Aneurysm of the umbilical artery	Intraabdominal cystic vascular mass at umbilical insertion
5. Hemorrhagic endovasculitis of the placenta	Histologic diagnosis
6. Chorionic vein thrombosis	
7. Placental and umbilical vein thrombosis	
8. Umbilical cord torsion	
D. Maternal causes	
1. Medication	
a. Maternal indomethacin use	Closure of the ductus leads to NIHF
2. Disease	
a. Mirror syndrome	Maternal edema, preeclampsia
b. Systemic disease	Maternal anemia, diabetes, hypoproteinemia
E. Miscellaneous causes	
a. Congenital neuroblastoma	Large tumor mass might be visible; large abdominal cysts may be confused with dilated bowel
b. Torsion of an ovarian cyst	Cystic structure in the lower abdomen
c. Sacrococcygeal teratoma	Cystic or solid tumor arising from the coccyx; may show intrapelvic or abdominal extension
F. Unknown causes	

ASD, atrial septal defect; VSD, ventricular septal defect; Ig, immunoglobulin; PUBS, percutaneous umbilical cord blood sampling; PCR, polymerase chain reaction; G6PD, glucose-6-phosphate dehydrogenase; MCV, mean corpuscular volume; NIHF, nonimmune hydrops fetalis.

(Modified from Holzgreve W, Holzgreve B, Curry JR: Non-immune hydrops fetalis: Diagnosis and management. Semin Perinat 1985; 95:52–67.)

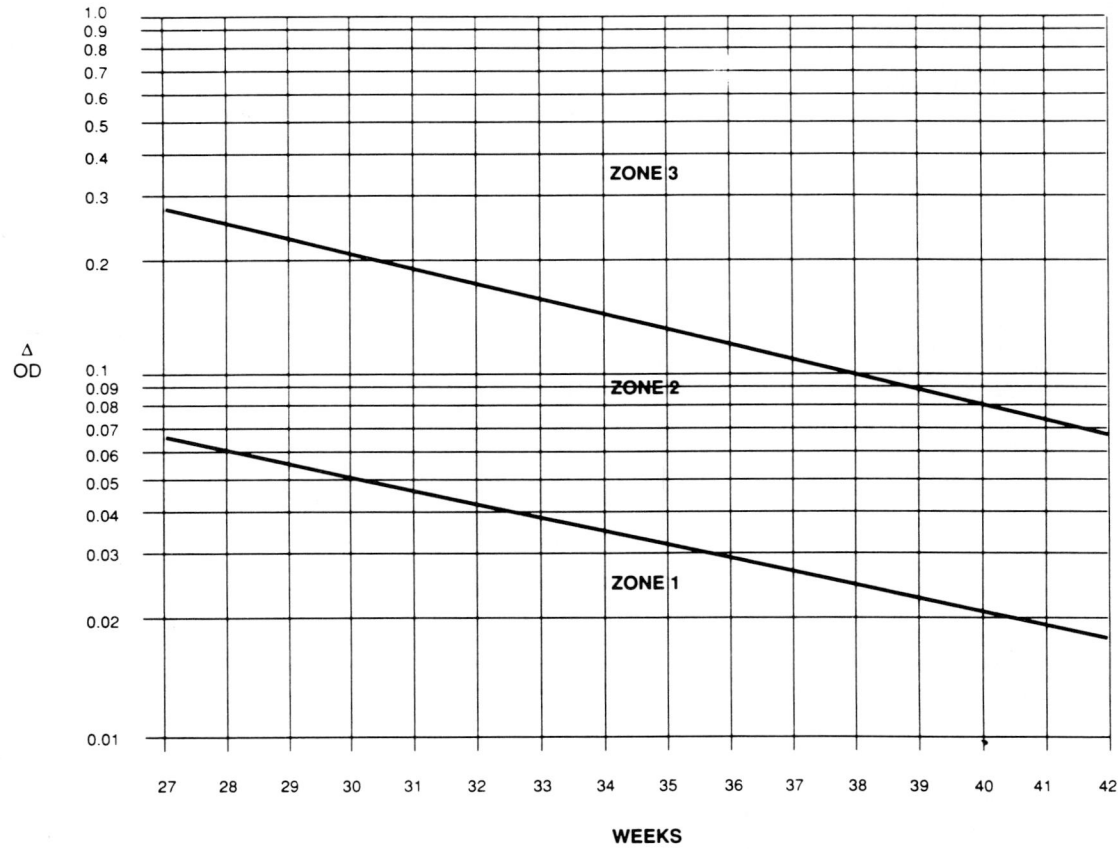

FIGURE 18-1. Liley's three-zone chart plotting normal range for ΔOD450 against gestational age. The closer the value falls to zone 3, the higher is the risk of fetal hydrops. (Liley AW: Liquor amnii analysis in management of pregnancy complicated by Rhesus sensitization. Am J Obstet Gynecol 1961; 82:1359–1370.)

Other Ultrasound Findings

A number of ultrasound findings have been advocated to be useful to predict fetal hydrops. The ultrasound features that have been investigated in predicting fetal anemia include increased umbilical vein, fetal hepatosplenomegaly, head circumference/abdominal circumference ratios, bowel wall thickening, right atrial or right ventricular cardiac enlargement, fetal heart rate testing, and Doppler velocimetry, to name a few. The significance of these findings is presented next.

In 1981, DeVore and colleagues reported dilation of the *umbilical vein* to be a predictor of severe anemia in Rh disease.[9] This initial report involved only 15 cases, however, and subsequent data have not supported the utility of this finding.

Hepatosplenomegaly is an early diagnostic finding in erythyroblastosis fetalis. Recently, Vintzileos and colleagues measured fetal liver length in a longitudinal plane from the right hemidiaphragm to the tip of the right lobe.[10] They noted a growth rate of greater than 5 mm per week in all severely affected fetuses. Once again, this study involved a limited sample size, and the technique has not been widely applied.

Nicolaides and colleagues evaluated a number of ultrasound parameters in patients with Rh disease immediately before fetal blood sampling.[11] They constructed normograms for *fetal head and abdominal circumferences, head/abdomen ratio, estimated fetal intraperitoneal volume, placental thickness,* and *umbilical vein diameter* from 410 healthy singleton pregnancies. Twelve of 50 isoimmunized patients exhibited hydrops, all with hemoglobin values less than 5 g/dl. Only four of an additional eight patients with severe anemia displayed any abnormal ultrasound findings. In addition, only 6 of 19 fetuses with hemoglobin values between 5 and 10 g/

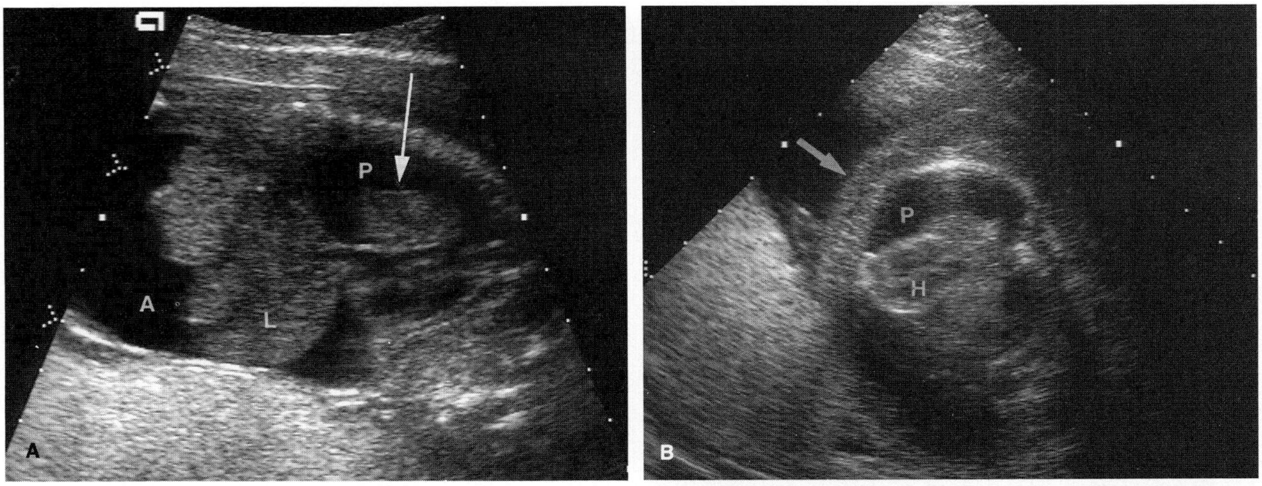

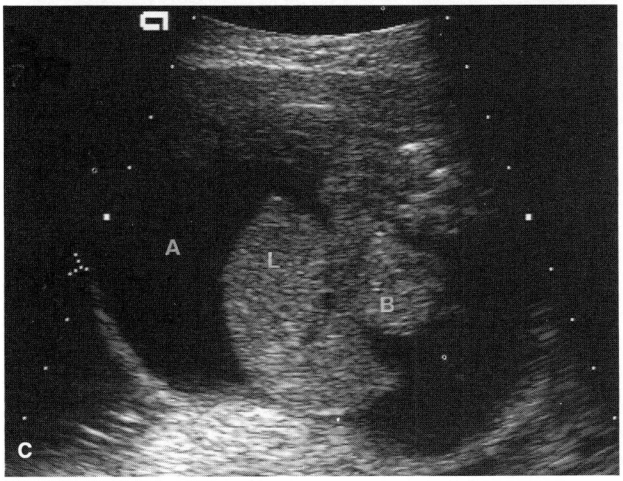

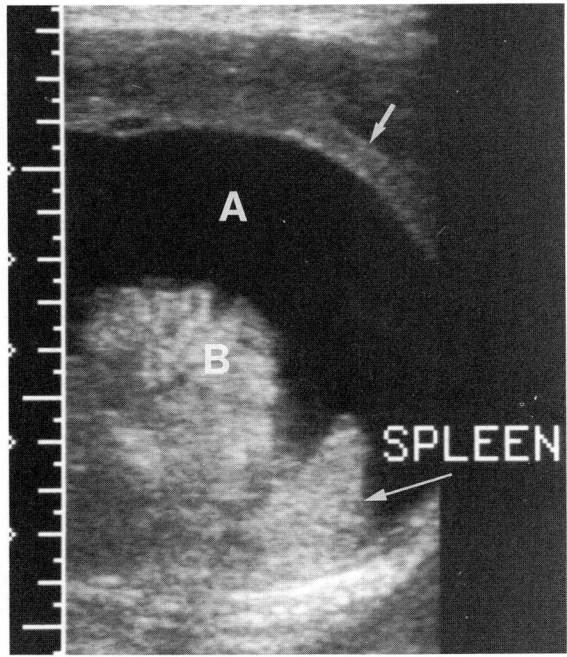

FIGURE 18-2. Fetus with hydrops of unknown cause. **(A)** Sagittal section shows ascites (A) and pleural effusions (P). The *arrow* points to the hypoplastic lung. L, liver. **(B)** Axial section of the thorax shows the heart (H) with pleural effusion (P). Note the cutaneous edema (*arrow*). **(C)** Axial section of the upper abdomen shows the liver (L), bowel (B), and massive ascites (A).

FIGURE 18-3. Immune hydrops. Fetus with Rh isoimmunization has cutaneous edema (*arrow*) and ascites (A). B, bowel. (Courtesy of John P. McGahan, MD, Sacramento, CA.)

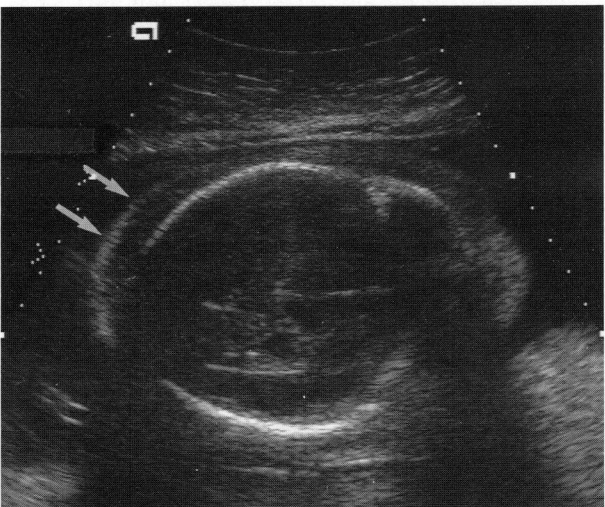

FIGURE 18-4.   Skin edema is often best visualized in the scalp, where the skin can be clearly seen displaced from the skull, as shown in this fetus with hydrops of an unknown cause (*arrows*).

dl had abnormal ultrasound findings. The investigators concluded that the role of ultrasound in these cases is limited to the search for hydrops. In a similar investigation, Chitkara and colleagues evaluated hydrops and prehydropic changes, which they defined as *hydramnios, placental thickening* (greater than 4 cm), or increased *umbilical vein diameter*.[8] Among eight cases with severe anemia (fetal hematocrit less than 15%), five displayed hydropic changes, one revealed hydramnios only, and the remaining two had completely normal evaluations. Eleven of 19 cases with hematocrits between 16% and 29% had completely normal scans as well. These authors suggested that hydramnios may be the earliest sonographic sign of fetal anemia, seen in two thirds of their patients undergoing serial scans (hematocrits, 14%–26%). These data support the earlier observation that progressive erythroblastosis fetalis usually follows

TABLE 18-6.   Classic Sonographic Progression of Findings in Hydrops Fetalis

Hydramnios
↓
Placental thickening (>4 cm)
↓
Hepatomegaly
↓
Ascites
↓
Overt hydrops

TABLE 18-7.   Early Sonographic Signs of Fetal Anemia

Pre-ascites (visualization of both sides of bowel wall before 32 weeks of gestation
Small pericardial effusion
Right atrial enlargement
Right ventricular enlargement
Hydramnios (new onset)

a consistent sonographic progression of hydramnios followed by placental thickening, hepatomegaly, ascites, and overt hydrops[12] (Table 18-6). Chitkara and colleagues caution, however, that the absence of hydramnios does not preclude the presence of fetal anemia.[8] It cannot be overemphasized that none of the above sonographic signs has been shown to be universally present before the development of severe anemia.

Despite these somewhat discouraging results, it is clear that ultrasound is an indispensable component of the modern management of the isoimmunized pregnancy. Severe anemia cannot be predicted in all cases, but several early sonographic signs of fetal anemia have been suggested (Table 18-7). Benacerraf and colleagues reported that visualization of both sides of the *bowel wall,* particularly in the second and early third trimester, may precede the detection of frank ascites by 24 to 48 hours.[13] With increasing interest and expertise in fetal echocardiography, it has been suggested that a *small pericardial effusion* or *right atrial* or *ventricular enlargement* may be an early sign of fetal anemia.

Frigoletto and colleagues described the combined use of frequent (every 24 to 72 hours) high-resolution targeted ultrasound and *biophysical testing* (nonstress fetal heart rate testing for reactivity and sonographic assessment of fetal breathing, body movement, tone, and amniotic fluid) in the successful, noninvasive management of 11 moderately anemic fetuses.[4] These authors emphasized the importance of intensive and frequent surveillance for severely isoimmunized pregnancies. In particular, it has been our experience that the pre-ascites finding (visualization of both sides of the bowel wall) is a useful marker in many cases. These early findings, however, typically precede frank hydrops and severe fetal anemia by only a few days at best. It is critical that these findings not be ignored or simply reevaluated sonographically in a week, but rather that perinatal consultation regarding invasive assessment (PUBS) or delivery be considered, depending on the gestational age.

Even though it is clearly out of the scope of

discussion for this chapter, it is important to note that a number of authors suggest that *antepartum fetal heart rate testing* can be extremely important in the evaluation of the potentially anemic fetus.[14-16] Spontaneous late decelerations, an intermittently sinusoidal pattern, and blunting of fetal heart rate variability have each been suggested as early signs of fetal anemia, preceding the development of hydrops fetalis. Nicolaides and colleagues, however, found a wide range of positive and negative predictive values with these findings, concluding that these changes do not allow for the accurate prediction of the severity of fetal anemia.[17]

Another modality that has been explored in an attempt to find a reliable noninvasive tool for the detection of fetal anemia is *Doppler flow velocity waveforms*. Rightmire and colleagues reported an inverse relation between fetal hematocrit and both descending thoracoaortic velocity and the umbilical arterial Pourcelot (resistance) index in a retrospective study of isoimmunized patients before their first fetal blood sampling.[18] Using these two indices, they were able to construct a formula that predicted hematocrit within 3.8% ± 3%. Copel and colleagues prospectively tested two formulas using pulsed Doppler assessments of umbilical artery Pourcelot index, peak aortic velocity, or both.[19] Statistical significance for one formula was noted, but the presence or absence of hydrops was the only factor responsible for the relation between fetal hematocrit and the formula. The most promising work has come from Mari and colleagues, who reported increased middle cerebral artery peak velocities (MCA-PV) in anemic fetuses.[19a] Early data suggested that using a cutoff of 0.75 multiple standard errors of estimation (MSEE) above the MCA-PV mean could identify anemic fetuses with a sensitivity of 97.5%, a specificity of 69.2%, a positive predictive value of 90.6%, and a negative predictive value of 90.0%. Although work continues in this area, including umbilical venous and inferior vena caval flow velocities, no practical approach has come into common use. Color flow mapping for the detection of *tricuspid regurgitation* has been helpful in distinguishing hydropic fetuses who are hemodynamically stable for a bolus intravascular transfusion from those who will not tolerate such a volume load.

Pitfalls

In reviewing the ultrasound findings, several artifacts must be considered that mimic fluid collections:

Pseudoascites: Fetal body fat in a macrosomic fetus may look like subcutaneous edema. Similarly, this artifact is seen when the abdominal wall musculature produces a hypoechoic rim around the abdomen (Fig. 18-5).

False pericardial effusion: The fetal myocardium is relatively hypoechoic and may occasionally suggest a pericardial effusion. There may also be a small amount of pericardial fluid noted in normal fetuses.

Nonascitic intraabdominal fluid: There may be fluid collections present that do not represent fetal edema but are fluid collections secondary to the rupture of the fetal renal calyx, fetal bladder, thoracic duct, or other viscus.

Normal fetal or hair subcutaneous fat: This may mimic scalp edema (Figs. 18-4 and 18-6).

Ultrasound continues to play a central role in the management of the isoimmunized pregnancy. It is critical that these extremely high-risk pregnancies be managed in tertiary centers with the expertise to assess the sometimes subtle sonographic and other biophysical findings associated with fetal anemia. The potential for rapid deterioration from an apparently normal fetus to one with frank hydrops underscores the importance of consistent and frequent evaluation in these cases.

Percutaneous Umbilical Cord Blood Sampling

The alternative of PUBS for fetal hematocrit determination is attractive from the standpoint of accu-

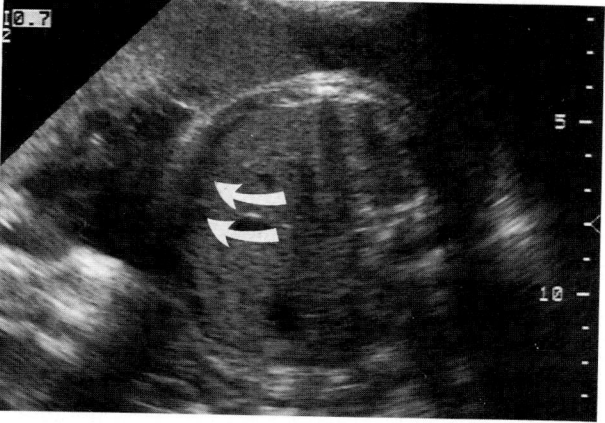

FIGURE 18-5. Pseudoascites. Transverse ultrasound of the abdomen shows hypoechoic rim at the edge of the abdomen (*arrows*), which should not be confused with true ascites.

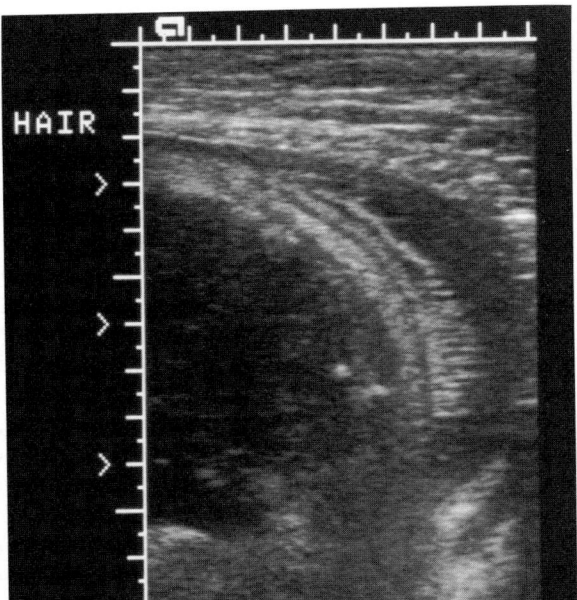

FIGURE 18-6. Echogenic fetal hair is observed posterior to the fetus, which may be misinterpreted as a nuchal thickening or scalp edema. (Courtesy of Michael Cronan, RDMS, Sacramento, CA.)

rate assessment.[20] Unfortunately, PUBS incurs fetal risks greater than those for amniocentesis, including a 1% to 2% mortality. In addition, there is a significant risk for enhancing the isoimmunization process due to the fetomaternal hemorrhage commonly associated with the procedure.[21] Beyond this, significant morbidity associated with PUBS includes fetal distress, trauma, fetomaternal

TABLE 18-8.   Equipment and Supplies for Percutaneous Umbilical Blood Sampling and Fetal Transfusion

High-resolution ultrasound machine
Sector or linear transducer (3.5–5 MHz)
Needle guide
22-gauge needle
Drugs for maternal sedation and fetal paralysis
Local anesthesia
Betadine
Sterile drape
Sterile probe cover
Sterile coupling gel
Heparinized blood tubes
Three-way stopcock

(Blake LC, McGahan JP: Percutaneous umbilical cord blood sampling and fetal transfusion. Semin Intervent Radiol 1992; 9:105–111.)

infection, preterm rupture of the membranes, and preterm labor. PUBS not only may be used for fetal hematocrit determination but also is useful for a number of other indications (Table 18-8).

Most cordocenteses are performed without maternal sedation and without fetal paralysis. The approach for PUBS may be transplacental or transamniotic and is usually into the site of insertion of the umbilical vein into the placenta (Fig. 18-7). A number of different locations have been used for the site of cord puncture, including the cord itself, intraabdominal vein, or fetal intrahepatic vein (Fig. 18-8). Cord insertion to the placenta is the best site for sampling but may not always be available, and a free-floating loop is sometimes used in patients with oligohydramnios because the cord is relatively fixed in position.[22]

The equipment and supplies needed for PUBS are listed in Table 18-8. The maternal abdomen is prepared and draped for the procedure, and the ultrasound transducer is placed into a sterile covering. Under continuous visualization, usually a 22-gauge needle is inserted directly into the umbilical vein. A firm push is usually necessary for the final placement of the needle into the vein. After proper needle placement, about 0.5 to 1 ml of blood is sampled and discarded. Then 1 to 4 ml of fetal blood is aspirated into a heparinized tube. This sample is immediately analyzed with a Coulter cell

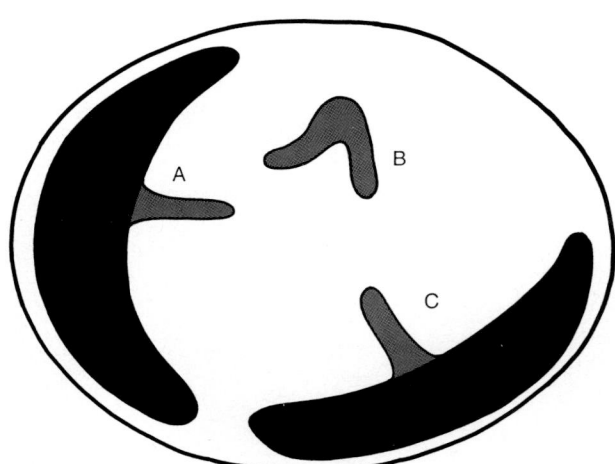

FIGURE 18-7. Potential access to umbilical cord for percutaneous umbilical cord blood sampling includes: **(A)** transplacental route into the umbilical cord, **(B)** transamniotic route into free loop of cord, or **(C)** transamniotic route into posterior cord insertion. (Modified from Blake LC, McGahan JP: Percutaneous umbilical cord blood sampling and fetal transfusion. Semin Intervent Radiol 1992; 9:105–111.)

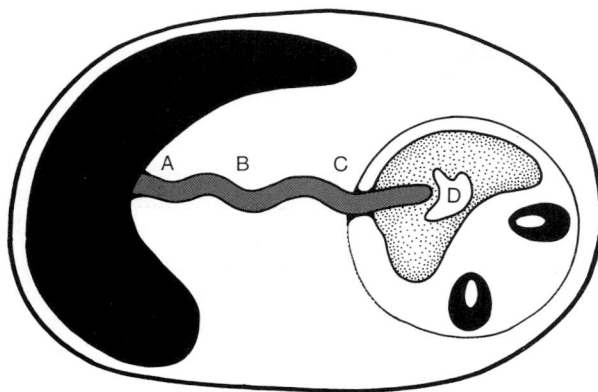

FIGURE 18-8. The most common site chosen for puncture of the fetal intravascular system is **(A)** origin of the umbilical cord from the placenta. However, other sites include **(B)** free-floating loop of cord and **(C)** insertion of cord into the fetal abdomen. Less commonly **(D)**, the fetal intrahepatic vein may be used.

counter to verify fetal origin. A Kleihauer-Betke stain can be done for confirmation of fetal blood cells. The needle is then removed, and the cord puncture site is visualized until bleeding stops.

Management With Fetal Transfusion

In cases of isoimmunization severe enough to effect hydrops, several transfusions may be needed throughout the pregnancy to get the fetus to a ges-

tational age at which delivery may be contemplated. After several transfusions, the fetal bone marrow is usually suppressed, and the entire fetal circulation is replaced by adult red cells. The fetal anemia can be immediately corrected by the transfusion, but a prolonged delay in the resolution of the hydrops may be noted.

When the fetal hematocrit is low, as determined by PUBS, or when there is development of fetal hydrops, intrauterine fetal transfusion is indicated. Previously, this was performed using the fetal intraperitoneal route, but much better results have been reported with direct intravascular infusion of packed red blood cells for fetal transfusion. Survival rates for fetuses managed in this manner have been as high as 90%, including fetuses with frank fetal hydrops.

The technique for fetal transfusion is similar to that previously described for PUBS (Fig. 18-9). Supplies needed for fetal transfusion are listed in Table 18-8. Fetal transfusions are commonly performed with fetal paralysis. Short-term fetal paralysis may be obtained by injection of pancuronium (0.1–0.3 mg/kg) based on estimated fetal weight.[23,24] These drugs may be injected into the fetal thigh or, more commonly, directly into the fetal vasculature. During the procedure, the fetal heart rate is monitored while a needle is guided into the umbilical vein. Fetal hematocrit is obtained, and a transfusion with packed red cells is performed to raise the fetal hematocrit to about

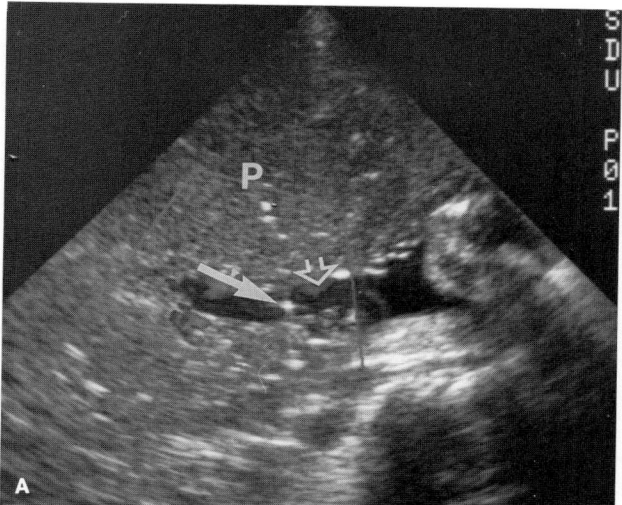
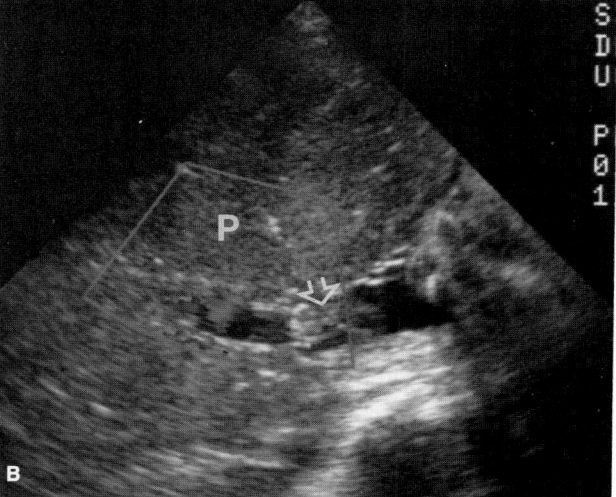

FIGURE 18-9. Fetal transfusion. **(A)** The echogenic needle tip (*arrow*) was placed, using the freehand technique, transplacentally into the umbilical vein (*open arrow*). **(B)** With injection of either saline or packed red blood cells, increased echoes are observed within the umbilical vein (*open arrow*) that flow toward the fetus. P, placenta. (Courtesy of John P. McGahan, MD, Sacramento, CA.)

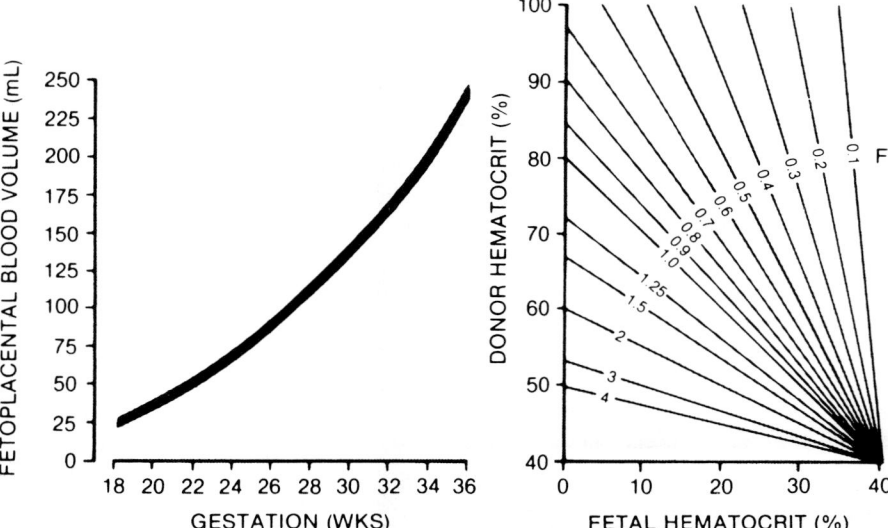

FIGURE 18-10. Fetal transfusion. Calculation of volume of blood necessary to achieve a postfetal hematocrit of about 40% is obtained by estimating the fetal blood volume based on gestation age. This is multiplied by the factor F obtained by knowing the donor hematocrit (usually 80%) and plotting this against the initial fetal hematocrit, which usually varies from 10% to 20%. (Nicolaides KH, Soothil PW, Rodeck CH, Clewel W: Rh disease: Intravascular fetal blood transfusion by cordocentesis. Fetal Ther 1986; 1:185.)

40%. A number of different charts and tables have been developed based on donor hematocrit, fetal hematocrit, and fetal placental blood volume obtained for various gestational ages (Fig. 18-10). Also, a guideline for estimated transfusion volume is

$$\text{Volume of packed red blood cells} =$$
$$(\text{desired Hct} - \text{actual Hct})$$
$$\times \text{estimated fetoplacental blood volume}$$
$$\times \text{estimated fetal weight (kg)}$$
$$\div \text{donor hematocrit}$$

The donor hematocrit is usually 80% (packed red blood cells) that are O- or type-matched. Once the umbilical vein is punctured and the initial hematocrit is obtained, saline may be injected, which appears echogenic in the vascular system. Flow must be toward the fetus, indicating umbilical vein, rather than away from the fetus, as would occur with injection in the umbilical artery (see Fig. 18-9). A posttransfusion hematocrit is obtained before removing the needle. It appears that fetal transfusion will continue to be an important tool in the treatment of fetal anemia.

NONIMMUNE FETAL HYDROPS

With the use of anti-D γ-globulin, the incidence of immune hydrops has decreased. Concomitantly, with the more widespread use of prenatal ultrasound, there has been increased detection of non-

immune fetal hydrops. Therefore, it is estimated that the occurrence of nonimmune fetal hydrops is greater than that of immune hydrops. The causes of nonimmune fetal hydrops number well over 100 and are listed in Table 18-5. They can be classified as focal fetal abnormalities, generalized fetal abnormalities, placental causes, or maternal causes (see Table 18-4). In about 15% of cases, no specific etiologic factor for fetal hydrops can be determined.

Ultrasound

Ultrasound has emerged as one of the primary tools for investigation into the severity and cause of nonimmune fetal hydrops. Because ultrasound is noninvasive, it is preferred before use of more invasive tests such as amniocentesis or PUBS. Furthermore, ultrasound may be able to pinpoint the exact cause of fetal hydrops. The following sections outline areas of importance in each organ system or region with regard to fetal hydrops. We first describe anatomic areas in which *focal fetal abnormalities* that cause fetal hydrops occur and then describe more *generalized fetal abnormalities*.

Focal Abnormalities
Cranium and Neck. Initial inspection of the skull is directed toward ruling out the presence of an encephalocele. When a normal skull is appreciated, the intracranial anatomy is examined, with attention paid to preservation of the midline anatomy and parenchymal tissue. Displacement of the midline with a mass affect may represent an intracra-

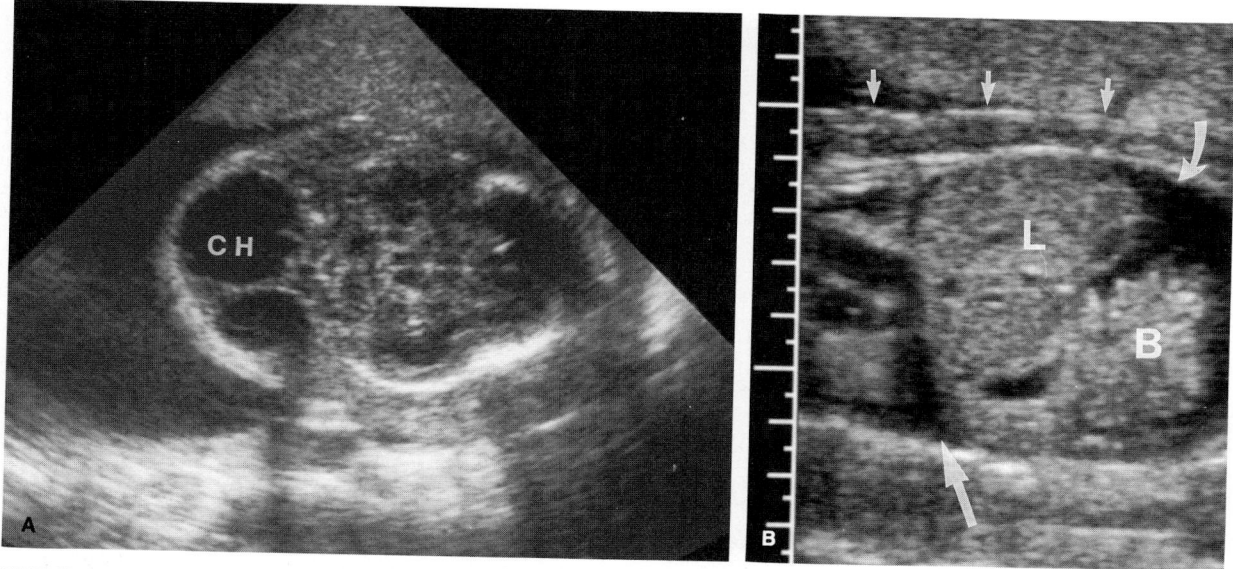

FIGURE 18-11. Fetal hydrops—cystic hygroma. **(A)** Axial scan of the head and neck region shows a cystic hygroma (CH) posterior to the occipital region. **(B)** Coronal ultrasound shows pleural effusion (*large arrow*), ascites (*curved arrow*), and skin edema (*small arrows*). L, liver; B, bowel. (Courtesy of John P. McGahan, MD, Sacramento, CA.)

nial hemorrhage or tumor. Cystic structures in the parenchyma may represent loss of brain tissue (porencephaly) or presence of an arteriovenous malformation. Pulsed Doppler and Doppler color flow mapping are useful in differentiating these two conditions. The presence of a midline facial cleft is suggestive of holoprosencephaly. The presence of fluid-filled structures of the neck may point to causes associated with cystic hygromas (Fig. 18-11), such as Turner's syndrome (Fig. 18-12) or Elejalde's syndrome.

Thorax. Inspection of the thorax for pleural effusions and masses is critical in the work-up of hydrops, especially when they are noted before the onset of generalized nonimmune hydrops. The presence of effusions may suggest the cause (eg, chylothorax), but it also points to the potential complication of pulmonary hypoplasia if the onset is early and persistent. Severe chylothorax and other abnormalities that raise intrathoracic pressure may cause hydrops by decreasing venous return[25] (Fig. 18-13). If a mass effect is seen, a me-

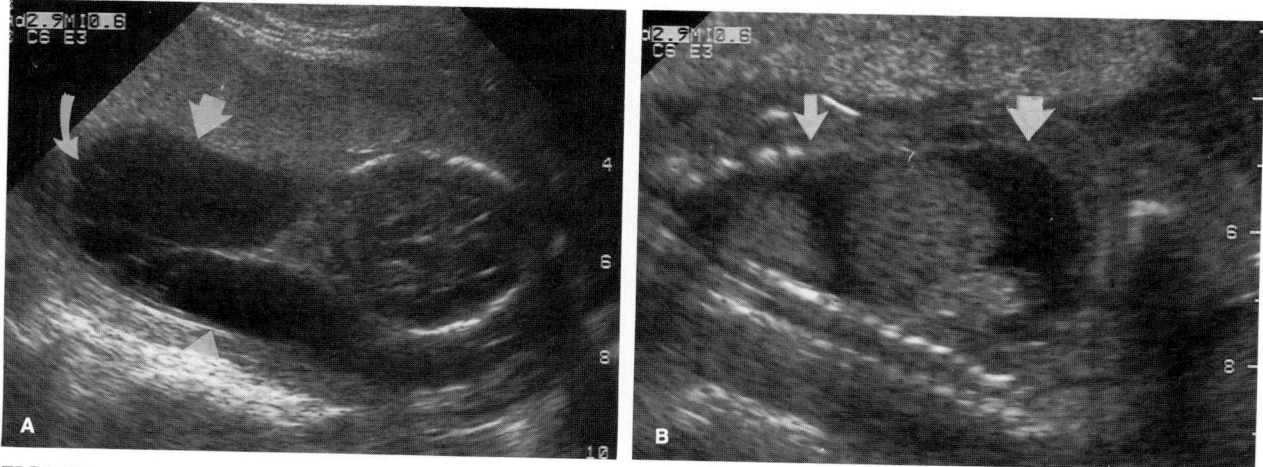

FIGURE 18-12. Hydrops in a fetus with Turner's syndrome. **(A)** *Arrows* outline a large cystic hygroma. **(B)** In the sagittal scan, the *smaller arrow* corresponds to a pleural effusion, while the *large arrow* indicates ascites.

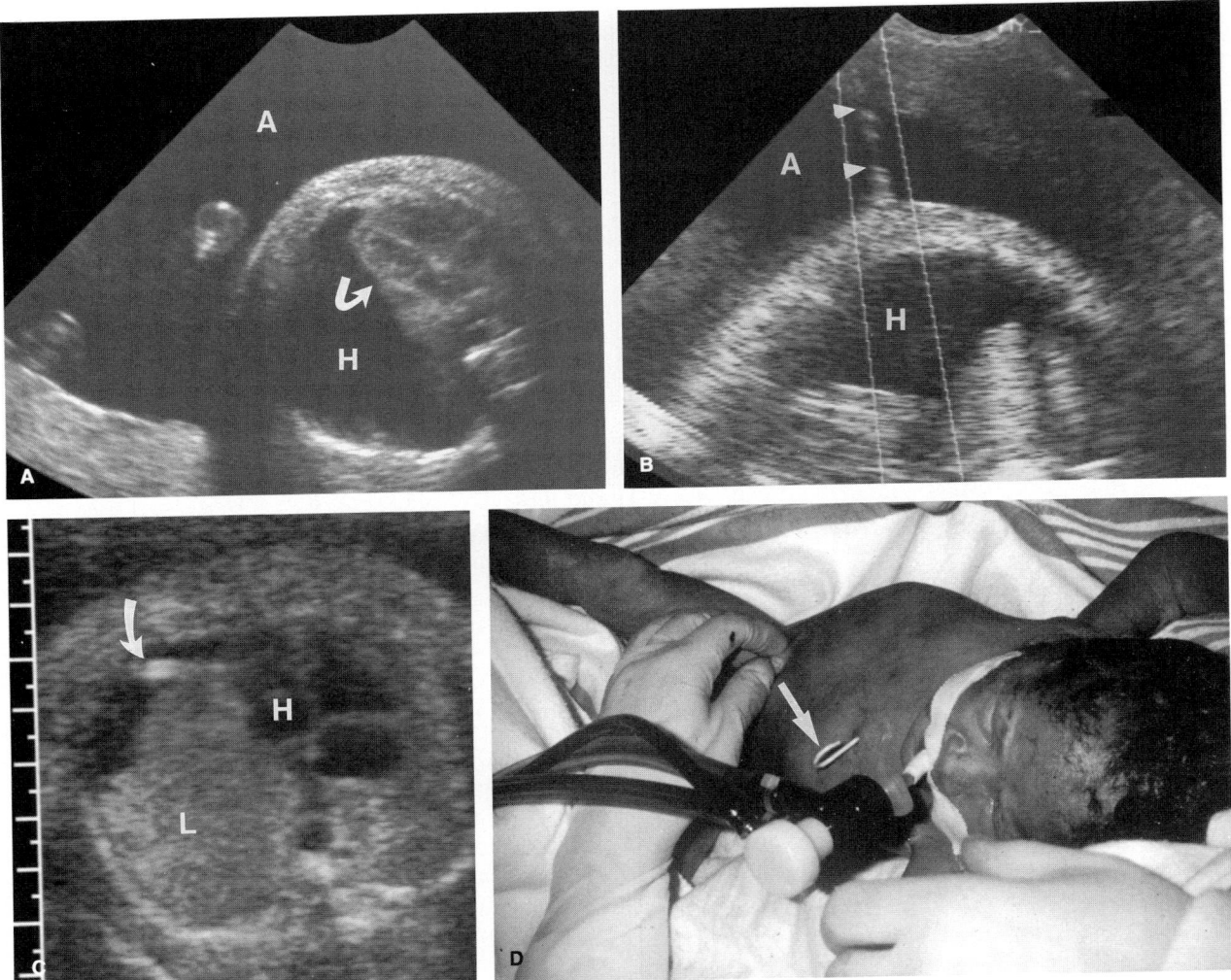

FIGURE 18-13.   Fetal hydrops: pleural effusion and intervention. (**A**) Transverse scan through the fetal thorax initially demonstrated an isolated pleural effusion (H). Subcutaneous fetal edema, ascites, and polyhydramnios (A) developed on this follow-up scan. (**B**) A fetal shunt (*arrowheads*) was placed into the hydrothorax (H). A, amniotic fluid. (**C**) Two days later, there is still cutaneous edema, but with the shunt tube in place (*curved arrow*), the hydrothorax is decreased. H, heart; L, lung. (**D**) Photograph of the newborn when there was fetal lung maturation shows shunt tube in place. (Slotnick RN, McGahan JP, Milio L, et al: Antenatal diagnosis and treatment of fetal bronco-pulmonary sequestration. Fetal Ther 1990; 5:33–39.)

diastinal tumor or pulmonary sequestration may be present. More commonly, shifting of the heart is caused by a diaphragmatic hernia, and the presence of the stomach bubble at the level of the heart is diagnostic. Finally, the presence of multiple cysts may represent congenital cystadenomatoid malformation of the lung. Although this may present with cysts smaller than the resolution of ultrasound, the most common types have cysts that are 1 to 2 cm. The presence of peristalsis can help differentiate between a diaphragmatic hernia

and cystadenomatoid malformation of the lung. All these anatomic abnormalities frequently effect a mediastinal shift, which may cause hydrops through direct compression of the lymphatics and major blood vessels.

A detailed inspection of the heart is required to look for anatomic and conduction defects. Fetal echocardiography is helpful in ruling out congestive heart failure in the fetus due to congenital heart defects or anemia. Numerous structural defects have been associated with hydrops. The hall-

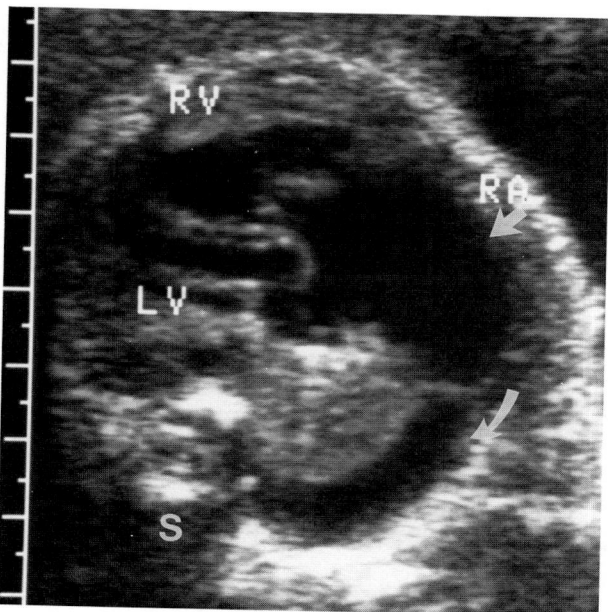

FIGURE 18-14. Fetus with Ebstein's anomaly who developed hydrops with pleural effusion (*curved arrow*). Note enlarged right atrium (RA). RV, right ventricle; LV, left ventricle; S, spine. (Courtesy of John P. McGahan, MD, Sacramento, CA.)

mark of these defects is atrioventricular regurgitation causing congestive heart failure (Figs. 18-14 and 18-15). Other anatomic lesions may also play a role. Both intracardiac and intrapericardial tumors may be involved. Rhabdomyomas are suggestive of tuberous sclerosis and should prompt a thorough evaluation of the mother and father. The three major categories of arrhythmia that cause hydrops can also be diagnosed by fetal echo. Supraventricular tachycardia and atrial flutter bring about failure through decreased filling times. Fetal heart block may also be identified and is associated with maternal anti-La and anti-Ro antibodies. Myocardial disease may also result from a fetal viral infection, such as with cytomegalovirus. This myocarditis results in inadequate ventricular function leading to congestive failure and hydrops.

Gastrointestinal. The presence of a fluid collection limited to the fetal abdomen is isolated fetal ascites. Fetal ascites frequently progresses to hydrops, depending on its cause. Examination of the abdomen should focus on the presence of cystic structures that represent dilated loops of bowel and bowel wall calcifications. The various bowel atresias are associated with polyhydramnios (and therefore hydrops), although the findings may

also be limited to ascites. The cause is thought to be related to decreased colloid osmotic pressure intravascularly because protein may be lost into the bowel. The presence of the bowel loops may help identify the location of the obstruction. The characteristic double-bubble sign is associated with duodenal atresia. Multiple loops of dilated bowel may represent a more distal atresia or an imperforate anus. If echogenic peritoneal plaques or calcifications are noted, there is a high incidence of cystic fibrosis. It is appropriate to offer mutation screening to the parents if an amniocentesis or chorionic villus sampling is not planned for fetal karyotype. If the mutation screening suggests that the parents are carriers of cystic fibrosis genes, then amniocentesis may allow confirmation of the disease state in the fetus.

Hepatic. Numerous hepatic causes of hydrops are known; however, most of these are not diagnosed prenatally because ultrasound findings are not helpful. When findings are present, they may be limited to hepatomegaly or hepatic cysts. When cysts are present, the kidneys should also be carefully examined to rule out cysts because polycystic disease of the kidneys may be associated with hepatic cysts.

Renal. The kidneys are evaluated for evidence of obstruction, malposition, maldevelopment, and function. Dilated renal pelvis and ureter suggest obstruction that may lead to ruptured bladder or kidney and urinary ascites. The presence of a pelvic kidney or a hypoplastic kidney has been associated with hydrops. Enlarged kidneys may represent polycystic kidneys, particularly if bilateral. Finally, fetal kidney disease may be identified by amniocentesis. Congenital nephrosis leads to an elevated amniotic fluid α-fetoprotein, which may be the only clue to this condition. Congenital nephrosis also leads to hypoalbuminemia and cardiac failure.

Generalized Abnormalities
Infection. Several infectious agents, particularly viral, have been associated with hydrops. The most common are cytomegalovirus, toxoplasmosis, and parvovirus. Although most of the viral agents are presumed to cause hydrops through hepatic injury leading to portal hypertension and hypoalbuminemia, parvovirus causes severe anemia by suppressing the fetal bone marrow. To diagnose an infectious cause of hydrops, a high index

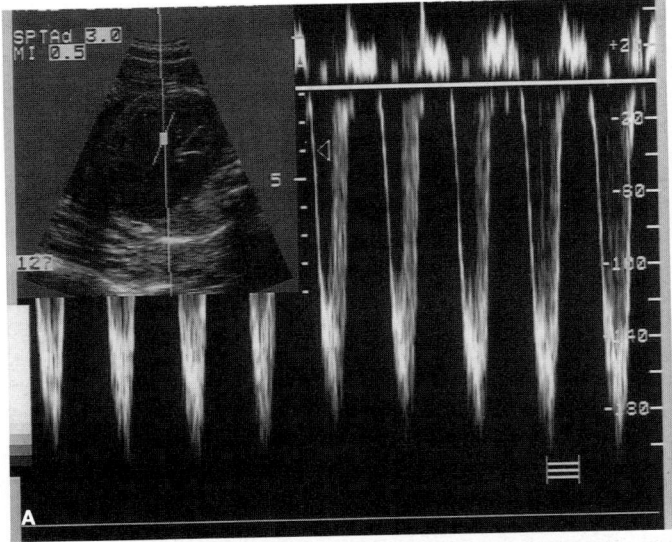

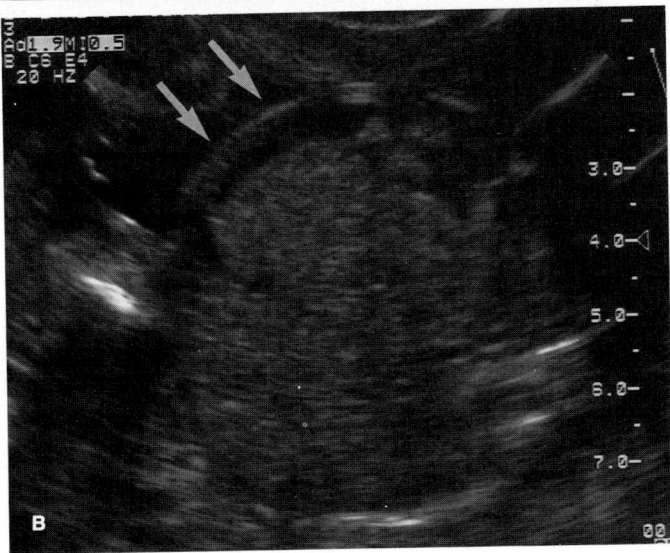

FIGURE 18-15. Fetal hydrops with tricuspid regurgitation (non-Ebstein). **(A)** Doppler cursor placed through the tricuspid valve reveals a large regurgitation. **(B)** Axial ultrasound of the abdomen shows ascites (*arrows*) in the same fetus.

of suspicion must be present. A history of a community parvovirus epidemic or other exposure may lead to maternal antibody testing. The presence of intracranial calcifications, microcephaly, or hydrocephaly may provoke cytomegalovirus and toxoplasmosis screening. The interpretation of maternal antibodies may be difficult, since IgM and IgG for these viruses do not always follow the standard curves for antibody appearance and disappearance. It is best to use reference laboratories to confirm positive findings from nonreference facilities. When antibodies are suggestive of recent exposure, fetal testing by amniocentesis or fetal blood sampling may be necessary to confirm fetal infection. Unfortunately, there is little or no ther-

apy available for most of these infections. In the case of toxoplasmosis, however, therapy directed at treatment of the fetus has been described by Daffos and colleagues.[26] Because the cause of hydrops in parvovirus infection is transient marrow suppression, fetal transfusions may be used to treat the hydrops until the marrow recovers.

Skeletal Dysplasias. The number of skeletal dysplasias associated with hydrops appears to grow yearly as new conditions are reported. Maldergem and colleagues compiled a listing of skeletal dysplasias reported to be associated with hydrops.[27] Some of these syndromes are well recognized, but others consist of a report of a few cases in the

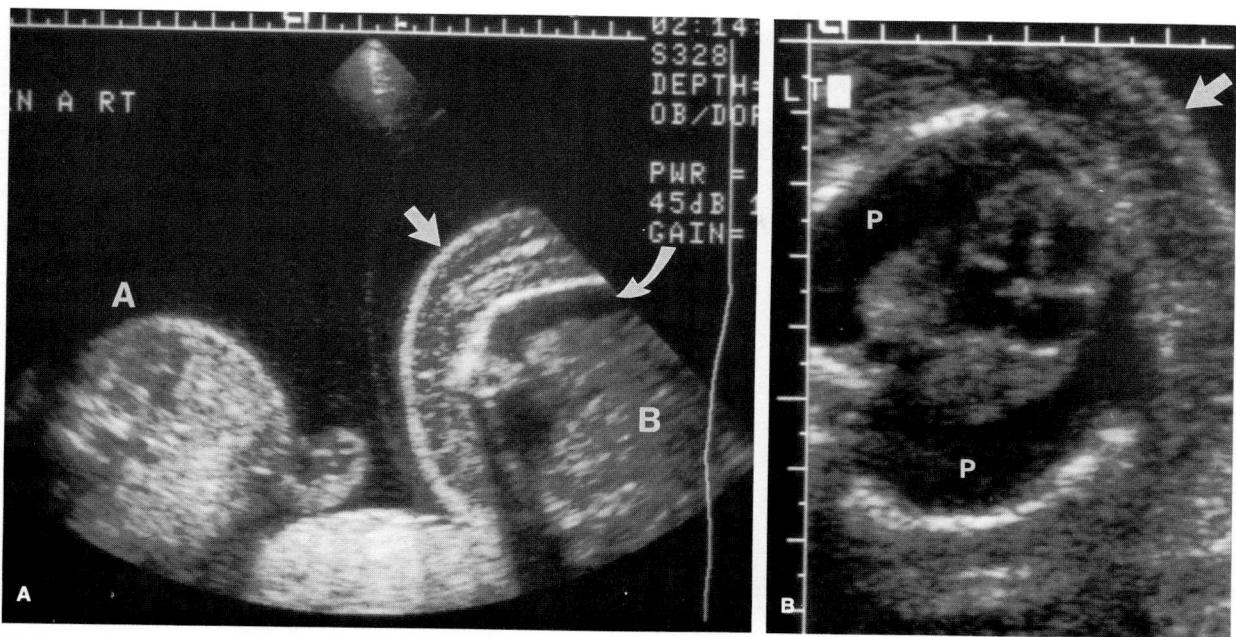

FIGURE 18-16. Twin-to-twin transfusion for hydrops fetalis. (**A**) Ultrasound shows smaller twin (A) and larger plethoric twin (B) with cutaneous edema (*arrow*) and pleural effusion (*curved arrow*). (**B**) Scan of the thorax of twin B shows bilateral pleural effusion (P) and cutaneous edema (*arrow*). (Courtesy of Michael Cronan, RDMS, Sacramento, CA.)

literature, and one cannot be sure whether they represent a new dysplasia or a variation on a better known one. The exact dysplasia is often determined postnatally. The examination of the skeleton should emphasize the long bones, with attention paid to shape, mineralization, and length. Both right and left sides should be studied. The skull should also be studied for facial abnormalities, such as frontal bossing, and the shape and size of the chest should be noted.

Metabolic Disorders. A number of metabolic diseases can present with fetal hydrops. Their rarity, however, and the expense of testing for all of them makes it difficult to screen for them without a family history.

Syndromes. Several fetal syndromes are associated with fetal hydrops. Other ultrasound findings frequently seen with these syndromes that may be helpful in establishing a diagnosis are listed in Table 18-5. Many chromosomal abnormalities are associated with hydrops. In some cases, the source of the hydrops is a related defect, while in others, such as Turner's syndrome (45,X karyotype), a defect in lymphatic development is thought to lead to hydrops. Finally, the rare finding of fetal hydrops

with maternal preeclampsia has been described. The *mirror syndrome* is so named because the maternal edema mimics the fetal.

Twins. Monochorionic pregnancies may be accompanied by twin-to-twin transfusion syndrome in which one fetus is anemic and the other is plethoric. The plethoric fetus can show frank evidence of hydrops, which is presented in more detail in Chapter 20 (Fig. 18-16).

Placenta and Cord. The placenta is often found to be enlarged in infants with hydrops, and some authors consider placentomegaly as a body compartment for the purposes of diagnosing hydrops. Moreover, some abnormalities of the placenta may lead to hydrops. Chorioangiomas may lead to hydrops through high-output failure (Fig. 18-17). Although it cannot be diagnosed prenatally, hemorrhagic endovasculitis has been associated with hydrops and has been reported as the only abnormality in some infants with hydrops. The umbilical cord has also been implicated as a cause of hydrops. Umbilical cord aneurysms, located intraabdominally at the cord insertion, umbilical vein thrombosis, cord tension, and true knots in the cord have all been associated with hydrops.

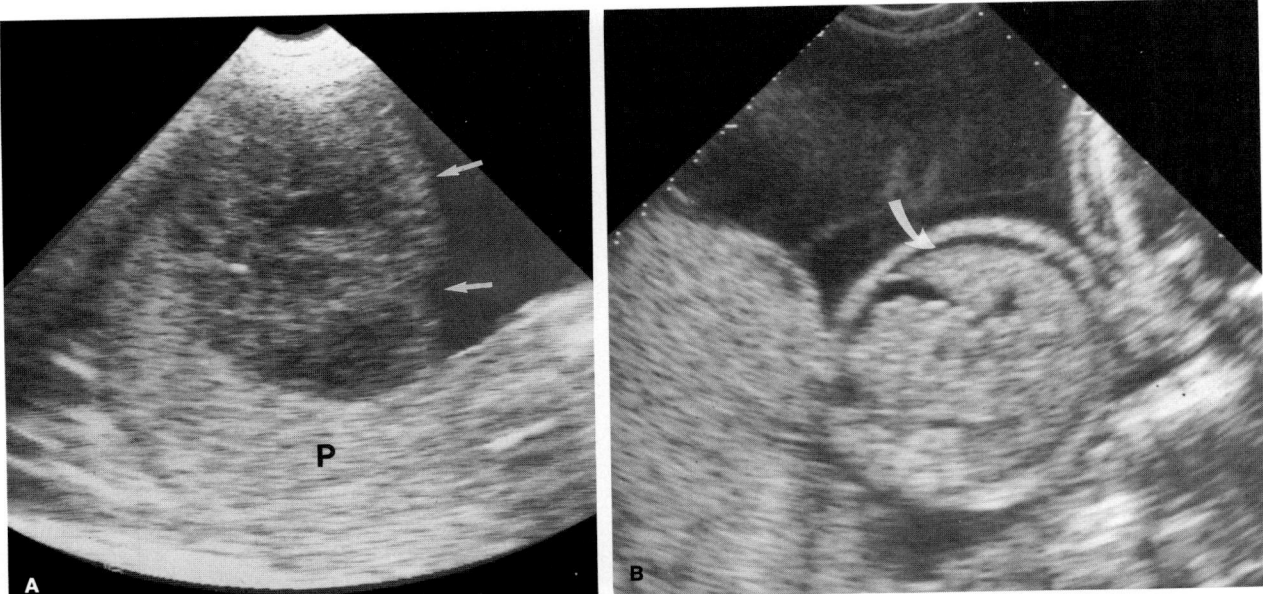

FIGURE 18-17.   Placental chorioangioma with fetal hydrops. (**A**) Axial ultrasound of the placenta shows well-demarcated placental chorioangioma. P, placenta. (**B**) Axial ultrasound of the abdomen shows small amount of abdominal ascites surrounding the liver (*arrow*) and bowel. (Courtesy of Larry Mack, MD, and Dale Cyr, RDMS, University of Washington, Seattle.)

Maternal Serologic Studies

Other causes of fetal anemia, such as a glucose-6-phosphate dehydrogenase or pyruvate kinase deficiency, congenital viral infection (eg, parvovirus B19), or α-thalassemia, may be diagnosed or strongly suspected based on maternal testing.

Invasive Fetal Testing

Nonimmune hydrops may be associated with a chromosomal abnormality when other anatomic defects are present or an isolated finding. Amniocentesis is the least invasive means of obtaining cells for cytogenic analysis (see Table 18-3). Fetal karyotyping from amniotic fluid usually takes 10 to 14 days to perform. Amniotic fluid may also be tested for the presence of certain viral causes of hydrops, such as cytomegalovirus, when that is appropriate. These analyses are primarily limited to viral cultures or rapid antigen detection methods when available. The development of DNA hybridization through polymerase chain reaction (PCR) is beginning to allow for the identification of the DNA for some viruses directly and rapidly. Although primarily available in the research setting, PCR can provide a useful diagnostic study to establish or confirm a viral cause for hydrops.

The cells grown in the genetics lab may be analyzed for the presence of metabolic disorders when appropriate family history is present, or hemoglobinopathies, if they are suspected. PUBS offers faster karyotype analysis as well as the opportunity to test the fetus directly. The fetal complete blood count is one of the most useful tests available. If anemia is present, the differential diagnosis is narrowed in scope. Antigen-specific fetal IgM (eg, anti-cytomegalovirus IgM or antitoxoplasmosis IgM) may be present after 20 weeks of gestation and point toward congenital infection. In some instances, such as toxoplasmosis, fetal antigen-specific IgA may be helpful. As PCR studies become available for more viruses, the identification of viral DNA in the fetus may become the quickest and most efficient means of identifying congenital viral infections. Until PCR becomes widely available, the diagnosis will be made through antigen and antibody tests. Before 20 weeks of gestation, although the fetus cannot produce IgM, elevated fetal liver indices or thrombocytopenia may suggest a viral cause. Metabolic testing is also available for fetal blood. Unfortunately, it is not practical to screen for all metabolic disease; thus, the tests chosen must be guided by a family history of disease. Although there are many causes of nonimmune hydrops, one may be limited to narrowing the diagnosis to a class of causes. In some instances, the cause of the hydrops cannot be diagnosed prenatally, and in other cases, it may not be diagnosed even at autopsy. Nonetheless, the autopsy is a crucial part of the work-up of the affected infant who dies because the findings may answer questions not only for this pregnancy but also for future ones.

Prognosis

The perinatal death rate has been reported to range from 40% to 90%. Although the major risk to the affected infant results from the cause of the hydrops, the hydrops itself can hold some risk. If there is polyhydramnios, the risk of preterm labor is increased, and severe hydramnios may require therapeutic amniocentesis if maternal breathing is impaired or intractable preterm labor occurs. When the hydrops is associated with pleural effusions, fetal pulmonary hypoplasia may ensue. To prevent this complication, invasive procedures, such as thoracentesis or thoracoamniotic shunting, may be necessary (see Fig. 18-13). Although the prognosis is varied depending on the cause, Carlson and colleagues have shown a 100% mortality rate for fetuses with a biventricular outer dimension that is greater than the 95th percentile on echocardiography during diastole.[28] Among fetuses with biventricular dimension below the 95th percentile, 86% survived. Additionally, the risk of other pregnancy complications, such as preeclampsia, appears to be increased.

Management

Management of hydrops is usually a balance between treating its cause and treating the symptom. Measures such as fetal transfusion or digitalization may be available to decrease the stimulus for the formation of hydrops. Likewise, therapies such as spiramycin, pyrimethamine, and sulfadiazine in the case of fetal toxoplasmosis, which treat the cause but might not have a direct affect on the hydrops, should also be used. In association with cause-directed therapy, or if the cause is unknown, the options are delivery for extrauterine evaluation and therapy or intrauterine thoracentesis or shunting when necessary to prevent pulmonary hypoplasia and hydrops (see Fig. 18-13). Delivery of the infant is usually reserved for cases with documented lung maturity, but in the face of an impending intrauterine demise, exceptions may be made.

REFERENCES

1. Machin GA: Hydrops revisitive: Literature review of 1,414 cases published in the 1980's. Am J Med Genet 1989; 34:366.
2. Santolaya J, Alley D, Jaffe R, Warsof SL: Antenatal classification of hydrops fetalis. Obstet Gynecol 1992; 79:256.
3. Liley AW: Liquor amnii analysis in the management of the pregnancy complicated by rhesus sensitization. Am J Obstet Gynecol 1961; 83:1359.
4. Frigoletto FD, Greene MF, Benacerraf BR, et al: Ultrasonographic fetal surveillance in the management of the isoimmunized pregnancy. N Engl J Med 1986; 315:430.
5. Nicolaides KH, Rodeck CH, Mibashan RS, Kemp JR: Have Liley charts outlived their usefulness? Am J Obstet Gynecol 1986; 155:90.
6. Bowman JM: The management of Rh-Isoimmunization. Obstet Gynecol 1978; 52:1.
7. Ananth U, Queenan JT: Does midtrimester OD 450 of amniotic fluid reflect severity of Rh disease? Am J Obstet Gynecol 1989; 161:47.
8. Chitkara U, Wilkins I, Lynch L, et al: The role of sonography in assessing severity of fetal anemia in Rh and Kell-isoimmunized pregnancies. Obstet Gynecol 1988; 71:393.
9. DeVore GR, Mayden K, Tortora M, et al: Dilation of the fetal umbilical vein in rhesus hemolytic anemia: A predictor of severe disease. Am J Obstet Gynecol 1981; 141:464.
10. Vintzileos AM, Campbell WA, Storlazzi E, et al: Fetal liver ultrasound measurements in isoimmunized pregnancies. Obstet Gynecol 1986; 68:162.
11. Nicolaides KH, Fontanarosa M, Gabbe SG, Rodeck CH: Failure of ultrasonographic parameters to predict the severity of fetal anemia in rhesus isoimmunization. Am J Obstet Gynecol 1988; 158:920.
12. Hobbins JC: Use of ultrasound in complicated pregnancies. Clin Perinatol 1980; 7:397.
13. Benacerraf BR, Frigoletto FD Jr: Sonographic sign for the detection of early fetal ascites in the management of severe isoimmune disease without intrauterine transfusion. Am J Obstet Gynecol 1985; 153:635.
14. Visser GHA: Antepartum sinusoidal and decelerative heart rate patterns in Rh disease. Am J Obstet Gynecol 1982; 143:538.
15. Porto M, Murata Y, Keegan KA, et al: Intermittent sinusoidal fetal heart rate pattern and moderate fetal anemia. Abstract No. 350. New Orleans: Society of Perinatal Obstetricians, February 1-4, 1989.
16. Milio LA, Arnold SA, Parer JT: The relationship between fetal heart rate variability and hematocrit in Rh isoimmunization. Abstract No. 14. Las Vegas: Society of Perinatal Obstetricians, February 3-6, 1988.
17. Nicolaides KH, Sadovsky G, Cetin E: Fetal heart rate patterns in red blood cell isoimmunized pregnancies. Am J Obstet Gynecol 1989; 161:351.

18. Rightmire DA, Nicolaides KH, Rodeck CH, Campbell S: Fetal blood velocities in Rh isoimmunization: Relationship to gestational age and to fetal hematocrit. Obstet Gynecol 1986; 68:233.

19. Copel JA, Grannum PA, Breen JJ, et al: Pulsed Doppler flow-velocity waveforms in the prediction of fetal hematocrit of the severely isoimmunized pregnancy. Am J Obstet Gynecol 1989; 161:341.

19a. Mari G, Adrignolo A, Abuhamad AZ, et al: Doppler ultrasound in the management of the pregnancy complicated by fetal anemia. Am J Obstet Gynecol 1993; 168:318.

20. Weiner CP, Williamson RA, Wenstrom KD, et al: Management of fetal hemolytic disease by cordocentesis. I. Prediction of fetal anemia. Am J Obstet Gynecol 1991; 165:546.

21. Nicolini U, Kochenour NK, Greco P, et al: Consequences of fetomaternal hemorrhage after intrauterine transfusion. Br Med J 1988; 297:1379.

22. Blake LC, McGahan JP: Percutaneous umbilical cord blood sampling and fetal transfusion. Semin Intervent Radiol 1992; 9:105–111.

23. Moise K, Carpenter R, Deter R, et al: The use of fetal neuromuscular blockade during intrauterine procedures. Am J Obstet Gynecol 1987; 157:874.

24. Copel J, Grannum P, Harrison D, et al: The use of intravenous pancuronium bromide to produce fetal paralysis during intravascular transfusion. Am J Obstet Gynecol 1988; 158:170.

25. Slotnick RN, McGahan JP, Milio L, et al: Antenatal diagnosis and treatment of fetal broncho-pulmonary sequestration. Fetal Ther 1990; 5:33–39.

26. Daffos F, Forestier F, Capella PM, et al: Prenatal management of 746 pregnancies at risk for congenital toxoplasmosis. N Engl J Med 1988; 318:271.

27. Maldergem LV, Jauniaux E, Fourneau C, Gillerot Y: Genetic causes of hydrops fetalis. Pediatrics 1992; 89:81.

28. Carlson DE, Platt LD, Medearis AL, Horenstein J: Prognostic indicators of the resolution of nonimmune hydrops fetalis and survival of the fetus. Am J Obstet Gynecol 1990; 163:1785.

John P. McGahan and Manuel Porto:
DIAGNOSTIC OBSTETRICAL ULTRASOUND.
© 1994 J.B. Lippincott Company.

Lyndon M. Hill

Chapter *19*

Fetal Skeletal Anomalies

Abnormalities of the fetal extremities are not rare. The numerous syndromes that may have an associated skeletal anomaly, however, generally mandate that once a skeletal abnormality is suspected, referral to an ultrasound specialist is necessary not only for confirmation but also to differentiate between the several possible diagnoses with similar skeletal manifestations.

Although many deformities may affect the fetal extremities, the list of abnormalities that can be detected by means of prenatal sonography is considerably shorter. For example, 70% of the skeletal dysplasias identified in the Latin American Collaborative Study of Congenital Malformations had one of four diagnoses: achondroplasia, thanatophoric dysplasia, achondrogenesis, or osteogenesis imperfecta.[1] The prevalence rate of skeletal dysplasias has been estimated to be between 2.4 and 4.7 per 10,000 births[1] (Table 19-1).

Measurement of the femur is an acknowledged part of the standard second- and third-trimester ultrasound examinations. This measurement alone results in the identification of most lethal skeletal abnormalities.[2] A thorough fetal anatomic survey that incorporates documentation of all the long

bones permits the detection of skeletal anomalies involving long bones other than the femur (Table 19-2).

This chapter does not attempt to be a compendium of all the known skeletal anomalies that have been diagnosed with antenatal sonography; rather, specific pitfalls encountered in the ultrasound evaluation of the fetal skeleton are detailed. In addition, a stepwise, logical approach to the evaluation of a suspected skeletal abnormality is presented with the intention of enabling the reader to categorize quickly any skeletal anomaly confronted.

SKELETAL DYSPLASIAS

Sonographic Assessment of the Normal Skeleton

During the eighth week from the last menstrual period, a hyaline cartilage outline of the future appendicular skeleton begins to appear. The primary ossification centers of a long bone are located in the center of the shaft (diaphysis) and appear be-

TABLE 19-1. Birth Prevalence Rates (per 10,000) for the Skeletal Dysplasias*

Diagnostic Groups	No.	Rate
True achondroplasia	16	0.46
Questionable achondroplasia (live births)	6	0.17
Questionable achondroplasia (still births)	11	0.31
Thanatophoric dysplasia	3	0.09
Achondrogenesis	1	0.03
Thanatophoric dysplasia or achondrogenesis	4	0.11
Osteogenesis imperfecta	15	0.43
Campomelic dysplasia	3	0.09
Chondroectodermal dysplasia	2	0.06
Chondrodysplasia punctata: Conradi-Hünermann syndrome	1	0.03
Chondrodysplasia punctata: rhizomelic type	1	0.03
Cleidocranial dysplasia	1	0.03
Diastrophic dysplasia	1	0.03
Fibrous dysplasia	1	0.03
Hypophosphatasia	1	0.03
Other, with specific diagnosis	0	0.00
Other, without specific diagnosis	13	0.37
TOTAL	80	2.29

* Data from the Latin American Collaborative Study of Congenital Malformations, which reported on 349,470 births from 1978 to 1983.

(Modified from Orioli IM, Castilla EE, Barbosa-Neto JG: The birth prevalence rates for the skeletal dysplasias. J Med Genet 1986; 23:328–332.)

tween weeks 7 and 12. Transabdominal and transvaginal sonography can clearly define the fetal skeleton even in the first trimester (Fig. 19-1). The secondary ossification centers located in the epiphyses are at the distal ends of the long bone. During bone growth, the epiphyseal plate intervenes between the epiphysis and the end of the diaphysis (ie, metaphysis). When the epiphyseal plate is replaced by bone, growth of the bone ceases (Fig. 19-2).

The classification of skeletal dysplasias historically was based on specific radiographic findings of the long bones and spine. Hence, skeletal dysplasias were categorized according to the part of the long bone that was most affected.

Another classification system divided long bone changes into rhizo (root or proximal), meso (middle), and acro (distal, ie, hands and feet) forms of shortening (Fig. 19-3). The skeletal dysplasias affecting the proximal long bones, however, frequently have meso and occasionally acro shortening as well. *Micromelia* refers to generalized shortening of all the extremities.

Numerous biometric studies have correlated the length of specific long bones with menstrual age[3–5]

(see Chapter 2). A fetal long bone length greater than 2 standard deviations below the mean for the patient's gestational age does not necessarily indicate the presence of a skeletal dysplasia. Other possibilities for short fetal long bone include a normal physiologic variation in bone length, intrauterine growth retardation, an abnormal karyotype, and a syndrome that may have a skeletal abnormality as part of its presentation.

Kurtz and coworkers showed that the number of millimeters that the femur length is below 2 standard deviations can be used to differentiate a constitutionally small fetus from a fetus with skeletal dysplasia.[6] They found that 15 of 16 fetuses with a femur length that was 1 to 4 mm below 2 standard deviations were normal at birth, whereas all 12 fetuses with a femur length that was 5 mm below 2 standard deviations in the second and third trimesters of pregnancy were affected by a skeletal dysplasia.

Interval Long Bone Growth

If a skeletal dysplasia is suspected early in the second trimester, a follow-up study to assess interval long bone growth should be performed. The growth rate of the long bones decreases before the absolute length falls below the criteria outlined previously for diagnosis of a skeletal dysplasia. Normal interval growth indicates that the short femur length is not due to a skeletal dysplasia.

When evaluating limb growth, the history of specific skeletal dysplasias must be taken into account. For example, osteogenesis imperfecta type II may manifest as a short femur length by 15 weeks' gestation. A fetus with heterozygous achondroplasia, however, may have a normal femur length until between 21 and 27 weeks' gestation.[7]

Fetal Ratios

The proportions between specific fetal body parts may help to confirm the diagnosis of a skeletal dysplasia and also provide important diagnostic clues to narrow the sonologist's differential diagnosis.

Foot length is not affected by most skeletal dysplasias and can therefore be used to assess gestational age.[8] The foot length is nearly equal to the femur length. Normal foot length measurements are presented in Chapter 2. Hence, a normal femur length/foot length ratio approaches unity. Because this ratio is minimally affected by gestational age,

TABLE 19-2. Nomogram of Normal Values of Fetal Long Bones Versus Menstrual Age With the 5th and 95th Percentiles*

Week	Tibia: Percentile			Fibula: Percentile			Femur: Percentile			Humerus: Percentile			Ulna: Percentile			Radius: Percentile		
	5th	50th	95th	5th	50th	95th	5th	50th	95th	5th	50th	95th	5th	50th	95th	5th	50th	95th
12	—	7	—	—	6	—	4	8	13	—	9	—	—	7	—	—	7	—
13	—	10	—	—	9	—	6	11	16	6	11	16	5	10	15	6	10	14
14	7	12	17	6	12	19	9	14	18	9	14	19	8	13	18	8	13	17
15	9	15	20	9	15	21	12	17	21	12	17	22	11	16	21	11	15	20
16	12	17	22	13	18	23	15	20	24	15	20	25	13	18	23	13	18	22
17	15	20	25	13	21	28	18	23	27	18	22	27	16	21	26	14	20	26
18	17	22	27	15	23	31	21	25	30	20	25	30	19	24	29	15	22	29
19	20	25	30	19	26	33	24	28	33	23	28	33	21	26	31	20	24	29
20	22	27	33	21	28	36	26	31	36	25	30	35	24	29	34	22	27	32
21	25	30	35	24	31	37	29	34	38	28	33	38	26	31	36	24	29	33
22	27	32	38	27	33	39	32	36	41	30	35	40	28	33	38	27	31	34
23	30	35	40	28	35	42	35	39	44	33	38	42	31	36	41	26	32	39
24	32	37	42	29	37	45	37	42	46	35	40	45	33	38	43	26	34	42
25	34	40	45	34	40	45	40	44	49	37	42	47	35	40	45	31	36	41
26	37	42	47	36	42	47	42	47	51	39	44	49	37	42	47	32	37	43
27	39	44	49	37	44	50	45	49	54	41	46	51	39	44	49	33	39	45
28	41	46	51	38	45	53	47	52	56	43	48	53	41	46	51	33	40	48
29	43	48	53	41	47	54	50	54	59	45	50	55	43	48	53	36	42	47
30	45	50	55	43	49	56	52	56	61	47	51	56	44	49	54	36	42	47
31	47	52	57	42	51	59	54	59	63	48	53	58	46	51	56	38	44	50
32	48	54	59	42	52	63	56	61	65	50	55	60	48	53	58	37	45	53
33	50	55	60	46	54	62	58	63	67	51	56	61	49	54	59	41	46	51
34	52	57	62	46	55	65	60	65	69	53	58	63	51	56	61	40	47	53
35	53	58	64	51	57	62	62	67	71	54	59	64	52	57	62	41	48	54
36	55	60	65	54	58	63	64	68	73	56	61	65	53	58	63	39	48	57
37	56	61	67	54	59	65	65	70	74	57	62	67	55	60	65	45	49	53
38	58	63	68	56	61	65	67	71	76	59	63	68	56	61	66	45	49	54
39	59	64	69	56	62	67	68	73	77	60	65	70	57	62	67	45	50	54
40	61	66	71	59	63	67	70	74	79	61	66	71	58	63	68	46	50	55

* All values are expressed in millimeters.

(Romero R, Athanassiadis AP, Jeanty P: Fetal skeletal anomalies. Radiol Clin North Am 1989; 28[1]:75–99.)

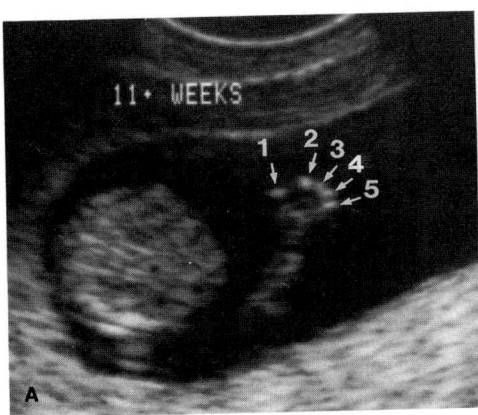
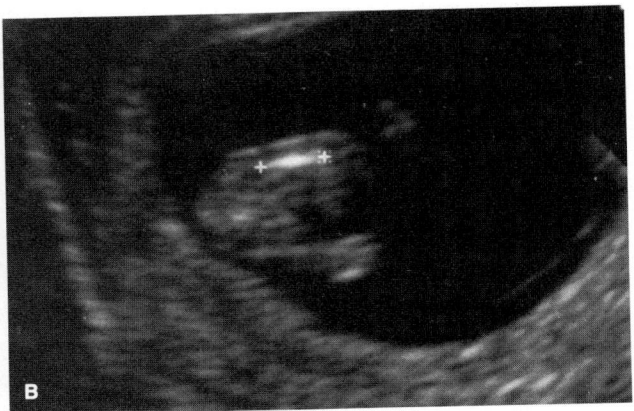

FIGURE 19-1.   Transvaginal examination of an 11-week gestation. (**A**) Five digits in the hand. (**B**) The graticules demarcate a 6-mm femur length.

it can be used even when a patient's dating parameters are in doubt.[9] In one series, the femur length/foot length ratio satisfactorily differentiated between 10 cases of skeletal dysplasia and 5 cases of intrauterine growth retardation[10] (Fig. 19-4).

The proportions between other body parts also are abnormal in skeletal dysplasias. For example, in the more severe skeletal dysplasias, abdominal and head circumference are frequently normal, while thoracic circumference is decreased. Consequently, the femur length/head circumference, head circumference/thoracic circumference, and abdominal circumference/thoracic circumference ratios have been shown to be the most reliable for the detection of severe skeletal dysplasia[11] (Fig. 19-5).

Additional Sonographic Signs

Polyhydramnios

Although its cause has not been established, polyhydramnios is frequently associated with skeletal abnormalities. The skeletal dysplasias most frequently associated with polyhydramnios are thanatophoric dwarfism (58%) and achondroplasia (27%).[12]

Degree of Skeletal Ossification

Acoustic shadowing is readily evident from the calvarium, ribs, and long bones of normal fetuses (Fig. 19-6). Diffuse hypomineralization suggests either hypophosphatasia, achondrogenesis type I, or osteogenesis imperfecta. Flattening of the fetal calvarium with the real-time transducer (Fig. 19-7) is an additional sonographic sign of hypomineralization.

Shape of the Calvarium

About 14% of thanatophoric dwarfs have a characteristic cloverleaf skull deformity (Fig. 19-8A,B), resulting from premature synostosis of the coronal and lambdoid sutures.[13] Hydrocephalus is an associated finding. Fetuses with homozygous achondroplasia may also have a cloverleaf skull. In the latter instance, however, both parents are achondroplastic dwarfs.

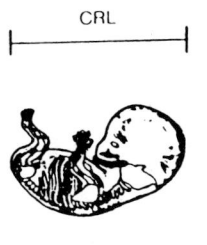
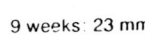
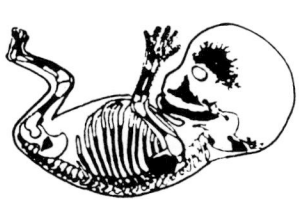
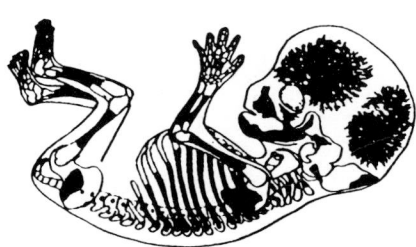

9 weeks: 23 mm   10 weeks: 39 mm   11 weeks: 49 mm

FIGURE 19-2.   Formation of ossification centers at 9, 10, and 11 weeks' gestation. Fetuses are actual size. (Hansmann M, Hackelöer B-J, Staudach A: Ultrasound Diagnosis in Obstetrics and Gynecology. New York: Springer-Verlag, 1985: 47.)

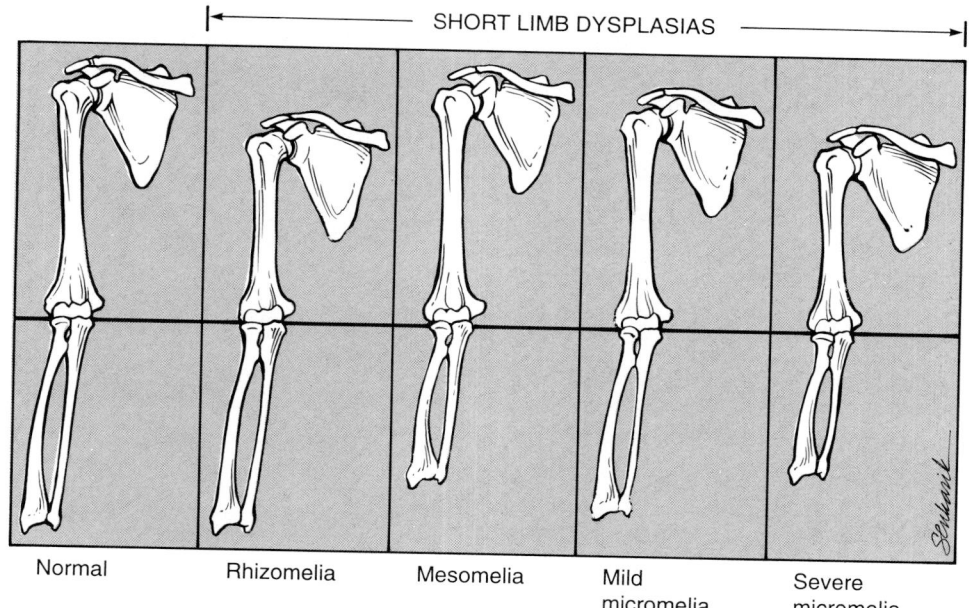

SHORT LIMB DYSPLASIAS

Normal   Rhizomelia   Mesomelia   Mild micromelia   Severe micromelia

FIGURE 19-3. Classification of long bone shortening as it affects rhizoid (proximal), mesal (middle), or micral (generalized) shortening of the extremities. (Modified from Levi CS, Reed MH, Harman CR: The fetal musculoskeletal system. In Rumack CM, Wilson SR, Sharboneau JW (eds): Diagnostic Ultrasound. St. Louis: Mosby Year Book, 1991: 849–869.)

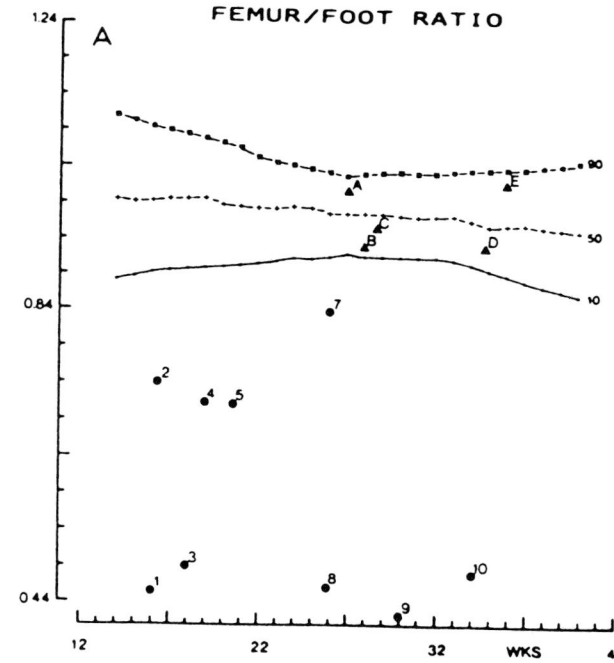

FEMUR/FOOT RATIO

FIGURE 19-4. Femur/foot ratios of 10 fetuses affected by skeletal dysplasia (●, 1–10) and 5 growth-retarded fetuses (▲, A–E). (Brons JTJ, Van der Harten JJ, Van Geijn HP, et al: Ratios between growth parameters for the prenatal ultrasonographic diagnosis of skeletal dysplasias. Eur J Obstet Gynecol Reprod Biol 1990; 34:37–46.)

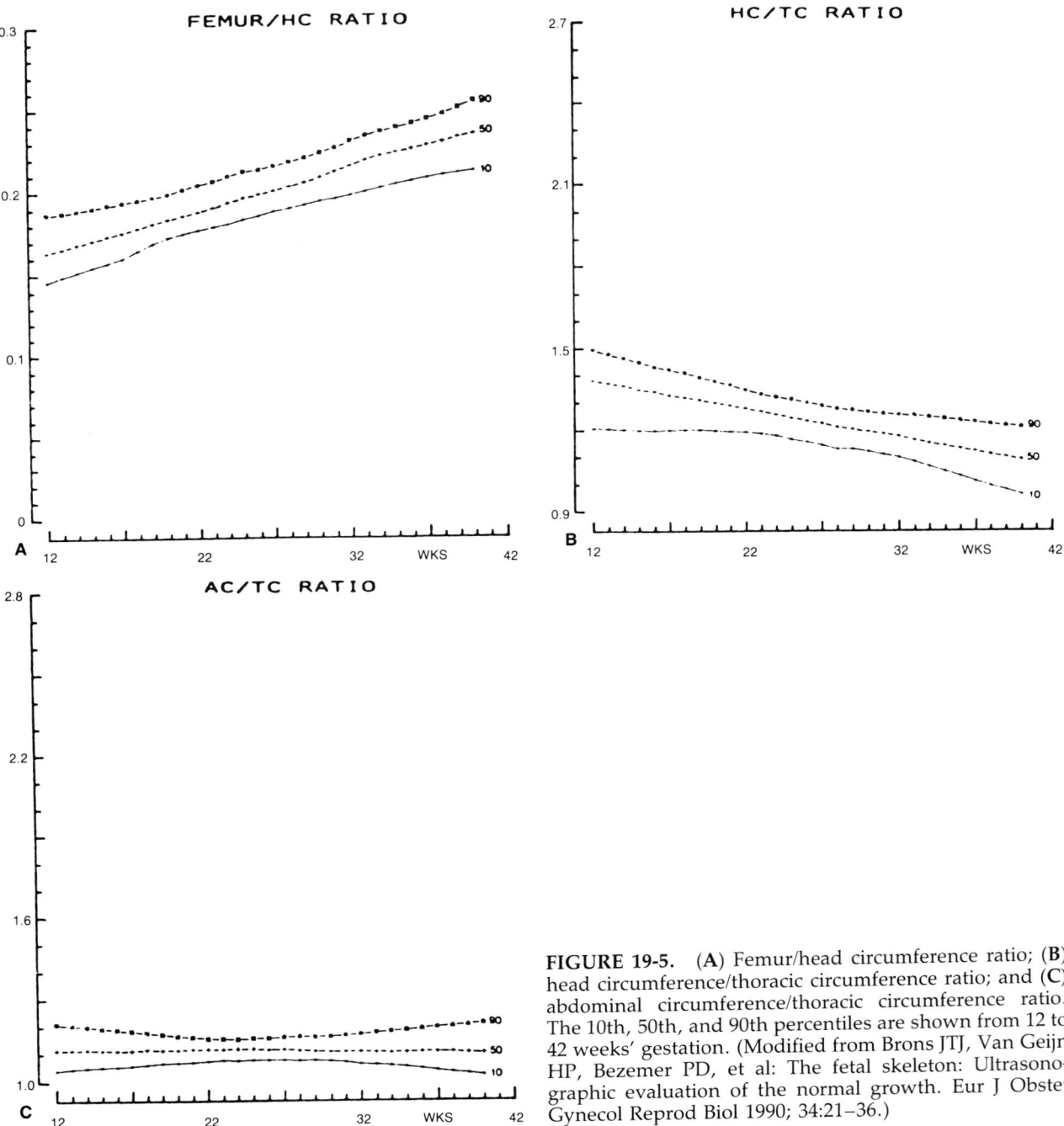

FIGURE 19-5. (**A**) Femur/head circumference ratio; (**B**) head circumference/thoracic circumference ratio; and (**C**) abdominal circumference/thoracic circumference ratio. The 10th, 50th, and 90th percentiles are shown from 12 to 42 weeks' gestation. (Modified from Brons JTJ, Van Geijn HP, Bezemer PD, et al: The fetal skeleton: Ultrasonographic evaluation of the normal growth. Eur J Obstet Gynecol Reprod Biol 1990; 34:21–36.)

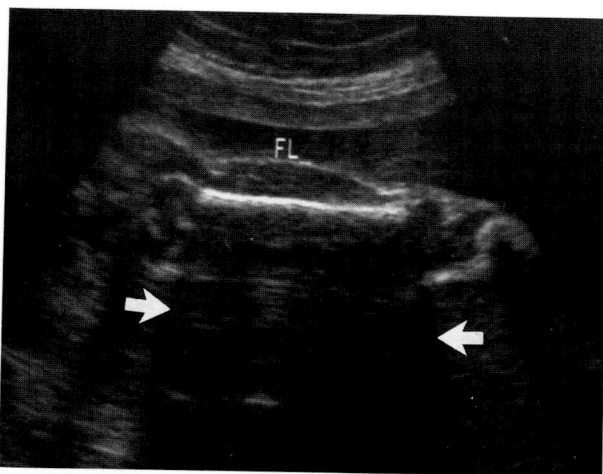

FIGURE 19-6. Femur length (FL) at 30 weeks' gestation. The *arrows* indicate acoustic shadowing from the diaphysis.

In its mild forms, the cloverleaf skull may simulate an encephalocele[14] (Fig. 19-9). The location and bilateralness of the deformity in question, however, can be used to separate encephalocele from a cloverleaf skull. A cloverleaf skull affects the temporal bones bilaterally, whereas encephaloceles are primarily midline in location. Frontal bossing is frequently present in fetuses with osteogenesis imperfecta (Fig. 19-10).

Fractures

The detection of rib or long bone fractures in association with severe micromelia suggests a diagnosis of osteogenesis imperfecta.

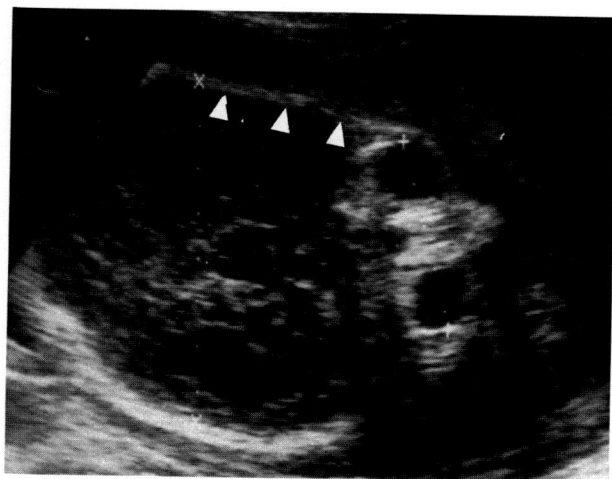

FIGURE 19-7. Osteogenesis imperfecta, type IIA. Flattening of the calvarium is evident with compression by the real-time transducer (*arrowheads*).

Long Bone Bowing

Camptomelic (bent-bow) dysplasia is characterized by ventral bowing of the long bones. Thanatophoric dysplasia and osteogenesis imperfecta also have bowed extremities.

Spinal Abnormalities

Hypomineralization of the spine is characteristic of achondrogenesis type II. In chondrodysplasia punctata, the spine is poorly developed with indistinct ossification centers.

Severe platyspondylisis (flattening of the vertebral bodies) is pathognomonic for thanatophoric dysplasia. A vertebral body height/vertebral interface ratio (Fig. 19-11) can be used to quantify platyspondylisis. Figure 19-12 illustrates the degree of vertebral flattening that may occur not only with thanatophoric dysplasia but also with achondroplasia.[15]

Polydactyly

The differential diagnosis for a skeletal dysplasia with polydactyly includes asphyxiating thoracic dystrophy, short-rib polydactyly syndrome (Figs. 19-13 and 19-14), and chondroectodermal dysplasia (Ellis-Van Creveld syndrome).[16]

Evaluation of the Fetal Chest

A number of the lethal skeletal dysplasias are associated with a narrowed chest, which may in the extreme result in pulmonary hypoplasia.

The circumference of the chest and heart at the level of the four-chamber view can be measured and compared (Fig. 19-15). Nomograms for thoracic circumference with respect to gestational age have been derived from cross-sectional data[17] (Table 19-3). A chest circumference of less than the 5th percentile has a positive predictive value of 94% for detecting pulmonary hypoplasia[18] (Fig. 19-16).

Sonographic Detection of Specific Skeletal Dysplasias

Thanatophoric Dysplasia

Thanatophoric dysplasia is a chondrodystrophy characterized by the disruption of growth plates and fibrous ossification.[19] It is the most common lethal skeletal dysplasia.

Opitz and Spranger suggested that there may be two types of thanatophoric dysplasia: (1) autosomal recessive, characterized by short, straight limbs and a cloverleaf skull, and (2) short and bowed long bones without a cloverleaf skull.[20] The

(*text continues on page 421*)

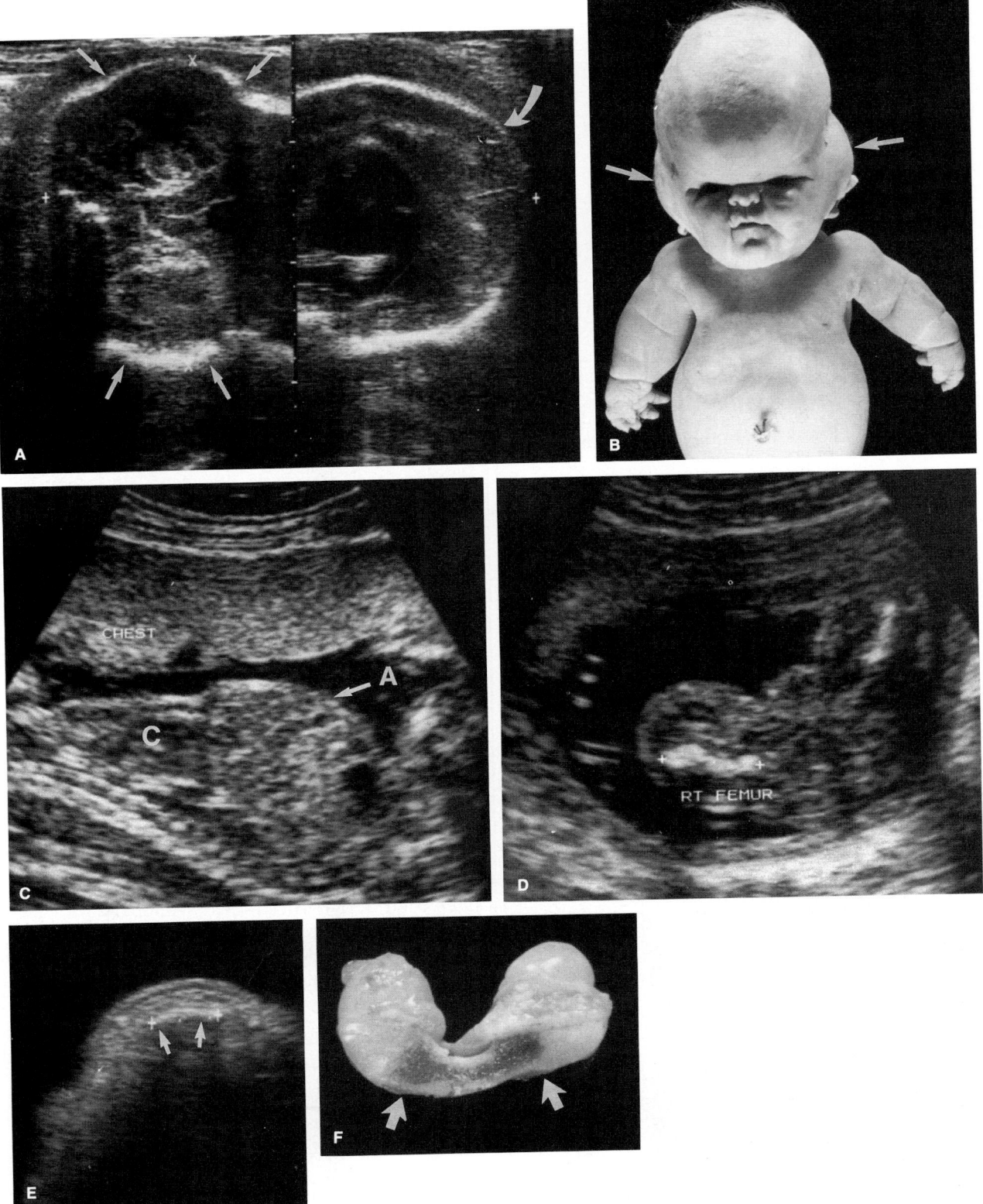

FIGURE 19-8. Thanatophoric dysplasia. (**A**) The typical cloverleaf skull deformity can be seen on antenatal sonography with bulging in the temporal regions (*arrows*) and frontal bossing (*curved arrows*). (**B**) Postnatal photograph of the cloverleaf skull pictured in **A** with bulging in upper regions (*arrows*) and marked frontal bossing. (**C**) Small chest (C) with protuberant abdomen (A). (**D**) Abnormally short femur. (**E**) Abnormally short and bowed ulna (*arrow*). (**F**) Postmortem shortened bowed femur (*arrows*).

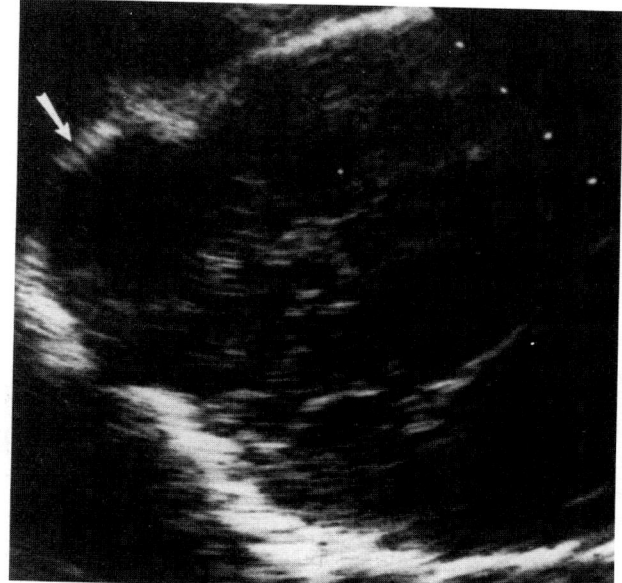

FIGURE 19-9. Cloverleaf skull. Axial scan in a 28-week fetus. Posterolateral bulging (*arrow*) covered by bright echoes that mimic bone but that on autopsy were only skin. Cloverleaf skull (Kleeblattschädel) simulating an encephalocele. (Stamm ER, Pretorius DH, Rumack CM, Manco-Johnson ML: Kleeblattschadel anomaly: In utero sonographic appearance. J Ultrasound Med 1987; 6:319.)

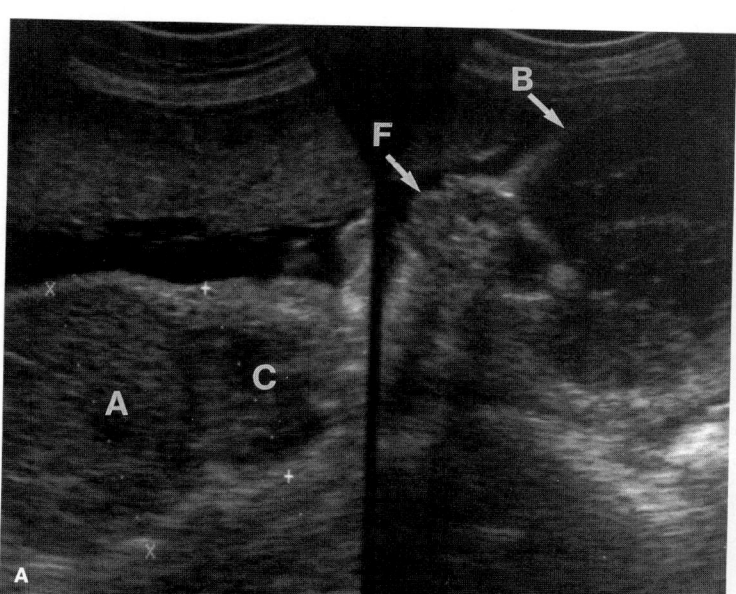
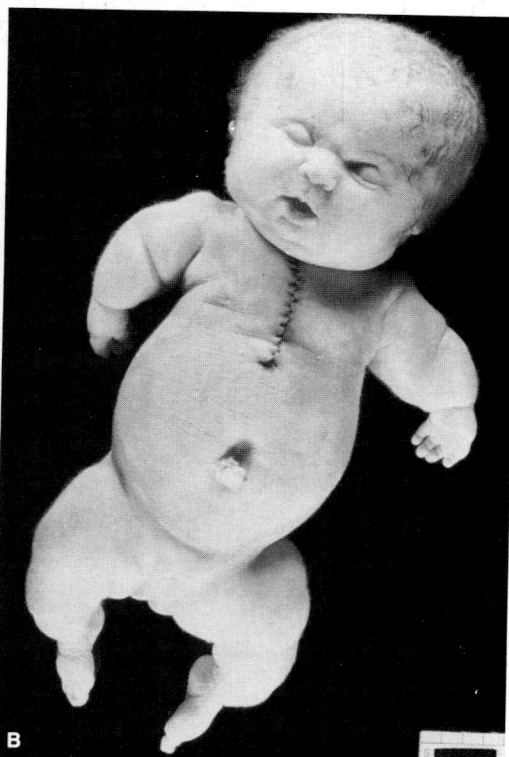

FIGURE 19-10. Osteogenesis imperfecta, type IIA. (**A**) Profile of a 31-week fetus with frontal bossing (B). Visualization of the gyral pattern within the near field of the fetal brain indicates hypomineralization of the calvarium. Also note small chest (C) and protuberant abdomen (A). F, face. (**B**) Postmortem photograph.

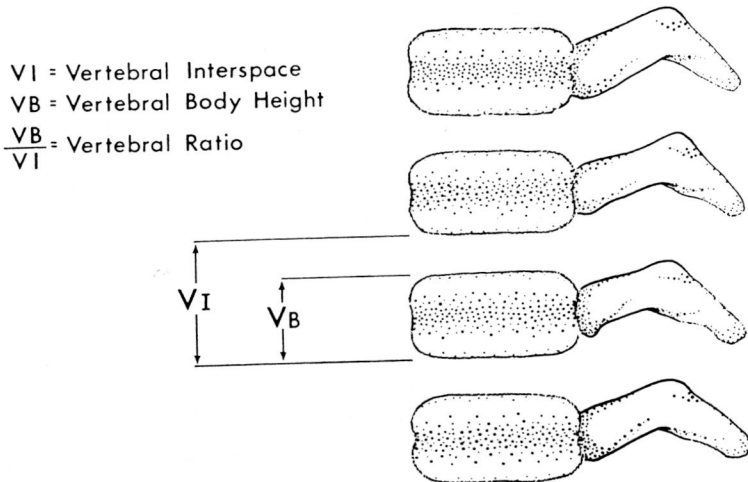

VI = Vertebral Interspace
VB = Vertebral Body Height
$\frac{VB}{VI}$ = Vertebral Ratio

FIGURE 19-11. Anatomic drawing of lumbar spine segments (lateral view) with definitions of vertebral ratio and vertebral interface. (Rouse GA, Filly RA, Toomey F, Grube GL: Short-limb skeletal dysplasias: Evaluation of the fetal spine with sonography and radiography. Radiology 1990; 174:177.)

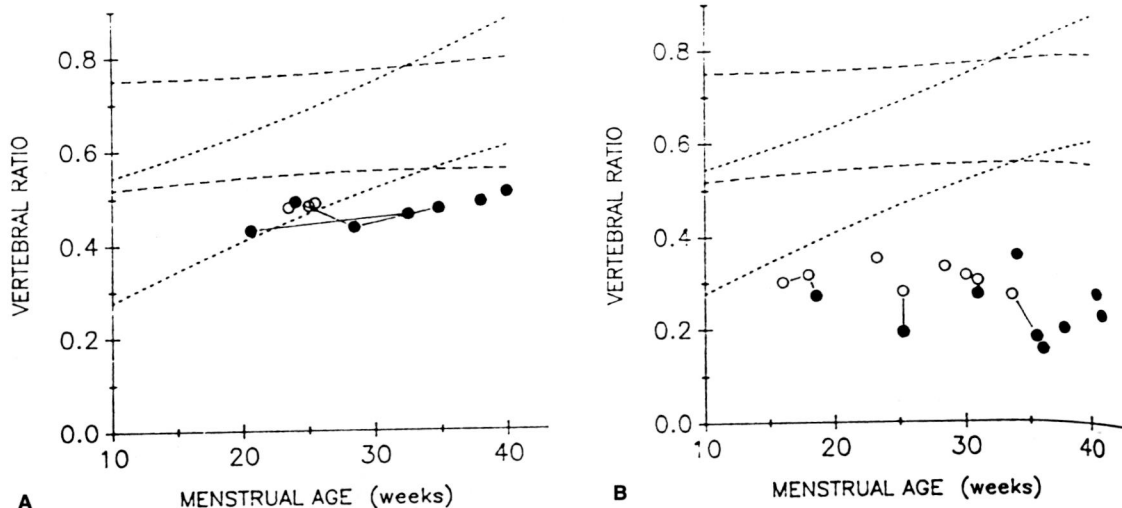

FIGURE 19-12. Sonographic (○) and radiographic (●) vertebral ratios observed in the second and third trimesters in (**A**) achondroplasia and (**B**) thanatophoric dwarfism. Two or more examinations of the same fetus are connected by lines. Also shown are 95% confidence bands obtained from normal sonographic data (*long dashes*) and normal radiographic data (*short dashes*). (Rouse GA, Filly RA, Toomey F, Grube GL: Short-limb skeletal dysplasias: Evaluation of the fetal spine with sonography and radiography. Radiology 1990; 174:177.)

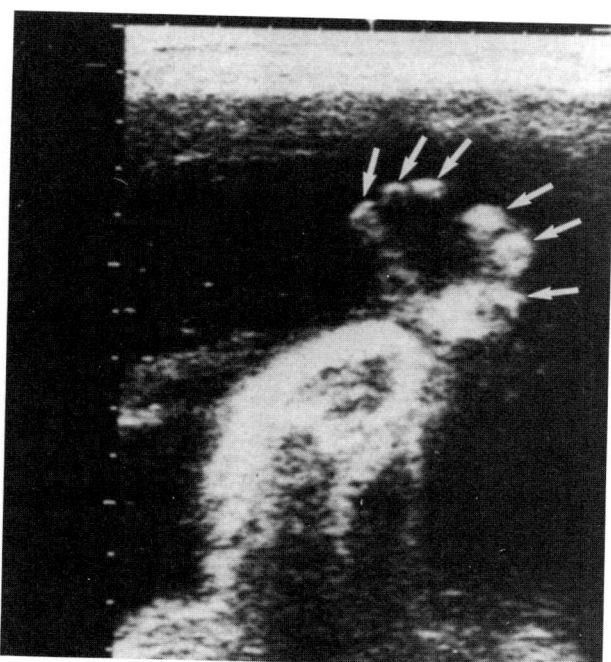

FIGURE 19-13. Ultrasound scan of a hand shows polydactyly (six fingers; *arrows*). (Meizner I, Bar-Ziv J: J Reprod Med 1989; 34:668.)

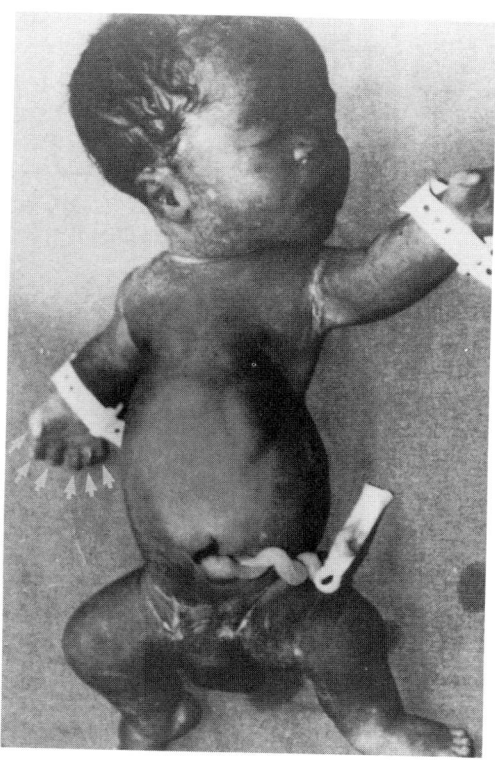

FIGURE 19-14. Neonate with short rib polydactyly syndrome, type I. Note small thoracic cage and protuberant abdomen. Polydactyly is evident (*arrows*). (Meizner I, Bar-Ziv J: J Reprod Med 1989; 34:668.)

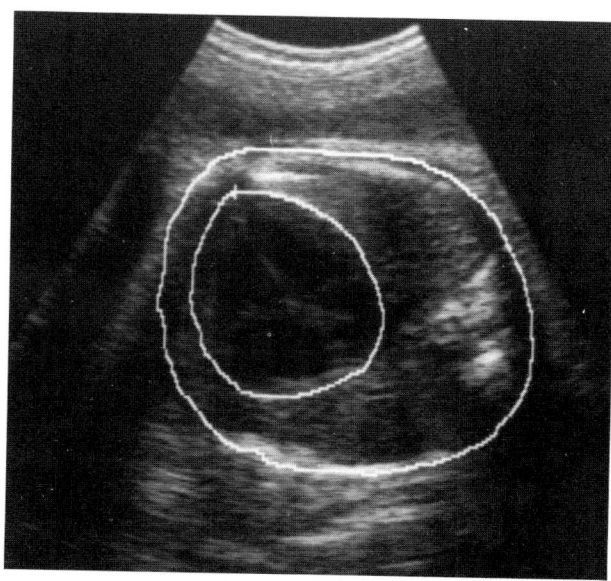

FIGURE 19-15. Outline for heart and chest circumferences at 33 weeks' gestation.

TABLE 19-3. Fetal Thoracic Circumference Measurements*

Gestational Age (wk)	No.	Predictive Percentiles								
		2.5	5	10	25	50	75	90	95	97.5
16	6	5.9	6.4	7.0	8.0	9.1	10.3	11.3	11.9	12.4
17	22	6.8	7.3	7.9	8.9	10.0	11.2	12.2	12.8	13.3
18	31	7.7	8.2	8.8	9.8	11.0	12.1	13.1	13.7	14.2
19	21	8.6	9.1	9.7	10.7	11.9	13.0	14.0	14.6	15.1
20	20	9.5	10.0	10.6	11.7	12.8	13.9	15.0	15.5	16.0
21	30	10.4	11.0	11.6	12.6	13.7	14.8	15.8	16.4	16.9
22	18	11.3	11.9	12.5	13.5	14.6	15.7	16.7	17.3	17.8
23	21	12.2	12.8	13.4	14.4	15.5	16.6	17.6	18.2	18.8
24	27	13.2	13.7	14.3	15.3	16.4	17.5	18.5	19.1	19.7
25	20	14.1	14.6	15.2	16.2	17.3	18.4	19.4	20.0	20.6
26	25	15.0	15.5	16.1	17.1	18.2	19.3	20.3	21.0	21.5
27	24	15.9	16.4	17.0	18.0	19.1	20.2	21.3	21.9	22.4
28	24	16.8	17.3	17.9	18.9	20.0	21.2	22.2	22.8	23.3
29	24	17.7	18.2	18.8	19.8	21.0	22.1	23.1	23.7	24.2
30	27	18.6	19.1	19.7	20.7	21.9	23.0	24.0	24.6	25.1
31	24	19.5	20.0	20.6	21.6	22.8	23.9	24.9	25.5	26.0
32	28	20.4	20.9	21.5	22.6	23.7	24.8	25.8	26.4	26.9
33	27	21.3	21.8	22.5	23.5	24.6	25.7	26.7	27.3	27.8
34	25	22.2	22.8	23.4	24.4	25.5	26.6	27.6	28.2	28.7
35	20	23.1	23.7	24.3	25.3	26.4	27.5	28.5	29.1	29.6
36	23	24.0	24.6	25.2	26.2	27.3	28.4	29.4	30.0	30.6
37	22	24.9	25.5	26.1	27.1	28.2	29.3	30.3	30.9	31.5
38	21	25.9	26.4	27.0	28.0	29.1	30.2	31.2	31.9	32.4
39	7	26.8	27.3	27.9	28.9	30.0	31.1	32.2	32.8	33.3
40	6	27.7	28.2	28.8	29.8	30.9	32.1	33.1	33.7	34.2

* Measurements in centimeters.

(Chitkara U, Rosenberg J, Chervenak FA, et al: Prenatal sonographic assessment of the fetal thorax: Normal values. Am J Obstet Gynecol 1987; 156:1069–1074.)

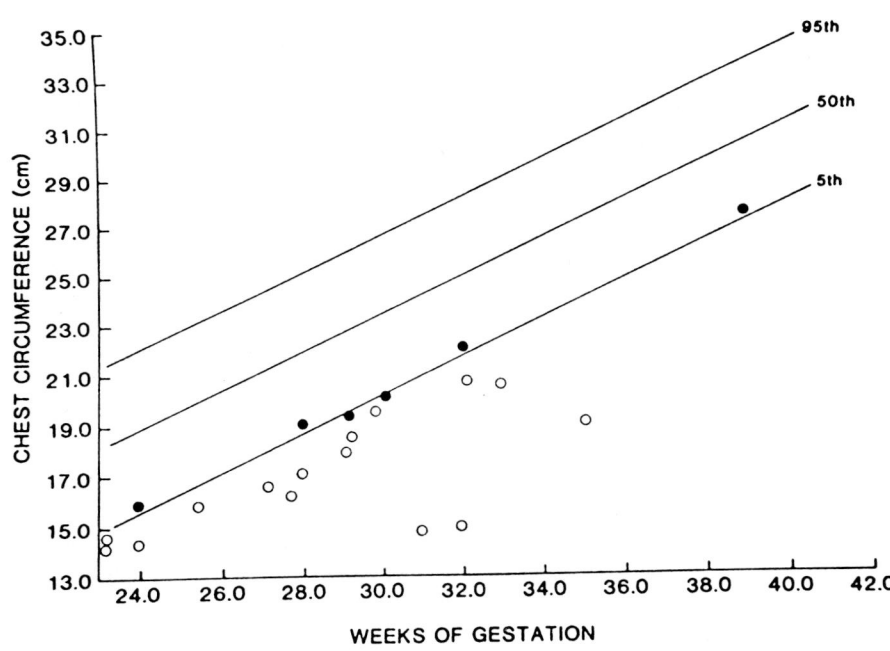

FIGURE 19-16. Chest circumference nomogram shows gestational age distribution of fetuses at (●) and below (○) the 5th percentile. One sixth of fetuses at the 5th percentile and 15 of 16 fetuses with a chest circumference below the 5th percentile had pulmonary hypoplasia. (Nimrod C, Nicholson S, Davies D, et al: Pulmonary hypoplasia testing in clinical obstetrics. Am J Obstet Gynecol 1988; 158:277–280.)

TABLE 19-4. Classification of Osteogenesis Imperfecta

Type*	Qualifying Suffixes	Course	Inheritance
I	Congenita tarda with blue sclerae	Usual onset in childhood or puberty; 96% of patients able to walk independently; deafness (35%) experienced as greatest handicap	AD (most frequent)
II	Perinatally lethal	Death before or shortly after birth	
A			AD (mostly new mutations, rarely AR)
B			AR, but possible new dominant mutations
C			AR
III	Progressively deforming	Progressive deformity of limbs and spine leading to severe handicap and often early death	AR, but possible new dominant mutations
IV	Congenita tarda with normal sclerae	Like type I but no deafness; dentinogenesis imperfecta	AD (most frequent)

* Types defined by Sillence DO, et al: Genetic heterogeneity in osteogenesis imperfecta. J Med Genet 1979; 16:101–116.
AD, autosomal dominant; AR, autosomal recessive.
(Modified from Brons JTJ, et al: Prenatal ultrasonographic diagnosis of osteogenesis imperfecta. Am J Obstet Gynecol 1988; 159:176.)

mode of inheritance of the latter type is unknown but is believed to be sporadic. Phenotypic characteristics of thanatophoric dysplasia that may be detected sonographically include: cloverleaf skull; hydrocephalus; micrognathia; bell-shaped, narrow thorax; apparent protuberance of the abdomen owing to the small chest; increased subcutaneous tissue; hypoplastic vertebral bodies; significant shortening and bowing of the long bones; polyhydramnios; and hydrops (see Fig. 19-8).

Osteogenesis Imperfecta

Osteogenesis imperfecta is genetically and prognostically a heterogeneous disorder that comprises both autosomal dominant and autosomal recessive entities. Molecular genetic and linkage studies have established that most patients with osteogenesis imperfecta are heterozygous for mutations in one of the genes that encode the chains for type I procollagen.[21] Lethal and nonlethal cases have been observed in the same family. In some of the milder cases, the bowed legs detected in the neonatal period straighten out spontaneously.

Sillence and colleagues classified osteogenesis imperfecta into four types based on genetic, phenotypic, and radiographic criteria[22]; type II was subsequently subdivided into three subgroups (Table 19-4). The age of onset and severity of skeletal malformations differ among the various types of osteogenesis imperfecta. Type IIA can be diagnosed at as early as 15 weeks' gestation. Hence, in

a pregnancy at risk for recurrence of osteogenesis imperfecta type II, a normal ultrasound examination after 17 weeks' gestation excludes a recurrence. Fetuses with type III osteogenesis imperfecta may have normal long bone measurements at 15 weeks' gestation; the onset of bone shortening and deformity may not become apparent until 19 to 22 weeks.[23] The late onset of type I and type IV makes prenatal diagnosis difficult; skeletal hypoechogenicity and limb bowing are frequently not detected until 24 to 32 weeks' gestation[24] (Fig. 19-17).

For families with a history of osteogenesis imperfecta, analysis of collagen synthesis by cells from a chorionic villus sampling can provide diagnostic information in the first trimester.[25]

The sonographic features of osteogenesis imperfecta type IIA include (Figs. 19-18 and 19-19):

- Severe micromelia that is apparent at an early gestational age
- Thickened long bones due to frequent fractures and secondary callus formation
- Hypomineralization of the skeleton as evidenced by a visualization of the brain in the near field and compressibility of the calvarium
- A chest circumference less than or equal to the 2.5th percentile
- The small size of the fetal chest, which makes the normal-size abdomen appear abnormally protuberant

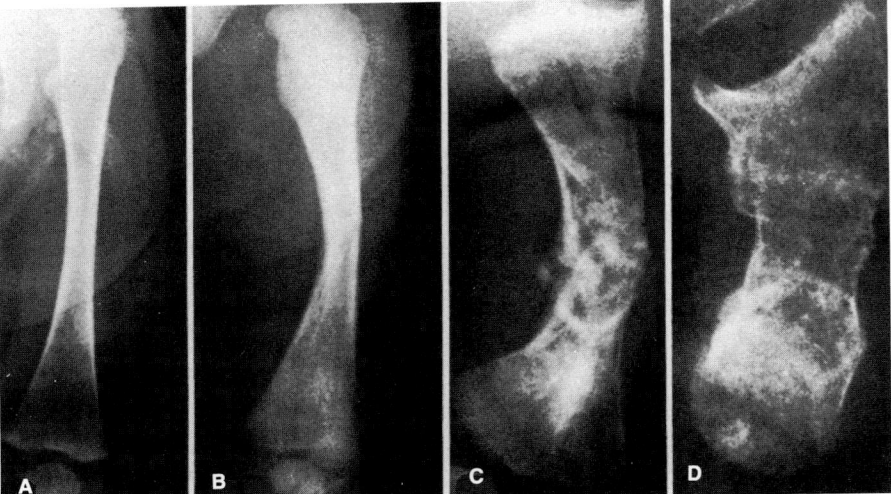

FIGURE 19-17. Increasing severity of femoral changes in osteogenesis imperfecta: (**A**) osteopenia, thin or normal shaft; (**B**) osteopenia, slightly bowed; (**C**) severely bowing and excessively mottled shaft, with or without fractures; (**D**) short, thick, telescoped shaft. (Spranger J, et al: Pediatr Radiol 1982; 12:21.)

Achondrogenesis

Achondrogenesis is a lethal, short-limbed dysplasia with autosomal recessive inheritance. Generalized cartilaginous disorganization results in a failure of ossification.

The degree of vertebral body and calvarial ossification and severity of micromelia have been used to categorize achondrogenesis into five subtypes.[26] For example, in type I (Parenti-Houston-Harris syndrome), poor ossification of the calvarium and rib fractures are present, whereas neither rib fractures nor poor calvarial ossification occurs in type II. In type IV, the vertebral bodies may be underdeveloped, but they are normally ossified.

The sonographic characteristics of this skeletal dysplasia vary with the type but may include micromelia, poor to absent spinal ossification, and normal or poor calvarial ossification. The severity of micromelia in achondrogenesis permits a sonographic diagnosis at as early as 15 to 19 weeks' gestation. A short trunk, protuberant abdomen, and redundant soft tissue are secondary findings that result from the primary defect of skeletal ossification. Polyhydramnios and fetal hydrops may be present.

Achondroplasia

Heterozygous achondroplasia is another of the more common skeletal dysplasias. Although 20% of cases are transmitted by means of autosomal dominant inheritance, the remaining 80% occur as spontaneous mutations.[27]

Sonographic findings in heterozygous achondroplasia include shortened extremities, large head, hydrocephalus due to obstruction at the level of the foramen magnum, kyphoscoliosis, and polyhydramnios. As pregnancy advances the disparity between head size and femur length continues to increase (Fig. 19-20). The gestational age at which the shortened limbs may be detected varies between 20.9 and 27.1 weeks.[7]

The characteristic head shape of achondroplastic dwarfs is due to the early synostosis of the cartilaginous bones of the skull base. The bones of the calvarium (derived from membranous bone) grow normally. As a result, the head becomes pear-shaped, with a large vault on a small base. In addition to being shortened, the femur and humerus are generally thick and enlarged at the ends. The chest cavity may be small, and the pelvis is narrowed.

Homozygous achondroplasia is a more severe form of achondroplasia. Respiratory insufficiency due to the extremely narrow chest uniformly results in an early neonatal death. As one would expect, an abnormally short femur is detected sooner (by about 1 month) in homozygous than in heterozygous achondroplasia.[28]

In hypochondroplasia, there are no changes in the skull, and the effect on the pelvis and long bones may not be apparent until the neonatal period. Prenatal sonographic detection of hypochondroplasia, however, is possible.[29] Hypochondroplasia is an autosomal dominant disorder.

Additional lethal and nonlethal skeletal malformations are outlined on Table 19-5.

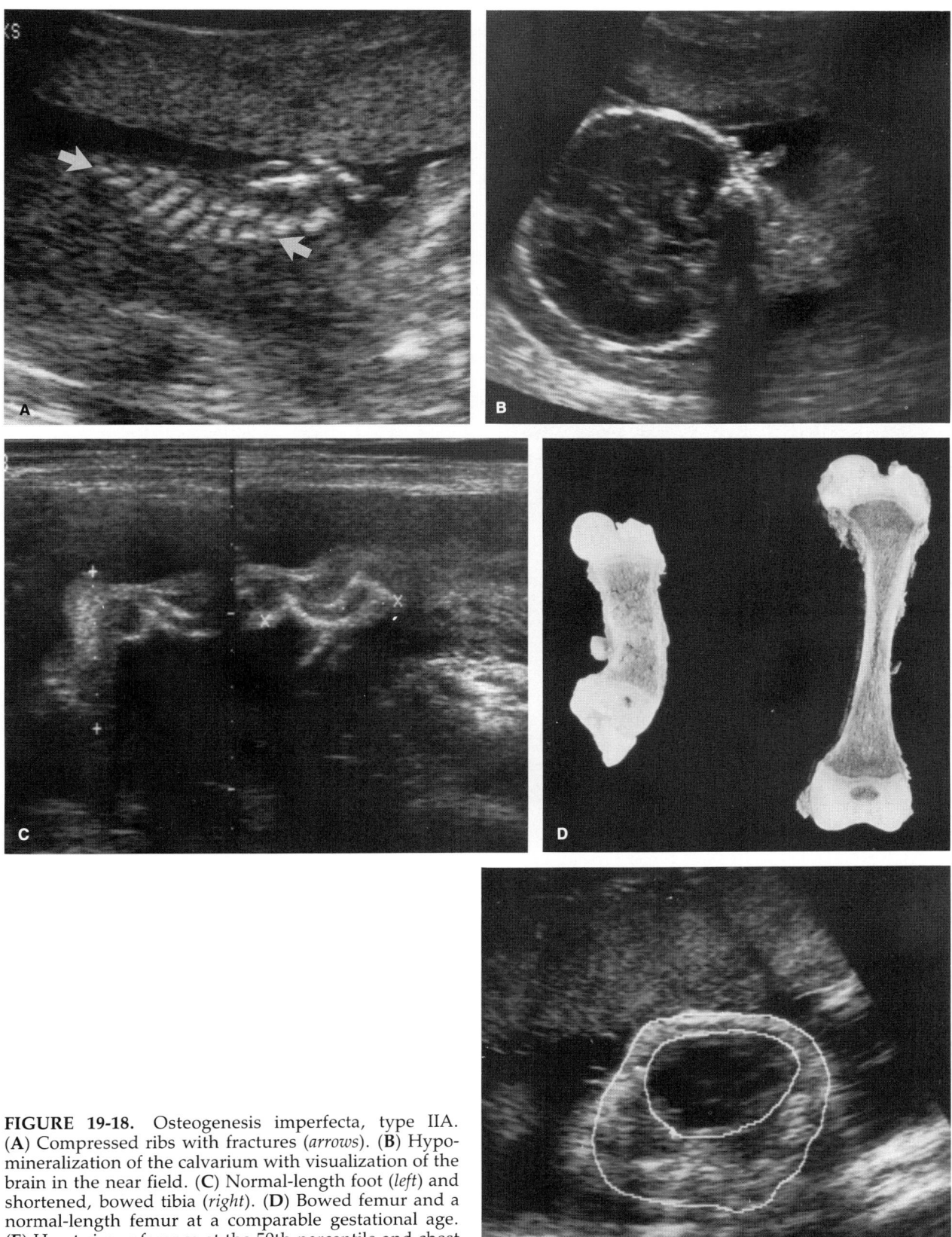

FIGURE 19-18. Osteogenesis imperfecta, type IIA. (**A**) Compressed ribs with fractures (*arrows*). (**B**) Hypomineralization of the calvarium with visualization of the brain in the near field. (**C**) Normal-length foot (*left*) and shortened, bowed tibia (*right*). (**D**) Bowed femur and a normal-length femur at a comparable gestational age. (**E**) Heart circumference at the 50th percentile and chest circumference less than the 2.5th percentile, indicating pulmonary hypoplasia.

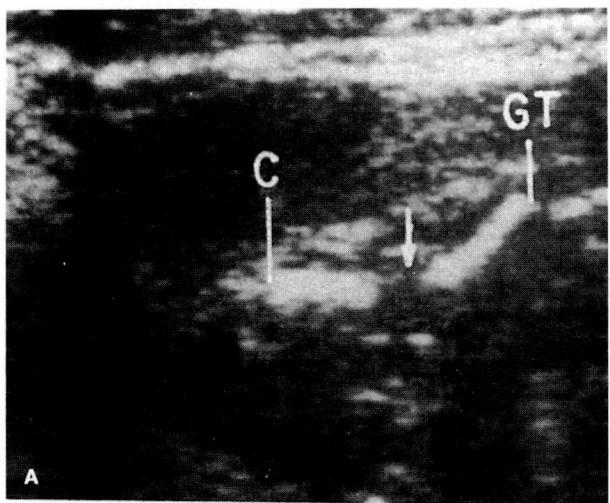

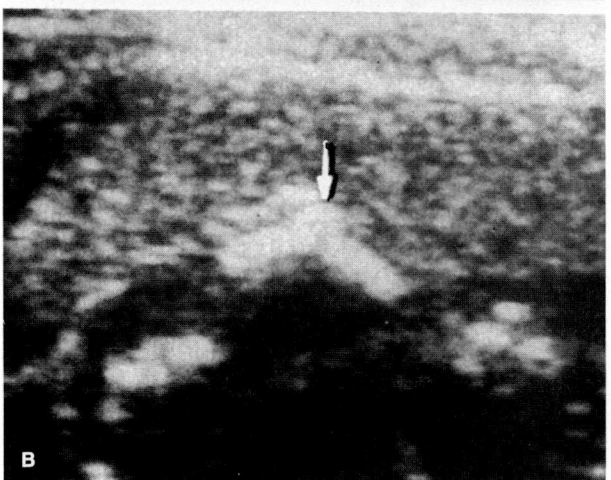

FIGURE 19-19. Osteogenesis imperfecta, dominant form. (**A**) Fracture in mid-shaft of right femur (*arrow*) at 20 weeks' gestation. Movement was noted at the fracture site. GT, greater trochanter; C, condyle. (**B**) Healed fracture with callus formation (*arrow*) and varus angulation at mid-shaft of right femur at 26 weeks' gestation. (Kurtz AB, Wapner RJ: Ultrasonographic diagnosis of second-trimester skeletal dysplasias: A prospective analysis in a high-risk population. J Ultrasound Med 1983; 2:99–106.)

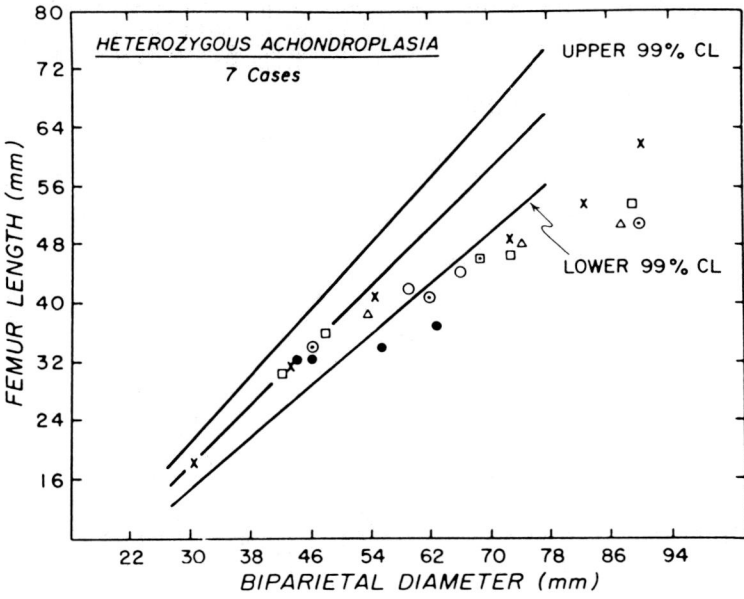

FIGURE 19-20. The femur lengths of seven fetal cases of heterozygous achondroplasia are plotted showing abnormal growth of the femurs when compared with the biparietal diameter. □, case 1; ⊡, case 2; ⊙, case 3; ○, case 4; △, case 5; ●, case 6; ×, case 7. (Kurth ABB, et al: J Ultrasound Med 1986; 5:137.)

TABLE 19-5. **Sonographic Detection of Rare Skeletal Malformations**

Skeletal Malformation	Inheritance	Sonographically Detectable Characteristics	Gestational Age at Diagnosis (wk)
Weyers' syndrome[43]	AR	Deficient ulnar and fibular rays with bilateral hydronephrosis	19
Jeune syndrome[44]	AR	Narrow thorax; short, deformed bones (involving mostly the ulna, radius, and fibula); polydactyly; renal dysplasia	18
Short-rib polydactyly syndrome type III[45]	AR	Shortened extremities; polydactyly of hands and feet; narrow chest; congenital heart disease; polyhydramnios	31
Chondroectodermal dysplasia (Ellis-Van Creveld syndrome)[16]	AR	Short limbs; narrow thorax; polydactyly; congenital heart disease	17
Chondrodysplasia Punctata			
Conradi-Hünermann syndrome[46]	AD	Punctate calcifications of epiphysis; mild, asymmetric shortening of the long bones; scoliosis; cataracts	17
Rhizomelic type[47]	AR	Severe shortening of extremities; early neonatal demise from recurrent infection	28
Camptomelic dysplasia[48]	AR	Short and bowed limbs; hypoplastic fibula; hypoplastic scapula; hypertelorism; micrognathia; club feet	18
Spondyloepiphyseal dysplasia congenita[49]	AR AD	Shortened extremities; lack of ossification of distal femoral and proximal tibial epiphyses; polyhydramnios	17
Hypophosphatasia[50]	AR	Underossification of the bony skeleton; limb shortening	27
Diastrophic dysplasia[51]	AR	Extreme shortening of the extremities; micrognathia; clubfeet; abduction of thumbs ("hitchhiker thumbs")	31
Spondylothoracic dysplasia[52]			
Type I (Jarcho-Levin syndrome)[53]	AR	Microcephaly; cleft palate; short thorax; disorganized vertebral bodies; protuberant abdomen; normal limb length; abdominal wall defects; usually fatal	16
Type II	AD	Milder involvement; nearly normal longevity	
Kniest's syndrome[54]	Sporadic AR, AD	Cataracts; cleft palate; platyspondyly; short femur	31
Antley-Bixler syndrome[55]	Sporadic AR	Long bone fractures; femoral bowing; midfacial hypoplasia; craniosynostosis; urogenital anomalies; polyhydramnios	25
Oromandibular limb hypogenesis syndrome[56]	Unknown	Polyhydramnios; micrognathia; clubfeet; hand anomalies; shortened long bones; pulmonary hypoplasia	37

AD, autosomal dominant; AR, autosomal recessive.

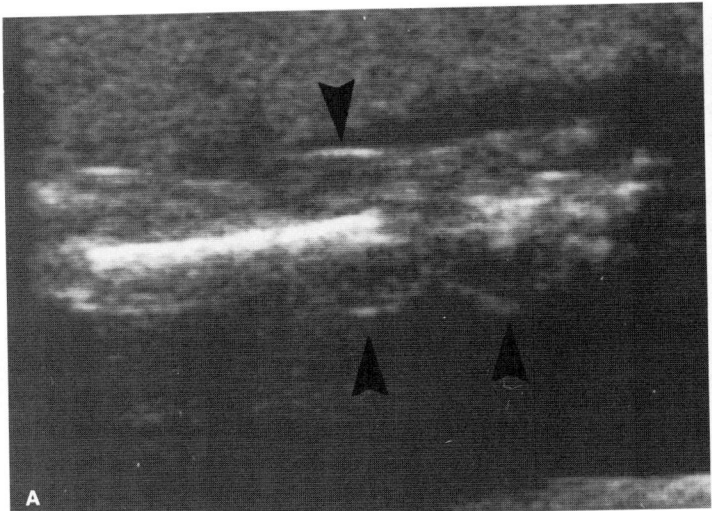

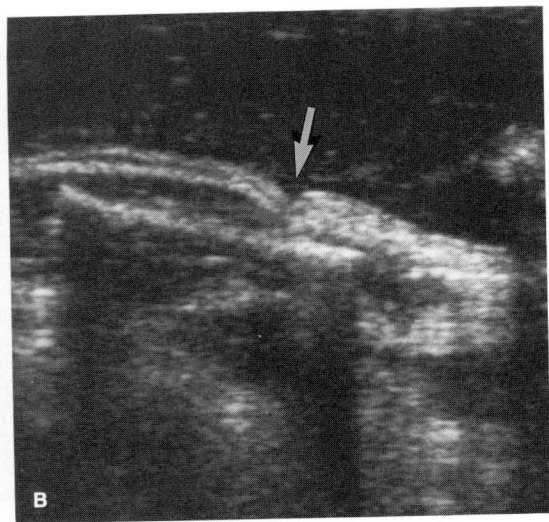

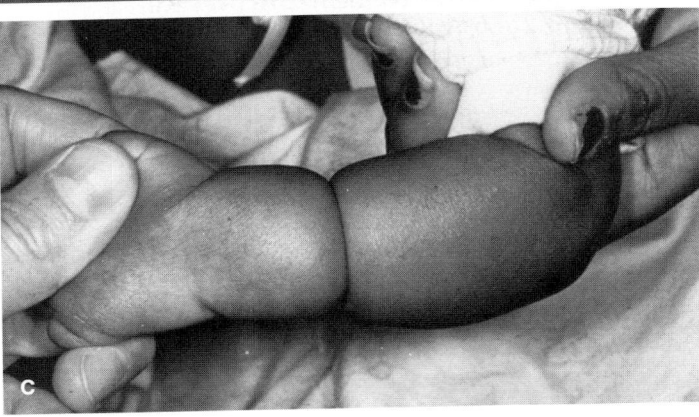

FIGURE 19-21. Forearm constriction band. **(A)** Left arm at 18.6 weeks' gestation. The subcutaneous edema around the hand and forearm was 7 mm in depth (*arrowheads*). **(B)** Left arm at 38.6 weeks' gestation. The point of constriction in the forearm is clearly delineated (*arrow*). **(C)** Left arm at 6 weeks' of age with a prominent constriction band. (Hill LM, et al: J Ultrasound Med 1988; 7 :293–295.)

OTHER SKELETAL ABNORMALITIES

Limb Reduction Defects

Malformations of the extremities can occur at different stages of development. Limb formation may be suppressed, normal growth and development may be impaired, or secondary destruction may occur after limb development.

The varied deformities associated with amniotic band syndrome are secondary to entanglement with mesodermic bands derived from the chorionic surface of the amnion after the latter has separated from the chorion.[30] Isacsohn and colleagues (Fig. 19-21) classified annular constrictions into five stages of severity: (1) the presence of a shallow groove, (2) encroachment on underlying subcutaneous tissue and muscle by the constriction band, (3) extension of the constriction band down to the bone, (4) pseudoarthrosis of underlying bone, and (5) intrauterine amputation.[31]

The frequency of limb reduction malformations is outlined in Table 19-6. The more common limb anomalies are defined in Table 19-7. Froster-Iskenius and Baird reported an incidence of 1 limb reduction defect in every 1692 live births.[32] Most limb reductions are thought to result from defects of development, but prenatal destruction of part of a limb can occur. Genetically determined disturbances of vascular or nervous tissue can result in intrauterine amputations that morphologically resemble the lesions found in the presence of amniotic bands.

TABLE 19-6. Types of Limb Defects

Site of Reduction	Total No. for Period (1952–1984)	Incidence per 10,000 Live Births* (1952–1984)
Amelia	17	0.1
Terminal transverse defects	223	1.8
Terminal longitudinal defects†	410	3.3
Intercalary defect	199	1.6
Preaxial hand defects	100	0.8
Postaxial hand defects	64	0.5
Radial defects	40	0.3
Ulnar defects	23	0.2
Other digital defects	119	1.0
Central ray defects	81	0.7
Preaxial foot defects	17	0.1
Postaxial foot defects	23	0.2
Central ray foot defects	27	0.2
Other foot defects	52	0.4
Humeral defects	10	0.1
Femoral defects	39	0.3
Tibial defects	25	0.2
Fibular defects	17	0.1

* These do not sum to the total birth incidence of limb defects because some cases had more than one defect.

† This includes several of the other categories shown.

(Froster-Iskenius UG, Baird PA: Limb reduction defects in over one million consecutive live births. Teratology 1989; 39:127–135.)

Three fourths of limb reduction abnormalities affect the upper limbs, and one fourth affect the lower limbs. Among the reduction sites, the radius is most frequently involved (Fig. 19-22). In the lower extremities, the fibula is the most frequently congenitally absent long bone. Unilateral absence of the tibia is not as frequent. Because the latter bone supports the body, its absence is more serious, and treatment is generally unsatisfactory.

Unilateral congenital femoral hypoplasia may result from a viral infection, focal ischemia, or irradiation during the period of limb bud development (4–8 weeks' gestation); familial occurrence has also been reported. The femur–fibula–ulna syndrome is characterized by a hypoplastic to absent femur in association with the absence of the fibula.[33] A variety of upper extremity anomalies are also present, including ulnar defects and the absence of fingers (Fig. 19-23).

In sirenomelia (mermaid syndrome), there is a fusion of the lower extremities. The degree of fusion can vary from a simple membrane fusing the two legs together to total fusion, with a single femur and fibula. Bilateral renal agenesis or bilateral renal cystic dysplasia results in oligohydramnios[34] (Fig. 19-24).

About half of cases with a limb reduction abnormality have additional defects. Most of these defects are in the muscular skeletal system, but the cardiovascular, genitourinary, and gastrointestinal systems may also be involved. Limb reduction defects have been associated with trisomies 13, 18, and 21.

(*text continues on page 430*)

TABLE 19-7. Nomenclature for Rib and Limb Anomalies

Achiria	absence of hands
Achiropody	absence of hands and feet
Acromelia	shortening of distal segments (hands, feet)
Adactyly (ectrodactyly)	absence of fingers or toes
Amelia (ectromelia)	absence of extremity
Apodia	absence of feet
Brachydactyly	abnormal shortness of fingers
Camptomelia (campomelia)	bent limb
Clinodactyly	in-curved finger
Diastrophic	distorted
Ectrodactyly	split hands
Equinus	extension of foot
Hemimelia	absence (complete or incomplete) of limb below knee or elbow
Mesomelia	shortening of middle segments (forearm, lower leg)
Micromelia	shortened limbs; dwarfism
Oligodactyly	partial lack of fingers
Paraxial	beside axis of limb
Phocomelia	deficient development of middle portions of limb with preservation of proximal and distal segments
Polydactyly	extra digits
Postaxial	posterior to axis of limb, ie, postaxial hexadactyly is six digits with extra digit along dorsal aspect of hand or foot
Rhizomelia	shortening of proximal segment (femur, humerus)
Symbrachydactyly	short, fused digits
Syndactyly	lack of differentiation between digits
Talipes	clubfoot
Varus	bent inward

(Adapted from Mahony BS: The fetal musculoskeletal system. In Callen PW [ed]: Ultrasonography in Obstetrics and Gynecology. Philadelphia: WB Saunders, 1988:137–164.)

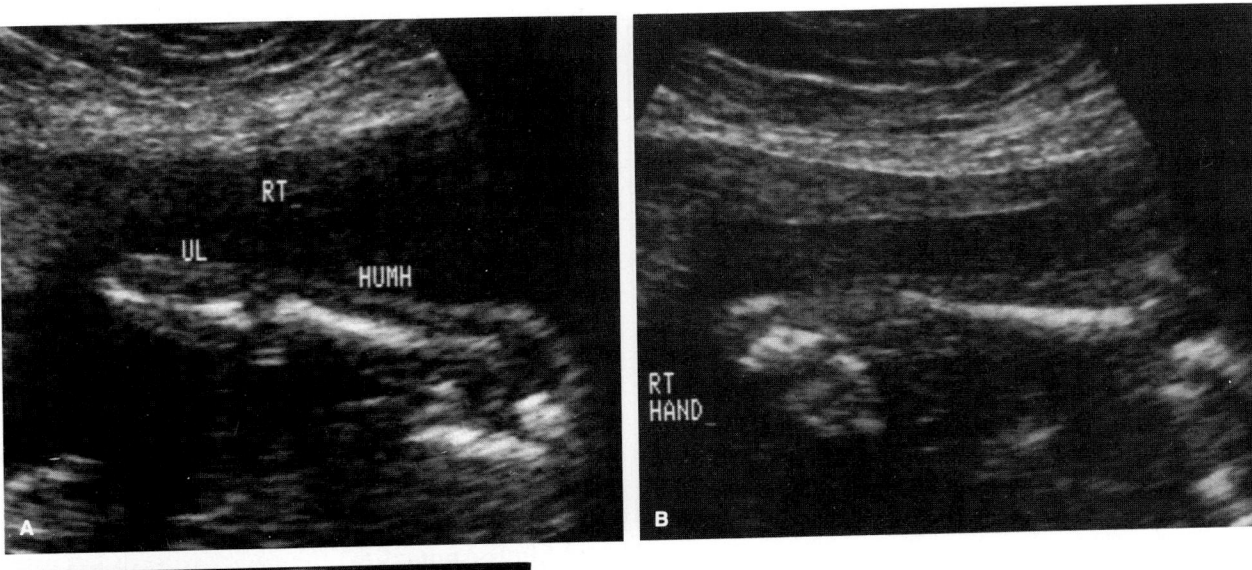

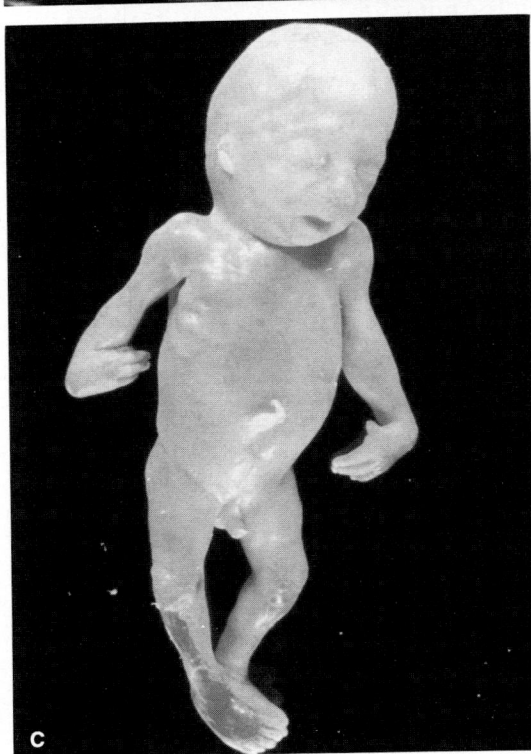

FIGURE 19-22. Right radial aplasia and ulnar hypoplasia in a fetus with trisomy 18. **(A)** Ulnar hypoplasia. Marked radial deviation has removed the hand from view. **(B)** Radial deviation of the hand. **(C)** Postmortem photograph confirming the prenatal findings.

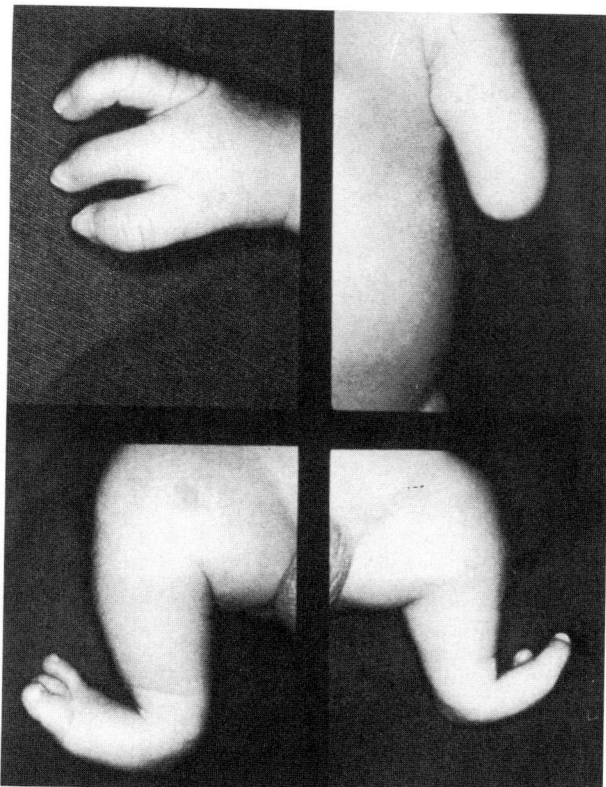

FIGURE 19-23. Photographs of the right and left side, upper and lower extremities. Peromelia of the left arm and two missing fingers of the right hand are evident. Absence of two toes from the right foot and three toes from the left foot can be seen. (Hirose K, et al: J Clin Ultrasound 1988; 16:199.)

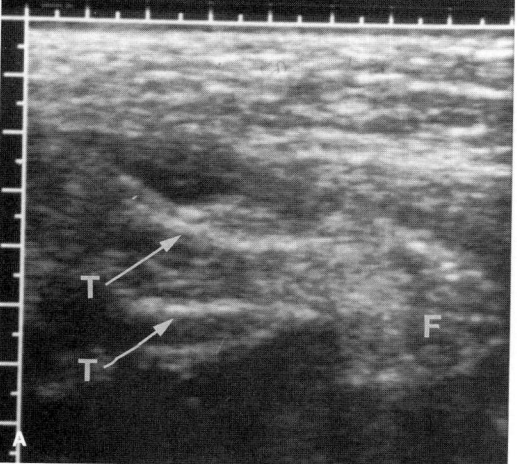

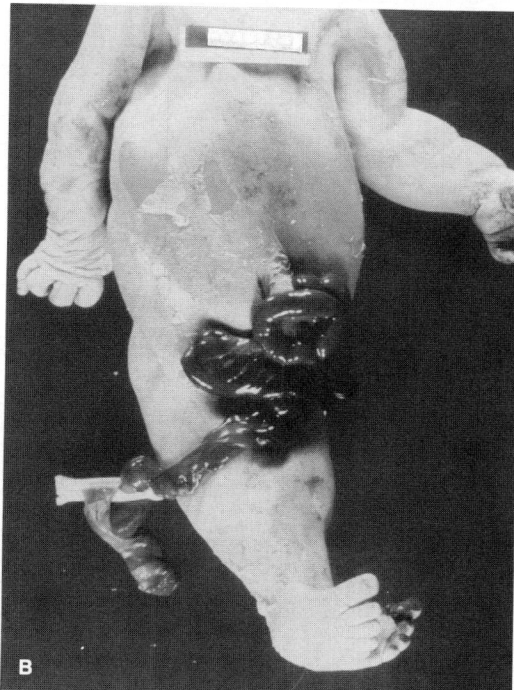

FIGURE 19-24. Sirenomelia. **(A)** Two tibias (T) are seen above fused feet (F). **(B)** Postmortem photograph confirms the prenatal finding.

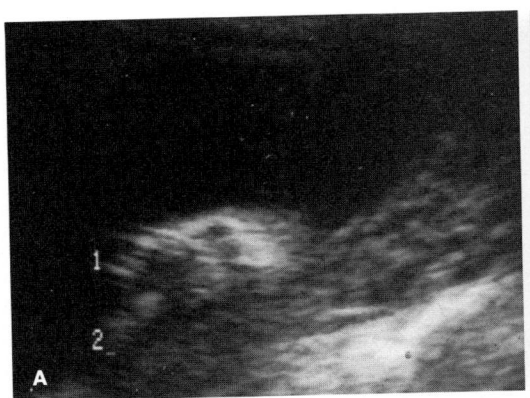
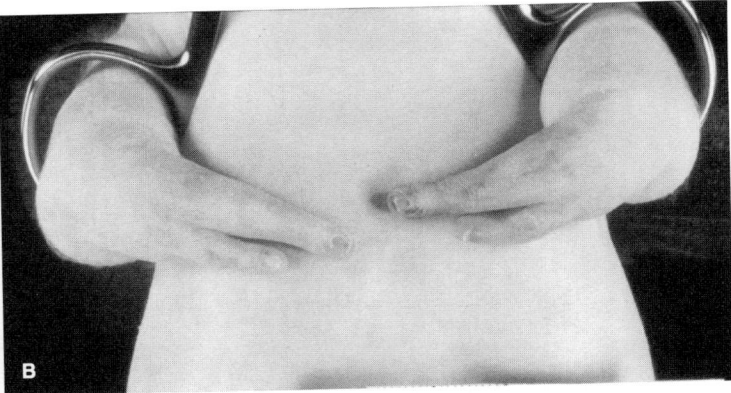

FIGURE 19-25. Ectrodactyly. **(A)** Ultrasound image shows fingers (1 and 2). **(B)** Hands at necropsy.

Malformation of the Hand

Although the causes of reduction malformations have been established, the mechanisms resulting in additional digits are more difficult to discern. Hexadactyly (six fingers or toes) is a relatively frequent anomaly; however, its prevalence varies with race and geographic location. The incidence in white and black children born in New York is 1 in 713.[35] Polydactyly with greater than six digits is rare and is usually associated with severe malformations.

One child in 65,000 is born without a hand.[36] The number of children born with serious deformities of the hand is much greater. Table 19-7 defines the more commonly observed hand malformations. They may occur as an isolated anomaly, are associated with a variety of syndromes, or result from a chromosomal abnormality (Fig. 19-25).

Clinodactyly is due to a shortening of the middle phalanx of the fifth finger. It is present in 60% of neonates with Down's syndrome[37] (Fig. 19-26).

Greater than half of fetuses with trisomy 18 have flexion deformities of the hands and overlapping fingers[38] (Fig. 19-27). This characteristic finding of trisomy 18 is not present before 14 weeks' gestation.

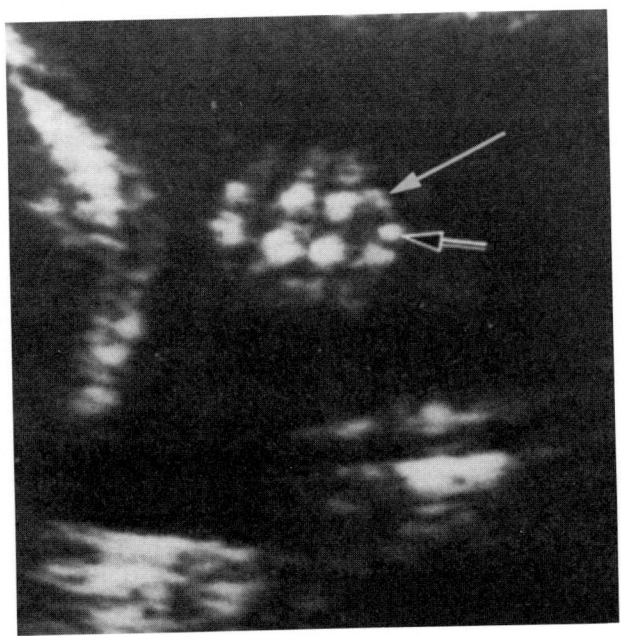

FIGURE 19-26. Clinodactyly. Image of fetal hand shows marked discrepancy between size of the middle phalanx of the fifth digit (*short arrow*) and size of the middle phalanx of the fourth digit next to it. Note also inward curve of the fifth finger (*long arrow*), which is abnormal. (Benacerraf BR, et al: Am J Obstet Gynecol 1988; 159:181.)

Clubfoot

A clubfoot is one of the most frequent congenital anomalies, occurring in between 1 in 250 and 1 in 1000 births.[39] In 95% of cases, the sole is turned medially so that the lateral aspect of the foot points to the ground (talipes equinovarus; Fig. 19-28). A calcaneovalgus deformity results when the foot is dorsiflexed and deviated laterally.

Many causes of clubfoot have been identified. An abnormal position in utero is an acknowledged external cause of clubfoot. Torpin, for example, reported a 32% incidence of clubfoot with prolonged oligohydramnios.[40] Other causes include abnormal bone formation, central nervous system malforma-

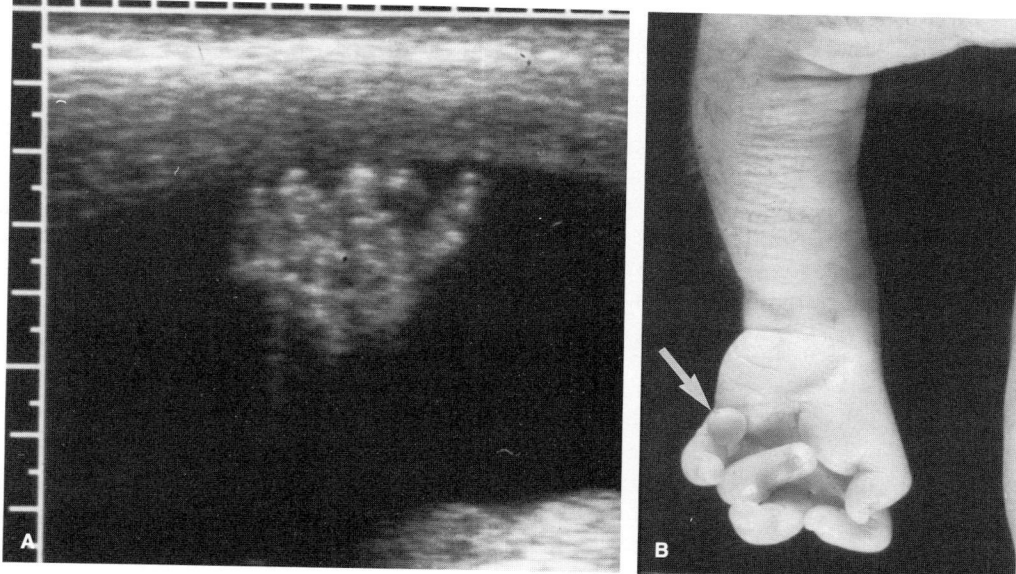

FIGURE 19-27.   Clenched fist associated with trisomy 18. **(A)** Ultrasound. **(B)** Hand at necropsy. Note accessory digit adjacent to fifth finger.

tions (eg, spina bifida), and muscular defects. Genetics is also important; about 15% of cases have a family history of clubfoot. With normal parents, the siblings of an affected girl or boy have a 5% and 2% chance, respectively, of having a clubfoot. If a parent also has a clubfoot, the risk approaches 25%.[41]

Most clubfeet are found in otherwise normal infants. Clubfoot also is associated with several syndromes, such as arthrogryposis, diastrophic dwarfism, Pena-Shokeir phenotype, and Larsen's syndrome. A clubfoot occurs in about 30% of fetuses with trisomy 18; it is less often associated with trisomy 13.[38]

Yamamoto reported a 10.3% incidence of malformations (eg, cleft lip or palate, congenital heart disease) associated with clubfoot.[42] The detection of a clubfoot in utero should therefore result in a careful anatomic survey in search of other congenital anomalies. The type and severity of other anomalies should then determine if a genetic amniocentesis is warranted.

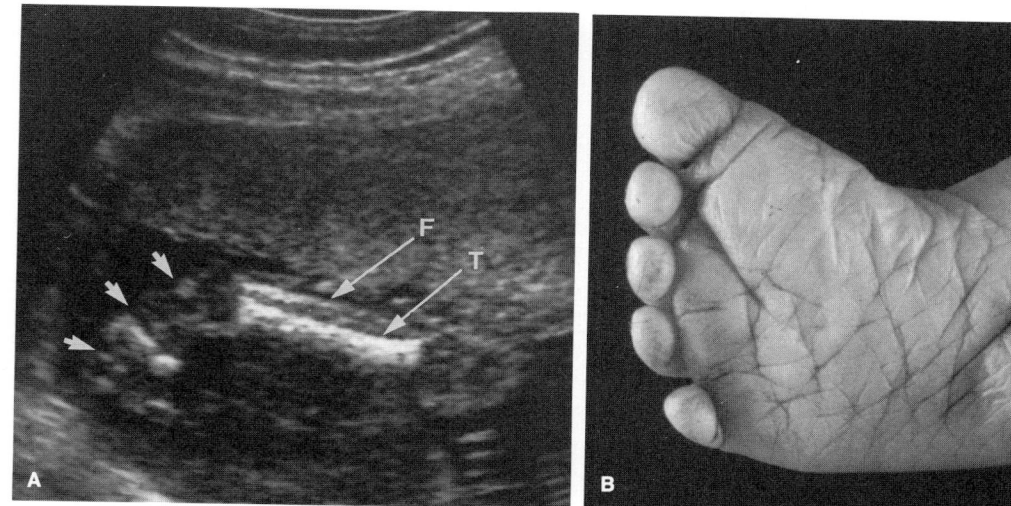

FIGURE 19-28.   Club foot. **(A)** Ultrasound showing tibia (T) and fibula (F) with turned-in foot (*arrows*). **(B)** Photograph after delivery.

CONCLUSION

Advances in ultrasound technology have permitted the sonologist and sonographer to examine the fetus in ever-increasing detail. The evaluation of a fetus with a suspected skeletal abnormality requires a thorough assessment of the extremities, cranium, spine, thorax, and abdomen. A knowledge of the other organ systems that may be involved is also helpful. The principles and sonographic techniques outlined in this chapter help to narrow the differential diagnosis. Because the ultrasound findings are not always pathognomonic, it is frequently impossible to diagnose the exact skeletal dysplasia. A significant percentage of fetuses with a skeletal dysplasia are stillborn or die in the early neonatal period. The antenatal ultrasound findings may be of great assistance to the perinatal pathologist in targeting the evaluation. A postmortem examination that includes karyotyping, photographs, complete body radiographs, and frequently bone histology is often necessary to provide appropriate recurrence risk figures to the parents.

REFERENCES

1. Orioli IM, Castilla EE, Barbosa-Neto JG: The birth prevalence ratios for the skeletal dysplasias. J Med Genet 1986; 23:328–332.
2. Hegge FN, Prescott GH, Watson PT: Utility of a screening examination of the fetal extremities during obstetrical sonography. J Ultrasound Med 1986; 5:639–45.
3. Hadlock FP, Harrist RB, Deter RL, Park SK: Fetal femur length as a predictor of menstrual age: Sonographically measured. AJR 1982; 138:875–878.
4. Jeanty P, Rodesch F, Delbeke D, Dumont JE: Estimation of gestational age from measurements of fetal long bones. J Ultrasound Med 1984; 3:75–79.
5. Hill LM, Guzick D, Thomas ML, Fries JK: Fetal radius length: A critical evaluation of race as a factor in gestational age assessment. Am J Obstet Gynecol 1989; 161:193–199.
6. Kurtz AB, Needleman L, Wapner RJ, et al: Usefulness of a short femur in the in utero detection of skeletal dysplasia. Radiology 1990; 177:197–200.
7. Kurtz AB, Filly RA, Wapner RJ, et al: In utero analysis of heterozygous achondroplasia: Variable time of onset as detected by femur length measurements. J Ultrasound Med 1986; 5:137–140.
8. Mercer BM, Sklar S, Shariatmadar A, et al: Fetal foot length as a predictor of gestational age. Am J Obstet Gynecol 1987; 156:350–355.
9. Campbell J, Henderson RGN, Campbell S: The fetal femur/foot length ratio: A new parameter to assess dysplastic limb reduction. Obstet Gynecol 1988; 72:181–184.
10. Brons JTJ, Van der Harten JJ, Van Geijn HP, et al: Ratios between growth parameters for the prenatal ultrasonographic diagnosis of skeletal dysplasias. Eur J Obstet Gynecol Reprod Biol 1990; 34:37–46.
11. Brons JTJ, Van Geijn HP, Bezemer PD, et al: The fetal skeleton: Ultrasonographic evaluation of the normal growth. Eur J Obstet Gynecol Reprod Biol 1990; 34:21–36.
12. Thomas RL, Hess LW, Johnson TRB: Prepartum diagnosis of limb-shortening defects with associated hydramnios. Am J Perinatol 1987; 4:293–299.
13. Mahony BS, Filly RA, Callen PW, Golbus MS: Thanatophoric dwarfism with the cloverleaf skull: A specific antenatal sonographic diagnosis. J Ultrasound Med 1985; 4:151–154.
14. Stamm ER, Pretorius DH, Rumack CM, Manco-Johnson ML: Kleeblattschadel anomaly: In utero sonographic appearance. J Ultrasound Med 1987; 6:319–324.
15. Rouse GA, Filly RA, Toomey F, Grube GL: Short-limb skeletal dysplasias: Evaluation of the fetal spine with sonography and radiography. Radiology 1990; 174:177–180.
16. Mahoney MJ, Hobbins JC: Prenatal diagnosis of chondroectodermal dysplasia (Ellis-Van Creveld syndrome) with fetoscopy and ultrasound. N Engl J Med 1977; 297:258–260.
17. Chitkara U, Rosenberg J, Chervenak FA, et al: Prenatal sonographic assessment of the fetal thorax: Normal values. Am J Obstet Gynecol 1987; 156:1069–1074.
18. Nimrod C, Nicholson S, Davies D, et al: Pulmonary hypoplasia testing in clinical obstetrics. Am J Obstet Gynecol 1988; 158:277–280.
19. Elejalde BR, de Elejalde MM: Thanatophoric dysplasia: Fetal manifestations and prenatal diagnosis. Am J Med Genet 1985; 22:669–683.
20. Opitz JM, Spranger JW (personal communication). In Elejalde BR, de Elejalde MM: Thanatophoric dysplasia: Fetal manifestations and prenatal diagnosis. Am J Med Genet 1985; 22:669–683.
21. Byers PH, Wallis GA, Willing MC: Osteogenesis imperfecta: Translation of mutation to phenotype. J Med Genet 1991; 28:433–442.
22. Sillence DO, Senn A, Danks DM: Genetic heterogeneity in osteogenesis imperfecta. J Med Genet 1979; 16:101–116.
23. Robinson LP, Worten NJ, Lachman RS, et al: Prenatal diagnosis of osteogenesis imperfecta type III. Prenat Diagn 1987; 7:7–15.
24. Chervenak FA, Romero R, Berkowitz RL, et al: Antenatal sonographic findings of osteogenesis imperfecta. Am J Obstet Gynecol 1982; 143:228–230.
25. Byers PH: Osteogenesis imperfecta: An update. Growth Genet Horm 1988; 4:1–5.
26. Mahony BS, Filly RA, Cooperberg PL: Antenatal sonographic diagnosis of achondrogenesis. J Ultrasound Med 1984; 3:333–335.

27. Tyson JE, Barnes AC, McKusick VA, et al: Obstetric and gynecologic considerations of dwarfism. Am J Obstet Gynecol 1970; 108:688–704.

28. Donnenfeld AE, Mennuti MT: Second trimester diagnosis of fetal skeletal dysplasias. Obstet Gynecol Surv 1987; 42:199–217.

29. Stoll C, Manini P, Bloch J, Roth M-P: Prenatal diagnosis of hypochondroplasia. Prenat Diagn 1985; 5:423–426.

30. Torpin R: Amniochorionic mesoblastic fibrous strings and amnionic bands. Am J Obstet Gynecol 1965; 91:65–75.

31. Isacsohn M, Aboulafia Y, Horwitz B, Ben-Hur N: Congenital annular constriction due to amniotic bands. Acta Obstet Gynecol Scand 1976; 55:179–182.

32. Froster-Iskenius UG, Baird PA: Limb reduction defects in over one million consecutive live births. Teratology 1989; 39:127–135.

33. Hirose K, Koyanagi T, Hara K, et al: Antenatal ultrasound diagnosis of the femur-fibula-ulna syndrome. J Clin Ultrasound 1988; 16:199–203.

34. Sirtori M, Ghidini A, Romero R, Hobbins JC: Prenatal diagnosis of sirenomelia. J Ultrasound Med 1989; 8:83–88.

35. Sesgin MZ, Stark BB: The incidence of congenital defects. Plast Reconstr Surg 1961; 27:26–27.

36. Birch-Jensen A: Congenital Deformities of the Upper Extremities. Copenhagen: Ejnan Munksgaard, 1949.

37. Benacerraf BR, Osathanondh R, Frigoletto FD: Sonographic demonstration of hypoplasia of the middle phalanx of the fifth digit: A finding associated with Down syndrome. Am J Obstet Gynecol 1988; 159:181–183.

38. Benacerraf BR, Miller WA, Frigoletto FD: Sonographic detection of fetuses with trisomies 13 and 18: Accuracy and limitations. Am J Obstet Gynecol 1988; 158:404–409.

39. Chervenak FA, Tortora M, Hobbins JC: Antenatal sonographic diagnosis of clubfoot. J Ultrasound Med 1985; 4:49–50.

40. Torpin R: Fetal Malformations Caused by Amnion Rupture During Gestation. Springfield, IL: Charles C Thomas, 1968.

41. Wynne-Davies R: Genetic and environmental factors in the etiology of talipes equinovarus. Clin Orthop 1972; 84:9–13.

42. Yamamoto H: A clinical genetic and epidemiologic study of congenital clubfoot. Jpn J Hum Genet 1979; 24:37–44.

43. Elejalde BR, de Elejalde MM, Booth C, et al: Prenatal diagnosis of Weyers syndrome (deficient ulnar and fibular rays with bilateral hydronephrosis). Am J Med Genet 1985; 21:439–444.

44. Elejalde BR, de Elejalde MM, Pansch D: Prenatal diagnosis of jeune syndrome. Am J Med Genet 1985; 21:433–438.

45. Meizner I, Bar-Ziv J: Prenatal ultrasonic diagnosis of short-rib polydactyly syndrome (SRPS) type III: A case report and a proposed approach to the diagnosis of SRPS and related conditions. J Clin Ultrasound 1985; 13:284–287.

46. Tuck SM, Slack J, Buckland J: Prenatal diagnosis of Conradi's syndrome: Case report. Prenat Diagn 1990; 10:195–198.

47. Duff P, Harlass FE, Milligan DA: Prenatal diagnosis of chondrodysplasia punctata by sonography. Obstet Gynecol 1990; 76:497–500.

48. Cordone M, Lituania M, Zampatti C, et al: In utero ultrasonographic features of campomelic dysplasia. Prenat Diagn 1989; 9:745–750.

49. Kirk JS, Comstock CH: Antenatal sonographic appearance of spondyloepiphyseal dysplasia congenita. J Ultrasound Med 1990; 9:173–175.

50. DeLange M, Rouse GA: Prenatal diagnosis of hypophosphatasia. J Ultrasound Med 1990; 9:115–117.

51. Gembruch U, Niesen M, Kehrberg H, Hansmann M: Diastrophic dysplasia: A specific prenatal diagnosis by ultrasound. Prenat Diagn 1988; 8:539–545.

52. Marks F, Hernanz-Schulman M, Horii S, et al: Spondylothoracic dysplasia: Clinical and sonographic diagnosis. J Ultrasound Med 1989; 8:1–5.

53. Romero R, Ghidini A, Eswara MS, et al: Prenatal findings in a case of spondylocostal dysplasia type I (Jarcho-Levin syndrome). Obstet Gynecol 1988; 71:988–991.

54. Bromley B, Miller W, Foster SC, Benacerraf BR: The prenatal sonographic features of Kniest syndrome. J Ultrasound Med 1991; 10:705–707.

55. Jacobson RL, St. John Dignon P, Miodovnik M, Siddiqi TA: Antley-Bixler syndrome. J Ultrasound Med 1992; 11:161–164.

56. Shechter SA, Sherer DM, Geilfuss CJ, et al: Prenatal sonographic appearance and subsequent management of a fetus with oromandibular limb hypogenesis syndrome associated with pulmonary hypoplasia. J Clin Ultrasound 1990; 18:661–665.

John P. McGahan and Manuel Porto:
DIAGNOSTIC OBSTETRICAL ULTRASOUND.
© 1994 J.B. Lippincott Company.

Carol B. Benson   Peter M. Doubilet

Chapter 20

Twin Pregnancy

The incidence of twins at delivery is about 1 in 80 to 90 pregnancies. Twins may be dizygotic, arising from fertilization of two separate ova, or monozygotic, resulting from division of a single fertilized ovum (Table 20-1). The frequency of monozygotic twins is the same in all populations, occurring at a rate of 3 to 5 per 1000 pregnancies delivered. In contrast, several factors influence the frequency of dizygotic twinning[1-3] (Table 20-2).

The incidence of monozygotic versus dizygotic twins in the United States is listed in Table 20-1. This is in contrast to the incidence of twinning in other portions of the world because dizygotic twins are affected by both heredity and environment. For instance, populations in Japan have a low birth prevalence of twins, in the range of 3 to 7 per 1000, whereas in areas of Africa, rates of twinning are in excess of 40 per 1000. Other factors associated with increased frequency of dizygotic twinning are listed in Table 20-2. For instance, 6% to 50% of pregnancies that follow ovulation induc-

tion therapy are dizygotic twin gestations, with the rate related to the particular drug therapies.[3]

PLACENTATION

Twin pregnancies may be categorized by placentation type based on *chorionicity*, the number of placentas, and *amnionicity*, the number of amniotic sacs (Table 20-3). The presence and composition of the dividing membrane between twins varies according to placentation type (Fig. 20-1). Placentation type of a twin gestation depends on the time at which twinning occurs. All dizygotic twins, which are separate from the time of ovulation and fertilization, implant separately and are dichorionic and diamniotic. Monozygotic twins divide at variable times after fertilization and, therefore, may have one of several placentation types[1,3] (Fig. 20-2; Table 20-4). Placentation for monozygotic twins is monochorionic–diamniotic in about two

TABLE 20-1. Twin Zygosity

Zygosity	Mechanism	Relative Frequency* (%)
Dizygotic	Fertilization of two ova	~70
Monozygotic	Single fertilized ovum divides	~30

* Frequency may vary depending on a variety of factors (see Table 20-2).

TABLE 20-2. Factors Influencing Frequency of Dizygotic Twins

Factor	Effect on Frequency
Race	Blacks > whites > Asians
Maternal family history	Increased if family history of dizygotic twins
Prior dizygotic twins	Increased in mothers with prior dizygotic twins
Maternal age	Increased with increasing age
Parity	Multiparous > nulliparous
Therapy for infertility	Increased with ovarian stimulation medication

thirds of cases and is dichorionic–diamniotic in about one third of cases. Only rarely, less than 1% of the time, do monozygotic twins have a mono-chorionic–monoamniotic placentation.

SONOGRAPHIC DIAGNOSIS OF TWINS AND PLACENTATION TYPE

The definitive diagnosis of twins can be made by identifying two fetuses with heartbeats, which can be accomplished beginning at about 6 weeks of gestation. Earlier diagnosis can be made in dichorionic gestations, at about 5.5 weeks, by identifying two gestational sacs, each containing a yolk sac.

Visualization of two intrauterine fluid collections without fetuses or yolk sacs before 5.5 weeks suggests a twin pregnancy. This last finding, however, is not definitive for twins because other entities may also present with two intrauterine fluid collections. A singleton pregnancy in a bicornuate uterus with fluid in the nongravid horn may mimic a twin gestation[4] (Fig. 20-3). A subchorionic hemorrhage may also appear as a second gestational sac.

The diagnosis of placentation type is important because the nature and frequency of pregnancy complications depend on chorionicity and amnionicity. Several sonographic features can be

used to determine placentation type[3,5] (Table 20-5). The definitive diagnosis of a diamniotic gestation can be made when a membrane is identified. Because the dividing membrane occasionally cannot be visualized, inability to demonstrate a membrane does not prove monoamnionicity. A monoamniotic gestation can be diagnosed only when there is both nonvisualization of a membrane and intermingling of the two umbilical cords.

The definitive diagnosis of a dichorionic gestation can be made if there are two placental masses or different fetal sexes. In the absence of these findings, membrane thickness can be used to predict chorionicity. A thick membrane suggests a dichorionic gestation, whereas a thin, wispy membrane suggests monochorionicity. Membrane thickness is highly accurate for predicting chorionicity in the first trimester (Figs. 20-1 and 20-4) and has predictive accuracy of 83% thereafter.[5]

COMPLICATIONS

Twin gestations have a higher rate of complications than do singletons both because some obstetrical complications that occur with singletons occur

(*text continues on page 438*)

TABLE 20-3. Placentation Types in Twin Pregnancies

Placentation Types	No. of Placentas	No. of Amniotic Sacs	No. of Layers in Dividing Membrane
Dichorionic, diamniotic	2	2	4
Monochorionic, diamniotic	1	2	2
Monochorionic, monoamniotic	1	1	No membrane

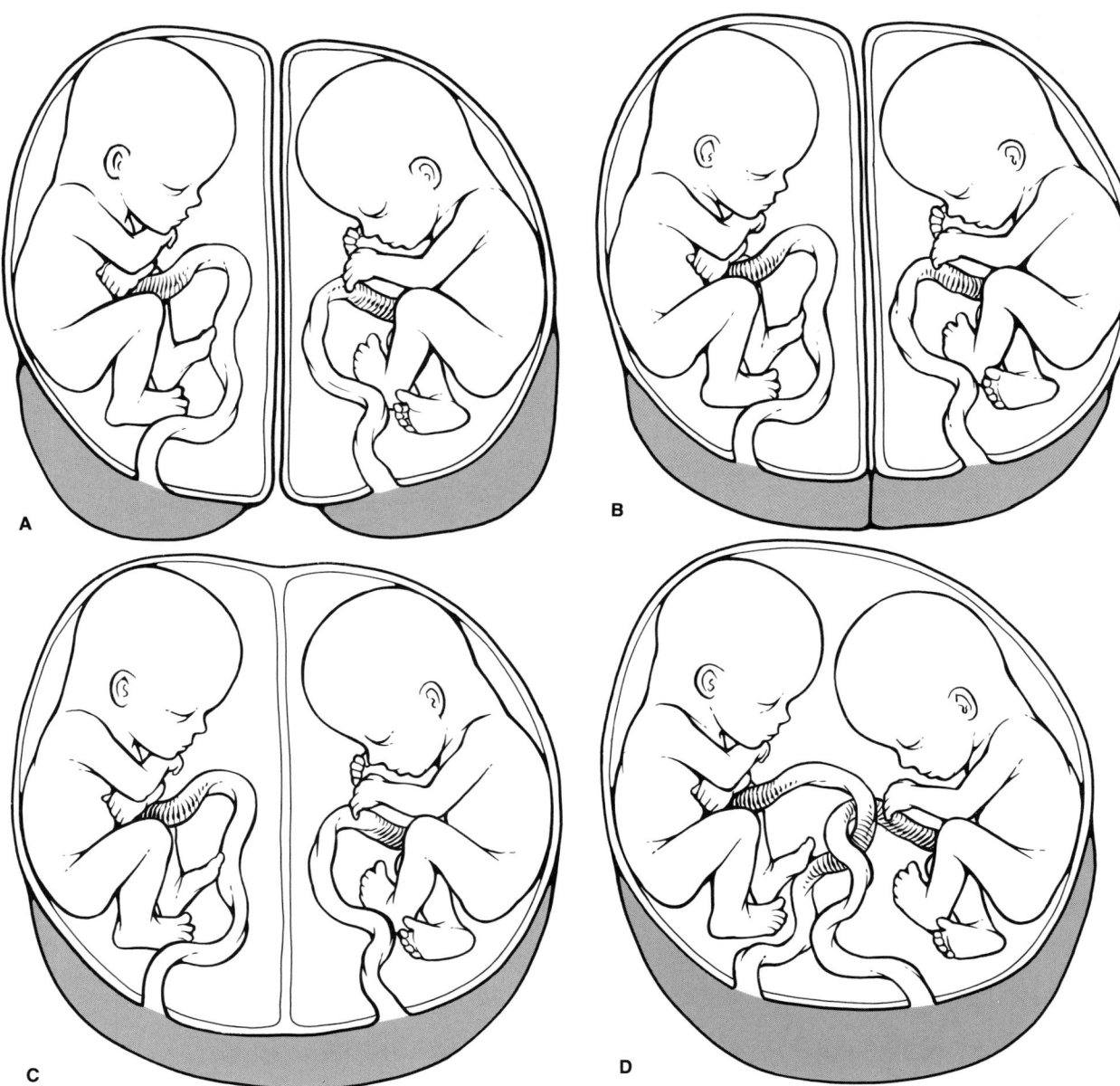

FIGURE 20-1.   Placentation types. **(A)** Dichorionic, diamniotic gestation with separate placentas. The membrane separating the twins is thick, with four layers: two chorionic and two amniotic membranes. **(B)** Dichorionic, diamniotic gestation with fused placentas. The membrane separating the twins is thick, with four layers. **(C)** Monochorionic, diamniotic gestation. The membrane separating the twins is thin, with two layers of amniotic membrane. **(D)** Monochorionic, monoamniotic gestation. No membrane separates the twins. The two umbilical cords intermingle in the single amniotic cavity. **(E)** Thick membrane. Sonogram demonstrates thick membrane (*arrow*) of a dichorionic, diamniotic gestation. The two placentas are clearly separate. **(F)** Thin membrane. Sonogram demonstrates thin, wispy membrane (*arrow*) of a monochorionic, diamniotic twin gestation.

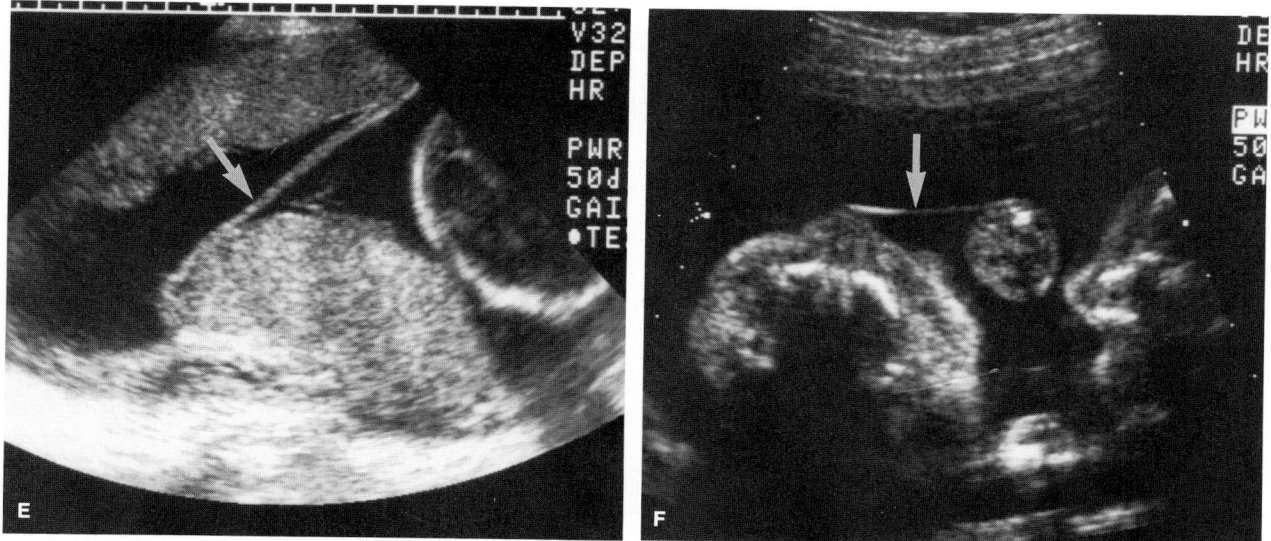

FIGURE 20-1. *(Continued)*

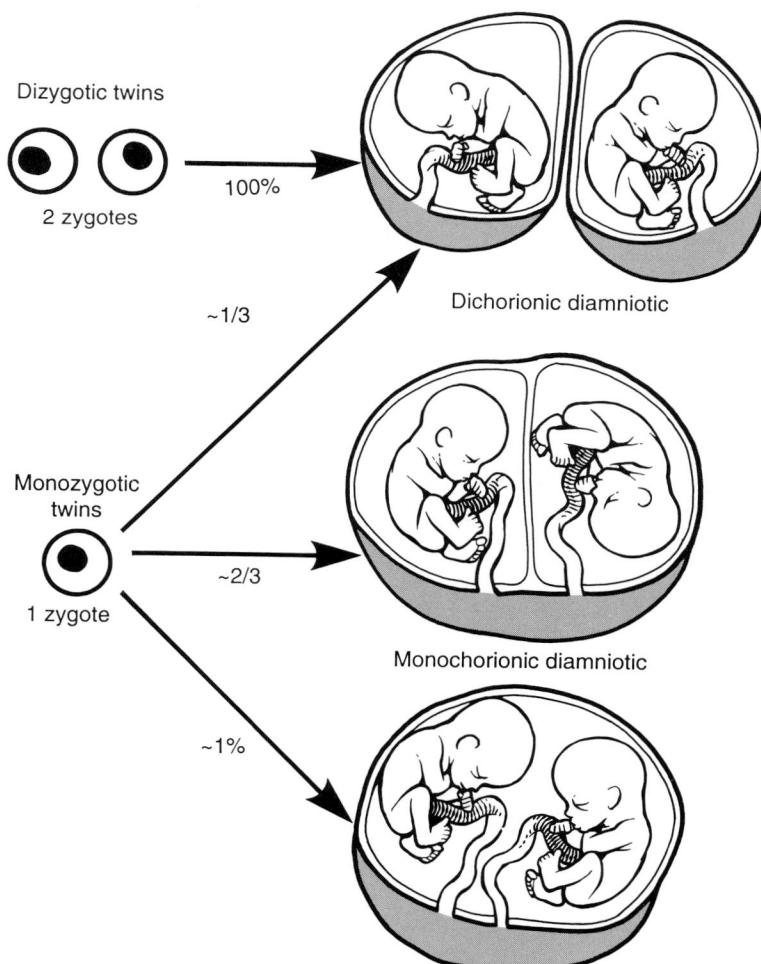

FIGURE 20-2. Monozygotic versus dizygotic placentation. All dizygotic twins
have dichorionic, diamniotic placentation.
Monozygotic twins may be of any placentation type; about two thirds are monochorionic, diamniotic.

TABLE 20-4. Zygosity and Time of Twinning Versus Placentation Type

Zygosity	Time of Twinning	Placentation Type
DZ	Ovulation	DC, DA
MZ	After fertilization	
	0–4 days (~ 1/3 of MZ twins)	DC, DA
	4–8 days (~ 2/3 of MZ twins)	MC, DA
	8–13 days (~ 1% of MZ twins)	MC, MA
	> 13 days (rare)	MC, MA, conjoined twins

DZ, dizygotic; MZ, monozygotic; DC, dichorionic; DA, diamniotic; MC, monochorionic; MA, monoamniotic.

TABLE 20-5. Distinguishing Sonographic Features of Placentation Type

Feature	Placentation Type		
	DC, DA	*MC, DA*	*MC, MA*
No. of placentas	2 (May be contiguous)	1	1
Fetal sex	Same or different	Same	Same
Membrane thickness	Thick	Thin, wispy	None
Umbilical cords	Separate	Separate	May be intermingled

DC, dichorionic; DA, diamniotic; MC, monochorionic; MA, monoamniotic.

more frequently with twins and because a number of complications are specific to twins (Table 20-6). All multiple gestations are prone to preterm delivery, with the attendant neonatal morbidity and mortality associated with prematurity, as well as a number of other general obstetrical complications. Monozygotic twins have an increased incidence of fetal anomalies, including anencephaly, hydrocephalus, holoprosencephaly, sirenomelia, and sacrococcygeal teratoma. These anomalies are often discordant, affecting only one of the twins, despite the fact that the two arise from a single fertilized egg (Fig. 20-5).

Complications specific to twins depend on placentation type.[3] The greater the degree of sharing of chorion and amnion, the higher is the potential for complications. Monochorionic twins may develop complications resulting from vascular anastomoses through the common placenta. Monoamniotic twins are also at high risk for cord entanglement and serious cord accidents within their common amniotic cavity.

Twin-to-Twin Transfusion Syndrome

Twin-to-twin transfusion syndrome results from unbalanced exchange of blood from one fetus (donor twin) to the other (recipient twin) across ar-

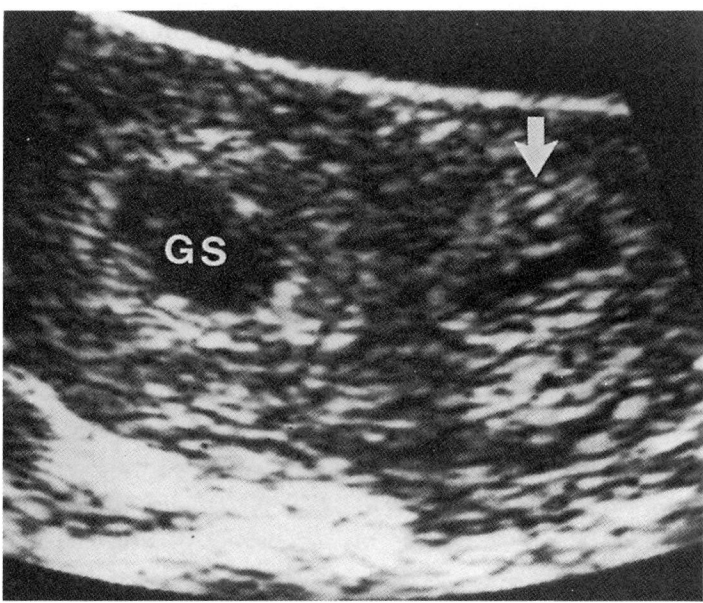

FIGURE 20-3. Bicornate uterus in a singleton pregnancy. Transverse scan of bicornate uterus at 6 weeks of gestation. In one horn of the uterus is an intrauterine gestational sac (GS), while the decidual reaction within the other horn is a pseudosac (*arrow*). (Chitkara UN, Berkowitz RL: Assessment of multiple pregnancy. In Chervenak FA, Isaacson VS, Campbell S [eds]: Ultrasound in Obstetrics and Gynecology. Boston: Little, Brown: 1993: 413–420.)

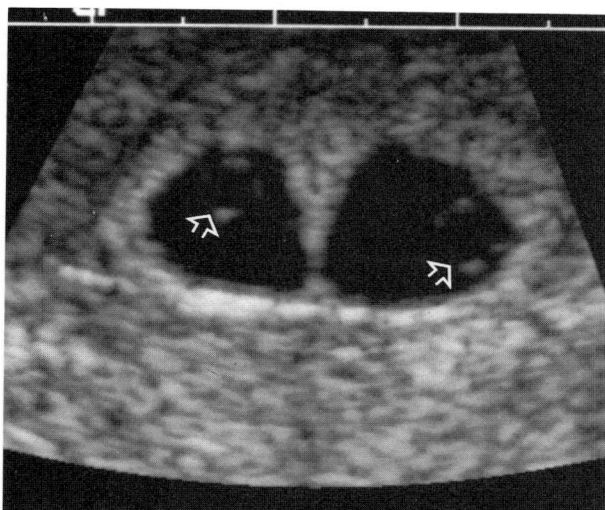

FIGURE 20-4. Dichorionic, diamniotic gestation. Transvaginal sonogram demonstrates two gestational sacs with thick separating membranes. A yolk sac is seen in each sac (*open arrows*).

TABLE 20-6.   Complications of Twin Gestations

Complications More Frequent in Twin than Singleton Gestations

Preterm delivery
Intrauterine growth retardation
Preeclampsia
Premature rupture of membranes
Placenta previa
Abruptio placentae
Postpartum hemorrhage
Cord accidents
Congenital anomalies (increased frequency in monozygotic twins)

Complications Specific to Twins

Twin-to-twin transfusion syndrome (monochorionic twins)
Acardiac twinning (monochorionic twins)
Co-twin demise with twin embolization syndrome (monochorionic twins)
Cord entanglement (monoamniotic twins)
Conjoined twins

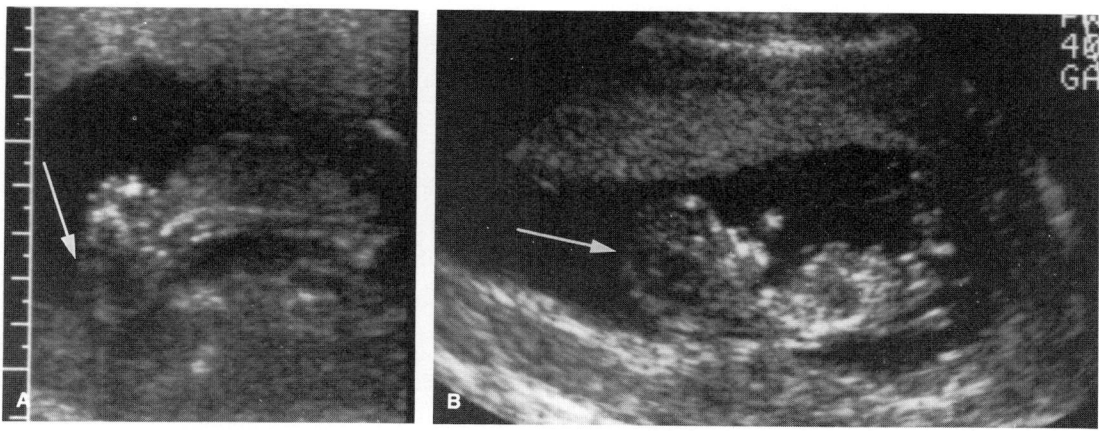

FIGURE 20-5.   Discordant anomaly in monozygotic twins. **(A)** Absent cranium in anencephalic twin A (*arrow*). **(B)** Twin B with normal cranium (*arrow*).

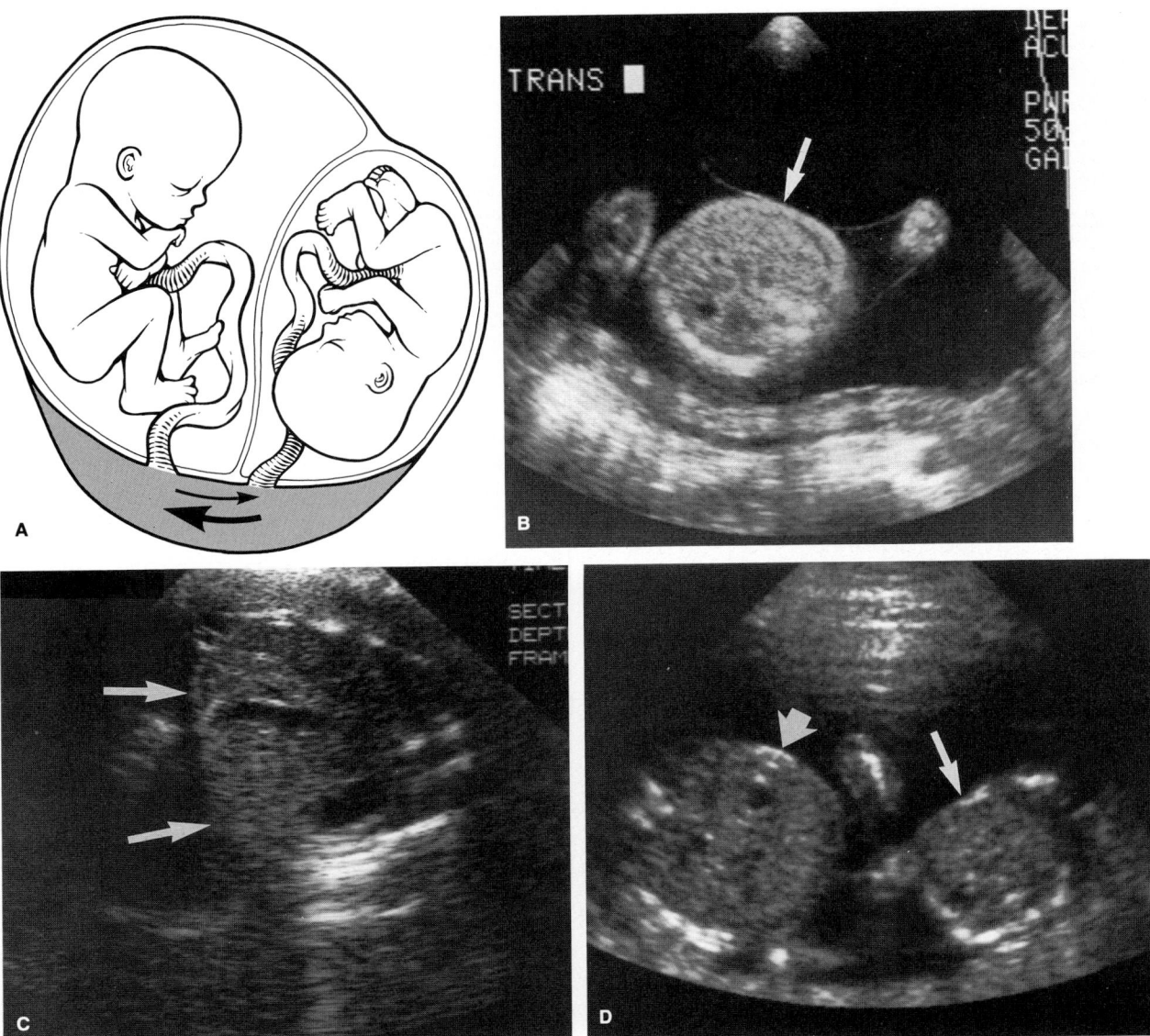

FIGURE 20-6. Twin-to-twin transfusion syndrome. **(A)** Arterial-to-venous anastomoses across the single placenta permit unbalanced exchange of blood between the twins, so that one becomes anemic and small and the other plethoric. The small, "donor" twin is surrounded by oligohydramnios, the larger, "recipient" twin by polyhydramnios. **(B)** Discrepant amniotic fluid volumes. Oligohydramnios surrounds the donor twin (*arrow*), while there is polyhydramnios in the recipient twin sac. (Benson CB, Doubilet PM: Sonography of multiple gestations. Radiol Clin North Am 1990; 28:149–161.) **(C)** Stuck twin. Sonogram demonstrates fetal abdomen (*arrows*) compressed against uterine wall by tightly applied membrane due to severe oligohydramnios. Severe polyhydramnios surrounds the co-twin. **(D)** Discordant fetal abdomens. Sonogram of twin abdomens shows donor twin abdomen (*long arrow*) is much smaller than recipient twin's (*short arrow*).

**TABLE 20-7.   Twin-to-Twin Transfusion Syndrome Versus
Intrauterine Growth Retardation of One Twin**

Diagnosis	Sonographic Features				
	EFW	AFV of Smaller	AFV of Larger	Hydrops in Larger	Chorionicity
Twin-to-twin transfusion syndrome	Discordant*	Oligohydramnios (may be "stuck")	Polyhydramnios	Sometimes	MC
Intrauterine growth retardation of one twin	Discordant*	Oligohydramnios	Normal	No	Any

* Difference in EFW at least 25% of larger EFW.

EFW, estimated fetal weight; AFV, amniotic fluid volume; MC, monochorionic.

tery-to-vein anastomoses in their common placenta. The sonographic features of twin-to-twin transfusion syndrome include discrepant amniotic fluid volumes and discordant fetal sizes[6–8] (Fig. 20-6). The anemic donor twin is small and has oligohydramnios. The oligohydramnios may be so severe that the donor twin is compressed against the uterine wall by the diamniotic membrane. When this occurs, the affected fetus is termed a *stuck twin* and has a poor prognosis. The polycythemic recipient twin usually is appropriate in size, has polyhydramnios, and may be hydropic. Discordance is best diagnosed when the difference in the estimated fetal weights between the twins is greater than 25% of the estimated weight of the larger twin.[9,10]

When discordant twins are encountered, the differential diagnosis is twin-to-twin transfusion syndrome versus intrauterine growth retardation of one, which can affect twins of any zygosity or placentation type[11] (Table 20-7). If the twins are dichorionic, the diagnosis must be intrauterine growth retardation of one. If the twins are monochorionic, the smaller twin has oligohydramnios, and the larger twin has polyhydramnios, twin-to-twin transfusion syndrome can be diagnosed.

Acardiac Twins

When large artery-to-artery and vein-to-vein anastomoses are present in a monochorionic twin gestation, the acardiac anomaly may occur. In such cases, one twin becomes the *pump twin,* supplying blood both to itself and to the acardiac co-twin. Blood flow in the co-twin is reversed in direction, with blood entering this twin through its umbilical artery and exiting through its umbilical vein. This leads to severe anomalies in the acardiac twin, including failure of development of a heart and poor or absent development of the upper extremities and head. The acardiac twin often has a two-vessel umbilical cord. The sonographic findings in acardiac twins are pathognomonic (Table 20-8; Fig. 20-7). The reversed direction of blood flow in the acardiac twin's umbilical vessels can be documented by Doppler.[12–14]

Conjoined Twins

Conjoined twins are rare, occurring in about 1 in 50,000 births. They are classified according to the location of conjoining (Fig. 20-8), with the most common sites being the anterior thoracic and abdominal walls. Conjoined twins are easily diagnosed by ultrasound, especially after the first trimester. Sonography is particularly useful for determining the location of conjoining and the extent of organ sharing (Figs. 20-9 and 20-10). This allows assessment of prognosis, surgical planning, and patient counseling before delivery.[15–18]

Demise of One Twin

When one twin dies in utero, the sonographic findings and risk to the co-twin depend on the chorionicity and the gestational age at the time of the demise (Table 20-9). When the demise occurs in the first trimester, the ultrasound appearance becomes that of a normal singleton pregnancy after several weeks, and the surviving co-twin is typically normal. This is sometimes referred to as the *vanishing twin phenomenon.* After demise later in

(*text continues on page 444*)

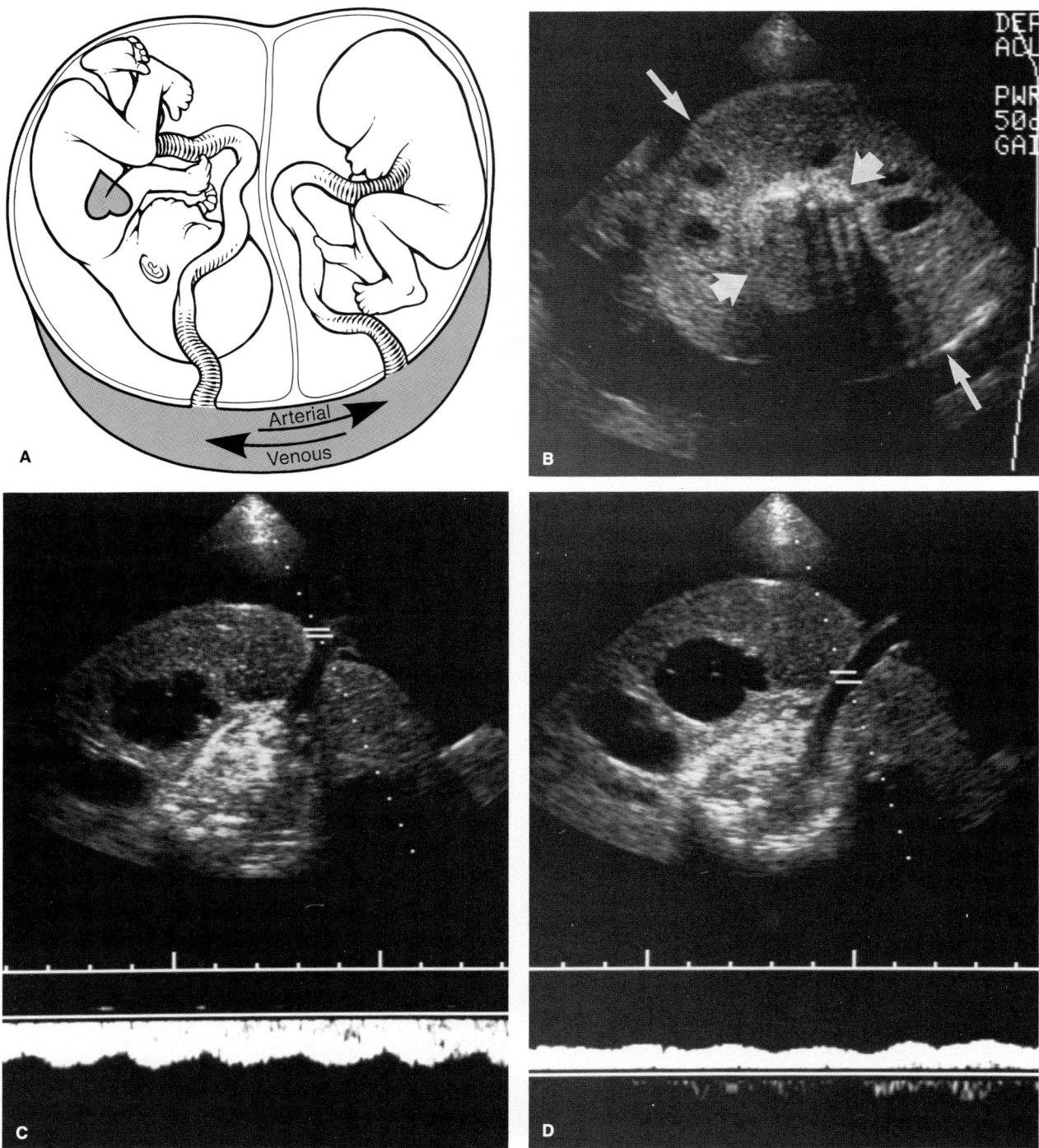

FIGURE 20-7.   Acardiac twinning. **(A)** Large artery-to-artery and vein-to-vein anastomoses across the common placenta result in reversed flow in the umbilical vessels, failure of development of the heart, and structural abnormalities in the acardiac twin. **(B)** Massive edema (*long arrows*) surrounds the acardiac twin abdomen (*short arrows*). **(C)** Umbilical artery Doppler demonstrates reversed flow in umbilical artery, toward the acardiac twin. **(D)** Umbilical vein Doppler demonstrates reversed flow in umbilical vein, away from the acardiac twin and toward the placenta. **(B–D:** Benson CB, Bieber FR, Genest DR, Doubilet PM: Doppler demonstration of reversed umbilical blood flow in an acardiac twin. J Clin Ultrasound 1989; 17:291–295.)

TABLE 20-8.   Sonographic Features of Acardiac Twinning

Acardiac Twin

Absent or rudimentary heart
Absent or malformed head
Absent or malformed upper extremities
Subcutaneous edema (often massive)
Two-vessel cord (common)
Reversed flow in umbilical artery (toward fetus)
  and vein (away from fetus)

Pump Twin

Normal or increased amniotic fluid
May be hydropic

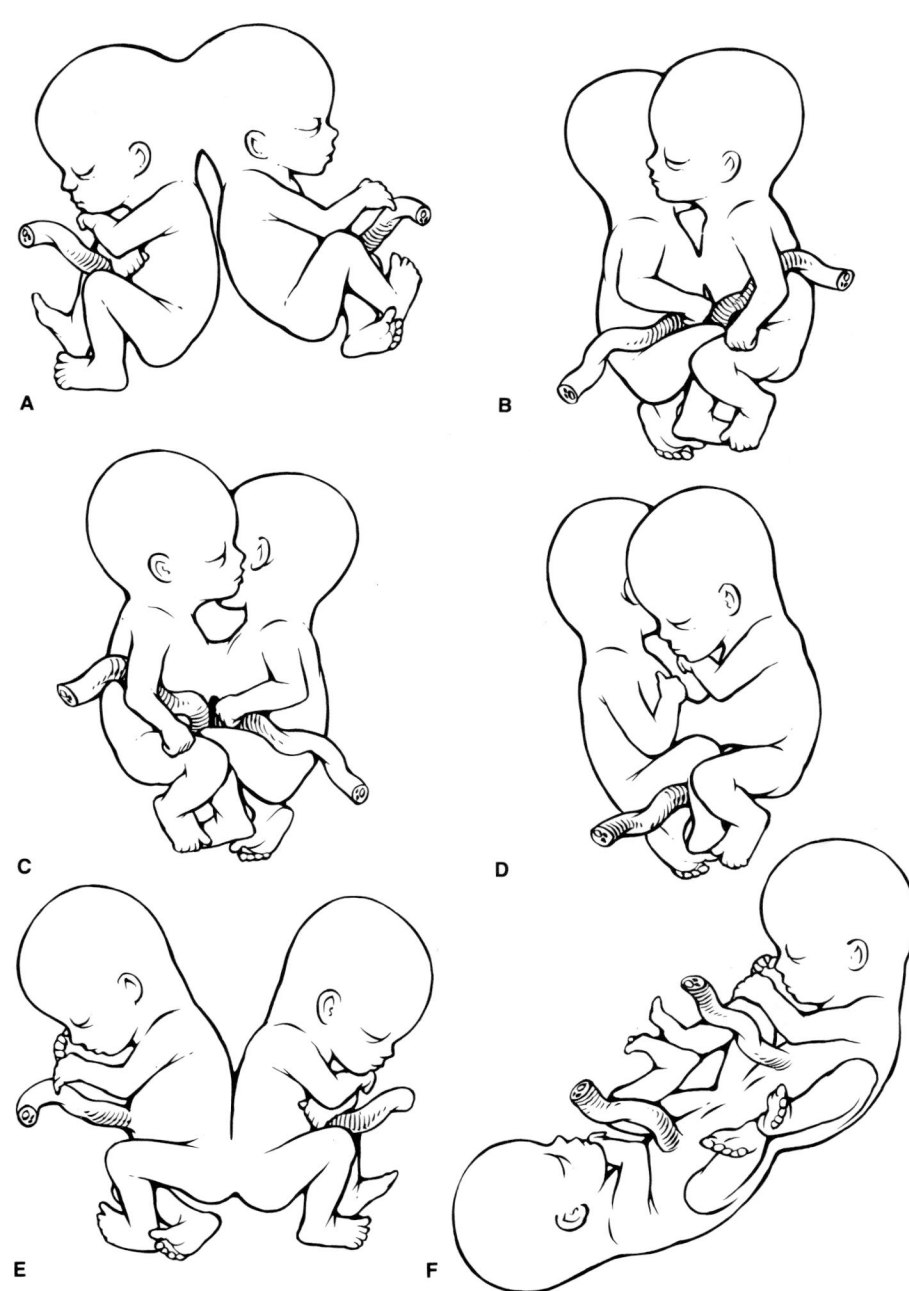

FIGURE 20-8. Most common forms of conjoined twins. Incomplete division of the fertilized ovum leads to conjoined twins with shared organs. **(A)** Craniopagus twins are joined at the head. **(B)** Xiphopagus twins are joined at the xiphoid. **(C)** Thoracopagus twins are joined at the thorax. **(D)** Omphalopagus twins are joined across the anterior abdomen. **(E)** Pygopagus twins are joined at the pelvis—facing away. **(F)** Ischiopagus twins are joined at the pelvis—opposed. (Modified from Mariona FG: Anomalies specific to multiple gestations. In Chervenak FA, Isaacson VS, Campbell S [eds]: Ultrasound in Obstetrics and Gynecology. Boston: Little, Brown, 1993: 1051–1062.)

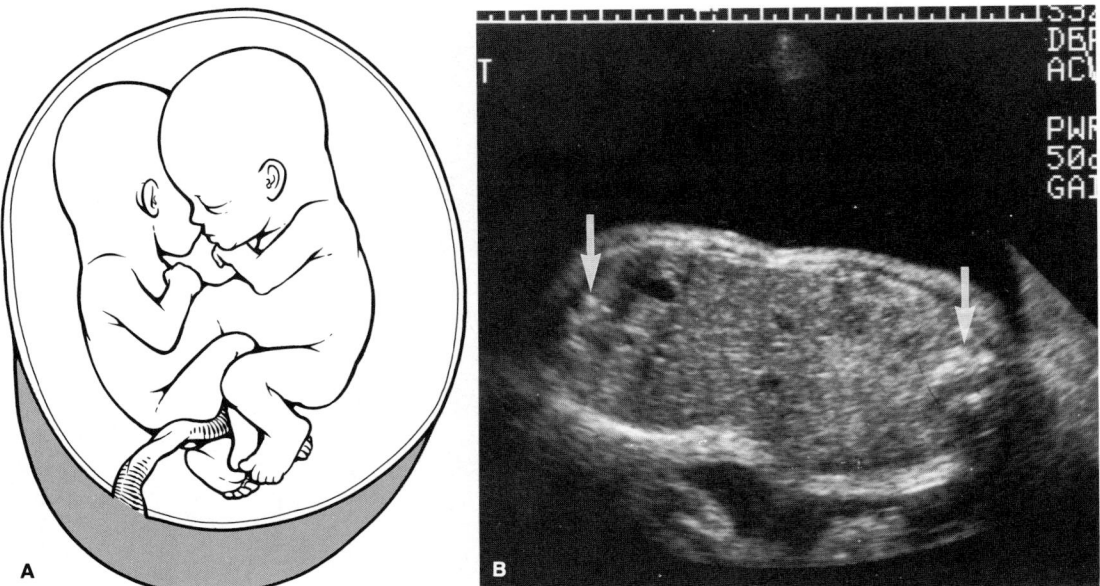

FIGURE 20-9. Omphalopagus twins. Transverse sonogram of conjoined twin abdomens demonstrates separate spines (*arrows*) with joining across anterior abdomen. (Benson CB, Doubilet PM: Sonography of multiple gestations. Radiol Clin North Am 1990; 28:149–161.)

gestation, the dead twin remains visible (Fig. 20-11). If the pregnancy is monochorionic, the surviving co-twin, while usually normal, rarely exhibits findings of twin embolization syndrome or disseminated intravascular coagulation. Twin embolization syndrome typically occurs after a second trimester demise of one twin. Emboli pass from the dead to the living twin through placental anastomoses and cause ischemia, infarction, or even death of the second twin.[3,19–23] Thromboembolic insults may result in porencephaly, hydranencephaly, or microcephaly (see Chapter 8). In addition, limb amputations, intestinal atresias, and even cardiac malformations have been attributed to thromboembolic insults. Because of the potential for twin embolization syndrome, selective termination of one twin is usually avoided when the gestation is monochorionic.

PROGNOSIS

Since complications of twinning vary with placentation type, the prognosis of a twin gestation depends on its chorionicity and amnionicity[1] (Table 20-10). Among twin pregnancies diagnosed in the first trimester with sonographic demonstration of two heartbeats, dichorionic twins have a better prognosis than monochorionic twins. Dichorionic

gestations result in two live-born infants more often, and complete pregnancy loss less often, than monochorionic gestations, with both groups having a similar frequency of live-born singletons.[19] Twins diagnosed later in pregnancy or at delivery have a higher perinatal mortality if they are monochorionic than if they are dichorionic (see Table 20-10). Monoamniotic twins have the highest perinatal mortality of all placentation types.[1]

GESTATIONAL AGE ASSESSMENT

Sonographic measurements of the fetuses in a twin gestation can be used to assign gestational age and to estimate and compare growth. In the second trimester, measurements of the fetal body parts are the same in twins as in singletons of the same gestational age (Table 20-11). In the third trimester, this remains true for the femur length, but data are conflicting concerning the biparietal diameter. Some studies have found no difference between twin and singleton biparietal diameter measurements, while others have found that biparietal diameter in twins lags behind that of singletons as the third trimester progresses. When dating twin gestations, therefore, singleton tables or formulas for femur length are accurate for dating throughout the second and third trimesters. Those for bi-

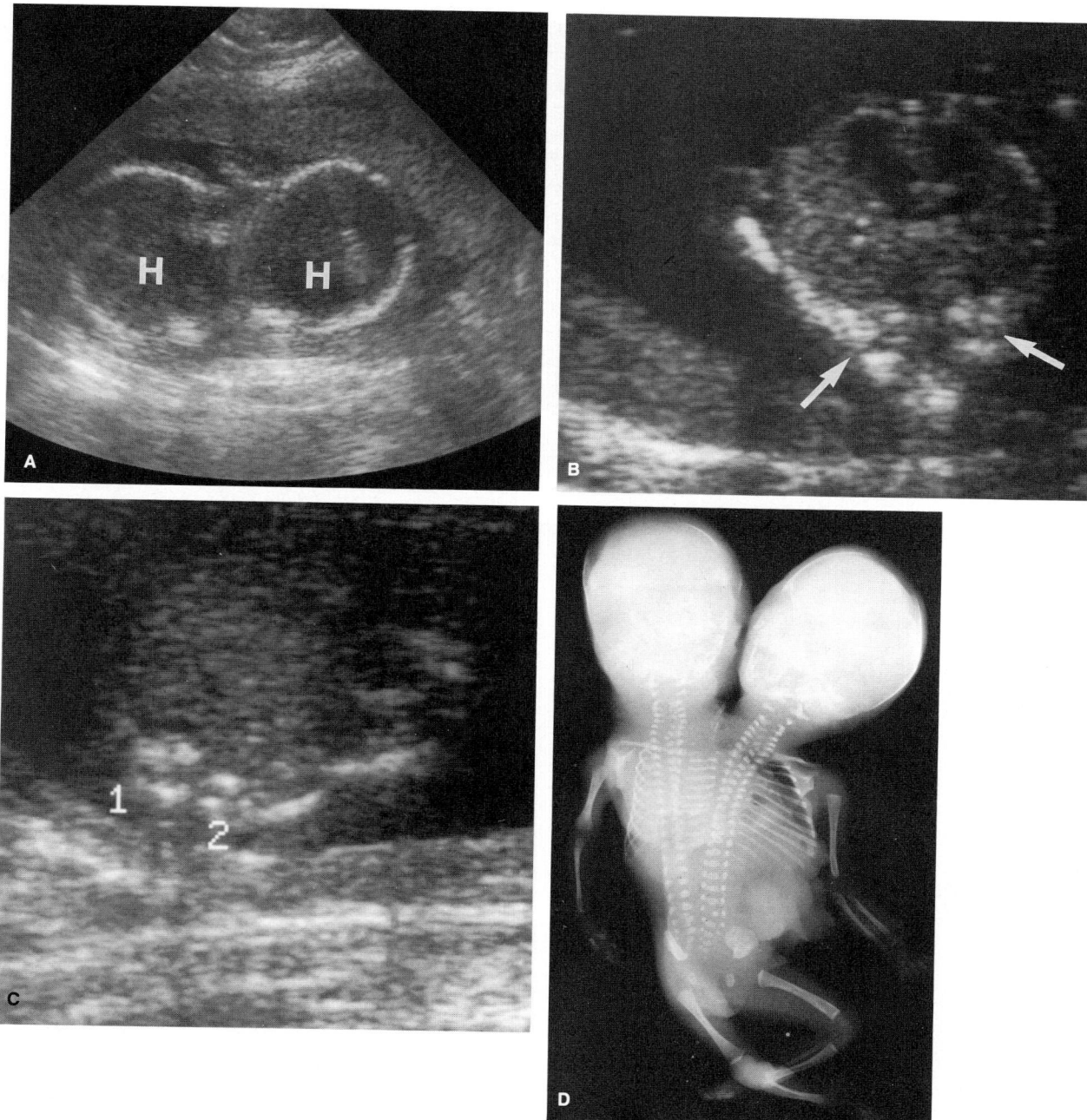

FIGURE 20-10.   Thoracoomphalopagus twins. **(A)** Ultrasound demonstrates two separate heads (H). **(B)** Scans demonstrate fusion of the two thoraces with two separate spines (*arrows*). **(C)** Scans show fusion of the abdomen with two separate spines (1 and 2). **(D)** Postnatal radiograph. (Courtesy of John P. McGahan, MD, Sacramento, CA.)

TABLE 20-9.   Demise of One Twin

Age at Demise	Sonographic Appearance		Risk to Surviving Co-Twin
	Early	*Late*	
< 6 weeks	Empty gestational sac	No evidence of prior twin	Minimal
6–13 weeks	Embryo or fetus with no heartbeat	No evidence of prior twin	Minimal
Second trimester	Fetus with no heartbeat	Fetus papyraceous	Minimal if DC; twin embolization syndrome if MC (rare)
Third trimester	Fetus with no heartbeat	Macerated fetus	Preterm labor; obstructed delivery; DIC if MC (rare)

DC, dichorionic; MC, monochorionic; DIC, disseminated intravascular coagulation.

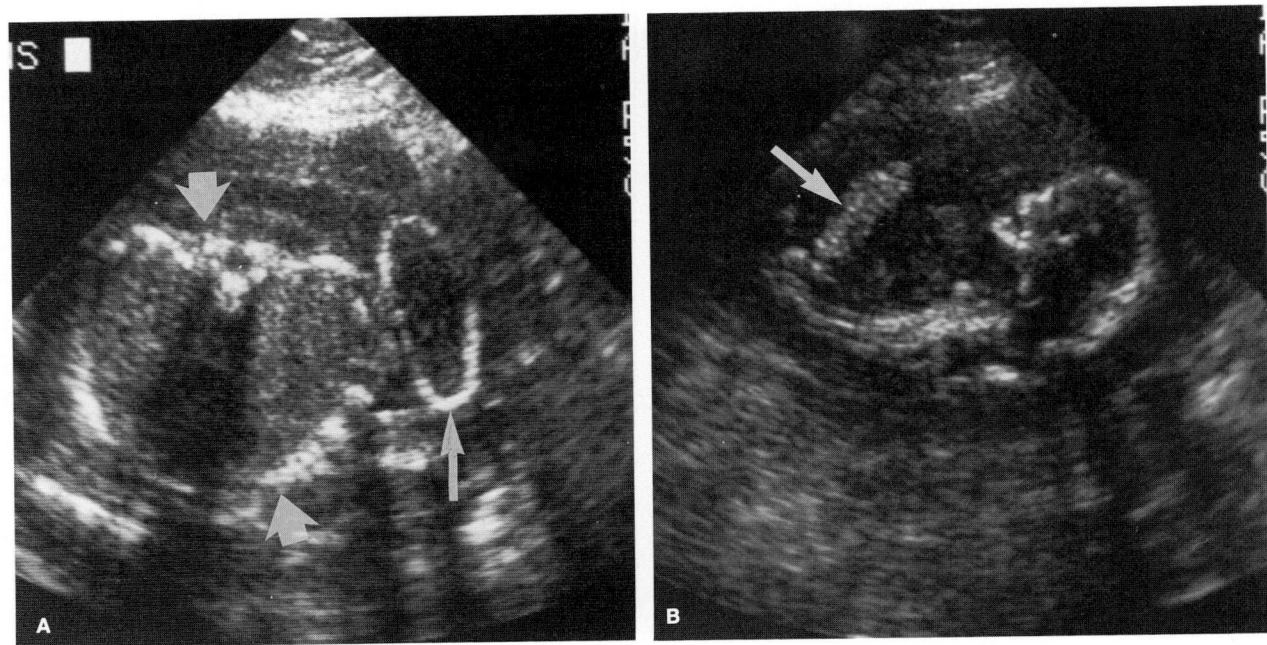

FIGURE 20-11.   Fetus papyraceus. **(A)** Head of paper-thin fetus (*long arrow*) is compressed against uterine wall by surviving co-twin (*short arrows*). **(B)** Longitudinal view of fetus papyraceus demonstrates head and spine still visible with echogenic (thrombosed) umbilical cord (*arrow*) extending anteriorly. (Benson CB, Doubilet PM: Sonography of multiple gestations. Radiol Clin North Am 1990; 28:149–161.)

TABLE 20-10.   Outcome of Twin Gestations

Twins With Heartbeats by First-Trimester Ultrasound

Placentation Type	Pregnancy Outcome—Live Births (%)			Live Birth Rate per Fetus
	Two	One	None	
DC, DA	83	12	5	89
MC, DA	56	11	33	61

Twins Diagnosed Later in Pregnancy

Placentation Type	Survival Rate Per Twin (%)
DC, DA	91
MC, DA	75
MC, MA	50

DC, dichorionic; DA, diamniotic; MC, monochorionic; MA, monoamniotic.

parietal diameter are accurate at least through the end of the second trimester. Twin-specific tables may be preferable when using biparietal diameter to assign gestational age in the third trimester.[3,24–27]

ULTRASOUND-GUIDED INVASIVE PROCEDURES

Ultrasound can be used to guide a number of procedures in multiple gestations. Twin amniocenteses are usually accomplished by two separate needle insertions, with injection of dye after the first insertion to confirm that the second needle has entered the second sac. When one fetus is abnormal, selective termination may be accomplished by guiding a needle into the fetal heart and injecting potassium chloride. A similar technique has been applied in multiple gestations of three or more fetuses to reduce the number of fetuses and thus enhance the survival chances of the remaining ones.[28] Such reduction procedures should be approached with caution and, in particular, should be avoided in monochorionic gestations.[29]

ULTRASOUND EXAMINATION

The sonographic examination of a twin pregnancy should consist of two separate singleton examinations, together with evaluation of a number of features that are specific to twin gestations (Table 20-12). The latter includes assessment of placentation type, comparison of two fetal sizes, and comparison of amniotic fluid volumes.

TABLE 20-11.   Measurements in Twin Versus Singleton Pregnancies

Measure	Second Trimester	Third Trimester
Biparietal diameter	Twin = singleton	Conflicting studies
Femur length	Twin = singleton	Twin = singleton
Abdominal circumference	Twin = singleton	Twin < singleton

TABLE 20-12.   Ultrasound of Twin Gestations

Fetal anatomic surveys
  If conjoined, assess extent of conjoining and organ sharing.
Fetal measurements
  Assign gestational age.
  Compare estimated fetal weights.
Fetal positions
Placental locations
Assess Chorionicity
  Number of placental masses
  Fetal sexes
  Membrane thickness
Assess amnionicity
  Presence of membrane
  Intermingling of cords
Compare amniotic fluid volumes
Guide procedures
  Amniocentesis
  Chorionic villous sampling
  Selective termination
  Multifetal pregnancy reduction

REFERENCES

1. Benirschke K, Kim CK: Multiple pregnancy, part I. N Engl J Med 1973; 288:1276–1284.

2. Benirschke K, Kim CK: Multiple pregnancy, part II. N Engl J Med 1973; 288:1329–1336.

3. Benson CB, Doubilet PM: Ultrasound of multiple gestations. Semin Roentgenol 1991; 26:50–61.

4. Chitkara UN, Berkowitz RL: Assessment of multiple pregnancy. In Chervenak FA, Isaacson VC, Campbell S (eds): Ultrasound in Obstetrics and Gynecology. Boston: Little, Brown, 1993: 413–420.

5. Townsend RR, Simpson GF, Filly RA: Membrane thickness in ultrasound prediction of chorionicity of twin gestations. J Ultrasound Med 1988; 7:327–332.

6. Brown DL, Benson CB, Driscoll SG, Doubilet PM: Twin-twin transfusion syndrome: Sonographic findings. Radiology 1989; 170:61–63.

7. Arts VFTh, Lohman AH: The vascular anatomy of monochorionic diamniotic twin placentas and the transfusion syndrome. Eur J Obstet Gynecol 1971; 3:85–93.

8. Pretorius DH, Manchester D, Barkin S, et al: Doppler ultrasound of twin transfusion syndrome. J Ultrasound Med 1988; 7:117–124.

9. Storlazzi E, Vintzileos AM, Campbell WA, et al: Ultrasonic diagnosis of discordant fetal growth in twin gestations. Obstet Gynecol 1987; 69:363–367.

10. Divon MY, Girz BA, Sklar A, et al: Discordant twins: A prospective study of the diagnostic value of real-time ultrasonography combined with umbilical artery velocimetry. Am J Obstet Gynecol 1989; 161:757–760.

11. Crane JP, Tomich PG, Kopt AM: Ultrasonic growth patterns in normal and discordant twins. Obstet Gynecol 1980; 55:678–683.

12. Benson CB, Bieber FR, Genest DR, Doubilet PM: Doppler demonstration of reversed umbilical blood flow in an acardiac twin. J Clin Ultrasound 1989; 17:291–295.

13. Benirschke K, Harper VDR: The acardiac anomaly. Teratology 1977; 15:311–316.

14. Pretorius DH, Leopold GR, Moore TR, et al: Acardiac twin report of Doppler sonography. J Ultrasound Med 1988; 7:413–416.

15. Fitzgerald EJ, Toi A, Cochlin DL: Conjoined twins: Antenatal ultrasound diagnosis and a review of the literature. Br J Radiol 1985; 58:1053–1056.

16. Sakala EP: Obstetric management of conjoined twins. Obstet Gynecol 1986; 67:21S–25S.

17. Kalchbrenner M, Weiner S, Templeton J, Losure TA: Prenatal ultrasound diagnosis of thoracopagus conjoined twins. J Clin Ultrasound 1987; 15:59–63.

18. Mariona FG: Anomalies specific to multiple gestations. In Chervenak FA, Isaacson VS, Campbell S (eds): Ultrasound in Obstetrics and Gynecology. Boston: Little, Brown, 1993: 1051–1062.

19. Benson CB, Doubilet PM: Outcome of twin gestations following sonographic demonstration of two heartbeats in the first trimester. Ultrasound Obstet Gynecol 1993; 3:343–345.

20. Landy HJ, Weiner S, Corson SL, et al: The "vanishing twin": Ultrasonographic assessment of fetal disappearance in the first trimester. Am J Obstet Gynecol 1986; 155:14–19.

21. Landy HJ, Weingold AB: Management of a multiple gestation complicated by an antepartum fetal demise. Obstet Gynecol Surv 1989; 44:171–176.

22. Jauniaux E, Elkazen N, Leroy F, et al: Clinical and morphologic aspects of the vanishing twin phenomenon. Obstet Gynecol 1988; 72:577–581.

23. Patten RM, Mack LA, Nyberg DA, Filly RA: Twin embolization syndrome: Prenatal sonographic detection and significance. Radiology 1989; 173:685–689.

24. Grumback K, Coleman BG, Arger PH, et al: Twin and singleton growth patterns compared using ultrasound. Radiology 1986; 158:237–241.

25. Socol ML, Tamura RK, Sabbagha RE, et al: Diminished biparietal diameter and abdominal circumference growth in twins. Obstet Gynecol 1984; 64:235–238.

26. Reece EA, Yarkoni S, Abdalla M, et al: A prospective longitudinal study of growth in twin gestations compared with growth in singleton pregnancies. I. The fetal head. J Ultrasound Med 1991; 10:439–443.

27. Reece EA, Yarkoni S, Abdalla M, et al: A prospective longitudinal study of growth in twin gestations compared with growth in singleton pregnancies. II. The fetal limbs. J Ultrasound Med 1991; 10:445–450.

28. Benson CB, Doubilet PM: Sonography of multiple gestations. Radiol Clin North Am 1990; 28:149–161.

29. Golbus MS: Selective termination. In Harrison MR, Golbus MS, Filly RA (eds): The Unborn Patient: Prenatal Diagnosis and Treatment. Philadelphia: WB Saunders, 1991: 166–171.

John P. McGahan and Manuel Porto:
DIAGNOSTIC OBSTETRICAL ULTRASOUND.
© 1994 J.B. Lippincott Company.

Lyndon M. Hill

Chapter 21

Chromosomal Abnormalities

The sonographer and sonologist are confronted with chromosomal abnormalities in fetuses considerably more frequently than is the neonatologist. Chromosomal abnormalities are present in 50% of first-trimester spontaneous abortions, 5% of stillbirths, and 0.5% of live births. This marked reduction in prevalence is due to the high rate of attrition as gestation advances. For example, the incidence of trisomy 21 at amniocentesis is about 33% higher than the estimate of live-born rates.[1] Fewer than 30% of trisomy 21, 5% of trisomy 18, and 3% of trisomy 13 fetuses survive to birth.[2] Maternal age–specific rates for chromosomal abnormalities found at chorionic villus sampling, at amniocentesis, and at birth are provided in Table 21-1.

This chapter provides a systematic approach to the sonographic evaluation of the anomalous fetus. In an attempt to narrow the differential diagnosis once a pattern of anomalies has been detected, specific criteria relative to each of the more common chromosomal abnormalities are provided. Since an ultrasound examination should not be carried out without pertinent maternal history, clinical information that will assist the sonographer and sonologist in evaluation of the fetus is also reviewed.

INDICATIONS FOR FETAL KARYOTYPING

Advanced Maternal Age

It is neither technically feasible nor appropriate to determine the chromosome complement of every fetus; however, well-established guidelines are available to assist couples in making an assessment of their risk for abnormal offspring.

The risk of carrying a fetus with an autosomal trisomy, XXY karyotype, or XXX karyotype significantly increases with maternal age. For the autosomal trisomies, this rise is followed by a leveling off at the upper end of the age range (Table 21-2). In contrast to the autosomal trisomies, there is a significant inverse relation with maternal age for cases of 45,X (discussed later). The greater the chromosomal abnormality, the greater is the chance that a spontaneous abortion will occur before the second trimester. Older mothers may

449

TABLE 21-1. Crude Maternal Age–Specific Rate for All Chromosomal Abnormalities

Maternal Age (y)	From Live-Born Studies (%)*		From Amniocenteses (%)†		From CVS (%)‡
	47, +21	All Chromosome Abnormalities	47, +21	All Chromosome Abnormalities	All Chromosome Abnormalities
33	0.16	0.29	0.24	0.48	—
34	0.20	0.36	0.30	0.66	—
35	0.26	0.49	0.40	0.76	0.78
36	0.33	0.60	0.52	0.95	0.80
37	0.44	0.77	0.67	1.20	2.58
38	0.57	0.97	0.87	1.54	3.82
39	0.73	1.23	1.12	1.89	2.67
40	0.94	1.59	1.45	2.50	3.40
41	1.23	2.00	1.89	3.23	6.11
42	1.56	2.56	2.44	4.00	8.05
43	2.00	3.33	3.23	5.26	5.15
44	2.63	4.17	4.00	6.67	10.00
45	3.33	5.26	5.26	8.33	7.14

All values expressed as percentages. CVS, chorionic villus sampling.

* Estimated live-born statistics.[76]

† Data compiled from 20,000 genetic amnioscenteses.[76]

‡ Data derived from 4,122 chorionic villus samplings, corrected for unconfirmed aberrations, especially mosaicism.[77]

(Hsu LYF: Prenatal diagnosis of chromosomal abnormalities through amniocentesis. In Milunsky A [ed]: Genetic Disorders and the Fetus: Diagnosis, Prevention and Treatment. Baltimore: Johns Hopkins University Press, 1992.)

spontaneously abort aneuploid conceptions more readily than younger mothers.[1]

The determination that 35 years of age or older at the time of delivery indicated *advanced maternal age* was made when only 5-year-interval risk figures were available. With 1-year-interval risk figures, more accurate, nondirective counseling is possible (Table 21-3).

Advanced Paternal Age

Previous studies suggested a relation between Down's syndrome and advanced paternal age.[3] More recent evidence is against a significant independent effect of increased paternal age on maternal age–specific rates for trisomy 18 and trisomy 21.[1]

Familial Chromosomal Abnormality

The risk that parents with a balanced structural rearrangement will have offspring with an unbalanced chromosome complement varies between 5% and 12%.

Previous Pregnancy With a Chromosomal Abnormality

There does not appear to be an increased risk of chromosomal abnormalities in future pregnancies after spontaneous abortions with trisomies that are always lethal in utero.[4] If a previous child has a noninherited chromosomal aberration (eg, trisomy 13, 18, or 21), the recurrence risk is between 1% and 2%.[5]

MATERNAL SERUM SCREENING FOR CHROMOSOMAL DEFECTS

Specific maternal serum triple-screen patterns have been associated with Down's syndrome[6] and trisomy 18; these include α-fetoprotein, unconjugated estriol, and human chorionic gonadotropin.[7]

Advanced maternal age and an abnormal maternal serum triple screen have been found to be independent risk factors for trisomy 21. Hence, using both parameters allows detection of a higher number of trisomy 21 fetuses than either parame-

TABLE 21-2. Crude Maternal Age–Specific Rates for Chromosomal Abnormalities in Pregnancies Monitored by Amniocentesis Because of Maternal Age ≥ 35 Years

Maternal Age (y)	No. of Pregnancies	Autosomal Aberrations (%)			Sex Chromosome Aberrations (%)	
		+21	*+18*	*+13*	*XXX*	*XXY*
35	5409	0.35	0.07	0.05	0.07	0.09
36	6103	0.57	0.08	0.03	0.08	0.08
37	6956	0.68	0.09	0.03	0.07	0.04
38	7926	0.81	0.15	0.04	0.08	0.08
39	7682	1.09	0.19	0.06	0.12	0.16
40	7174	1.23	0.25	0.12	0.06	0.15
41	4763	1.47	0.36	0.17	0.15	0.29
42	3156	2.19	0.63	0.19	0.28	0.35
43	1912	3.24	0.78	0.05	0.31	0.31
44	1015	2.95	0.49	—	0.49	0.39
45	508	4.53	0.39	0.20	0.39	0.98
46	232	8.19	0.43	—	0.43	1.29
>46	129	2.33	0.77	—	1.55	1.55
≥35	52,965	1.16	0.23	0.07	0.12	0.16

Values expressed as rate per 1000 pregnancies.

(Modified from Ferguson-Smith MA, Yates JRW: Maternal age specific rates for chromosome aberrations and factors influencing them: Report of a collaborative European study on 52,965 amniocenteses. Prenat Diagn 1984; 4:5–44.)

ter alone.[8] The screening of all women with either advanced maternal age or an age-adjusted triple screen, indicating an increase risk for Down's syndrome, would detect about 60% of Down's syndrome fetuses but would require the testing (ie, amniocentesis) of 4% to 8% of normal pregnancies.[9]

Ultrasound has an important role to play in any maternal serum triple-screen protocol. Accurate fetal dating is obviously necessary to properly interpret any maternal serum triple screen value. With an expected detection rate at my institution of about 95% for open neural tube defects, a targeted ultrasound examination has become the primary means of evaluating abnormally high maternal serum triple screens. Although a thorough review of this topic is beyond the scope of this chapter, Table 21-4 illustrates the likelihood of either a neural tube defect or a ventral wall defect given different maternal screening α-fetoprotein values and a negative ultrasonographic examination of 95% sensitivity. The reliability of an ultrasound examination to detect trisomy 21 and trisomy 18 is reviewed in subsequent sections of this chapter.

SONOGRAPHIC DETECTION OF CHROMOSOMAL ABNORMALITIES

No single anomaly is pathognomonic for a given chromosomal abnormality. Fetuses with an abnormal karyotype, however, are usually characterized by multiple malformations. Consequently, a careful anatomic survey with the delineation of several abnormalities may provide the astute sonographer or sonologist with sufficient clues to reduce the differential diagnosis. For example, the incidence of a two-vessel umbilical cord is increased with Turner's syndrome, trisomy 13, and trisomy 18, but not with trisomy 21. Hence, the detection of a cystic hygroma and a two-vessel umbilical cord would suggest the former chromosomal abnormalities rather than trisomy 21.

Although virtually any organ system may be affected, abnormal facial features (eg, cleft lip or palate, micrognathia, microphthalmia, low-set and misshapen ears) and digital anomalies (eg, overlapping fingers, clinodactyly, polydactyly, syndactyly) suggest the presence of a trisomic fetus.

Abnormally short ears have been noted in chil-

TABLE 21-3.   Risk of Having a Live-Born Child With Down's Syndrome by 1-Year Maternal Age Intervals From Ages 20 to 49 Years

Maternal Age (y)	Risk of Down's Syndrome
20	1/1923
21	1/1695
22	1/1538
23	1/1408
24	1/1299
25	1/1205
26	1/1124
27	1/1053
28	1/990
29	1/935
30	1/885
31	1/826
32	1/725
33	1/592
34	1/465
35	1/365
36	1/287
37	1/225
38	1/177
39	1/139
40	1/109
41	1/85
42	1/67
43	1/53
44	1/41
45	1/32
46	1/25
47	1/20
48	1/16
49	1/12

(Simpson JL: Antenatal diagnosis of cytogenetic abnormalities. Clin Obstet Gynecol 1981; 24:1023.)

dren with various aneuploidies. Lettieri and associates established a nomogram for ear length between 14 and 25 weeks' gestation; 10 of 14 aneuploidy fetuses (71%) had an ear length at or below the 10th percentile.[10]

The gestational ages at which specific fetal organs can be visualized sonographically have been established. A knowledge of the gestational age window during which a specific anomaly appears, as well as an understanding of an abnormality's natural history or evolution, is essential for appropriate fetal assessment. For example, the resolution of a first-trimester cystic hygroma does not indicate that the fetus is chromosomally normal.[11] Because of the high association between cystic hy-

gromas and chromosomal abnormalities, karyotyping should always be recommended[12] (Fig. 21-1).

The sonographic evaluation of congenital anomalies may be approached from two perspectives. First, the sonographer or sonologist should be familiar with the prevalence of chromosomal abnormalities given a particular sonographic finding. Second, the examiner should be aware of the typical clinical, pathologic, and sonographic features of the more common chromosomal abnormalities. A working knowledge of both scenarios provides maximal flexibility not only for diagnostic purposes but also for subsequent family counseling.

SPECTRUM OF AUTOSOMAL TRISOMIES

Since 60% of live-born infants with chromosomal abnormalities are trisomic,[13] this chapter emphasizes the sonographic detection of these specific chromosomal anomalies. A fetus may be trisomic for either an entire chromosome or only a portion of a chromosome (*partial trisomy*). Mosaicism of a trisomic cell line may occur. Each of these trisomic fetuses may present with different or similar sonographic manifestations. In addition, phenotypic variation may occur among fetuses with identical autosomal chromosomal abnormalities.

Trisomy for all chromosomes except chromosome 1 have been described. Thirty-one percent of all trisomies are trisomy 16.[2] Most trisomic fetuses do not survive into the second trimester. Infants with trisomy 8[14] or 9[15] are sufficiently rare to qualify for case reports and therefore are not reviewed here. The following sections will focus on the three trisomies that are most frequently seen in the neonatal period: trisomies 13, 18, and 21.

Trisomy 13 (Patau's Syndrome)

Although the incidence of this autosomal trisomy is about 1 in 5000 births,[16] 1.1% of spontaneously aborted fetuses are trisomy 13.[17] The congenital malformations associated with trisomy 13 were first described in 1960 by Patau and associates.[18]

Since most series of trisomic fetuses are relatively small, the types of abnormalities detected and their reported incidence should be considered neither definitive nor accurate. Rather, the organ systems that are most frequently involved should be noted. Table 21-5 lists the sonographically detectable abnormalities from one report of nine trisomy 13 fetuses.

TABLE 21-4. Risks of Open Spina Bifida and Ventral Wall Defects by Population Incidence and Maternal Serum AFP in Patients Who Had a Negative Ultrasonographic Examination of 95% Sensitivity*

AFP Multiples of Median	Ventral Wall Defect Only	Prior Incidence of Open Spina Bifida per 1000†								
		0.1	0.2	0.4	0.8	1.0	2.0	3.5	5.0	25.0
2.0	3600.0	18000.0	9000.0	4500.0	2300.0	1800.0	900.0	510.0	360.0	71.0
	16000.0	**79000.0**	**39000.0**	**20000.0**	**9800.0**	**7900.0**	**3900.0**	**2200.0**	**1600.0**	**310.0**
	69000.0	340000.0	170000.0	86000.0	43000.0	34000.0	17000.0	9800.0	6800.0	1300.0
2.5	1500.0	4700.0	2400.0	1200.0	590.0	470.0	240.0	140.0	95.0	19.0
	6300.0	**21000.0**	**10000.0**	**5100.0**	**2600.0**	**2100.0**	**1000.0**	**590.0**	**410.0**	**81.0**
	28000.0	90000.0	45000.0	22000.0	11000.0	9000.0	4500.0	2600.0	1800.0	350.0
3.0	590.0	1500.0	740.0	370.0	190.0	150.0	75.0	43.0	31.0	6.8
	2600.0	**6500.0**	**3200.0**	**1600.0**	**810.0**	**650.0**	**320.0**	**190.0**	**130.0**	**26.0**
	11000.0	28000.0	14000.0	700.0	3500.0	2800.0	1400.0	800.0	560.0	110.0
3.5	250.0	530.0	270.0	130.0	68.0	54.0	28.0	16.0	12.0	3.1
	1100.0	**2300.0**	**1200.0**	**580.0**	**290.0**	**230.0**	**120.0**	**67.0**	**47.0**	**10.0**
	4700.0	10000.0	5100.0	2500.0	1300.0	1000.0	510.0	290.0	200.0	41.0
4.0	110.0	210.0	110.0	54.0	28.0	22.0	12.0	7.1	5.2	1.8
	470.0	**930.0**	**460.0**	**230.0**	**120.0**	**94.0**	**47.0**	**27.0**	**19.0**	**4.6**
	2000.0	4000.0	2000.0	1000.0	510.0	400.0	200.0	120.0	81.0	17.0
4.5	50.0	93.0	47.0	24.0	13.0	10.0	5.6	3.6	2.8	1.4
	210.0	**400.0**	**200.0**	**100.0**	**51.0**	**41.0**	**21.0**	**12.0**	**9.0**	**2.6**
	930.0	1800.0	880.0	440.0	220.0	180.0	88.0	51.0	36.0	7.8
5.0	24.0	44.0	22.0	12.0	6.3	5.3	3.1	2.2	1.9	1.2
	100.0	**190.0**	**94.0**	**48.0**	**24.0**	**20.0**	**10.0**	**6.3**	**4.7**	**1.7**
	440.0	810.0	410.0	200.0	100.0	82.0	42.0	24.0	17.0	4.2

* The left-hand column gives risks of ventral wall defect and the other columns give risks of open spina bifida for various prior population incidences. At each level of maternal serum AFP and prior probability of open spina bifida, three figures are given. The upper figure assumes that ultrasonography provides no information beyond maternal serum AFP ($\gamma = 0$); the lower figure assumes ultrasonography is completely independent of maternal serum AFP ($\gamma = 1$); and the middle figure in boldface type assumes $\gamma = 0.5$ and is our best estimate of any individual woman's true risk.

† With prior incidence of open spina bifida per 1,000 is a theoretical risk expressed for different populations. The risk values obtained on this chart are expressed as 1 divided by the value. For instance, at two multiples of the median AFP the risk of a ventral wall defect would be 1/16,000. Similarly, for 5 multiples of the median the risk of a ventral wall defect would be 1/100.

AFP, α-fetoprotein.

(Thornton JG, et al: Tables for estimation of individual risks of fetal neural tube and ventral wall defects, incorporating prior probability, maternal α-fetoprotein levels, and ultrasonographic examination results. Am J Obstet Gynecol 1991; 164:154–160.)

When compared with other autosomal trisomies, fetuses with trisomy 13 tend to have more severe craniofacial (hypotelorism, eye anomalies, cleft lip and palate) and brain (holoprosencephaly) abnormalities (Figs. 21-2 and 21-3).

About half of all fetuses with alobar holoprosencephaly have trisomy 13[19] (Fig. 21-4).

Because of the high prevalence rate of congenital heart disease, fetal echocardiography plays an important role in the evaluation of the fetus suspected of having an autosomal trisomy. Although fetal karyotyping is the definitive test, it does not predict normal cardiac anatomy. Since there is an association between extracardiac malformations and congenital heart disease, fetal echocardiography should be obtained whenever a major structural abnormality is detected.[20]

The number and severity of congenital anomalies associated with trisomy 13 is highly variable. Monozygotic trisomy 13 twins with discordant major anomalies have been reported.[21] Cases with trisomy 13 mosaicism may have a near-normal phenotype or the full pattern of congenital anomalies seen in trisomy 13.[16]

Patau and colleagues originally noted a relation between trisomy 13 and fetal growth retardation.[18] Subsequent ultrasound studies have confirmed the

(text continues on page 457)

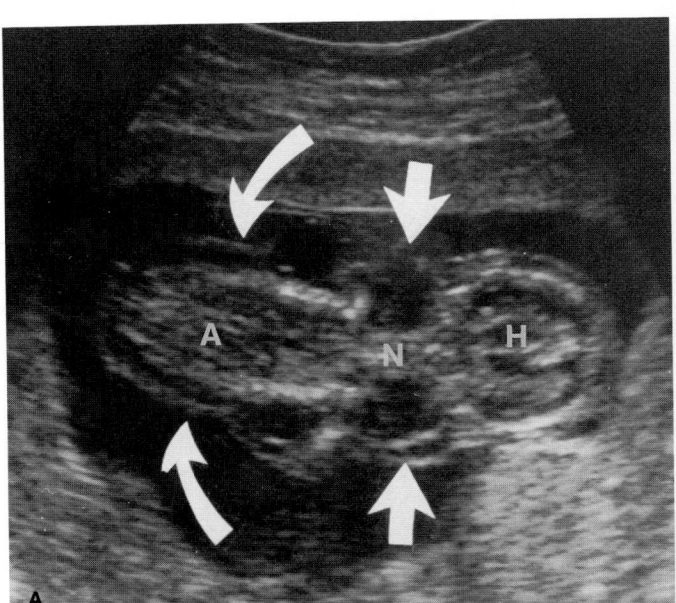
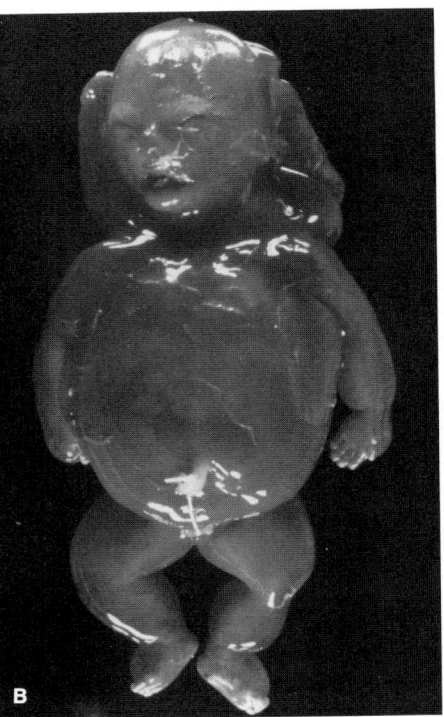

FIGURE 21-1.   Trisomy 21 fetus with cystic hygroma. **(A)** Eleven-week fetus with congenital lymphangiectasia. Straight arrow indicates cystic hygroma around neck (N); curved arrows indicate anasarca of the abdomen (A). **(B)** Photograph of the pathologic specimen. The cystic hygroma and diffuse edema are evident.

TABLE 21-5.   Sonographically Detectable Abnormalities in Nine Trisomy 13 Features

Abnormality	% Affected	Abnormality	% Affected
Head and face		Cardiovascular system	
Microcephaly	55	Any heart defect	77
Hypoplastic or absent nose	55	Tetralogy of Fallot	33
Cleft lip and palate	55	Ventricular septal defect and atrial septal defect	22
Small eyes	44	Isolated ventricular septal defect	22
Low-set ears	33	Mitral valve atresia	11
Hypotelorism	33	Respiratory system	
Holoprosencephaly	22	Pulmonary hypoplasia	33
Abnormally shaped ears	11	Gastrointestinal system	
Cyclopia	11	Umbilical hernia or omphalocele	11
Encephalocele	11	Urogenital system	
Neck		Small penis	50
Edema	11	Horseshoe kidney	22
Extremities		Enlarged kidneys (unexplained)	11
Postaxial polydactyly (hands)	77	Hydronephrosis	11
Postaxial polydactyly (feet)	11	Meningomyelocele or myelocele	20

(Modified from Kalousek DK, Fitch N, Paradice BA: Pathology of the Human Embryo and Previable Fetus: An Atlas. New York: Springer-Verlag, 1990: 190.)

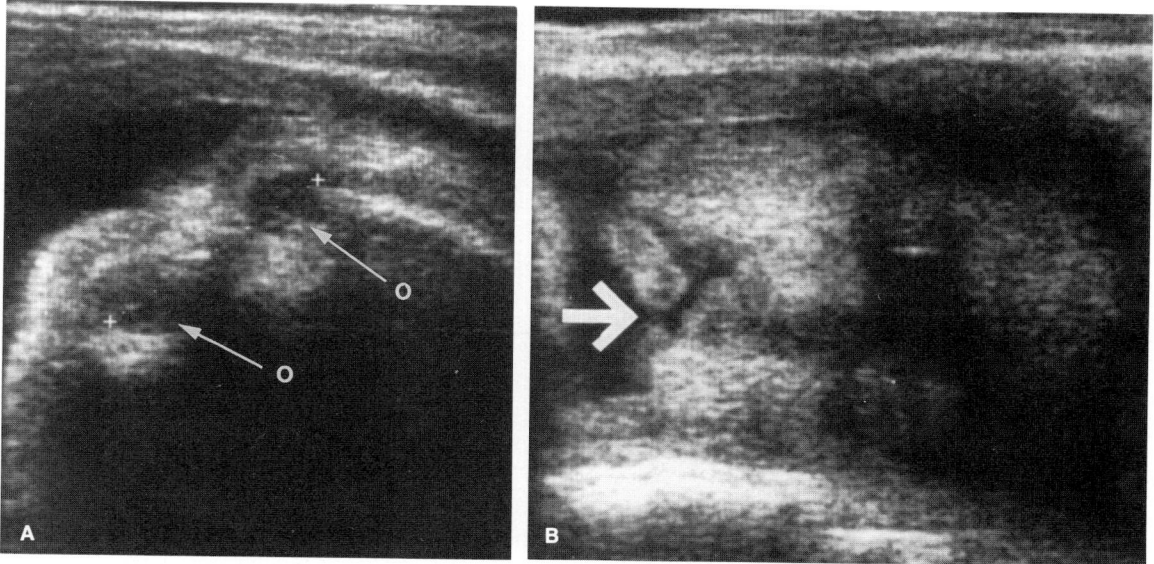

FIGURE 21-2. Facial abnormalities with trisomy 13. **(A)** Axial ultrasound of hypotelorism as marked by cursers. O, orbits. **(B)** Coronal ultrasound showing midline facial cleft (*arrow*). The forehead of the fetus is to the right.

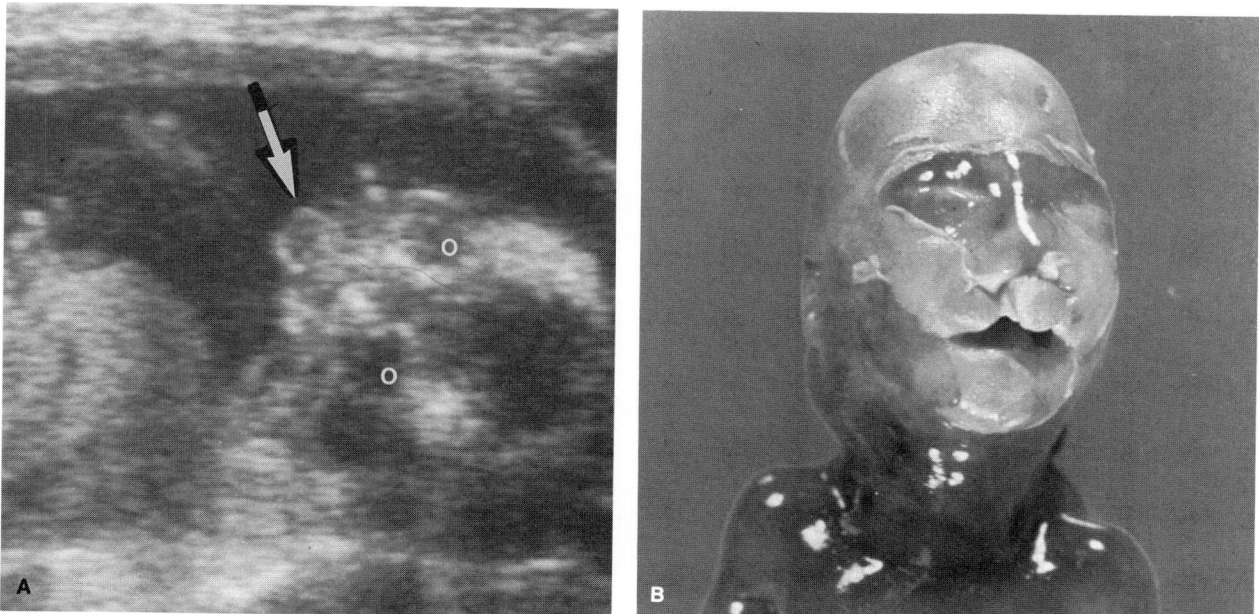

FIGURE 21-3. Facial abnormalities with trisomy 13: bilateral cleft lip and palate. **(A)** Coronal ultrasound shows echogenic premaxillary protrusion (*arrow*), which is noted to occur with bilateral cleft lip and palate. O, orbit. **(B)** Corresponding autopsy specimen.

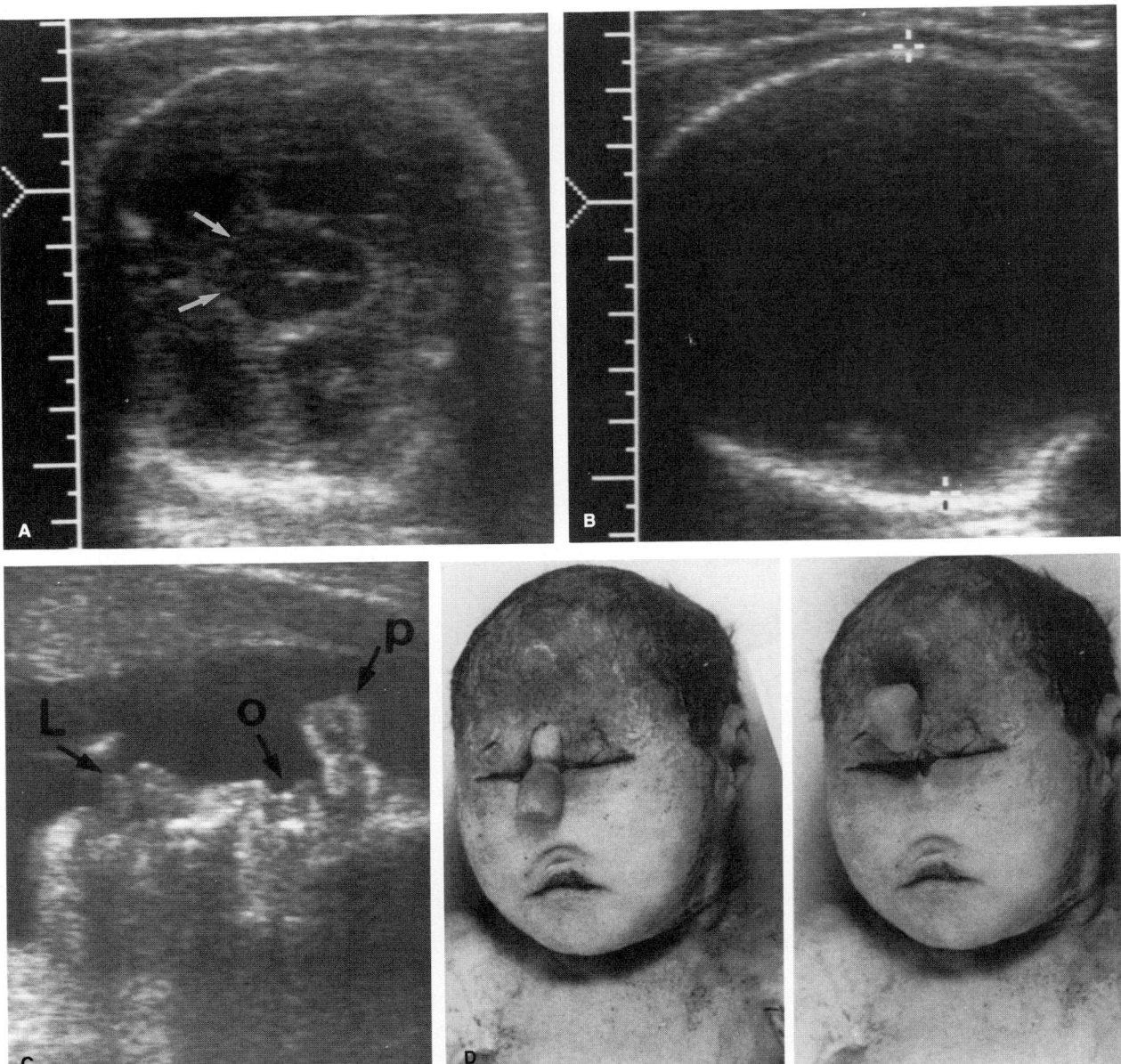

FIGURE 21-4. Trisomy 13 fetus with holoprosencephaly. **(A)** Axial ultrasound of the brain shows fused thalami (*arrows*). **(B)** Axial ultrasound demonstrates a monoventricular cavity with absence of midline structures. **(C)** Sagittal view of the facial features, including fused orbits (O), proboscis (P), and the lips (L). **(D)** Another fetus with trisomy 13 (ethmocephaly); proboscis (*left*) covers a facial slit (*right*). (Dimmick JE, Kalousek DK: Development Pathology of the Embryo and Fetus. Philadelphia: JB Lippincott, 1992: 358.)

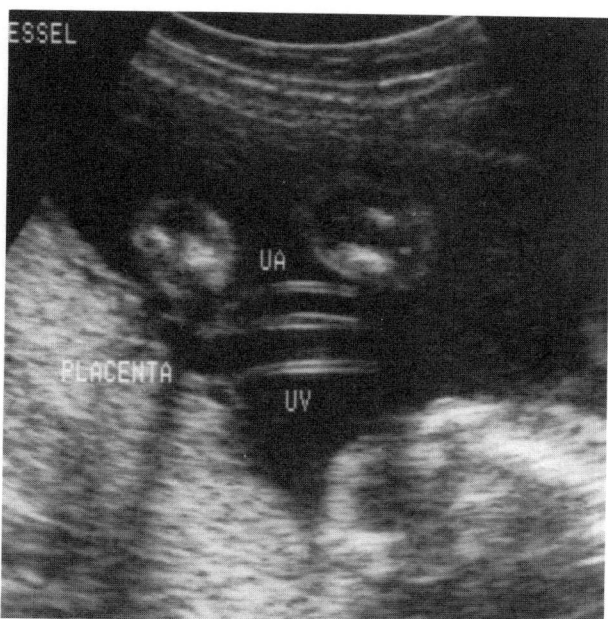

FIGURE 21-5.   Two-vessel umbilical cord (UA, umbilical artery; UV, umbilical vein).

presence of early symmetric intrauterine growth retardation with this autosomal trisomy.[22] The mean birthweight for trisomy 13 neonates is 2600 g.[23]

The presence of a single umbilical artery (Fig. 21-5) and abnormalities in amniotic fluid volume are also increased with trisomy 13[24] (Table 21-6).

Trisomy 18 (Edwards's Syndrome)

After Down's syndrome, trisomy 18 is the next most common chromosomal abnormality found in

TABLE 21-6.   Prevalence of Single Umbilical Artery and Abnormalities of Amniotic Fluid Volume in 16 Trisomy 13, 31 Trisomy 18, and 17 Trisomy 21 Neonates

	Cases (%)		
Abnormality	Trisomy 13	Trisomy 18	Trisomy 21
Single umbilical artery	19	29	0.2–1
Polyhydramnios	12	29	18
Oligohydramnios	6	—	—

(Modified from Tyson RW, Kalousek DK: Chromosomal abnormalities in stillbirth and neonatal death. In Dimmick JE, Kalousek DK: Developmental Pathology of the Embryo. Philadelphia: JB Lippincott, 1992.)

TABLE 21-7.   Sonographically Detectable Abnormalities in 24 Trisomy 18 Fetuses

Abnormality	% Affected
Head and face	
Micrognathia	29
Low-set ears	25
Triangular face	21
Cleft lip and/or palate	12
Small mouth	8
Prominent occiput	4
Absence of external ear	4
Neck	
Cystic hygroma, edema	25
Extremities	
Fingers two and five overlap three and four	50
Rocker-bottom feet	33
Clinodactyly of the fifth finger	21
Clubfeet	17
Joint contractures	12
Duplicated or absent thumb	12
Short arms	8
Central nervous system	
Choroid plexus cysts	30[39]
Meningomyelocele	4
Cardiovascular system	
Any heart defect	96
Aortic coarctation	21
Ventricular septal defect	19
Atrial septal defect	17
Persistent left superior vena cava	17
Hypoplastic left ventricle	4
Atrioventricular canal	4
Respiratory system	
Pulmonary hypoplasia	12
Gastrointestinal system	
Omphalocele	33
Diaphragmatic eventration or hernia	20
Urogenital system	
Horseshoe kidney	33
Kidney hypoplasia	8
Dilated ureter	8
Enlarged kidney	4
Small penis	4

(Modified from Kalousek DK, Fitch N, Paradice BA: Pathology of the Human Embryo and Previable Fetus: An Atlas. New York: Springer-Verlag, 1990: 188.)

the newborn population, occurring once in every 3000 live births.[24] About 1% of spontaneous abortions and 1% of stillbirths are trisomic for chromosome 18.[2] Although an additional chromosome 18 is present in over 80% of trisomy 18 fetuses, 10%

(text continues on page 461)

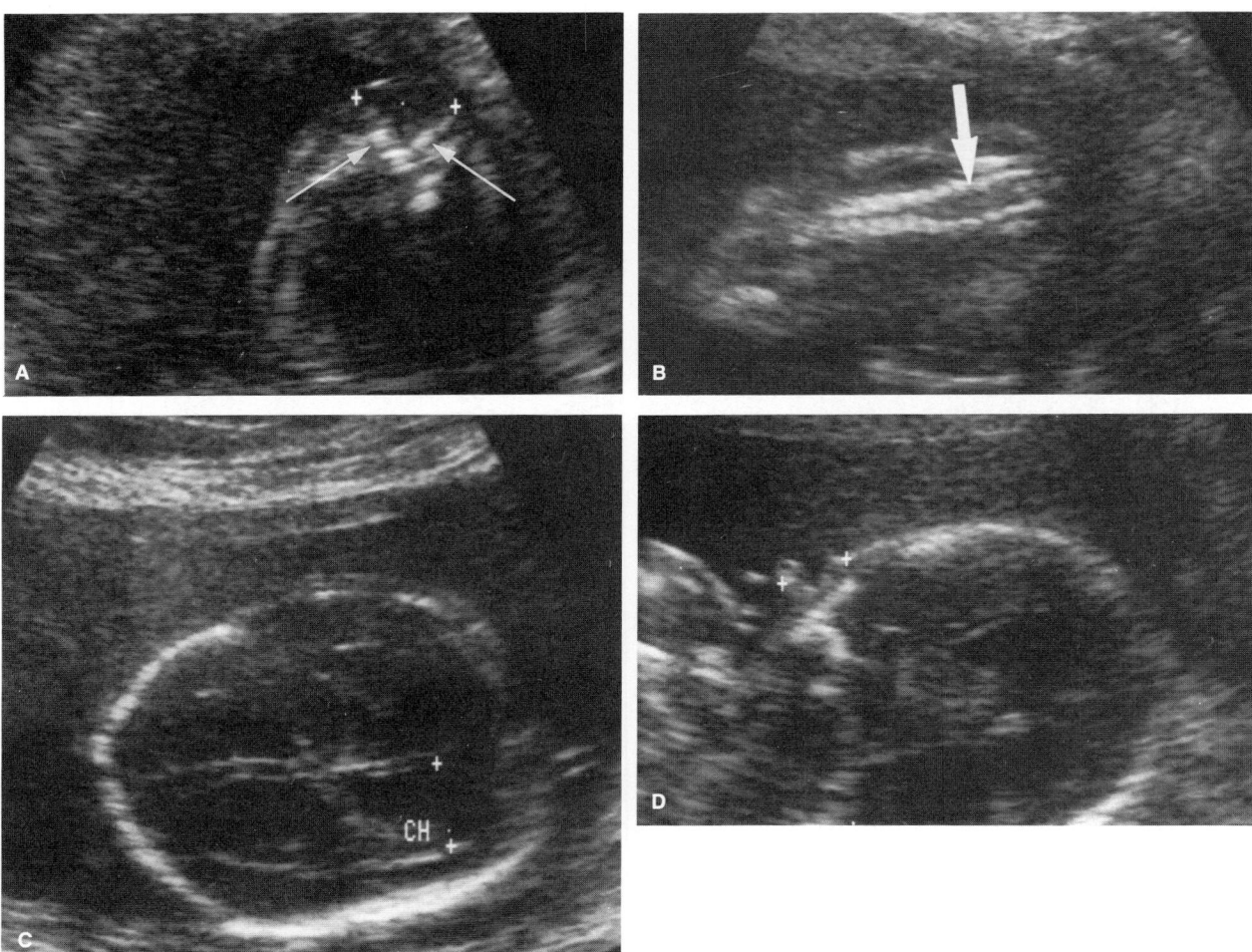

FIGURE 21-6. Features of trisomy 18. **(A)** Transverse ultrasound shows splaying of the ossification centers of the lumbar spine (*arrows*), with the *graticules* indicating an open neural tube defect. **(B)** Coronal view of the spinal column illustrates splaying of the ossification centers (*arrow*) at the level of the defect. **(C)** Ventriculomegaly is demonstrated by dilation of the atria of the lateral ventricles (*graticules*) measuring 14 mm. The choroid plexus (CH) is dangling in the lateral ventricle. **(D)** Coronal ultrasound of the head demonstrates low-set, irregularly shaped ears (*graticules*). **(E)** Polyhydramnios. A single vertical pocket of amniotic fluid measures 10 cm. **(F)** Ultrasound of the forearm shows marked radial deviation of the right hand. H, humerus. **(G)** Because of the marked radial deviation, the hand is not visualized when the ulna is viewed longitudinally. UL, ulna; HUMH, humerus. **(H)** Fetus at autopsy.

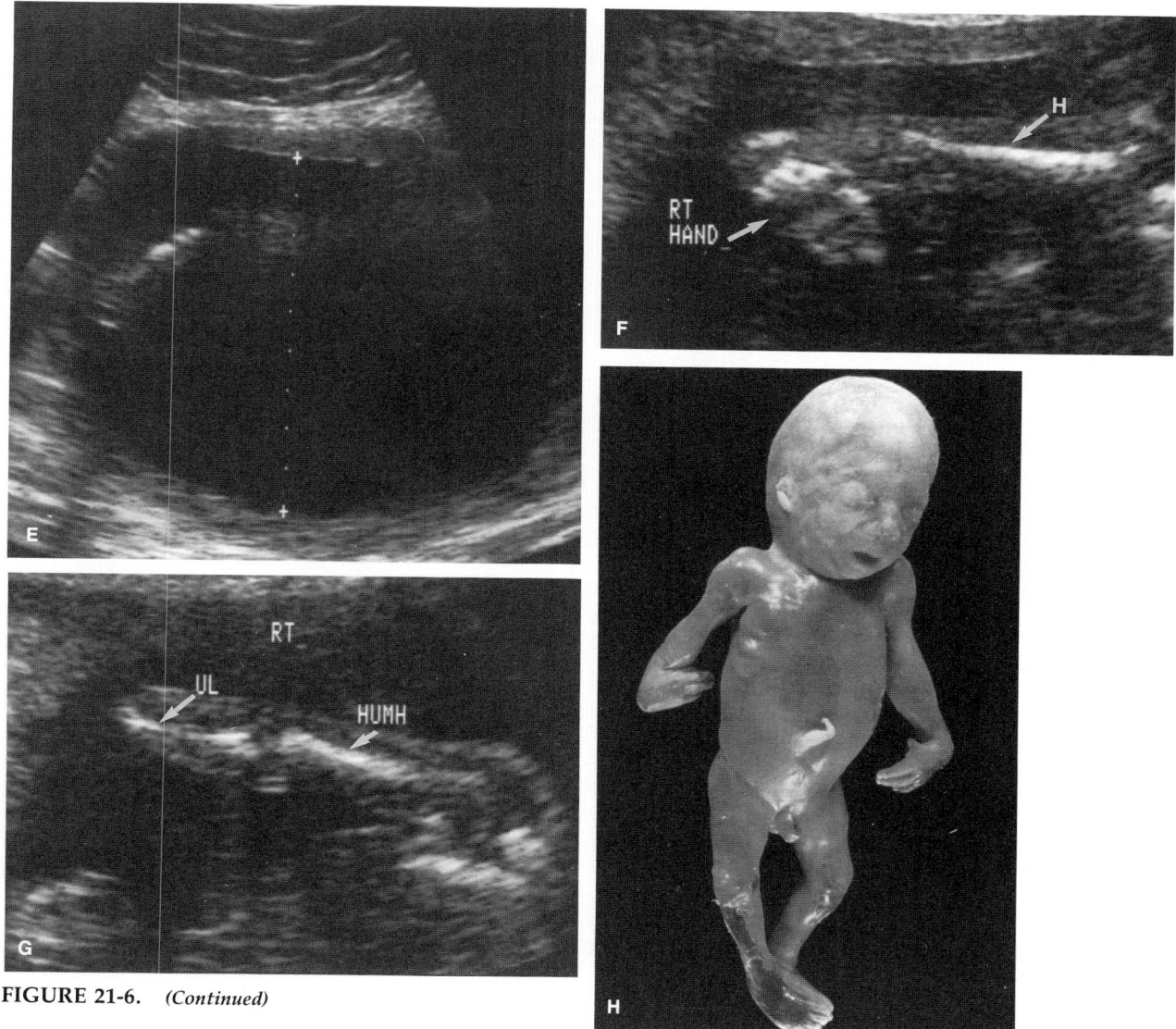

FIGURE 21-6.   *(Continued)*

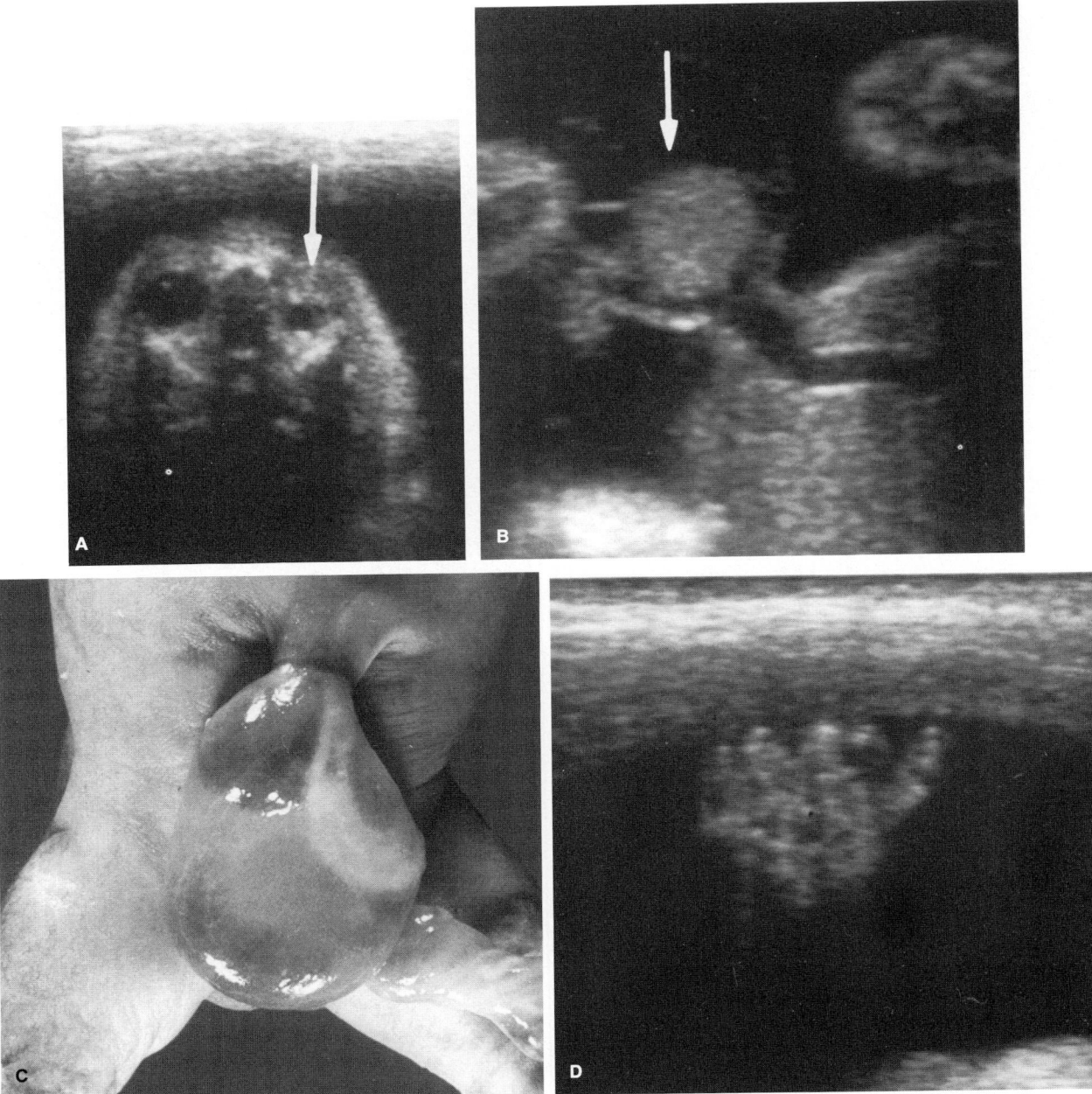

FIGURE 21-7. Features of trisomy 18. **(A)** Microphthalmos (*arrow*). There is marked discrepancy in the size of the two orbits indicative of microphthalmos. **(B)** Omphalocele-containing bowel (*arrow*) originating at the site of origin of the umbilical cord. **(C)** Omphalocele at autopsy. **(D)** Clenched fist. **(E)** Clenched fist at autopsy. **(F)** Horseshoe kidney at autopsy with ureters and bladder.

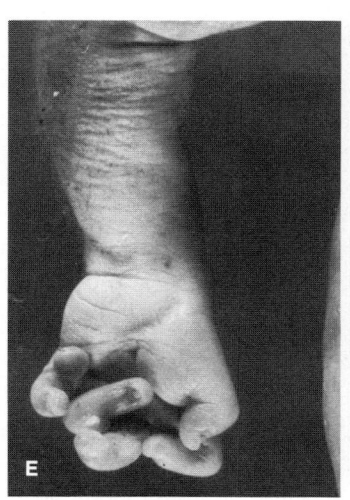
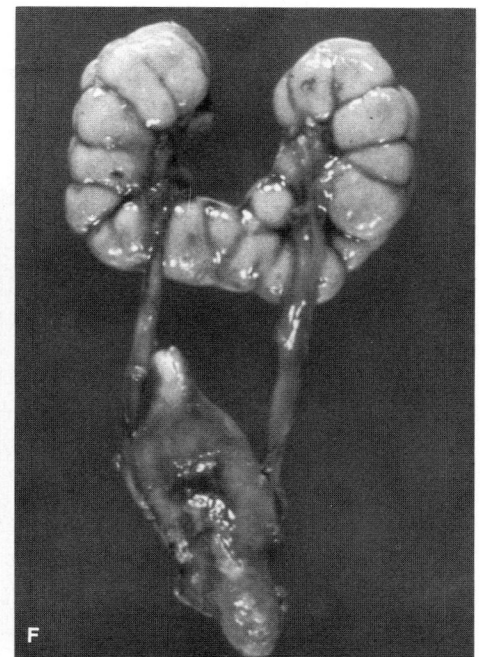

FIGURE 21-7.   *(Continued)*

are mosaic, and 5% result from a translocation.[25] As anticipated, neonates with mosaic trisomy 18 are less severely affected and survive longer than neonates with an extra chromosome 18.[26]

The congenital malformations associated with trisomy 18 were first reported in 1960 by Edwards and associates.[27] Over 130 abnormalities have been described in infants with trisomy 18.[28] Table 21-7 lists the sonographically detectable abnormalities from one study of 24 trisomy 18 fetuses (Figs. 21-6 and 21-7).

As with trisomy 13, the pattern of congenital abnormalities may suggest a diagnosis of trisomy 18.

Polyhydramnios is present with trisomy 18 in 29% to 62% of cases (see Table 21-6).

In one series of 31 neonates and stillborn fetuses with trisomy 18, 87% were growth retarded.[28] Before 24 weeks of gestation, however, the incidence of growth retardation with trisomy 18 was only 28%.[29] Even first-trimester growth delay (crown-to-rump length at 5 days shorter than expected) in trisomy 18 has been reported.[30] The mean birthweight of trisomy 18 fetuses is 2300 g.[19]

The combination of symmetric intrauterine growth retardation and polyhydramnios should suggest the possibility of a chromosomal abnormality, specifically trisomy 18. Approximately 21%

of fetuses with trisomy 18 have intrauterine growth retardation and polyhydramnios.[29]

Fifty to 70% of trisomy 18 fetuses have overlapping of the fingers (digits two and five overlapping three and four; see Fig. 21-7D,E). Occasionally, only one hand has overlapping of the fingers. Other skeletal abnormalities, such as clubfeet (Fig. 21-8) or rocker-bottom feet, and limb reduction abnormalities (see Fig. 21-6F,G) may also occur with trisomy 18.[19]

About half of trisomy 18 fetuses have a strawberry-shaped skull (flattening of the occiput with pointing of the frontal bones; Fig. 21-9) on the standard biparietal diameter (BPD) view. Nicolaides and colleagues hypothesized that the pointing of the frontal bones is due to hypoplasia of the face and frontal cerebral lobes; hypoplasia of the hindbrain would result in flattening of the occiput.[31]

The neuropathologic changes associated with trisomy 18 tend to be variable and hence are not diagnostic. Hydrocephalus with or without meningomyelocele (see Fig. 21-6A–C), agenesis of the corpus callosum, and a small cerebellum are among the central nervous system malformations that are potentially detectable with antenatal ultrasonography.[32,33] In the presence of a small cerebellum, the cisterna magna appears prominent.

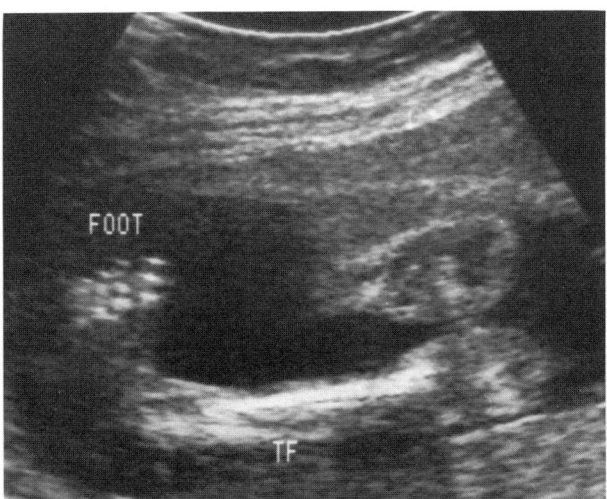

FIGURE 21-8. Clubfoot. When scanning through the tibia and fibula (TF), the bones of the feet should appear perpendicular to the scan plane rather than angled medially, as in this case.

Several reports have been made of second-trimester choroid plexus cysts in fetuses with trisomy 18 or 21[34,35] (Fig. 21-10). Twinning and associates reviewed the literature in 1991 and found 222 cases of choroid plexus cysts associated with 13 cases of

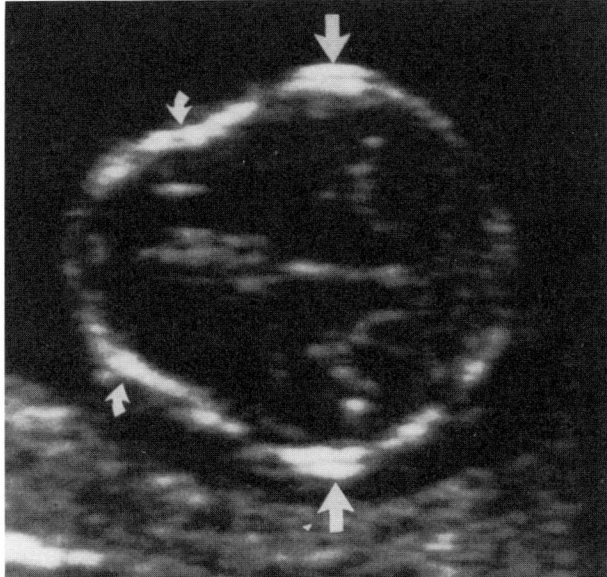

FIGURE 21-9. Strawberry cranium. Axial scan of the cranium demonstrates a wide occipitoparietal diameter (*large arrows*) and a narrow frontal diameter (*curved arrows*). (Nyberg DA, Kramer D, Resta RG, et al: Prenatal sonographic findings of trisomy 18: Review of 47 cases. J Ultrasound Med 1993; 2:103.)

trisomy 18 and two cases of trisomy 21—an overall incidence of 5.8% for trisomy 18 and 0.9% for trisomy 21.[36] Fitzsimmons and associates found choroid plexus cysts in 10 of 14 (70%) trisomy 18 fetuses younger than 26 weeks of gestational age.[37] Since this was an autopsy study, it undoubtedly overestimated the detection rate of choroid plexus cysts at sonography. Two antenatal studies visualized choroid plexus cysts in about 30% of fetuses with trisomy 18.[38,39] Choroid plexus cysts invariably resolve by 24 weeks' gestation.

All fetuses with choroid plexus cysts should have a careful anatomic survey to look for additional sonographic signs of trisomy 18. Most of the larger studies report that additional major malformations are detected sonographically in about 80% to 90% of trisomy 18 fetuses.[29,40] If one assumes a frequency of trisomy 18 in the general population of 1 in 3000 births, the probability of trisomy 18 in a fetus with isolated choroid plexus cysts has been calculated to be 1 in 477.[38] Some groups continue to recommend amniocentesis for isolated choroid plexus cysts.[41]

Twenty-nine percent of trisomy 18 fetuses have a single umbilical artery (see Table 21-6).

Although second- and third-trimester umbilical cord cysts have been associated with trisomy 18,[42] first-trimester umbilical cord cysts that generally resorb by 12 weeks' gestation are not associated with chromosomal abnormalities.

Congenital heart disease is nearly always present with trisomy 18 (see Table 21-7). Polyvalvular dysplasia is a characteristic feature of trisomy 18 and is present in about 60% of cases.[17] The valvular tissue is thickened and redundant; the pulmonary valve is most frequently affected. Polyvalvular dysplasia is frequently mild, however, and therefore is extremely difficult to diagnosis antenatally. In the neonate with trisomy 18, patent ductus arteriosus is common.[43] Endocardial cushion defects, mitral atresia, double-outlet right ventricle, and dextrocardia have also been described with trisomy 18.[28] Although ventricular septal defects have been reported to occur in between 19%[44] and 81%[28] of fetuses with trisomy 18, they are frequently difficult to identify in the early part of the second trimester.

Marion and associates developed a clinical scoring system to aid in the neonatal diagnosis of trisomy 18.[45] Specific congenital abnormalities are given points depending on the frequency with which they are present in trisomy 18. A similar attempt to evaluate the fetus is possible by means of antenatal sonography. In two separate series of

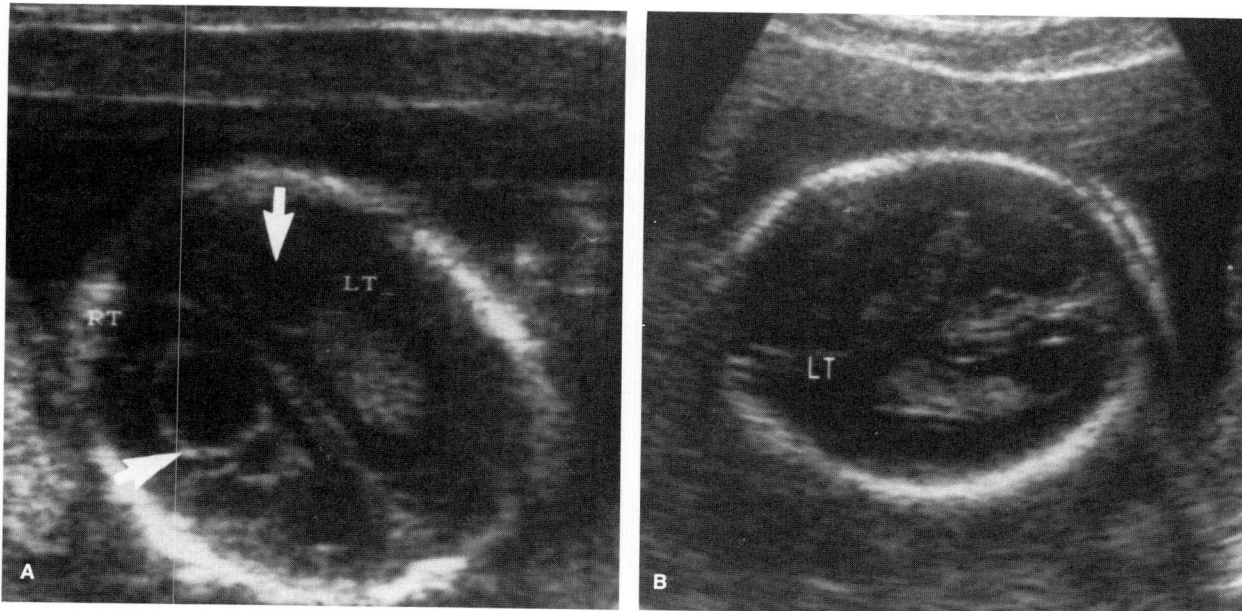

FIGURE 21-10. Bilateral choroid plexus cysts. **(A)** At 17.4 weeks of gestation, bilateral choroid plexus cysts are present (*arrows*). **(B)** Three weeks later, the choroid plexus cysts have resolved. LT, left choroid.

trisomy 18 fetuses,[29,40] prenatal sonographic findings were detected in about 80% of cases and in all 18 fetuses examined after 24 weeks' gestation.[29] Benacerraf and colleagues reported that 12 of 15 fetuses (80%) with trisomy 18 had one or more of the following sonographically detectable abnormalities: polyhydramnios (4), congenital heart disease (4), diaphragmatic hernia (3), and omphalocele (2).[40] Eleven of the 12 fetuses with trisomy 18 had abnormalities of the hands or feet. Nyberg and associates reported extremity abnormalities in 29 of 35 (83%) trisomy 18 fetuses.[29]

A maternal serum triple screen with α-fetoprotein, unconjugated estriol, and human chorionic gonadotropin at or below 0.75, 0.60, and 0.55 multiples of the median, respectively, identifies between 40% and 95% of trisomy 18 fetuses, with a false-positive rate of 0.5%.[7] Perhaps maternal age, maternal serum triple screen, and the sonographic features of trisomy 18 can be incorporated into a scoring system that quantifies a specific patient's risk of carrying a fetus with trisomy 18.

Trisomy 21 (Down's Syndrome)

Trisomy 21 is the most frequent autosomal chromosomal abnormality, occurring once in every 660 live births.[19] John Langdon Down first described the characteristic features of trisomy 21 in 1866.[46]

The major abnormalities associated with Down's syndrome appear to be due to the genes localized at the q22 band of chromosome 21. Cases of trisomy 21 are generally sporadic. There is a 1% recurrence risk for women under age 30; the recurrence risk for older women is no greater than the risk associated with their age. Ninety-five percent of cases are due to an extra chromosome 21. About 3% to 5% of Down's syndrome cases are due to translocation; 2% to 3% are mosaics.[23]

The phenotypic characteristics of trisomy 21 are to a certain extent gestational age dependent. For example, spontaneously aborted trisomy 21 fetuses between 8 and 14 weeks' gestation have either an increased nuchal thickness or generalized edema; by 16 to 22 weeks' gestation, the incidence of this abnormality decreases to about 22%.[47] Nuchal thickness should be measured sonographically at the level of the thalami, but angled slightly posterior to include the cerebellum. The distance from the external surface of the occipital bone to the external surface of the skin is measured (Fig. 21-11). The correct plane should include the cavum, the cerebral peduncles, and the cerebellar hemispheres (see Chapter 9). A nuchal skinfold thickness of 6 mm or greater is abnormal (see Fig. 9-2).[48] Benacerraf and colleagues reported that a thickened nuchal fold is present in 40% to 70% of fetuses with Down's syndrome in women over 35

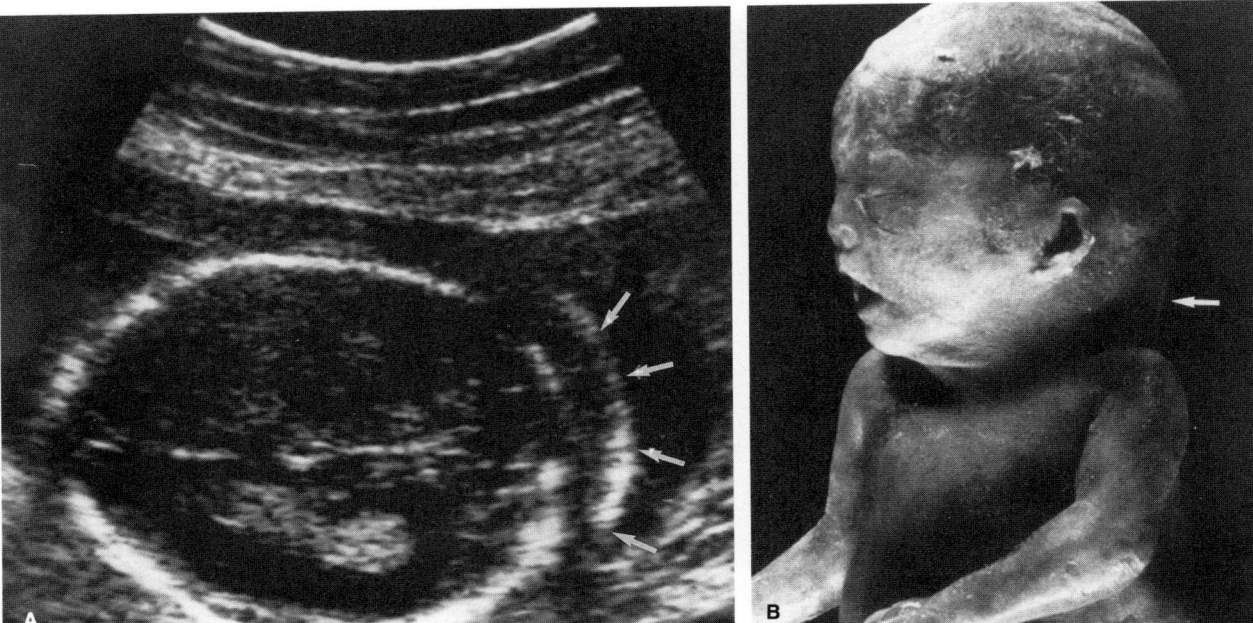

FIGURE 21-11.   Nuchal folds in fetus with trisomy 21. **(A)** Thickened nuchal fold (*arrows*). See Figure 9-2 for correct plane to detect nuchal thickening. **(B)** Photograph of the pathologic specimen illustrating thickened nuchal fold (*arrow*).

years of age.[49] Fetuses with a thickened nuchal fold and no other indications for an amniocentesis (ie, normal maternal serum triple screen, 34 years or age or younger) have a 22% incidence of trisomy 21.

The femur length and humeral length of Down's syndrome fetuses tend to be shorter than those of matched controls.[50] Several authors have attempted to take advantage of these findings by comparing the femur or humeral length with either the BPD or the expected long bone measurement for gestational age.[51]

Using a cutoff of 1.5 standard deviations above the mean for the BPD/femur length ratio, Lockwood and colleagues were able to detect 50% to 70% of fetuses with Down's syndrome, with a false-positive rate of 6%.[52] Nyberg and associates, however, reported a sensitivity of only 31.1% for the detection of Down's syndrome with either a short femur or a short humerus.[50] When both a short femur and a short humerus were required, sensitivity was reduced to 17.8%.

Differences in the normal values for both the BPD/femur length ratio (Table 21-8) and the measured/expected femur length ratio among centers indicate that reported cutoff values are not universally applicable. When institutional norms are established, the BPD/femur length ratio appears to

have a positive predictive value for the detection of Down's syndrome (Table 21-9) that is comparable to that for a maternal age of 35 to 36 years.[53]

Although the incidence of intrauterine growth retardation is increased with trisomy 21 (29%), it is

TABLE 21-8.   Comparison of the Biparietal Diameter/Femur Length Ratio Cutoff Values From Three Institutions

Gestational Age (wk)	BPD/FL Ratio		
	New Haven	*Boston*	*Pittsburgh*
15	1.93	1.77	1.94
16	1.93	1.66	2.03
17	1.76	1.61	1.90
18	1.74	1.54	1.70
19	1.68	1.51	1.70
20	1.58	1.48	1.60
21	1.54		1.59
22	1.47		1.58

* Mean + 1.5 SD.

BPD, biparietal diameter; FL, femur length.

(Hill LM, Guzick D, Belfar H, et al: The current role of sonography in the detection of Down syndrome. Obstet Gynecol 1989; 74:620.)

TABLE 21-9.   Results Obtained in 22 Fetuses With Down's Syndrome Using the Biparietal Diameter/Femur Length Ratio From Different Populations

City of Investigation	Sensitivity (%)	Specificity (%)	Positive Predictive Value	
			*General Population**	*Age 35†*
Pittsburgh	36.4	93.4	1/174	1/46
New Haven	22.7	90.6	1/294	1/112
Boston	71.4	57.1	1/427	1/163

* Prevalence of Down's syndrome: 1 in 1000.

† Prevalence of Down's syndrome: 1 in 270.

(Hill LM, Guzick D, Belfar H, et al: The current role of sonography in the detection of Down syndrome. Obstet Gynecol 1989; 74:620.)

significantly less frequent than with either trisomy 13 (50%) or trisomy 18 (87%).[28]

Ten percent of trisomy 21 fetuses have no external abnormalities; an additional 29% may have only a single palmar crease (Fig. 21-12), with or without clinodactyly of the fifth fingers (Fig. 21-13A–C). If clinodactyly is detected sonographically, the parents should be examined; autosomal dominant clinodactyly is more common than clinodactyly associated with Down's syndrome.

Anomalies that are most frequently associated with Down's syndrome before 20 weeks' gestation include cystic hygroma, nuchal thickening, and hyperechogenic bowel[54] (see Fig. 21-13D). Small bowel is considered to be hyperechogenic when its echogenicity approaches that of bone.[54]

Internal congenital malformations also occur less frequently with Down's syndrome than with either trisomy 13 or trisomy 18. Table 21-10 outlines the autopsy findings in 17 stillborn fetuses with trisomy 21.[28]

Congenital heart disease is common in fetuses with trisomy 21. The incidence of congenital heart disease is higher in the second trimester than at term because fetuses with severe heart disease are stillborn. About 40% of trisomy 21 fetuses with congenital heart disease have atrioventricular septal defects[55] (endocardial cushion defects; Fig. 21-14).

Thirty percent of fetuses with duodenal atresia (Fig. 21-15) have Down's syndrome; only 15% of trisomy 21 fetuses have duodenal atresia.[19] Occasionally, duodenal atresia can be diagnosed between 18 and 20 weeks' gestation. This specific abnormality is generally not diagnosed, however, until after 24 weeks of gestational age.[56]

The incidence of polyhydramnios with trisomy 21 is frequently secondary to the presence of duodenal atresia (Table 21-11).

The frequency of detecting congenital abnormalities with Down's syndrome increases with menstrual age.[54]

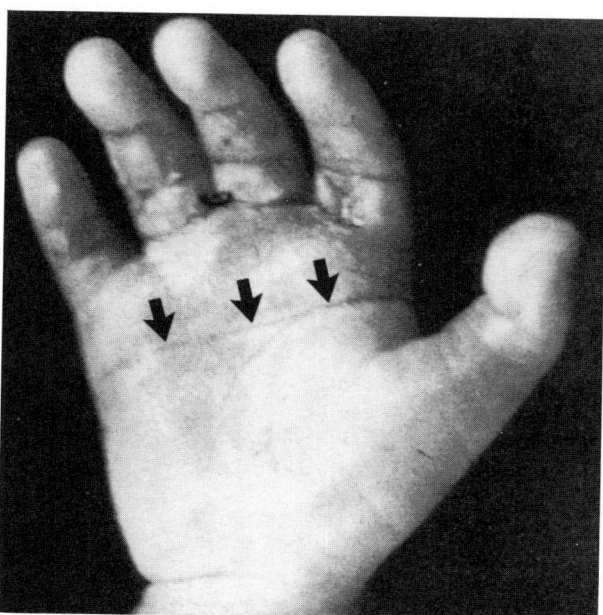

FIGURE 21-12.   Simian crease (*arrows*) in 23-week fetus with trisomy 21. (Winter RM, Knowles SAS, Bieber FR, Baraitser M: The Malformed Fetus and Stillbirth: A Diagnostic Approach. New York: Wiley, 1988: 71.)

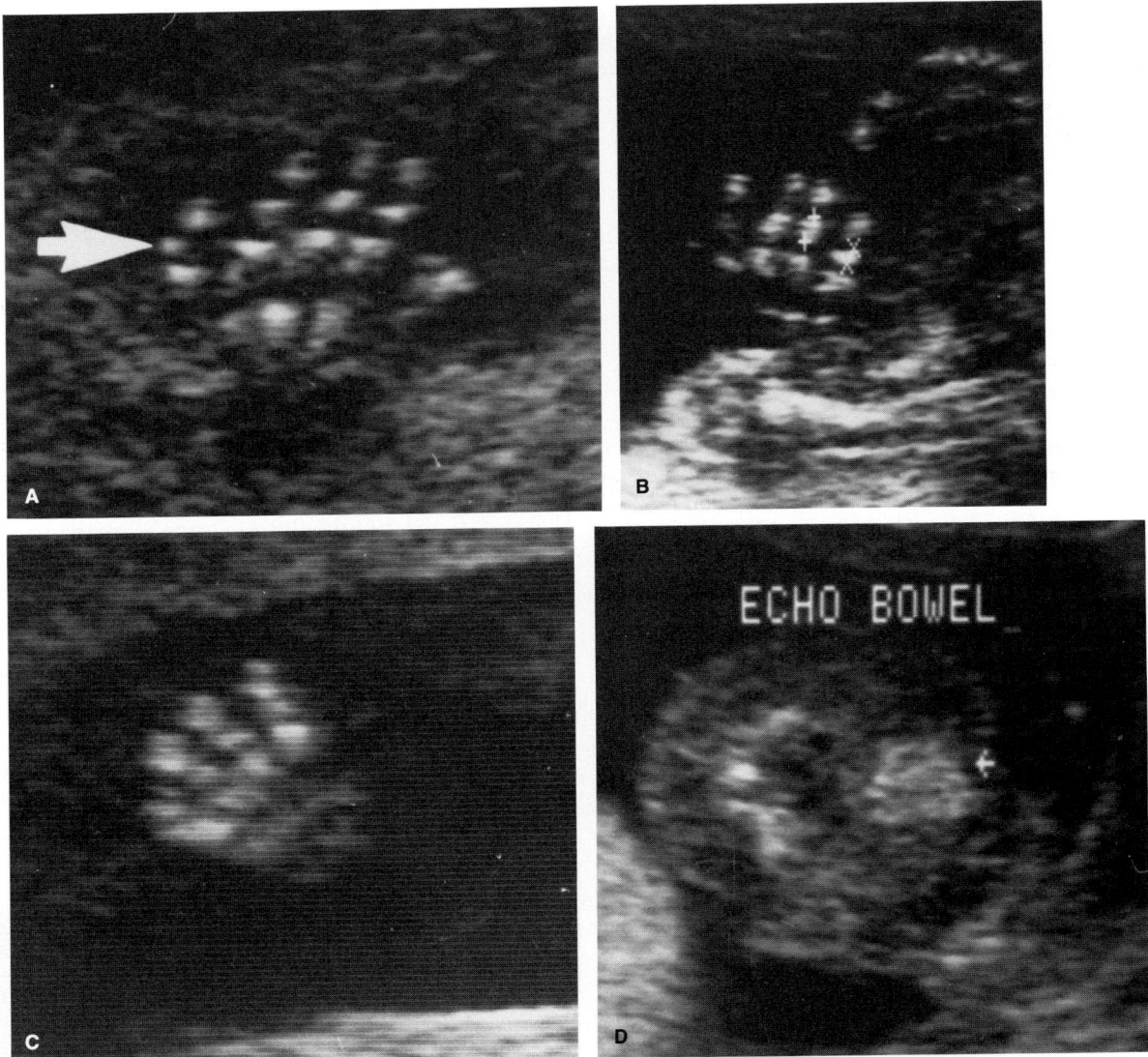

FIGURE 21-13.   Abnormalities in trisomy 21. **(A)** Clinodactyly of the fifth finger with hypoplasia of the middle phalanx (*arrow*). **(B)** Normal fifth (×) and fourth (+) middle phalanges in another fetus. **(C)** Short stubby fingers in another fetus with trisomy 21 (compare with the normal hand in **B**). **(D)** Echogenic small bowel (*arrow*) in fetus with trisomy 21.

TABLE 21-10. Sonographically Detectable Abnormalities in 17 Stillborns With Trisomy 21

Abnormality	% Affected
Body	
Hydrops	29
Cystic hygroma	5
Head and face	
Protuberant tongue	18
Low-set ears	6
Extremities	
Clinodactyly	59
Single palmar crease	59
Bilateral	41
Unilateral	18
Short fingers	18
Syndactyly	6
Gap between first and second toes	6
Cardiovascular system	
Endocardial cushion defect	12
Ventricular septal defect	12
Atrial septal defect	12
Pulmonary stenosis	6
Respiratory system	
Pulmonary hypoplasia	18
Gastrointestinal system	
Duodenal atresia	18
Imperforate anus	6

Cystic hygromas are congenital malformations of the lymphatic system. Although they are most commonly found in the nuchal region, cystic hygromas may also occur in the anterior neck, chest wall, axilla, or groin.

Nuchal hygromas generally extend from the upper portion of the occipital bone caudally and medially to the sternocleidomastoid muscle. They consist of two symmetric cavities completely separated by a midline nuchal ligament. Each cavity of the hygroma is subdivided by incomplete septa (Fig. 21-17A).

The fetal lymphatic vessels drain into the paired jugular lymph sacs, which in turn drain into the internal jugular veins. A cystic hygroma forms when the connection between the jugular lymph sac and jugular veins fails to develop. Consequently, the jugular lymph sacs increase in size, and lymph accumulates within the tissues. Nonimmune hydrops eventually develops (see Fig. 21-17B,C). If the jugular lymphatic sacs and the jugular veins subsequently develop a connection, or if an alternate route of drainage develops, the hygroma regresses and the peripheral edema resolves.[62] The neonate in the latter instance has redundant neck skin and perhaps residual puffiness of the hands and feet.

Turner's Syndrome (45,X Karyotype)

A syndrome consisting of small stature, sexual infantilism, webbed neck, and cubitus valgus was first described by Turner in 1938.[57]

In 45,X, 78% of cases involve the paternal X. As with the other chromosomal abnormalities reviewed, fetuses who are mosaic XO or who are missing only part of one X (X-isochromosome) generally have fewer abnormalities.[58]

Less than 1% of 45 monosomy conceptus survive to the neonatal period.[59] Previable fetuses with monosomy X characteristically have a triad of nuchal cystic hygroma, generalized edema, and aortic coarctation.[60]

The declining rate of 45,X with maternal age suggests an increasing tendency of the 45,X conceptus to abort early.

Seventy percent of fetuses with cystic hygroma in the second or third trimester (Fig. 21-16) have Turner's syndrome, 15% have other chromosomal abnormalities, and 15% are karyotypically normal.[61] Other chromosomal abnormalities associated with cystic hygroma include trisomy 13, trisomy 18, and trisomy 21.[11]

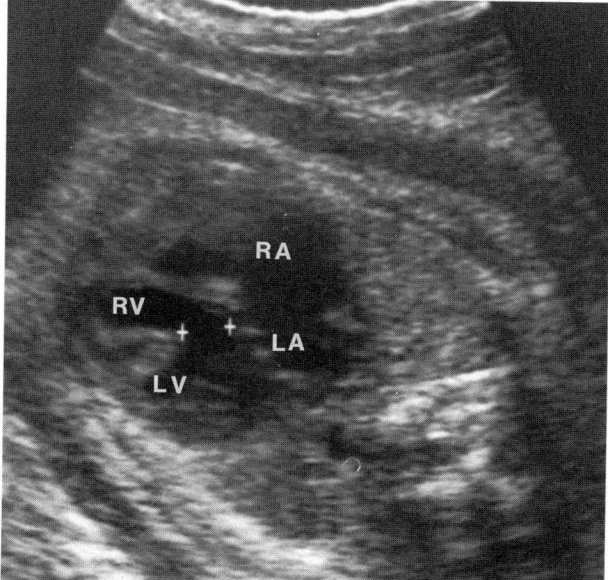

FIGURE 21-14. Trisomy 21. Endocardial cushion defect. The graticules demarcate a large ventricular septal defect. The lower portion of the atrial septum is also absent. RA, right atrium; LA, left atrium; RV, right ventricle; LV, left ventricle.

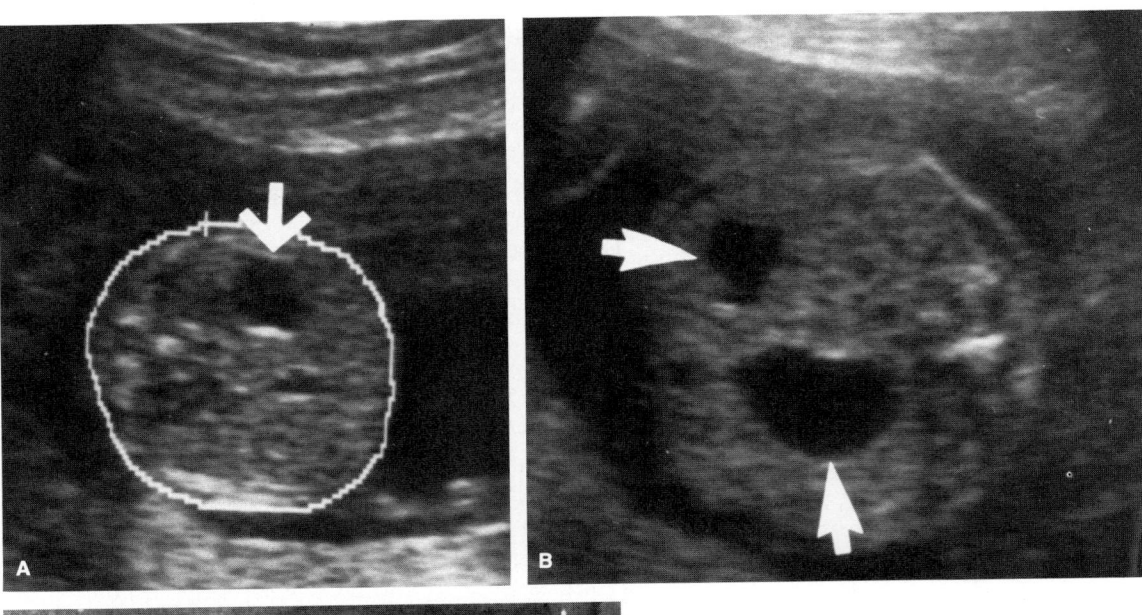

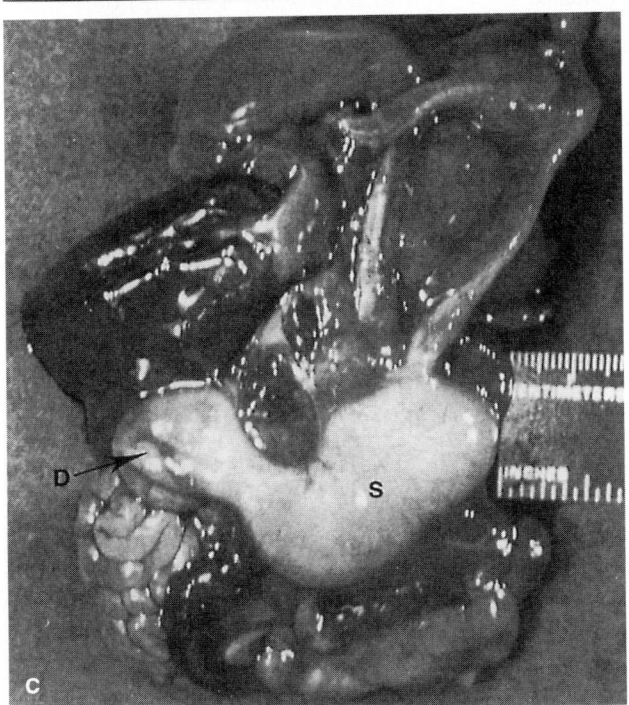

FIGURE 21-15. Duodenal atresia. **(A)** Abdominal circumference with a normal stomach bubble (*arrow*) at 17 weeks. **(B)** The double-bubble of duodenal atresia (*arrows*) is at 23 weeks. **(C)** Autopsy of 23-week fetus with a distended duodenum (D) proximal to an atretic area. S, stomach. (Winter RM, Knowles SAS, Bieber FR, Baraitser M: The Malformed Fetus and Stillbirth: A Diagnostic Approach. New York: Wiley, 1988: 71.)

The advent of transvaginal sonography has permitted the first-trimester diagnosis of a nuchal translucency (3 mm or greater) that is distinct from the skin line of the posterior neck. This finding is associated with a 35% incidence of chromosomal abnormalities.[63] Bronshtein and associates divided first-trimester cystic hygromas into nonseptated (ie, nuchal translucency) and septated.[64] In the former group, the hygromas tended to resorb, and the fetuses were karyotypically normal; the four cystic hygromas ending in fetal death and associated with aneuploidy were septated.

In contrast to fetuses with second-trimester cystic hygromas, the distribution of chromosomal aberrations is distinctly different with nuchal translucencies. The frequency of trisomies 13, 18, and 21 and of chromosomal rearrangements is increased, but the incidence of Turner's syndrome is reduced

TABLE 21-11.   Conditions Associated With Cystic Nuchal Hygromas

Chromosomal Disorders

XO
XXY
Trisomy 13
Trisomy 18
Trisomy 21
deletion (13q)
deletion (18p)
deletion (6q)

Single Gene Syndromes

Robert's syndrome (autosomal recessive)
Familial neck webbing (autosomal dominant)
Noonan's syndrome
Lethal multiple pterygium syndrome

Teratogenic Disorders

Fetal alcohol syndrome

from 70% with second-trimester cystic hygromas to 13.2% in fetuses with first-trimester nuchal translucency.[65] This implies that the underlying cause of nuchal cystic hygroma is different between fetuses with Turner's syndrome and those with other aneuploidies.

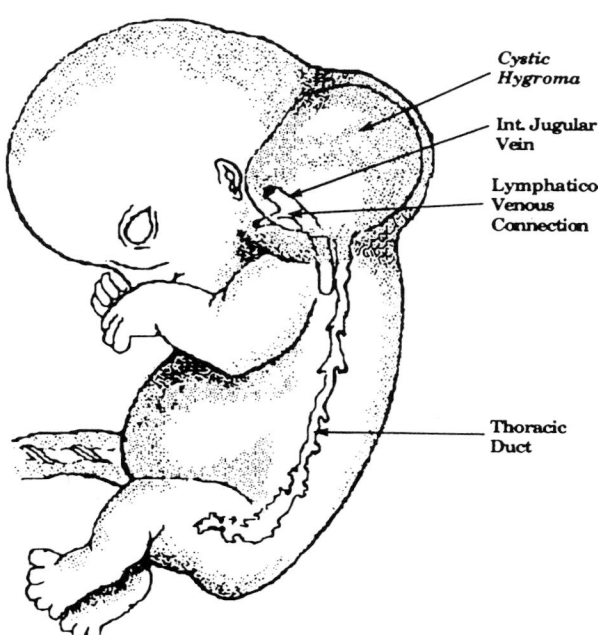

FIGURE 21-16.   Nuchal mass (cystic hygroma) typically seen in abnormal development of the fetal lymphatic system. (Johnson MP, et al: Am J Obstet Gynecol 1993; 168:156.)

Cystic hygromas have also been described with the other conditions outlined in Table 21-11.

Over 20% of fetuses with Turner's syndrome have a cardiac defect, 70% of which are aortic coarctation.[58] Garden and colleagues hypothesized that encroachment by the dilated lymphatic ducts on the ascending aorta produces flow changes in the heart that result in the high incidence of cardiac anomalies.[66] When there is a discrepancy between the size of the ventricles, with the left ventricle being smaller than normal, coarctation of the aorta should be considered along with hypoplastic left heart and tetralogy of Fallot[67] (see Fig. 21-17D).

Renal abnormalities, specifically horseshoe kidneys, are the only other anomalies associated with Turner's syndrome that might be detected sonographically.[58]

If the fetus with Turner's syndrome survives to the neonatal period, long-term survival is generally good. The congenital lymphedema usually recedes during the first few years of life. Although the ovaries are normal in early fetal life, they rapidly degenerate, so that by adolescence there is little functioning ovarian tissue remaining. Patients with Turner's syndrome have a relatively short stature; their verbal IQ is normal.[58]

Triploidy

Triploidy results from an extra haploid set of chromosomes at fertilization. The extra set of chromosomes is usually from the father.

Triploidy is a random event that is unrelated to maternal age.[68] It accounts for 20% of all chromosomally abnormal spontaneous abortions. There is about 1 triploid neonate for every 10,000 births.[69]

The placentas of triploid fetuses are characteristically partial hydatidiform moles (70%); the remaining placentas are microscopically normal. Jacobs and colleagues reported that when the extra set of chromosomes was paternal, a partial hydatidiform mole resulted; if the extra set was maternal, the placenta was small and microscopically normal.[69] The presence of a normal placenta undoubtedly contributes to fetal survival.[62]

A markedly elevated maternal serum α-fetoprotein has been associated with fetal triploidy.[70] The presence of a large placental surface area with increased vascularity permits the ready transfer of proteins from the fetal to the maternal circulation.[71]

Lack of appropriate growth of the crown-to-rump length has been reported with triploid fetuses.[72,73] In those pregnancies that reach the sec-

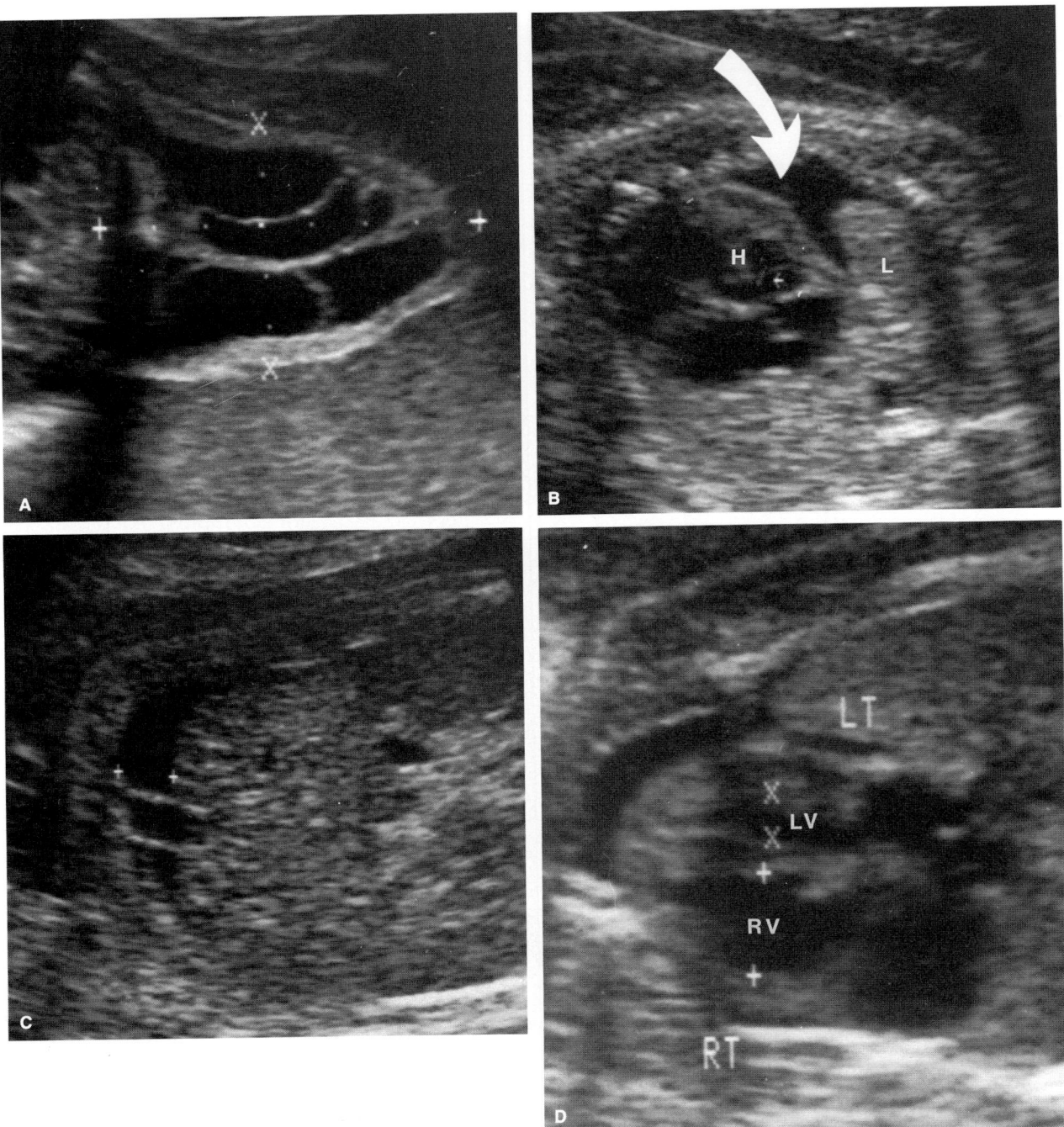

FIGURE 21-17. Turner's syndrome in a 32-week fetus. **(A)** Cystic hygroma (*graticules*) with a midline nuchal ligament. Each hygroma cavity is subdivided by incomplete septa. **(B)** Transverse ultrasound of fetal chest shows pleural effusion (*curved arrow*). L, lung; H, heart. **(C)** Transverse ultrasound of fetal abdomen shows ascites (*graticules*). **(D)** Small left ventricle (LV); the right ventricle (RV) is an appropriate size for the patient's gestational age. These findings are consistent with aortic coarctation. RT, right; LT, left.

TABLE 21-12.   Sonographically Detectable Abnormalities in 11 Triploid Fetuses

Abnormality	% Affected	Abnormality	% Affected
Head and face		Cardiovascular system	
Large head	75	Any heart defect	66
Cleft palate	50	Atrial septal and ventricular septal defects	25
Low-set ears	25	Ventricular septal defect, isolated	25
Cleft lip	16	Atrioventricular canal	16
Microphthalmia	8	Aortic stenosis	16
Large ears	8	Single ventricle	8
Neck		Double-outlet right ventricle	8
Edema	16	Respiratory system	
Extremities		Hypoplastic lungs	66
Syndactyly between the third and fourth fingers	58	Central nervous system	
		Neural tube defect	16
Clinodactyly of the fifth finger	16	Holoprosencephaly	8
Syndactyly between the toes	50	Urogenital system	
		Hypoplastic kidney	8
		Horseshoe kidney	8

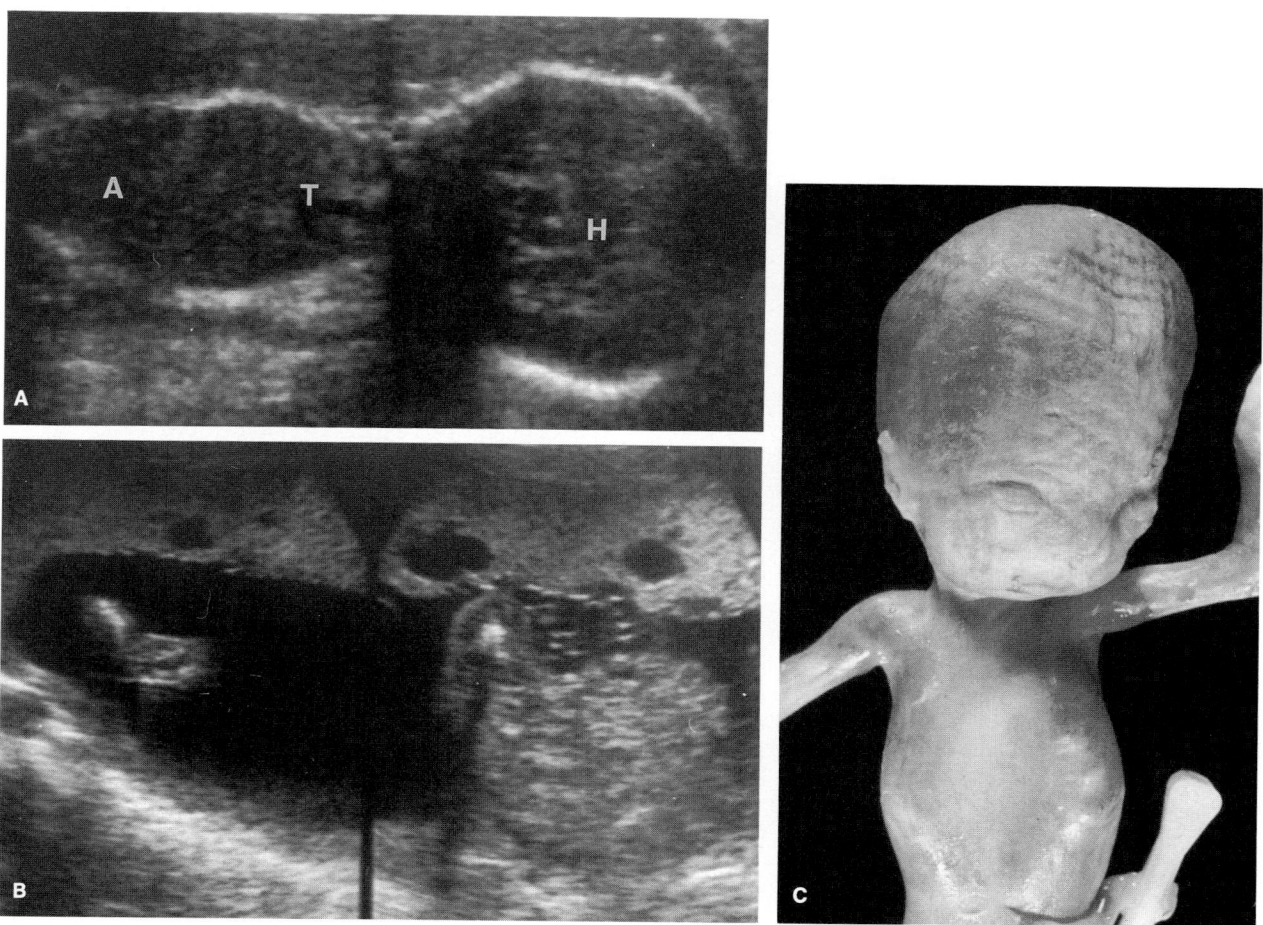

FIGURE 21-18.   Sonographic findings with triploidy. **(A)** Intrauterine growth retardation with extreme head (H) to body disproportion. T, thorax; A, abdomen. **(B)** Hydropic placenta. **(C)** Fetal autopsy with triploidy; note the marked disproportion between the fetal head and body as well as the micrognathia. (Crane JP, et al: Antenatal ultrasound findings in fetal triploidy syndrome. J Ultrasound Med 1985; 4:519.)

ond trimester, early-onset growth retardation with extreme head/body ratio disproportion is characteristic. Table 21-12 indicates the sonographically detectable abnormalities in triploid fetuses (Fig. 21-18).

Abnormalities in amniotic fluid volume, polyhydramnios, and oligohydramnios have been reported with triploidy.[74]

CONCLUSION

Accurate prenatal diagnosis of fetal anomalies is essential to make appropriate management decisions. Traditionally, an autopsy has been the ultimate diagnostic tool for fetal anomaly detection. This chapter implies that a careful anatomic survey can be used for the same purpose and in some instances may replace necropsy. The accuracy of an ultrasound examination in the detection of fetal anomalies, however, is affected by oligohydramnios, fetal demise, and the presence of multiple anomalies—all of which occur more frequently in the presence of a chromosomal abnormality. It cannot be emphasized too strongly that a thorough fetal autopsy is important not only to confirm the prenatal diagnosis but also to delineate associated or additional anomalies for syndrome identification. Tissue should be submitted for cytogenic analysis at the time of autopsy if this analysis was not performed prenatally.[75]

REFERENCES

1. Ferguson-Smith MA, Yates JRW: Maternal age specific rates for chromosome aberrations and factors influencing them: Report of a collaborative European study on 52965 amniocenteses. Prenat Diagn 1984; 4:5–44.
2. Jacobs PA, Hassold JT: Chromosome abnormalities: Origin and etiology in abortions and live births. In Vogel F, Sperling (eds): Human Genetics. Berlin: Springer-Verlag, 1987: 233–244.
3. Matsunga E, Tonomura A, Oishi H, Kikuchi Y: Reexamination of paternal age effect in Down's syndrome. Hum Genet 1978; 40:259–268.
4. Warburton D, Kline J, Stein Z, et al: Does the karyotype of a spontaneous abortion predict the karyotype of a subsequent abortion? Evidence from 273 women with two karyotyped spontaneous abortions. Am J Hum Genet 1987; 41:465–483.
5. Stene J, Stene E, Mikkelsen M: Risk for chromosome abnormality at amniocentesis following a child with a non-inherited chromosome aberration. Prenat Diagn [special issue] 1984; 4:81–95.

6. Haddow JE, Palomaki GE, Knight GJ, et al: Prenatal screening for Down's syndrome with use of maternal serum markers. N Engl J Med 1992; 327:588–593.
7. Palomaki GE, Knight GJ, Haddow JE, et al: Prospective intervention trial of a screening protocol to identify fetal trisomy 18 using maternal serum alpha-fetoprotein, unconjugated oestriol, and human chorionic gonadotropin. Prenat Diagn 1992; 12:925–930.
8. Palomaki GE, Haddow JE: Maternal serum alpha-fetoprotein, age, and Down syndrome risk. Am J Obstet Gynecol 1987; 156:460–463.
9. Doran T, Cadesky K, Wong P, et al: Maternal serum alpha-fetoprotein and fetal autosomal trisomies. Am J Obstet Gynecol 1986; 154:277–281.
10. Lettieri L, Rodis JF, Vintzileos AM, et al: Ear length in second-trimester aneuploid fetuses. Obstet Gynecol 1993; 81:57–60.
11. Hill LM, Macpherson T, Rivello D, Peterson C: The spontaneous resolution of cystic hygromas and early fetal growth delay in fetuses with trisomy 18. Prenat Diagn 1991; 11:673–677.
12. Johnson MP, Johnson A, Holzgreve W, et al: First-trimester simple hygroma: Cause and outcome. Am J Obstet Gynecol 1993; 168:156–161.
13. Bell JA, Bell JR, Pearn JH: Diagnostic trends in childhood chromosome abnormalities and their implications: A total population eight-year survey from Queensland, Australia. Birth Defects 1987; 23:307–314.
14. Riccardi VM: Trisomy 8: An international study of 70 patients. Birth Defects 1977; 13:171–184.
15. Anneren G, Sedin G: Case report: Trisomy 9 syndrome. Acta Paediatr Scand 1981; 70:125–128.
16. Jones KL: Smith's Recognizable Patterns of Human Malformation, 4th ed. Philadelphia: WB Saunders, 1988: 16–25.
17. Kalousek DK, Fitch N, Paradice BA: Pathology of the Human Embryo and Previable Fetus: An Atlas. New York: Springer-Verlag, 1990: 190.
18. Patau K, Smith DW, Therman E, et al: Multiple congenital anomaly caused by an extra chromosome. Lancet 1960; 1:790–793.
19. Donnenfeld AE, Mennuti MT: Sonographic findings in fetuses with common chromosome abnormalities. Clin Obstet Gynecol 1988; 31:80–96.
20. Fogel M, Capel JA, Cullen MT, et al: Congenital heart disease and fetal thoracoabdominal anomalies: Associations in utero and the importance of cytogenetic analysis. J Perinatol 1991; 8:411–416.
21. Naor N, Amir Y, Cohen T, Davidson S: Trisomy 13 in monozygotic twins discordant for major congenital anomalies. J Med Genet 1987; 24:500–502.
22. Dicke JM, Crane JP: Sonographic recognition of major malformations and aberrant fetal growth in trisomic fetuses. J Ultrasound Med 1991; 18:433–438.
23. Simpson JL, Golbus MS: Genetics in Obstetrics and Gynecology, 2nd ed. Philadelphia: WB Saunders, 1992: Chapter 5.

24. Wladimiroff JW, Stewart PA, Reuss A, Sachs ES: Cardiac and extra-cardiac anomalies as indicators for trisomies 13 and 18: A prenatal ultrasound study. Prenat Diagn 1989; 9:515–520.

25. Kalousek DK, Fitch N, Paradice BA: Pathology of the Human Embryo and Previable fetus: An Atlas. New York: Springer-Verlag, 1990: 186.

26. Eaton FP, Kontras SB, Sommer A, Wehe A: Longterm survival in trisomy 18: New chromosomal and malformation syndromes. Birth Defects 1975; 11:327–328.

27. Edwards JH, Harnden DG, Cameron AH, et al: A new trisomic syndrome. Lancet 1960; 1:787–789.

28. Tyson RW, Kalousek DK: Chromosomal abnormalities in stillbirth and neonatal death. In Dimmick JE, Kalousek DK (eds): Developmental Pathology of the Embryo. Philadelphia: JB Lippincott, 1992.

29. Nyberg DA, Kramer D, Resta RG, et al: Prenatal sonographic findings of trisomy 18: Review of 47 cases. J Ultrasound Med 1993; 2:103–113.

30. Lynch L, Berkowitz RL: First trimester growth delay in trisomy 18. Am J Perinatol 1989; 6:237–239.

31. Nicolaides KH, Salvesen DR, Snijdens RJM, Gosden CM: Strawberry-shaped skull in fetal trisomy 18. Fetal Diagn Ther 1992; 7:132–137.

32. Hill LM, Marchese S, Peterson C, Fries J: The effect of trisomy 18 on transverse cerebellar diameter. Am J Obstet Gynecol 1991; 165:72–75.

33. Sumi S: Brain malformations in the trisomy 18 syndrome. Brain 1970; 93: 821–830.

34. Chitkara U, Cogswell C, Norton K, et al: Choroid plexus cysts in the fetus: A benign anatomic variant or pathological entity? Obstet Gynecol 1988; 72:185–189.

35. Benacerraf BR, Laboda LA: Cyst of the fetal choroid plexus: A normal variant? Am J Obstet Gynecol 1989; 160:319–321.

36. Twinning P, Zuccollo J, Clewes J, Swallow J: Fetal choroid plexus cysts: A prospective study and review of the literature. Br J Radiol 1991; 64:98–102.

37. Fitzsimmons J, Wilson D, Pascoe-Mason J, et al: Choroid plexus cysts in fetuses with trisomy 18. Obstet Gynecol 1989; 73:257–260.

38. Benacerraf BR, Harlow B, Frigoletto F Jr: Are choroid plexus cysts an indication for second trimester amniocentesis? Am J Obstet Gynecol 1990; 162:1001–1006.

39. Thorpe-Beeston JG, Gosden CM, Nicolaides KH: Choroid plexus cysts and chromosomal defects. Br J Radiol 1990:63:783–786.

40. Benacerraf BR, Miller WA, Frigoletto FD: Sonographic detection of fetuses with trisomies 13 and 18: Accuracy and limitations. Am J Obstet Gynecol 1988; 158:404–409.

41. Achiron R, Barkai G, Bat-Miriam K, Mashiach S: Fetal lateral ventricle choroid plexus cysts: The dilemma of amniocentesis. Obstet Gynecol 1991; 78:815–818.

42. Jauniaux E, Donner C, Thomas C, et al: Umbilical cord pseudocyst in trisomy 18. Prenat Diagn 1988; 8:557–563.

43. Musewe NN, Alexander DJ, Teshima I, et al: Echocardiographic evaluation of the spectrum of cardiac anomalies associated with trisomy 13 and trisomy 18. J Am Coll Cardiol 1990; 15:673–677.

44. Kalousek DK, Fitch N, Paradice BA: Pathology of the Human Embryo and Previable Fetus: An Atlas. New York: Springer-Verlag, 1990: 188.

45. Marion RW, Chitayat D, Hutcheon RG, et al: Trisomy 18 score: A rapid, reliable diagnostic test for trisomy 18. Pediatrics 1988; 113:45–48.

46. Penrose LS, Smith GF: Down's anomaly. London: Churchill, 1966.

47. Kalousek DK, Fitch N, Paradice BA: Pathology of the Human Embryo and Previable Fetus: An Atlas. New York: Springer-Verlag, 1990: 181–182.

48. Benacerraf BR, Frigoletto FD: Soft tissue nuchal-fold in the second-trimester fetus: Standards for normal measurements compared with those in Down syndrome. Am J Obstet Gynecol 1987; 157:1146–1149.

49. Benacerraf BR, Laboda LA, Frigoletto FD: Thickened nuchal fold in fetuses not at risk for aneuploidy. Radiology 1992; 184:239–242.

50. Nyberg DA, Resta RG, Luthy DA, et al: Humerus and femur length shortening in the detection of Down's syndrome. Am J Obstet Gynecol 1993; 168:534–538.

51. Benacerraf BR, Gelman R, Frigoletto FD: Sonographic identification of second-trimester fetuses with Down's syndrome. N Engl J Med 1987; 317:1371–1376.

52. Lockwood C, Benacerraf B, Krinsky A, et al: A sonographic screening method for Down syndrome. Am J Obstet Gynecol 1987; 157:803–808.

53. Hill LM, Guzick D, Belfar H, et al: The current role of sonography in the detection of Down syndrome. Obstet Gynecol 1989; 74:620–623.

54. Nyberg DA, Resta RG, Luthy DA, et al: Prenatal sonographic findings of Down syndrome: Review of 94 cases. Obstet Gynecol 1990; 76:370–377.

55. Spicer RL: Cardiovascular disease in Down syndrome. Pediatr Clin North Am 1984; 31:1331–1343.

56. Nyberg DA: Intra-abdominal abnormalities. In Diagnostic Ultrasound of Fetal Anomalies: Text and Atlas. Chicago: Year Book Medical Publishers, 1990: Chapter 10.

57. Turner HH: A syndrome of infantilism, congenital webbed neck, and cubitus valgus. Endocrinology 1938; 23:566–574.

58. Smith DW: Recognizable Patterns of Human Malformation. Philadelphia: WB Saunders, 1982: 72–75.

59. Hook EB, Warburton D: The distribution of chromosomal genotypes associated with Turner's syndrome: Livebirth prevalence rates and evidence for diminished fetal mortality and severity in genotypes associated with structural X abnormalities or mosaicism. Hum Genet 1983; 64:24–27.

60. Kalousek D, Seller D: Differential diagnosis of pos-

terior cervical hygroma in previable fetuses. Am J Med Genet 1987; 3(Suppl): 83–92.

61. Pons JC, Diallo AA, Eydoux P, et al: Chorionic villus sampling after first trimester diagnosis of fetal cystic hygroma colli. Eur J Obstet Gynecol Reprod Biol 1989; 33:141–146.

62. Mostello DJ, Bofinger MK, Siddiqi TA: Spontaneous resolution of fetal cystic hygromas and hydrops in Turner syndrome. Obstet Gynecol 1989; 73:862–865.

63. Nicolaides KH, Azar G, Byrne D, et al: Fetal nuchal translucency: Ultrasound screening for chromosomal defects in first trimester pregnancy. Br Med J 1992; 304:867–869.

64. Bronshtein M, Rottem S, Yoffe N, Blumenfeld Z: First-trimester and early second-trimester diagnosis of nuchal cystic hygroma by transvaginal sonography: Diverse prognosis of the septated from the nonseptated lesion. Am J Obstet Gynecol 1989; 161:78–82.

65. Johnson MP, Johnson A, Holzgreve W, et al: First trimester simple hygroma: Cause and outcome. Am J Obstet Gynecol 1993; 168:156–161.

66. Garden AS, Benzie RJ, Miskin M, Gardner HA: Fetal cystic hygroma colli: Antenatal diagnosis, significance and management. Am J Obstet Gynecol 1986; 154:221–225.

67. Benacerraf BR, Saltzman DH, Sanders SP: Sonographic sign suggesting the prenatal diagnosis of coarctation of the aorta. J Ultrasound Med 1989; 8:65–69.

68. Doshi N, Surti U, Szulman AE: Morphologic anomalies in triploid liveborn fetuses. Hum Pathol 1983; 14:716–723.

69. Jacobs PA, Szulman AG, Funkhouser J, et al: Hu-

man triploidy relationship between parental origin of the additional complement and development of partial hydatidiform mole. Ann Human Genet 1982; 46:223–231.

70. Pircon RA, Towers CV, Porto M, et al: Maternal serum alpha-fetoprotein and fetal triploidy. Prenat Diagn 1989; 9:701–707.

71. Kazazian LC, Baramki TA, Thomas RL: Triploid fetus: An important consideration in the evaluation of very high maternal serum alpha-fetoprotein. Prenat Diagn 1989; 9:27–30.

72. Edwards MT, Smith WL, Hanson J, Yousef MA: Prenatal sonographic diagnosis of triploidy. J Ultrasound Med 1986; 5:279–281.

73. Benacerraf BR: Intrauterine growth retardation in the first trimester associated with triploidy. J Ultrasound Med 1988; 7:153–154.

74. Blackburn WR, Miller WP, Superneau DW, et al: Comparative studies of infants with mosaic and complete triploidy: An analysis of 55 cases. Birth Defects 1982; 18:251–274.

75. Shen-Schwarz S, Neish C, Hill LM: Antenatal ultrasound for fetal anomalies: Importance of perinatal autopsy. Pediatr Pathol 1989; 9:1–9.

76. Schreinemachers DM, Cross PK, Hook EB: Rates of trisomies 21, 18, 13 and other chromosome abnormalities in about 20,000 prenatal studies compared with estimated rates in live births. Hum Genet 1982; 61:318.

77. Mikkelsen M, Aymé S: Chromosomal findings in chorionic villi: A collaborative study. In Vogel F, Sperling K (eds): Proceedings of the 7th International Congress of Human Genetics. Berlin: Springer, 1987:598.

John P. McGahan and Manuel Porto:
DIAGNOSTIC OBSTETRICAL ULTRASOUND.
© 1994 J.B. Lippincott Company.

Appendix

Guidelines for Performance of the Antepartum Obstetrical Ultrasound Examination*

These guidelines have been developed for use by practitioners performing obstetrical ultrasound studies. A limited examination may be performed in clinical emergencies or used as a follow-up to a complete examination. In some cases, an additional and/or specialized examination may be necessary. While it is not possible to detect all structural congenital anomalies with diagnostic ultrasound, adherence to the following guidelines will maximize the possibility of detecting many fetal abnormalities.

EQUIPMENT

These studies should be conducted with real-time scanners, using an abdominal and/or vaginal approach. A transducer of appropriate frequency (3 MHz or higher abdominally, 5 MHz or higher vaginally) should be used. A static scanner (3 to 5 MHz) may be used but should not be the sole method of examination. The lowest possible ultrasonic exposure settings should be used to gain the necessary diagnostic information.

Comment: Real-time is necessary to reliably confirm the presence of fetal life through observation of cardiac activity, respiration, and active movement. Real-time studies simplify evaluation of fetal anatomy as well as the task of obtaining fetal measurements. The choice of frequency is a trade-off between beam penetration and resolution. With modern equipment, 3- to 5-MHz abdominal transducers allow sufficient penetration in nearly all patients, while providing adequate resolution. During early pregnancy, a 5-MHZ abdominal or a 5- to 7-MHz vaginal transducer may provide adequate penetration and produce superior resolution.

* From American Institute of Ultrasound in Medicine: Guidelines for Performance of the Antepartum Obstetrical Ultrasound Examination, 1991, with permission.

DOCUMENTATION

Adequate documentation of the study is essential for high quality patient care. This should include a permanent record of the ultrasound images, incorporating whenever possible the measurement parameters and anatomical findings proposed in the following sections of this document. Images should be appropriately labeled with the examination date, patient identification, and, if appropriate, image orientation. A written report of the ultrasound findings should be included in the patient's medical record regardless of where the study is performed.

GUIDELINES FOR FIRST TRIMESTER SONOGRAPHY

Overall Comment: Scanning in the first trimester may be performed either abdominally or vaginally. If an abdominal scan is performed and fails to provide definitive information concerning any of the following guidelines, a vaginal scan should be performed whenever possible.

1. The location of the gestational sac should be documented. The embryo should be identified and the crown–rump length recorded.

   Comment: The crown–rump length is an accurate indicator of fetal age. Comparison should be made to standard tables. If the embryo is not identified, characteristics of the gestational sac, including mean diameter of the anechoic space to determine fetal age and analysis of the hyperechoic rim, should be noted. During the late first trimester, biparietal diameter and other fetal measurements may also be used to establish fetal age.

2. Presence or absence of fetal life should be reported.

   Comment: Real-time observation is critical in this diagnosis. It should be noted that fetal cardiac activity may not be visible prior to seven weeks abdominally and frequently at least one week earlier vaginally as determined by crown–rump length. Thus, confirmation of fetal life may require follow-up evaluation.

3. Fetal number should be documented.

   Comment: Multiple pregnancies should be reported only in those instances where multiple embryos are seen. Due to variability in fusion between the amnion and chorion, the appearance of more than one sac-like structure in early pregnancy is often noted and may be confused with multiple gestation or amniotic band.

4. Evaluation of the uterus (including cervix) and adnexal structures should be performed.

   Comment: This will allow recognition of incidental findings of potential clinical significance. The presence, location, and size of myomas and adnexal masses should be recorded.

GUIDELINES FOR SECOND AND THIRD TRIMESTER SONOGRAPHY

1. Fetal life, number, and presentation should be documented.

   Comment: Abnormal heart rate and/or rhythm should be reported. Multiple pregnancies require the reporting of additional information: placental number, sac number, comparison of fetal size, and when visualized, fetal genitalia and presence or absence of an interposed membrane.

2. An estimate of the amount of amniotic fluid (increased, decreased, normal) should be reported.

   Comment: While this evaluation is subjective, there is little difficulty in recognizing the extremes of amniotic fluid volume. Physiologic variation with stage of pregnancy must be taken into account.

3. The placental location, appearance, and its relationship to the internal cervical os should be recorded.

   Comment: It is recognized that placental position early in pregnancy may not correlate well with its location at the time of delivery.

4. Assessment of gestational age should be accomplished using a combination of biparietal diameter (or head circumference) and femur length. Fetal growth and weight (as opposed to age) should be assessed in the third trimester and requires the addition of abdominal diameters or circumferences. If previous studies have been performed, an estimate of the appropriateness of interval change should be given.

Comment: Third trimester measurements may not accurately reflect gestational age. Initial determination of gestational age should therefore be performed prior to the third trimester whenever possible. If one or more previous studies have been performed, the gestational age at the time of the current examination should be based on the earliest examination that permits measurement of crown–rump length, biparietal diameter, head circumference, and/or femur length by the equation: current fetal age = initial embryo/fetal age + number of weeks from first study. The current measurements should be compared with norms for the gestational age based on standard tables. If previous studies have been performed, interval change in the measurements should be assessed.

4A. Biparietal diameter at a standard reference level (which should include the cavum septi pellucidi and the thalamus) should be measured and recorded.

> *Comment:* If the fetal head is dolichocephalic or brachycephalic, the biparietal diameter alone may be misleading. On occasion, the computation of the cephalic index, a ratio of the biparietal diameter to fronto-occipital diameter, is needed to make this determination. In such situations, the head circumference or corrected biparietal diameter is required.

4B. Head circumference is measured at the same level as the biparietal diameter.

4C. Femur length should be measured routinely and recorded after the 14th week of gestation.

> *Comment:* As with biparietal diameter, considerable biological variation is present late in pregnancy.

4D. Abdominal circumference should be determined at the level of the junction of the umbilical vein and portal sinus.

> *Comment:* Abdominal circumference measurement may allow detection of growth retardation and macrosomia—conditions of the late second and third trimester. Comparison of the abdominal circumference with the head circumference should be made. If the abdominal measurement is below or above that expected for a stated gestation, it is recommended that circumferences of the head and body be measured and the head circumference/abdominal circumference ratio be reported. The use of circumferences is also suggested in those instances where the shape of either the head or body is different from that normally encountered.

5. Evaluation of the uterus and adnexal structures should be performed.

> *Comment:* This will allow recognition of incidental findings of potential clinical significance. The presence, location, and size of myomas and adnexal masses should be recorded.

6. The study should include, but not necessarily be limited to, the following fetal anatomy: cerebral ventricles, four-chamber view of the heart (including its position within the thorax), spine, stomach, urinary bladder, umbilical cord insertion site on the anterior abdominal wall, and renal region.

> *Comment:* It is recognized that not all malformations of the above-mentioned organ systems (such as the spine) can be detected using ultrasonography. Nevertheless, a careful anatomical survey may allow diagnosis of certain birth defects which would otherwise go unrecognized. Suspected abnormalities may require a specialized evaluation.

Master List of Growth Landmarks, Growth Measurements, Fetal Weight, and Fetal Ratios

GROWTH LANDMARKS/PARAMETERS

Endovaginal sonographic findings from 3.5 to 6.5 menstrual weeks (Table 1-1)

Expected hCG levels for increasing mean sac measurements (Table 2-1)

Gestational age, hCG levels, and transvaginal ultrasound findings (Table 2-2)

MENSTRUAL AGE COMPARISON WITH FETAL MEASUREMENTS (UNLESS SPECIFIED OTHERWISE)

Abdominal circumference (compared with other growth parameters) (Appendix Table I)

Abdominal circumference (Table 2-8)

Abdominal circumference—standard deviations (Table 5-11)

Biocular distance (Table 10-1)

Biparietal diameter (Table 2-5)

BPD (compared with other growth parameters) (Appendix Table I)

Cerebellar diameter (Table 2-13)

Clavicular length (Table 2-10)

Crown-rump length (Table 2-4)

Femur length (compared with other growth parameters) (Appendix Table I)

Femur length (Table 2-9)

Femur length—5th and 95th percentile (Table 19-2)

Fibula—5th and 95th percentile (Table 19-2)

Foot length (Table 2-12)

Head circumference (compared with other growth parameters) (Appendix Table I)

Head circumference (Table 2-7)

Head circumference—standard deviations (Table 8-16)

Humeral length (Table 2-9)

Humerus—5th and 95th percentile (Table 19-2)

Interocular distance (Table 10-1)
Kidney diameter (Table 17-11)
Kidney length (Table 17-10)
Kidney measurements compared to abdominal measurements (Table 17-12)
Mean predicted gestational sac size (Table 2-3)
Ocular diameter (Table 10-1)
Radius—5th and 95th percentile (Table 19-2)
Thigh circumference (Table 2-11)
Thoracic circumference (Table 11-2)
Thoracic length (Appendix Table II)
Tibia—5th and 95th percentile (Table 19-2)
Tibial length (Table 2-9)
Ulna—5th and 95th percentile (Table 19-2)
Ulna length (Table 2-9)
Umbilical artery—systolic to diastolic ratio (Table 5-8)

RATIOS OF FETAL MEASUREMENTS

Head circumference to abdominal circumference ratio (Table 8-17)

Femur length to head circumference ratio (Table 8-18)
Thoracic circumference to abdominal circumference ratio (Table 11-3)
Thoracic circumference to head circumference ratio (Table 11-3)
Thoracic circumference to humoral length ratio (Table 11-3)
Thoracic circumference to femur length (Table 11-3)

FETAL WEIGHTS BASED UPON VARIOUS FETAL MEASUREMENTS

Femur length and abdominal circumference (Appendix Table III)
BPD and abdominal circumference (Appendix Table IV)
Fetal weight throughout pregnancy (Table 5-13)

TABLE I. Predicted Fetal Measurements at Specific Menstrual Age

Menstrual Age (wk)	Biparietal Diameter (cm)	Head Circumference (cm)	Abdominal Circumference (cm)	Femur Length (cm)
12.0	1.7	6.8	4.6	0.7
12.5	1.8	7.5	5.3	0.9
13.0	2.1	8.2	6.0	1.1
13.5	2.3	8.9	6.7	1.2
14.0	2.5	9.7	7.3	1.4
14.5	2.7	10.4	8.0	1.6
15.0	2.9	11.0	8.6	1.7
15.5	3.1	11.7	9.3	1.9
16.0	3.2	12.4	9.9	2.0
16.5	3.4	13.1	10.6	2.2
17.0	3.6	13.8	11.2	2.4
17.5	3.8	14.4	11.9	2.5
18.0	3.9	15.1	12.5	2.7
18.5	4.1	15.8	13.1	2.8
19.0	4.3	16.4	13.7	3.0
19.5	4.5	17.0	14.4	3.1
20.0	4.6	17.7	15.0	3.3
20.5	4.8	18.3	15.6	3.4
21.0	5.0	18.9	16.2	3.5
21.5	5.1	19.5	16.8	3.7
22.0	5.3	20.1	17.4	3.8

(continued)

TABLE I. (*Continued*)

Menstrual Age (wk)	Biparietal Diameter (cm)	Head Circumference (cm)	Abdominal Circumference (cm)	Femur Length (cm)
22.5	5.5	20.7	17.9	4.0
23.0	5.6	21.3	18.5	4.1
23.5	5.8	21.9	19.1	4.2
24.0	5.9	22.4	19.7	4.4
24.5	6.1	23.0	20.2	4.5
25.0	6.2	23.5	20.8	4.6
25.5	6.4	24.1	21.3	4.7
26.0	6.5	24.6	21.9	4.9
26.5	6.7	25.1	22.4	5.0
27.0	6.8	25.6	23.0	5.1
27.5	6.9	26.1	23.5	5.2
28.0	7.1	26.6	24.0	5.4
28.5	7.2	27.1	24.6	5.5
29.0	7.3	27.5	25.1	5.6
29.5	7.5	28.0	25.6	5.7
30.0	7.6	28.4	26.1	5.8
30.5	7.7	28.8	26.6	5.9
31.0	7.8	29.3	27.1	6.0
31.5	7.9	29.7	27.6	6.1
32.0	8.1	30.1	28.1	6.2
32.5	8.2	30.4	28.6	6.3
33.0	8.3	30.8	29.1	6.4
33.5	8.4	31.2	29.5	6.5
34.0	8.5	31.5	30.0	6.6
34.5	8.6	31.8	30.5	6.7
35.0	8.7	32.2	30.9	6.8
35.5	8.8	32.5	31.4	6.9
36.0	8.9	32.8	31.8	7.0
36.5	8.9	33.0	32.3	7.1
37.0	9.0	33.3	32.7	7.2
37.5	9.1	33.5	33.2	7.3
38.0	9.2	33.8	33.6	7.4
38.5	9.2	34.0	34.0	7.4
39.0	9.3	34.2	34.4	7.5
39.5	9.4	34.4	34.8	7.6
40.0	9.4	34.6	35.3	7.7

(From Hadlock FP, Deter RL, Harrist RB, et al: Estimating fetal age: Computer-assisted analysis of multiple fetal growth parameters. Radiology 1984; 152:497–501. Used by permission.)

TABLE II. Fetal Thoracic Length Measurements*

Gestational Age (wk)	No.	Predictive Percentiles								
		2.5	5	10	25	50	75	90	95	97.5
16	6	0.9	1.1	1.3	1.6	2.0	2.4	2.8	3.0	3.2
17	22	1.1	1.3	1.5	1.8	2.2	2.6	3.0	3.2	3.4
18	31	1.3	1.4	1.7	2.0	2.4	2.8	3.2	3.4	3.6
19	21	1.4	1.6	1.8	2.2	2.7	3.0	3.4	3.6	3.8
20	20	1.6	1.8	2.0	2.4	2.8	3.2	3.6	3.8	4.0
21	30	1.8	2.0	2.2	2.6	3.0	3.4	3.7	4.0	4.1
22	18	2.0	2.2	2.4	2.8	3.2	3.6	3.9	4.1	4.3
23	21	2.2	2.4	2.6	3.0	3.4	3.8	4.1	4.3	4.5
24	27	2.4	2.6	2.8	3.1	3.5	3.9	4.3	4.5	4.7
25	20	2.6	2.8	3.0	3.3	3.7	4.1	4.5	4.7	4.9
26	25	2.8	2.9	3.2	3.5	3.9	4.3	4.7	4.9	5.1
27	24	2.9	3.1	3.3	3.7	4.1	4.5	4.9	5.1	5.3
28	24	3.1	3.3	3.5	3.9	4.3	4.7	5.0	5.4	5.4
29	24	3.3	3.5	3.7	4.1	4.5	4.9	5.2	5.5	5.6
30	27	3.5	3.7	3.9	4.3	4.7	5.1	5.4	5.6	5.8
31	24	3.7	3.9	4.1	4.5	4.9	5.3	5.6	5.8	6.0
32	28	3.9	4.1	4.3	4.6	5.0	5.4	5.8	6.0	6.2
33	27	4.1	4.3	4.5	4.8	5.2	5.6	6.0	6.2	6.4
34	25	4.2	4.4	4.7	5.0	5.4	5.8	6.2	6.4	6.6
35	20	4.4	4.6	4.8	5.2	5.6	6.0	6.4	6.6	6.8
36	23	4.6	4.8	5.0	5.4	5.8	6.2	6.5	6.8	7.0
37	22	4.8	5.0	5.2	5.6	6.0	6.4	6.7	7.0	7.1
38	21	5.0	5.2	5.4	5.8	6.2	6.6	6.9	7.1	7.3
39	7	5.2	5.4	5.6	6.0	6.4	6.8	7.1	7.3	7.5
40	6	5.4	5.6	5.8	6.1	6.5	6.9	7.3	7.5	7.7

* Measurements in centimeters.

(From Chitkara U, Rosenberg J, Chervenak FA, et al: Prenatal sonographic assessment of the fetal thorax: Normal values. Am J Obstet Gynecol 1987; 156:1069–1074. Used by permission.)

TABLE III   Estimates of Fetal Weight (in Grams) Based on Abdominal Circumference and Femur Length

Femur Length (cm)	Abdominal Circumference (cm)									
	20.0	*20.5*	*21.0*	*21.5*	*22.0*	*22.5*	*23.0*	*23.5*	*24.0*	*24.5*
4.0	663	691	720	751	783	816	851	887	925	964
4.1	680	709	738	769	802	836	871	907	946	986
4.2	697	726	757	788	821	855	891	928	967	1007
4.3	715	745	776	808	841	875	912	949	988	1029
4.4	734	764	795	827	861	896	933	971	1010	1051
4.5	753	783	815	847	882	917	954	993	1033	1074
4.6	772	803	835	868	903	939	976	1015	1056	1098
4.7	792	823	856	889	924	961	999	1038	1079	1122
4.8	812	844	877	911	947	984	1022	1062	1103	1146
4.9	833	865	899	933	969	1007	1046	1086	1128	1171
5.0	855	887	921	956	993	1031	1070	1111	1153	1197
5.1	877	910	944	980	1016	1055	1095	1136	1179	1223
5.2	899	933	967	1004	1041	1080	1120	1162	1205	1250
5.3	922	956	992	1028	1066	1105	1146	1188	1232	1277
5.4	946	981	1016	1053	1091	1131	1172	1215	1259	1305
5.5	971	1005	1041	1079	1118	1158	1199	1242	1287	1333
5.6	995	1031	1067	1105	1144	1185	1227	1271	1316	1362
5.7	1021	1057	1094	1132	1172	1213	1255	1299	1345	1392
5.8	1047	1084	1121	1160	1200	1242	1285	1329	1375	1422
5.9	1074	1111	1149	1188	1229	1271	1314	1359	1406	1454
6.0	1102	1139	1178	1217	1258	1301	1345	1390	1437	1485
6.1	1130	1168	1207	1247	1289	1331	1376	1421	1469	1518
6.2	1160	1198	1237	1278	1319	1363	1408	1454	1501	1551
6.3	1189	1228	1268	1309	1351	1395	1440	1487	1535	1585
6.4	1220	1259	1299	1341	1384	1428	1473	1520	1569	1619
6.5	1251	1291	1332	1373	1417	1461	1507	1555	1604	1655
6.6	1284	1324	1365	1407	1451	1496	1542	1590	1640	1691
6.7	1317	1357	1399	1441	1486	1531	1578	1626	1676	1728
6.8	1351	1391	1433	1477	1521	1567	1615	1663	1713	1765
6.9	1385	1427	1469	1513	1558	1604	1652	1701	1752	1804
7.0	1421	1463	1506	1550	1595	1642	1690	1740	1791	1843
7.1	1458	1500	1543	1588	1633	1681	1729	1779	1830	1883
7.2	1495	1538	1581	1626	1673	1720	1769	1819	1871	1924
7.3	1534	1577	1621	1666	1713	1761	1810	1861	1913	1966
7.4	1573	1616	1661	1707	1754	1802	1852	1903	1955	2009
7.5	1614	1657	1702	1749	1796	1845	1895	1946	1999	2053
7.6	1655	1699	1745	1791	1839	1888	1939	1990	2043	2098
7.7	1698	1742	1788	1835	1883	1933	1983	2035	2089	2144
7.8	1741	1786	1833	1880	1928	1978	2029	2082	2135	2191
7.9	1786	1832	1878	1926	1975	2025	2076	2129	2183	2238
8.0	1832	1878	1925	1973	2022	2073	2124	2177	2232	2287
8.1	1879	1926	1973	2021	2071	2121	2173	2227	2281	2337
8.2	1928	1974	2022	2070	2120	2171	2224	2277	2332	2388
8.3	1978	2024	2072	2121	2171	2223	2275	2329	2384	2440

Abdominal Circumference (cm)										
25.0	*25.5*	*26.0*	*26.5*	*27.0*	*27.5*	*28.0*	*28.5*	*29.0*	*29.5*	*30.0*
1006	1048	1093	1139	1188	1239	1291	1346	1403	1463	1525
1027	1070	1115	1162	1211	1262	1315	1371	1429	1489	1551
1049	1093	1138	1186	1235	1287	1340	1396	1454	1515	1578
1071	1116	1162	1209	1259	1311	1365	1422	1480	1541	1605
1094	1139	1185	1234	1284	1336	1391	1448	1507	1568	1632
1118	1163	1210	1259	1309	1362	1417	1474	1534	1596	1660
1142	1187	1235	1284	1335	1388	1444	1501	1561	1623	1688
1166	1212	1260	1310	1361	1415	1471	1529	1589	1652	1717
1191	1237	1286	1336	1388	1442	1498	1557	1618	1681	1746
1216	1263	1312	1363	1415	1470	1527	1585	1647	1710	1776
1243	1290	1339	1390	1443	1498	1555	1615	1676	1740	1806
1269	1317	1367	1418	1471	1527	1584	1644	1706	1770	1837
1296	1344	1395	1447	1500	1556	1614	1674	1737	1801	1868
1324	1373	1423	1476	1530	1586	1645	1705	1768	1833	1900
1352	1401	1452	1505	1560	1617	1675	1736	1799	1865	1933
1381	1431	1482	1535	1591	1648	1707	1768	1832	1897	1966
1411	1461	1513	1566	1622	1679	1739	1801	1864	1931	1999
1441	1491	1544	1598	1654	1712	1772	1834	1898	1964	2033
1472	1523	1575	1630	1686	1744	1805	1867	1932	1999	2068
1503	1555	1608	1663	1719	1778	1839	1902	1966	2034	2103
1535	1587	1641	1696	1753	1812	1873	1936	2002	2069	2139
1568	1620	1674	1730	1788	1847	1908	1972	2038	2105	2175
1602	1654	1709	1765	1823	1882	1944	2008	2074	2142	2212
1636	1689	1744	1800	1858	1919	1981	2045	2111	2180	2250
1671	1724	1779	1836	1895	1956	2018	2082	2149	2218	2289
1707	1760	1816	1873	1932	1993	2056	2121	2188	2256	2328
1743	1797	1853	1911	1970	2031	2094	2160	2227	2296	2367
1780	1835	1891	1949	2009	2070	2134	2199	2267	2336	2408
1819	1873	1930	1988	2048	2110	2174	2240	2307	2377	2449
1857	1913	1970	2028	2089	2151	2215	2281	2348	2418	2490
1897	1953	2010	2069	2130	2192	2256	2322	2391	2461	2533
1938	1994	2051	2110	2171	2234	2299	2365	2433	2504	2576
1979	2035	2093	2153	2214	2277	2342	2408	2477	2547	2620
2021	2078	2136	2196	2258	2321	2386	2453	2521	2592	2665
2065	2122	2180	2240	2302	2365	2431	2498	2566	2637	2710
2109	2166	2225	2285	2347	2411	2476	2543	2612	2683	2756
2154	2211	2270	2331	2393	2457	2523	2590	2659	2730	2803
2200	2258	2317	2378	2440	2504	2570	2638	2707	2778	2851
2247	2305	2365	2426	2488	2553	2618	2686	2755	2827	2899
2295	2353	2413	2474	2537	2602	2668	2735	2805	2876	2949
2344	2403	2463	2524	2587	2652	2718	2785	2855	2926	2999
2394	2453	2513	2575	2638	2702	2769	2837	2906	2977	3050
2446	2504	2565	2626	2690	2754	2821	2889	2958	3029	3102
2498	2557	2617	2679	2743	2807	2874	2942	3011	3082	3155

(continued)

TABLE III (*Continued*)

Femur Length (cm)	Abdominal Circumference (cm)								
	30.5	31.0	31.5	32.0	32.5	33.0	33.5	34.0	34.5
4.0	1590	1658	1729	1802	1879	1959	2042	2129	2220
4.1	1617	1685	1756	1830	1907	1987	2071	2158	2249
4.2	1644	1712	1783	1858	1935	2016	2100	2187	2279
4.3	1671	1740	1812	1886	1964	2045	2129	2217	2308
4.4	1699	1768	1840	1915	1993	2075	2159	2247	2339
4.5	1727	1797	1869	1944	2023	2105	2189	2278	2370
4.6	1756	1826	1898	1974	2053	2135	2220	2309	2401
4.7	1785	1855	1928	2004	2084	2166	2251	2340	2432
4.8	1814	1885	1959	2035	2115	2197	2283	2372	2464
4.9	1845	1916	1990	2066	2146	2229	2315	2404	2497
5.0	1875	1947	2021	2098	2178	2261	2347	2437	2530
5.1	1906	1978	2053	2130	2210	2294	2380	2470	2563
5.2	1938	2010	2085	2163	2243	2327	2413	2503	2597
5.3	1970	2043	2118	2196	2277	2360	2447	2537	2631
5.4	2003	2076	2151	2229	2311	2395	2482	2572	2665
5.5	2036	2109	2185	2264	2345	2429	2516	2607	2700
5.6	2070	2143	2220	2298	2380	2464	2552	2642	2736
5.7	2104	2178	2254	2333	2415	2500	2587	2678	2772
5.8	2139	2213	2290	2369	2451	2536	2624	2714	2808
5.9	2175	2249	2326	2405	2488	2573	2660	2751	2845
6.0	2211	2286	2363	2442	2525	2610	2698	2789	2883
6.1	2248	2323	2400	2480	2562	2647	2736	2827	2921
6.2	2285	2360	2438	2518	2600	2686	2774	2865	2959
6.3	2323	2398	2476	2556	2639	2725	2813	2904	2998
6.4	2362	2437	2515	2595	2678	2764	2852	2943	3037
6.5	2401	2477	2555	2635	2718	2804	2892	2983	3077
6.6	2441	2517	2595	2675	2759	2844	2933	3024	3118
6.7	2481	2557	2636	2716	2800	2885	2974	3065	3159
6.8	2523	2599	2677	2758	2841	2927	3016	3107	3200
6.9	2564	2641	2719	2800	2884	2969	3058	3149	3242
7.0	2607	2683	2762	2843	2927	3012	3101	3192	3285
7.1	2650	2727	2806	2887	2970	3056	3144	3235	3328
7.2	2694	2771	2850	2931	3014	3100	3188	3279	3372
7.3	2739	2816	2895	2976	3059	3145	3233	3323	3416
7.4	2785	2861	2940	3021	3105	3190	3278	3369	3461
7.5	2831	2908	2987	3068	3151	3236	3324	3414	3507
7.6	2878	2955	3034	3115	3198	3283	3371	3461	3553
7.7	2926	3003	3081	3162	3245	3331	3418	3508	3600
7.8	2974	3051	3130	3211	3294	3379	3466	3555	3647
7.9	3024	3100	3179	3260	3343	3427	3514	3604	3695
8.0	3074	3151	3229	3310	3392	3477	3564	3653	3744
8.1	3125	3202	3280	3360	3443	3527	3614	3702	3793
8.2	3177	3253	3332	3412	3494	3578	3664	3752	3843
8.3	3230	3306	3384	3464	3546	3630	3716	3803	3893

(From Hadlock FP, Harrist RB, Carpenter RJ, et al: Sonographic estimation of fetal weight. Radiology 1984; 150:535–540. Used by permission.)

63	563	583	603	624	645	667	690	714	738	764	790	817	845
64	580	600	620	641	663	686	709	733	758	784	811	838	867
65	597	617	638	659	682	705	728	753	778	805	832	860	889
66	614	635	656	678	701	724	748	773	799	826	853	882	911
67	632	653	675	697	720	744	769	794	820	848	876	905	935
68	651	672	694	717	740	765	790	816	842	870	898	928	958
69	670	691	714	737	761	786	811	838	865	893	922	952	983
70	689	711	734	758	782	807	833	860	888	916	946	976	1,008
71	709	732	755	779	804	830	856	883	912	941	971	1,002	1,033
72	730	763	777	801	827	853	880	907	936	965	996	1,027	1,060
73	751	775	799	824	850	876	904	932	961	991	1,022	1,054	1,087
74	773	797	822	847	874	901	928	957	987	1,017	1,049	1,081	1,114
75	796	820	845	871	898	925	954	983	1,013	1,044	1,076	1,109	1,143
76	819	844	870	896	923	951	980	1,009	1,040	1,072	1,104	1,137	1,172
77	843	868	894	921	949	977	1,007	1,037	1,068	1,100	1,133	1,167	1,202
78	868	894	920	947	975	1,004	1,034	1,065	1,096	1,129	1,162	1,197	1,232
79	893	919	946	974	1,003	1,032	1,062	1,094	1,126	1,159	1,193	1,228	1,264
80	919	946	973	1,002	1,031	1,061	1,091	1,123	1,156	1,189	1,224	1,259	1,296
81	946	973	1,001	1,030	1,060	1,090	1,121	1,153	1,187	1,221	1,256	1,292	1,329
82	974	1,001	1,030	1,059	1,089	1,120	1,152	1,185	1,218	1,253	1,288	1,325	1,363
83	1,002	1,030	1,059	1,089	1,120	1,151	1,183	1,217	1,251	1,286	1,322	1,359	1,397
84	1,032	1,060	1,090	1,120	1,151	1,183	1,216	1,249	1,284	1,320	1,356	1,394	1,433
85	1,062	1,091	1,121	1,151	1,183	1,216	1,249	1,283	1,318	1,355	1,392	1,430	1,469
86	1,093	1,122	1,153	1,184	1,216	1,249	1,283	1,318	1,354	1,390	1,428	1,467	1,507
87	1,125	1,155	1,186	1,218	1,250	1,284	1,318	1,353	1,390	1,427	1,465	1,505	1,545
88	1,157	1,188	1,220	1,252	1,285	1,319	1,354	1,390	1,427	1,465	1,504	1,543	1,584
89	1,191	1,222	1,254	1,287	1,321	1,356	1,391	1,428	1,465	1,503	1,543	1,583	1,625
90	1,226	1,258	1,290	1,324	1,358	1,393	1,429	1,456	1,504	1,543	1,583	1,624	1,666
91	1,262	1,294	1,327	1,361	1,396	1,432	1,468	1,506	1,544	1,584	1,624	1,666	1,708
92	1,299	1,332	1,365	1,400	1,435	1,471	1,508	1,546	1,586	1,626	1,667	1,709	1,752
93	1,337	1,370	1,404	1,439	1,475	1,512	1,550	1,588	1,628	1,668	1,710	1,753	1,796
94	1,376	1,410	1,444	1,480	1,516	1,554	1,592	1,631	1,671	1,712	1,755	1,798	1,842
95	1,416	1,450	1,486	1,522	1,559	1,597	1,635	1,675	1,716	1,758	1,800	1,844	1,889
96	1,457	1,492	1,528	1,565	1,602	1,641	1,680	1,720	1,762	1,804	1,847	1,892	1,937
97	1,500	1,535	1,572	1,609	1,647	1,686	1,726	1,767	1,809	1,852	1,895	1,940	1,986
98	1,544	1,580	1,617	1,654	1,693	1,733	1,773	1,815	1,857	1,900	1,945	1,990	2,037
99	1,589	1,625	1,663	1,701	1,740	1,781	1,882	1,864	1,907	1,951	1,996	2,042	2,089
100	1,635	1,672	1,710	1,749	1,789	1,830	1,871	1,914	1,958	2,002	2,048	2,094	2,142

(continued)

TABLE IV (Continued)

BPD (mm)	AC (mm)												
	220	225	230	235	240	245	250	255	260	265	270	275	280
31	395	412	431	450	470	491	513	536	559	584	610	638	666
32	405	423	441	461	481	502	525	548	572	597	624	651	680
33	415	433	452	472	493	514	537	560	585	611	638	666	693
34	425	444	463	483	504	526	549	573	598	624	652	680	710
35	436	455	475	495	517	539	562	587	612	638	666	695	725
36	447	466	486	507	529	552	575	600	626	653	681	710	740
37	458	478	498	519	542	565	589	614	640	667	696	725	756
38	470	490	510	532	554	578	602	628	654	682	711	741	772
39	482	502	523	545	568	592	616	642	669	697	727	757	789
40	494	514	536	558	581	606	631	657	684	713	743	773	806
41	506	527	549	572	595	620	645	672	700	729	759	790	828
42	519	540	562	585	609	634	660	688	716	745	776	807	841
43	532	554	576	600	624	649	676	703	732	762	793	825	859
44	545	567	590	614	639	665	692	719	749	779	810	843	877
45	559	581	605	629	654	680	708	736	765	796	828	861	896
46	573	596	620	644	670	696	724	753	783	814	846	880	915
47	588	611	635	660	686	713	741	770	801	832	865	899	934
48	602	626	650	676	702	730	758	788	819	851	884	919	954
49	617	641	666	692	719	747	776	806	837	870	903	938	975
50	633	657	683	709	736	765	794	824	856	889	923	959	996
51	649	674	699	726	754	783	812	843	876	909	944	980	1,017
52	665	690	717	744	772	801	831	863	895	929	964	1,001	1,039
53	682	708	734	762	790	820	851	883	916	950	986	1,023	1,061
54	699	725	752	780	809	839	870	903	936	971	1,007	1,045	1,084
55	717	743	771	799	828	859	891	924	958	993	1,030	1,068	1,107
56	735	762	789	818	848	879	911	945	979	1,015	1,052	1,091	1,131
57	753	780	809	838	869	900	933	966	1,001	1,038	1,075	1,114	1,155
58	772	800	829	858	889	921	954	989	1,024	1,061	1,099	1,139	1,180
59	792	820	849	879	911	943	977	1,011	1,047	1,085	1,123	1,163	1,205
60	811	840	870	900	932	965	999	1,035	1,071	1,109	1,148	1,189	1,231
61	832	861	891	922	955	988	1,023	1,058	1,095	1,134	1,173	1,214	1,257
62	853	882	913	945	977	1,011	1,046	1,083	1,120	1,159	1,199	1,241	1,284

63	874	904	935	967	1,001	1,035	1,071	1,107	1,145	1,185	1,226	1,268	1,311
64	896	927	958	991	1,025	1,059	1,096	1,133	1,171	1,211	1,253	1,295	1,339
65	919	950	982	1,015	1,049	1,084	1,121	1,159	1,198	1,238	1,280	1,323	1,368
66	942	973	1,006	1,039	1,074	1,110	1,147	1,185	1,225	1,266	1,308	1,352	1,397
67	965	997	1,030	1,065	1,100	1,136	1,174	1,213	1,253	1,294	1,337	1,381	1,427
68	990	1,022	1,056	1,090	1,126	1,163	1,201	1,241	1,281	1,323	1,367	1,411	1,458
69	1,015	1,048	1,082	1,117	1,153	1,190	1,229	1,269	1,310	1,353	1,397	1,442	1,489
70	1,040	1,074	1,108	1,144	1,181	1,219	1,258	1,298	1,340	1,383	1,427	1,473	1,521
71	1,066	1,100	1,135	1,171	1,209	1,247	1,287	1,328	1,370	1,414	1,459	1,505	1,553
72	1,093	1,128	1,163	1,200	1,238	1,277	1,317	1,358	1,401	1,445	1,491	1,538	1,586
73	1,121	1,156	1,192	1,229	1,267	1,307	1,348	1,390	1,433	1,478	1,524	1,571	1,620
74	1,149	1,184	1,221	1,259	1,297	1,338	1,379	1,421	1,465	1,511	1,557	1,605	1,655
75	1,178	1,214	1,251	1,289	1,328	1,369	1,411	1,454	1,499	1,544	1,592	1,640	1,690
76	1,207	1,244	1,281	1,320	1,360	1,401	1,444	1,487	1,533	1,579	1,627	1,676	1,727
77	1,238	1,275	1,313	1,352	1,393	1,434	1,477	1,522	1,567	1,614	1,663	1,712	1,764
78	1,269	1,306	1,345	1,385	1,426	1,468	1,512	1,557	1,603	1,650	1,699	1,749	1,801
79	1,301	1,339	1,378	1,418	1,460	1,503	1,547	1,592	1,639	1,687	1,737	1,787	1,840
80	1,333	1,372	1,412	1,453	1,495	1,538	1,583	1,629	1,676	1,725	1,775	1,826	1,879
81	1,367	1,406	1,446	1,488	1,531	1,575	1,620	1,666	1,714	1,763	1,814	1,866	1,919
82	1,401	1,441	1,482	1,524	1,567	1,612	1,657	1,704	1,753	1,803	1,854	1,906	1,960
83	1,436	1,477	1,518	1,561	1,605	1,650	1,696	1,744	1,793	1,843	1,895	1,948	2,002
84	1,473	1,513	1,555	1,599	1,643	1,689	1,735	1,784	1,833	1,884	1,936	1,990	2,045
85	1,510	1,551	1,594	1,637	1,682	1,728	1,776	1,825	1,875	1,926	1,979	2,033	2,089
86	1,548	1,589	1,633	1,677	1,722	1,769	1,817	1,866	1,917	1,969	2,022	2,077	2,134
87	1,586	1,629	1,673	1,717	1,764	1,811	1,859	1,909	1,960	2,013	2,067	2,122	2,179
88	1,626	1,669	1,714	1,759	1,806	1,854	1,903	1,953	2,005	2,058	2,113	2,169	2,226
89	1,667	1,711	1,756	1,802	1,849	1,897	1,947	1,998	2,050	2,104	2,159	2,216	2,274
90	1,709	1,753	1,799	1,845	1,893	1,942	1,992	2,044	2,097	2,151	2,207	2,264	2,322
91	1,752	1,797	1,843	1,890	1,938	1,988	2,039	2,091	2,144	2,199	2,255	2,313	2,372
92	1,796	1,841	1,888	1,936	1,984	2,035	2,086	2,139	2,193	2,248	2,305	2,363	2,423
93	1,841	1,887	1,934	1,982	2,032	2,083	2,135	2,188	2,242	2,298	2,356	2,414	2,475
94	1,887	1,934	1,982	2,030	2,080	2,132	2,184	2,238	2,293	2,350	2,407	2,467	2,527
95	1,935	1,982	2,030	2,080	2,130	2,182	2,235	2,289	2,345	2,402	2,460	2,520	2,582
96	1,984	2,031	2,080	2,130	2,181	2,233	2,287	2,342	2,398	2,456	2,515	2,575	2,637
97	2,033	2,082	2,131	2,181	2,233	2,286	2,340	2,396	2,452	2,510	2,570	2,631	2,693
98	2,085	2,133	2,183	2,234	2,286	2,340	2,395	2,451	2,508	2,567	2,627	2,688	2,751
99	2,137	2,186	2,237	2,288	2,341	2,395	2,450	2,507	2,565	2,624	2,684	2,746	2,810
100	2,191	2,241	2,292	2,344	2,397	2,452	2,507	2,564	2,623	2,682	2,743	2,806	2,870

(continued)

TABLE IV (Continued)

BPD (mm)	AC (mm)												
	285	290	295	300	305	310	315	320	325	330	335	340	345
31	696	726	759	793	828	865	903	943	985	1,029	1,075	1,123	1,173
32	710	742	774	809	844	882	921	961	1,004	1,048	1,094	1,143	1,193
33	725	757	790	825	861	899	938	979	1,022	1,067	1,114	1,163	1,214
34	740	773	806	841	878	916	956	998	1,041	1,087	1,134	1,183	1,235
35	756	789	823	858	896	934	975	1,017	1,061	1,107	1,154	1,204	1,256
36	772	805	840	876	913	953	993	1,036	1,080	1,127	1,175	1,226	1,278
37	788	822	857	893	931	971	1,012	1,056	1,101	1,147	1,196	1,247	1,300
38	805	839	874	911	950	990	1,032	1,076	1,121	1,168	1,218	1,269	1,323
39	822	856	892	930	969	1,009	1,052	1,096	1,142	1,190	1,240	1,292	1,346
40	839	874	911	949	988	1,029	1,072	1,117	1,163	1,212	1,262	1,315	1,369
41	857	892	929	968	1,008	1,049	1,093	1,138	1,185	1,234	1,285	1,338	1,393
42	875	911	948	987	1,028	1,070	1,114	1,159	1,207	1,256	1,308	1,361	1,417
43	893	930	968	1,007	1,048	1,091	1,135	1,181	1,229	1,279	1,331	1,385	1,442
44	912	949	987	1,027	1,069	1,112	1,157	1,204	1,252	1,303	1,355	1,410	1,467
45	932	969	1,008	1,048	1,090	1,134	1,179	1,226	1,275	1,326	1,380	1,435	1,492
46	951	989	1,028	1,069	1,112	1,156	1,202	1,249	1,299	1,351	1,404	1,460	1,518
47	971	1,010	1,049	1,091	1,134	1,178	1,225	1,273	1,323	1,375	1,430	1,486	1,545
48	992	1,031	1,071	1,113	1,156	1,201	1,248	1,297	1,348	1,401	1,455	1,512	1,571
49	1,013	1,052	1,093	1,135	1,179	1,225	1,272	1,322	1,373	1,426	1,482	1,539	1,599
50	1,034	1,074	1,115	1,158	1,203	1,249	1,297	1,347	1,399	1,452	1,508	1,566	1,626
51	1,056	1,096	1,138	1,181	1,226	1,273	1,322	1,372	1,425	1,479	1,535	1,594	1,655
52	1,078	1,119	1,161	1,205	1,251	1,298	1,347	1,398	1,451	1,506	1,563	1,622	1,683
53	1,101	1,142	1,185	1,229	1,276	1,323	1,373	1,425	1,478	1,533	1,591	1,651	1,713
54	1,124	1,166	1,209	1,254	1,301	1,349	1,399	1,452	1,506	1,562	1,620	1,680	1,742
55	1,148	1,190	1,234	1,279	1,327	1,376	1,426	1,479	1,534	1,590	1,649	1,710	1,773
56	1,172	1,215	1,259	1,305	1,353	1,402	1,454	1,507	1,562	1,619	1,678	1,740	1,803
57	1,197	1,240	1,285	1,331	1,380	1,430	1,482	1,535	1,591	1,649	1,709	1,770	1,835
58	1,222	1,266	1,311	1,358	1,407	1,458	1,510	1,564	1,621	1,679	1,739	1,802	1,866
59	1,248	1,292	1,338	1,386	1,435	1,486	1,539	1,594	1,651	1,710	1,770	1,834	1,899
60	1,274	1,319	1,366	1,414	1,464	1,515	1,569	1,624	1,682	1,741	1,802	1,866	1,932
61	1,301	1,346	1,393	1,442	1,493	1,545	1,599	1,655	1,713	1,773	1,835	1,899	1,965
62	1,328	1,374	1,422	1,471	1,522	1,575	1,630	1,686	1,745	1,805	1,868	1,932	1,999

63	1,356	1,403	1,451	1,501	1,552	1,606	1,661	1,718	1,777	1,838	1,901	1,967	2,034
64	1,385	1,432	1,481	1,531	1,583	1,637	1,693	1,751	1,810	1,872	1,935	2,001	2,069
65	1,414	1,462	1,511	1,562	1,615	1,669	1,725	1,784	1,844	1,906	1,970	2,037	2,105
66	1,444	1,492	1,542	1,594	1,647	1,702	1,759	1,817	1,878	1,941	2,006	2,073	2,142
67	1,474	1,523	1,574	1,626	1,679	1,735	1,792	1,852	1,913	1,976	2,042	2,109	2,179
68	1,505	1,555	1,606	1,658	1,713	1,769	1,827	1,887	1,949	2,012	2,078	2,147	2,217
69	1,537	1,587	1,639	1,692	1,747	1,803	1,862	1,922	1,985	2,049	2,116	2,184	2,255
70	1,570	1,620	1,672	1,726	1,781	1,839	1,898	1,959	2,022	2,087	2,154	2,223	2,295
71	1,603	1,654	1,706	1,761	1,817	1,875	1,934	1,996	2,059	2,125	2,193	2,262	2,334
72	1,636	1,688	1,741	1,796	1,853	1,911	1,971	2,044	2,098	2,164	2,232	2,302	2,375
73	1,671	1,723	1,777	1,832	1,890	1,948	2,009	2,072	2,137	2,203	2,272	2,343	2,416
74	1,706	1,759	1,813	1,869	1,927	1,987	2,048	2,111	2,176	2,244	2,313	2,384	2,458
75	1,742	1,795	1,850	1,906	1,965	2,025	2,087	2,151	2,217	2,265	2,354	2,426	2,501
76	1,779	1,833	1,888	1,945	2,004	2,065	2,127	2,192	2,258	2,326	2,397	2,469	2,544
77	1,816	1,871	1,927	1,985	2,044	2,105	2,168	2,233	2,300	2,369	2,440	2,513	2,588
78	1,855	1,910	1,966	2,025	2,085	2,146	2,210	2,275	2,343	2,412	2,484	2,557	2,633
79	1,894	1,949	2,006	2,065	2,126	2,188	2,252	2,318	2,386	2,456	2,528	2,602	2,679
80	1,934	1,990	2,048	2,107	2,168	2,231	2,296	2,362	2,431	2,501	2,574	2,649	2,725
81	1,975	2,031	2,089	2,149	2,211	2,275	2,340	2,407	2,476	2,547	2,620	2,695	2,773
82	2,016	2,073	2,132	2,193	2,255	2,319	2,385	2,462	2,522	2,594	2,667	2,743	2,821
83	2,059	2,116	2,176	2,237	2,300	2,364	2,431	2,499	2,569	2,641	2,715	2,791	2,870
84	2,102	2,160	2,220	2,282	2,345	2,410	2,477	2,546	2,617	2,689	2,764	2,841	2,920
85	2,146	2,205	2,266	2,328	2,392	2,457	2,525	2,594	2,665	2,739	2,814	2,891	2,970
86	2,192	2,251	2,312	2,375	2,439	2,505	2,573	2,643	2,715	2,789	2,864	2,942	3,022
87	2,238	2,298	2,359	2,423	2,488	2,554	2,623	2,693	2,765	2,840	2,916	2,994	3,074
88	2,285	2,346	2,408	2,472	2,537	2,604	2,673	2,744	2,817	2,892	2,968	3,047	3,128
89	2,333	2,394	2,457	2,521	2,587	2,655	2,725	2,796	2,869	2,944	3,021	3,101	3,182
90	2,382	2,444	2,507	2,572	2,639	2,707	2,777	2,849	2,923	2,998	3,076	3,155	3,237
91	2,433	2,495	2,559	2,624	2,691	2,760	2,830	2,903	2,977	3,053	3,131	3,211	3,293
92	2,484	2,547	2,611	2,677	2,744	2,814	2,885	2,958	3,032	3,109	3,187	3,268	3,350
93	2,536	2,599	2,664	2,731	2,799	2,869	2,940	3,014	3,089	3,166	3,245	3,326	3,409
94	2,590	2,653	2,719	2,786	2,854	2,925	2,997	3,070	3,146	3,224	3,303	3,384	3,468
95	2,644	2,709	2,774	2,842	2,911	2,982	3,054	3,129	3,205	3,283	3,362	3,444	3,528
96	2,700	2,765	2,831	2,899	2,969	3,040	3,113	3,188	3,264	3,343	3,423	3,505	3,589
97	2,757	2,822	2,889	2,958	3,028	3,099	3,173	3,248	3,325	3,404	3,484	3,567	3,651
98	2,815	2,881	2,948	3,018	3,088	3,160	3,234	3,309	3,387	3,466	3,547	3,630	3,715
99	2,874	2,941	3,009	3,078	3,149	3,222	3,296	3,372	3,450	3,529	3,611	3,694	3,779
100	2,935	3,002	3,070	3,140	3,211	3,285	3,359	3,436	3,514	3,594	3,676	3,759	3,845

(continued)

TABLE IV *(Continued)*

BPD (mm)	AC (mm)										
	350	355	360	365	370	375	380	385	390	395	400
31	1,225	1,279	1,336	1,396	1,458	1,523	1,591	1,661	1,735	1,812	1,893
32	1,246	1,301	1,358	1,418	1,481	1,546	1,615	1,686	1,761	1,838	1,920
33	1,267	1,323	1,381	1,441	1,504	1,570	1,639	1,711	1,786	1,865	1,946
34	1,289	1,345	1,403	1,464	1,528	1,595	1,664	1,737	1,812	1,891	1,973
35	1,311	1,367	1,426	1,488	1,552	1,619	1,689	1,762	1,839	1,918	2,001
36	1,333	1,390	1,450	1,512	1,577	1,645	1,715	1,789	1,865	1,945	2,029
37	1,356	1,413	1,474	1,536	1,603	1,670	1,741	1,815	1,893	1,973	2,057
38	1,379	1,437	1,498	1,561	1,627	1,696	1,768	1,842	1,920	2,001	2,086
39	1,402	1,461	1,523	1,586	1,653	1,722	1,794	1,870	1,948	2,030	2,115
40	1,426	1,486	1,548	1,612	1,679	1,749	1,822	1,898	1,977	2,059	2,145
41	1,451	1,511	1,573	1,638	1,706	1,776	1,849	1,926	2,005	2,088	2,174
42	1,475	1,536	1,599	1,664	1,733	1,804	1,878	1,954	2,035	2,118	2,205
43	1,500	1,562	1,625	1,691	1,760	1,832	1,906	1,984	2,064	2,148	2,236
44	1,526	1,588	1,652	1,718	1,788	1,860	1,935	2,013	2,094	2,179	2,267
45	1,552	1,614	1,679	1,746	1,816	1,889	1,964	2,043	2,125	2,210	2,298
46	1,579	1,641	1,706	1,774	1,845	1,918	1,994	2,073	2,156	2,241	2,330
47	1,605	1,669	1,734	1,803	1,874	1,948	2,024	2,104	2,187	2,273	2,363
48	1,633	1,697	1,763	1,832	1,904	1,976	2,055	2,136	2,219	2,306	2,396
49	1,661	1,725	1,792	1,861	1,934	2,009	2,086	2,167	2,251	2,339	2,429
50	1,689	1,754	1,821	1,891	1,964	2,040	2,118	2,200	2,284	2,372	2,463
51	1,718	1,783	1,851	1,922	1,995	2,071	2,150	2,232	2,317	2,406	2,498
52	1,747	1,813	1,882	1,953	2,027	2,103	2,183	2,266	2,351	2,440	2,532
53	1,777	1,843	1,913	1,984	2,059	2,136	2,216	2,299	2,386	2,475	2,568
54	1,807	1,874	1,944	2,016	2,091	2,169	2,250	2,333	2,420	2,510	2,604
55	1,838	1,906	1,976	2,049	2,124	2,203	2,284	2,368	2,456	2,546	2,640
56	1,869	1,938	2,008	2,082	2,158	2,237	2,319	2,403	2,491	2,582	2,677
57	1,901	1,970	2,041	2,115	2,192	2,272	2,354	2,439	2,528	2,619	2,714
58	1,934	2,003	2,075	2,150	2,227	2,307	2,390	2,475	2,564	2,657	2,752
59	1,966	2,037	2,109	2,184	2,262	2,342	2,426	2,512	2,602	2,694	2,790
60	2,000	2,071	2,144	2,219	2,298	2,379	2,463	2,550	2,640	2,733	2,829
61	2,034	2,105	2,179	2,255	2,334	2,416	2,500	2,588	2,678	2,772	2,869
62	2,069	2,140	2,215	2,291	2,371	2,453	2,538	2,626	2,717	2,811	2,909

63	2,104	2,176	2,251	2,328	2,408	2,491	2,577	2,665	2,757	2,851	2,949
64	2,140	2,213	2,288	2,366	2,446	2,530	2,616	2,705	2,797	2,892	2,991
65	2,176	2,250	2,326	2,404	2,485	2,569	2,656	2,745	2,838	2,933	3,032
66	2,213	2,287	2,364	2,443	2,524	2,609	2,696	2,786	2,879	2,975	3,075
67	2,251	2,326	2,403	2,482	2,564	2,649	2,737	2,827	2,921	3,018	3,117
68	2,290	2,365	2,442	2,522	2,605	2,690	2,778	2,869	2,964	3,061	3,161
69	2,329	2,404	2,482	2,563	2,646	2,732	2,821	2,912	3,007	3,104	3,205
70	2,368	2,444	2,523	2,604	2,688	2,774	2,863	2,955	3,050	3,149	3,250
71	2,409	2,485	2,564	2,646	2,730	2,817	2,907	2,999	3,095	3,193	3,295
72	2,450	2,527	2,607	2,689	2,773	2,861	2,951	3,044	3,140	3,239	3,341
73	2,491	2,569	2,649	2,732	2,817	2,905	2,996	3,089	3,186	3,285	3,386
74	2,534	2,612	2,693	2,776	2,862	2,950	3,041	3,135	3,232	3,332	3,435
75	2,577	2,656	2,737	2,821	2,907	2,996	3,088	3,183	3,279	3,380	3,483
76	2,621	2,700	2,782	2,866	2,953	3,042	3,134	3,229	3,327	3,428	3,531
77	2,666	2,746	2,828	2,912	3,000	3,090	3,182	3,277	3,376	3,477	3,581
78	2,711	2,792	2,874	2,959	3,047	3,137	3,230	3,326	3,425	3,526	3,631
79	2,757	2,838	2,921	3,007	3,095	3,186	3,279	3,376	3,475	3,576	3,681
80	2,804	2,886	2,969	3,056	3,144	3,235	3,329	3,426	3,525	3,627	3,733
81	2,852	2,934	3,018	3,105	3,194	3,286	3,380	3,477	3,577	3,679	3,785
82	2,901	2,983	3,068	3,155	3,244	3,336	3,431	3,529	3,629	3,732	3,838
83	2,950	3,033	3,118	3,206	3,296	3,388	3,483	3,581	3,682	3,785	3,891
84	3,001	3,084	3,169	3,257	3,348	3,441	3,536	3,634	3,735	3,839	3,945
85	3,052	3,135	3,221	3,310	3,401	3,494	3,590	3,688	3,790	3,894	4,000
86	3,104	3,188	3,274	3,363	3,454	3,548	3,644	3,743	3,845	3,949	4,056
87	3,157	3,241	3,328	3,417	3,509	3,603	3,700	3,799	3,901	4,005	4,113
88	3,210	3,295	3,383	3,472	3,565	3,659	3,756	3,855	3,958	4,063	4,170
89	3,265	3,351	3,438	3,528	3,621	3,716	3,813	3,913	4,015	4,120	4,228
90	3,321	3,407	3,495	3,585	3,678	3,773	3,871	3,971	4,074	4,179	4,287
91	3,377	3,464	3,552	3,643	3,736	3,832	3,930	4,030	4,133	4,239	4,347
92	3,435	3,522	3,611	3,702	3,795	3,891	3,989	4,090	4,193	4,299	4,408
93	3,494	3,581	3,670	3,761	3,855	3,951	4,050	4,151	4,254	4,361	4,469
94	3,553	3,641	3,738	3,822	3,916	4,013	4,111	4,213	4,316	4,423	4,532
95	3,614	3,701	3,791	3,884	3,978	4,075	4,174	4,275	4,379	4,486	4,595
96	3,675	3,763	3,854	3,946	4,041	4,138	4,237	4,339	4,443	4,550	4,659
97	3,738	3,826	3,917	4,010	4,105	4,202	4,302	4,404	4,508	4,615	4,724
98	3,803	3,890	3,981	4,074	4,170	4,267	4,367	4,469	4,573	4,680	4,790
99	3,866	3,956	4,047	4,140	4,236	4,333	4,433	4,536	4,640	4,747	4,857
100	3,932	4,022	4,113	4,207	4,303	4,400	4,501	4,603	4,708	4,815	4,924

(From Shepard MJ, Richard VA, Berkowitz RL, et al: An evaluation of two equations for predicting fetal weight by ultrasound. Am J Obstet Gynecol 1982; 142:47–54.)

Index

Page numbers in italics *indicate illustrations; those followed by* t *indicate tabular material.*

ISBN 0-397-51320-8